Ophthalmology: Current and Future Developments

(Volume 4)

(Contemporary Scleral Lenses: Theory and Application)

Edited by

Melissa Barnett
University of California, Davis, Sacramento, California, USA

&

Lynette K. Johns
The New England College of Optometry, Boston, Massachusetts, USA

Bentham Science Publishers Ltd.
Executive Suite Y - 2
PO Box 7917, Saif Zone
Sharjah, U.A.E.
Email: subscriptions@benthamscience.org

BENTHAM SCIENCE

CONTENTS

FOREWORD

The re-emergence of the scleral lens – in its modern design – is a recent technological and medical advancement in the care of patients with distorted and diseased corneas. These devices are capable of providing a phenomenal improvement of vision with remarkable comfort. The improvement in quality of life these devices offer cannot be minimized.

When healthcare makes significant advances, the need for education on such developments is vital, so that more healthcare practitioners become trained in employing an innovation and, as a result, more people benefit. It is in this context that *Contemporary Scleral Lenses: Theory and Application* is a most welcome and valuable addition to the literature. This text is edited and written by two eminent clinicians and scholars in the field of scleral lenses, Drs. Melissa Barnett and Lynette Johns. They are aided by some of the most distinguished practitioners in this modality. These experts have between themselves a great number of years of experience with scleral lens management of complex corneas, which they generously share with the reader.

A review of the content of this text reveals that this volume is remarkably comprehensive. It is carefully authored and referenced and starts with an exceptionally interesting historical chapter. The reader will be taken through lens design and optics but also the topography of the ocular surface. A complete chapter is dedicated to relevant instrumentation used in a scleral lens practice. Several chapters are devoted to the assessment of ocular health, lens fit and complications. All chapters are richly illustrated by carefully selected images. This makes *Contemporary Scleral Lenses: Theory and Application* a most useful educational tool. Optimal scleral lens fitting is carefully described along with potential complications. Integrated throughout the text are thoughtful and useful problem solving recommendations.

As we become more accustomed to scleral lenses in anterior segment management, we realize that scleral lenses do not need to be limited to the abnormal eye. They indeed may be utilized for the normal eye. An entire chapter addresses this indication.

The comprehensive design of this book describes everything from the beginning to the end and from the simplest to the most complex. Therefore, it makes an appreciated information source for the student or the novice. However, this text book with its wealth of information, the number of clinical pearls and the quality of illustrations offer even the experienced and most seasoned scleral lens practitioners valuable information and opportunities to learn.

Drs. Barnett and Johns are to be congratulated on the completion of their exceptionally useful and impressive text, *Contemporary Scleral Lenses: Theory and Application*, which is arriving at a time when we have a relative lack of educational material. This text book will most certainly find a place in my personal library and computer.

Jan P. G. Bergmanson
Brien A. Holden Professor of Optometry
Texas Eye Research and Technology Center
University of Houston College of Optometry
4901 Calhoun Rd, Houston, Texas 77204
USA

PREFACE

Contemporary Scleral Lenses: Theory and Application covers a vast array of scleral lens topics to inspire novice practitioners and provide valuable pearls to experienced practitioners. From the fascinating history of scleral lenses and how they evolved to the modern scleral lenses used in clinical practice today, this book highlights major advances in scleral lenses. The description of basic lens structure, optics and customizable features combined with the characterization of ocular surface shape intricacies allow the reader to conceptualize and appreciate the unique fitting relationship of a scleral lens. Scleral lens fitting had long been described as an art, however cutting edge information on technology in the scleral lens practice emphasizes the evolving scientific and objective approach to scleral lens fitting.

Examination flow, evaluation and documentation can help even the expert scleral lens practitioner. For those interested in setting up a scleral lens practice, an entire chapter is dedicated to recruiting and marketing the scleral lens practice. For the student and novice practitioner, a chapter is solely dedicated to scleral lens care and handling. There are a variety of complex medical and ocular indications for scleral lenses that are described in detail. These patients require many different specialists for their ocular and systemic care, and the unique perspective from esteemed corneal specialists regarding collaborative care of the scleral lens patient is included in this book. Utilization of scleral lenses for patients with regular corneas is gaining popularity and is also covered.

The purpose of this book is to aid the student, new and proficient practitioners to fit, evaluate, identify and manage scleral lens complications. We hope that this text will help practitioners to grow their scleral lens practice, collaborate with other practitioners and, most importantly, help patients to improve their vision, rehabilitate their ocular surface and improve their quality of life.

The future of scleral lenses requires exploring the intricacies of this modality. There is so much research that needs to be done with scleral lenses. Multiple authors provide their opinions and strategies when facing unique challenges of scleral lenses that are not described in publications elsewhere. We hope that this text will inspire further scleral lens research and publications.

We are honored to have this opportunity to publish this text. We thank you for reading and learning about this modality, which in turn helps patients improve their lives with scleral lenses. We hope that *Contemporary Scleral Lenses: Theory and Application* is a welcome reference that assists you in implementing scleral lenses into your practice.

ACKNOWLEDGEMENTS

It was an incredibly daunting thought to even imagine writing a book on contemporary scleral lenses. Many thanks and sincere gratitude to Matthew Kennedy and his wife Rebecca Kennedy, OD who encouraged us to undertake this project.

The unremitting encouragement and sacrifice of our families made it possible to devote the endless hours and years to complete this text. We would especially like to thank Todd, Alex and Drew Erickson and Khaled Imad for their unwavering love and support as we embarked on this formidable, yet incredible journey.

It is not possible to write this text without a collaborative effort. We are so appreciative of the support of our global scleral lens community to come together, cheer us on and contribute to this text. This work would not have been possible without the assistance of our authors. Many thanks to our authors: Bruce Baldwin, Jan Bergmanson, Tim Bowden, Patrick Caroline, Karen Carrasquillo, Gregory DeNaeyer, Barry Eiden, Karolien Elving-Kokke, Damon Ezekiel, Don Ezekiel, Deborah Jacobs, Jason Jedlicka, Randy Kojima, Carina Koppen, Jennifer Li, Michael J. Lipson, Jason Marsack, Jennifer McMahon, Brooke Messer, Langis Michaud, Henny Otten, Young Kee Park, Ken Pullum, Perry Rosenthal, Muriel Schornack, Jeffrey Sonsino, Mindy Toabe, Eef van der Worp, Esther-Simone Visser, Reints Visser, Maria K. Walker, Stephanie Woo and Geunyoung Yoon.

Melissa Barnett
University of California, Davis
Sacramento, CA, USA
E-mail: drbarnett@ucdavis.edu

&

Lynette K. Johns
The New England College of Optometry
Boston, Massachusetts, USA
E-mail: johnsl@neco.edu

List of Contributors

Brooke Messer	Cornea and Contact Lens Institute of Minnesota, Edina, MN, USA
Bruce Baldwin	Department of Ophthalmology, University of North Carolina, Chapel Hill, NC, USA
Carina Koppen	Faculty of Medicine and Health Sciences, University of Antwerp, Antwerp, Belgium Department of Ophthalmology, Antwerp University Hospital, Edegem (Antwerp), Belgium
Damon J. Ezekiel	Ezekiel Eyes, Nedlands, WA, Australia
Deborah S. Jacobs	BostonSight, Needham, MA, USA Massachusetts Eye & Ear, Boston, MA, USA
Eef van der Worp	University of Maastricht, Masstricht, The Netherlands École d'optométrie, de l'Université de Montréal, Montréal, QC, Canada Pacific University College of Optometry, Forest Grove, OR, USA
Esther-Simone Visser	Visser Contactlenzenpraktijk B.V., EJ Nijmegen, The Netherlands
Geunyoung Yoon	Flaum Eye Institute, Institute of Optics, Center for Visual Science, Biomedical Engineering, University of Rochester, USA,
Gregory DeNaeyer	Arena Eye Surgeons, Columbus, OH, USA
Henny M. Otten	Visser Contactlenzenpraktijk B.V., EJ Nijmegen, The Netherlands
Jason Marsack	College of Optometry, University of Houston, Houston, TX, USA
Jason Jedlicka	School of Optometry, Indiana University, Bloomington, IN, USA
Jeffrey Sonsino	Optique, PLLC, Nashville, TN, USA
Jennifer Anne McMahon	Great Western Hospitals NHS FT, Swindon, UK
Jennifer Y. Li	University of California, Davis, Sacramento, CA, USA
Karen G. Carrasquillo	BostonSight, Needham, MA, USA
Karolien Elving-Kokke	Visser Contactlenzenpraktijk B.V., EJ Nijmegen, The Netherlands
Langis Michaud	École d'optométrie, de l'Université de Montréal, Montréal, QC, Canada
Lynette K. Johns	The New England College of Optometry, Boston, MA, USA
Maria K. Walker	College of Optometry, University of Houston, Houston, TX, USA
Melissa Barnett	University of California, Davis, Sacramento, CA, USA
Michael J. Lipson	Department of Ophthalmology and Visual Science, University of Michigan, Northville Health Center, Northville, MI, USA
Mindy Toabe	MetroHealth Medical Center, Cleveland, OH, USA
Muriel Schornack	Department of Ophthalmology, The Mayo Clinic, College of Medicine, Rochester, MN, USA
Patrick Caroline	Pacific University College of Optometry, Forest Grove, OR, USA

Perry Rosenthal	Harvard Medical School, Boston, MA, USA Boston Eye Pain Foundation, Boston, MA, USA
Randy Kojima	Pacific University College of Optometry, Forest Grove, OR, USA
Stephanie Woo	Havasu Eye Center, Lake Havasu City, AZ, USA,
S. Barry Eiden	North Suburban Vision Consultants, Ltd, Keratoconus Specialists of Illinois, Deerfield, IL, USA
Timothy J. Bowden†	Bowden & Lowe, Kent, UK
Young Kee Park	YK Eye Clinic, Seoul, South Korea

PROLOGUE

Our introduction to scleral lenses would not have been possible without the innovation and insight of the four unique pioneers who were the first to utilize and describe modern scleral lenses using gas permeable materials: Don Ezekiel, Perry Rosenthal, Rients Visser, and Ken Pullum. We are honored that each contributed to this text. Please enjoy the personal recounts of their individual experiences with scleral lenses.

DON EZEKIEL

Our pathology lecturer in the optometry course was an ophthalmologist Ken Bardon Brown. Ken studied in London and worked with Joseph Dallos. He told of his experiences with fitting glass scleral lenses and of their benefits for patients. My father who was an optometrist spoke of optometry's future with the need to specialise and not be another optometrist. So contact lenses became my specialty. Soon after I graduated, I went to Sydney and spent a month with a prominent optometrist and long time editor of the Australian journal, Loyd Hewitt, learning his technique of fitting scleral lenses. In 1963, after being recently married, we travelled to London to further my knowledge in contact lenses. While there I passed the "Fellow of the Association of Contact Lens Practitioners" (FACLP) and the "Diploma of Contact Lens Practice"(DCLP) exams.

After graduation I worked at Perth's major hospital which gave me an introduction to Moorfields Eye hospital and to Frederick Ridley (pioneer of IOLs) who was head of the contact lens clinic. He encouraged me to spend sessions at the outpatients clinic where scleral lenses were fitted to a range of eye conditions that I had only previously read about in text books. Among the specialists I met and became friends with were Montague Ruben (a register at the time) and Norman Bier, the most prominent contact lens practitioner at the time in London and author of the very best book on fitting contact lenses.

I applied for a position at Hamblin's contact lens centre in New Cavendish street under contact lens pioneer Joseph Dallos. I was told he was difficult to work with, but for me he was a wonderful teacher and father figure. He only fitted glass scleral lenses. Dallos and Bier reported at the same time that fenestrating a lens allowed for all day lens wear without Sattler's veiling. Dallos told me how he worked out how to take a mould of an eye and how he came to fenestrate a lens.

Dallos, Bier and Ruben all advised and talked me into making my own lenses (another story!) As Dallos emphasised that only then could I be sure to supply my patients with lenses with accurate details. (Don't trust what you are given!). He also emphasised that it will allow you to develop and innovate new designs and lenses. My wife never forgave them!!

On my return to Perth, I started a specialty contact lens practice to make lenses for my patients. A group of ophthalmologists who had worked and trained at Moorfield's in London included Professor Ida Mann who was responsible for getting Dallos to London where he established the first contact lens clinic at Moorfield's. Incidentally, Professor Mann and I actually lived in the same suburb. These London trained ophthalmologists living in Perth were familiar with the benefits of scleral lenses for patients and referred patients specifically for scleral lenses. Among the patients were a constant stream of babies who had cataracts surgery. I would go into theatre, take a mould (invariably a good impression of the lower canthus with minimal cornea impression!) There had to be a easier and better way.

I now had a small laboratory making lenses for my patients. All corneal lens patients were fitted with GP lenses so why were we using PMMA for scleral lenses? We were using Boston materials so I flew to Boston (if you take a globe the world and pass a needle through the centre from Perth you come out just past Boston. I could not be further away).

The owners of Polymer Technology were Perry Rosenthal and Lou Major. I met with them and asked that they supply me with large GP blanks to make scleral lenses. Perry's response was that "No one fits scleral lenses anymore!" I told him he was wrong. Lou who was responsible for the manufacture of the materials eventually promised to make large GP blanks. Nothing happened! Every week I sent at least two telex messages asking for the blanks. Lou told me later of the growing pile of telex requests on his desk, so he eventually made the blanks for me.

Initially I refitted happy scleral lens patients with GP scleral lenses. All found them to be more comfortable to wear. Was it the oxygen permeability or the surface quality of the material that resulted in a more comfortable lens that could be worn all day? GP materials are heat sensitive so all lenses are lathe turned and not made from moulds taken from patients casts. Although Dallos was first to describe taking an impression of the eye, in the time I worked with him, he never took an impression of an eye. After fitting a patient, he made a duplicate of the lens. These he stored/arranged the lenses on three shelves as small, medium and large. He would look at a patients eye and select what he thought was a close fit and modify the lens from there. The first preformed scleral lens?

From my experiences with scleral lenses I worked out the most common lens parameters and from these we made standard paediatric scleral lenses in two diameters. Babies would be referred and we fit them with these lenses. (All with the power of +30.00D). As the child grew, we would modify the lens power on the same lens as needed. A paper on the lens was published in Contact Lens Spectrum some years ago on the Paediatric GP Scleral lens.

I was fitting scleral patients with all interesting conditions with GP scleral lenses with good results. All lenses were fenestrated. This resulted in the original paper I read at the annual BCLA meeting in Harrogate. Irving Fatt reported on the meeting and on my paper. He reported that the consensus from the meeting was that "no one thought the results were valid or believable as there would not be sufficient oxygen transmission through the lens to make the use of the GP material of any benefit." I subsequently read a paper and presented a video on my fitting technique at a meeting of the ISCLS in France. This included patients with a range of optical conditions that only a scleral lens would satisfy. Irving Fatt was at the meeting. He commented that I was clearly getting results. If I sent him lenses and lens designs, he would make calculations of the oxygen transmissions through the lens. His calculations reported that the eye received five times more oxygen to the cornea that the cornea required.

I gave all of my collection of old contact lenses and antique optical equipment including a bench to manufacture glass scleral lenses, numerous scleral fitting sets including a glass fitting set from Feinbloom (including some of his moulds), and original Czech lenses in their original glass vials) to Pat Caroline at Pacific University, together with all the correspondence from Irving Fatt and other pioneers that I corresponded with. It seems like I collected and kept everything that is now of historical value. Pat visited me in Perth and we went through the collection and correspondence. I lost count of the times he said "Oh my God."

Soon after the paper was published, Perry Rosenthal called and visited me in Perth. I showed him patients with a range of conditions who had been fitted with GP scleral lenses. We went to the lab and I showed him how we made lenses. No secrets. No patents. It is a wonderful lens for patients that was not readily available and any person interested in the lens was welcome to all the knowledge and technology. Perry saw the results and the rest is history.

It is very satisfying for me that scleral lenses are now being widely available for patients for whom it is often the only option to achieve vision and comfort. Dallos would be pleased.

Almost all readily available GP scleral lenses now available are sealed. I have only fitted fenestrated scleral lenses. The argument that this lens is more difficult to fit as the lens settles might be true, but now with the lens fitting sets incorporating designs of keratoconic and reverse geometry preformed lenses, it is not difficult to find a fitting lens and to estimate the amount of lens settling at the initial consultation. It is not rocket science.

The continual flushing system of tears from behind the lens and the ease of inserting a non-sealed lens, especially for the paediatric patient, results in a lens that is worn comfortably for the full day without any problems. A lens that allows the exchange of tears and the removal of debris from beneath the lens results in a healthy lens for the cornea. I believe the GP scleral lenses in the near future will be fit for our patients with normal corneas.

The use of gas permeable materials was a logical progression. For me it seems that the stars crossed. I was fortunate to have patients referred to me specifically for scleral lenses and to have a facility to make whatever lens that I wanted.

Getting the materials was the first hurdle. The hardest hurdle to overcome was getting practitioners to understand that fitting the scleral lens was not difficult. It is often a much needed and the only lens option for patients to obtain optimal vision with all day wearing comfort.

PERRY ROSENTHAL

In 1986 I was referred a patient whose only seeing eye had undergone a traumatic rupture that, after its repair, was characterized by a large anterior staphyloma and 8 diopters of astigmatism. Its vision was not correctable to functional levels with spectacles and surgery was contraindicated. Moreover, his distorted cornea was incapable of supporting a rigid corneal contact lens. I then recalled Don Ezekiel's pioneering work on fitting fenestrated gas-permeable scleral lenses, but the distorted shape of his cornea made it impossible to prevent the air bubbles from intruding on the visual axis. The only remaining option for restoring functional vision was to fit his eye with a non-fenestrated scleral lens. Coincidentally, at Polymer Technology, we had recently developed a new generation of rigid polymers with gas-permeability properties adequate to avoid the need to augment the supply of corneal oxygen with air bubbles during scleral lens wear and I fitted this eye with the first non-fenestrated gas-permeable scleral lens. The result was 20/30 vision, all day wearing and excellent tolerance. I remember thinking that it couldn't be that easy and it wasn't: my efforts to fit the next several patients was stymied by the development of lens suction. However, because the success of my first patient proved the potential viability of non-fenestrated GP scleral lenses, I embarked on what turned out to be a multiyear scleral lens design development program that was ultimately based on the use of mathematical spline functions. This turned out to be the breakthrough for fitting these devices.

RIENTS VISSER

From the day I started my contact lens practice back in 1970, I have been fitting contact lenses and scleral lenses for patients with a variety of medical conditions. I have always been driven by the question, "How can I help patients who don't have any options for treating their ocular and visual problems?"

In the beginning, I would see patients who had been wearing scleral lenses for a long time, in some cases more than 30 years. These patients had been wearing scleral lenses that were made of gas-impermeable materials such as glass or polymethyl methacrylate (PMMA), which was introduced later. Moreover, the indications for fitting patients with scleral lenses have changed over the years. When I started my contact lens practice, I saw patients with corneal scarring due to wounds inflicted during the Second World War or corneal scars resulting from tuberculosis or measles. Unfortunately, though, I also frequently saw opaque, vascularized corneas with corneal edema that resulted from severe hypoxia associated with wearing glass or PMMA scleral lenses for years; some of these patients even needed corneal transplantation. Advanced keratoconus and exposure keratitis were also frequent indications for scleral lenses.

Because PMMA scleral lenses produce an unacceptable level of corneal hypoxia, in the late sixties I designed and fitted PMMA corneal contact lenses, and later hydrogel lenses. However, I still prescribed scleral lenses (albeit with limited wearing time) for managing certain corneal conditions for which other lens types and treatments were not feasible. In these cases, I hand-molded thermoplastic PMMA scleral lenses and fitted these lenses to the patient's eye.

The report of the first successful use of gas-permeable haptic lenses by Donald Ezekiel [1] in 1983 was—for me—a new starting point in fitting scleral lenses, as these lenses significantly reduced the risk of hypoxic complications. After reading this publication, I immediately commissioned Polymer Technology to produce gas-permeable buttons for scleral lenses; in 1985, they delivered on this request, and Equalens II buttons were available for scleral lenses, marking the beginning of a very exciting chapter in my scleral lens practice. We quickly saw highly promising results by combining this highly gas-permeable material with our preformed scleral lens fitting methods, yielding good lens tolerance and providing safe and effective treatment [2, 3]. Importantly, wearing time also increased considerably. Later work by other scleral lens fitters confirmed that scleral lenses made of highly gas-permeable materials perform better [4, 5].

The 1990s was a landmark decade in the modern era of scleral contact lens design. First, a front-surface cylinder—with a haptic truncation that provided stabilization—was introduced to improve vision [6]. Next, a breakthrough—the back-surface toric scleral lens—was introduced by our team in collaboration with the Dutch contact lens company Procornea in Eerbeek, the Netherlands [7-9]. Importantly, studies of scleral shape supported our own clinical experience with back-surface toric lenses by demonstrating that the shape of the anterior sclera is often asymmetrical (*i.e.*, one or more segments of the sclera are either steeper or flatter than other scleral segments) [10, 11]. Moreover, these studies revealed that the shape of the cornea-scleral junction and the anterior sclera is often tangential rather than curved, driving the development of bitangential-shaped scleral lenses in a joint endeavor with the Dutch contact lens company NKL Contactlenzen in Emmen, the Netherlands [12]. The introduction of back-surface toric scleral lenses now enabled practitioners to achieve a more precise scleral lens fitting and resulted in greater patient satisfaction. Furthermore, the high stability of these toric scleral lenses enabled the use of front-surface cylinders and the ability to provide other optical corrections such as bifocal, prism, and aberration corrections.

The process of fitting scleral lenses requires more than simply using your hands and your head; you also need to use your heart. The ability to regain visual acuity, often after years of suffering with poor vision, helps get patients back to work and back into society; this is what has driven me for four decades and continues to drive me every day.

Helping patients is—of course—at the heart of what we do. But we cannot stop there. Continuing to develop new and improved fitting techniques and teaching colleagues through practical courses and lectures help ensure that scleral lenses and scleral lens practice will continue to improve.

KEN PULLUM

Most people make forward, backward or sideways career moves. In all honesty, most of mine were divine interventions by my GA (guardian angel). There have been quite a few, and for as long as I can remember, but the first to impact on my time in optometry was before I entered public exams at school, although I did not appreciate the effect of that one for a few years. This was in the days before everyone went swanning off on the gap year between leaving school and going to university. I thought the organisation VSO (Voluntary Service Overseas) had obvious adventurous attractions. I put in a completely inadequate application which was rejected, even after I appealed and asked them to reconsider. VSO helpfully suggested I would have more to offer as a graduate in a few years time.

My father was a manufacturing optician and set up a small business making spectacles for some of the local ophthalmic opticians, the correct UK term at the time for the professional group later undergoing a makeover and a rename as optometrists. There was no other careers advice at all. No-one could accuse me of being one of the star pupils, and there were quite a few times when I nearly gave up, or when the City University gave upon me. I just salvaged an indifferent degree, notably when I handed in the whole years second year course work two weeks before the end of year exams in the subject I found the most difficult. The tutor was livid pink, but deep down was a kindly man and recognised undergraduates' frailties. Maybe he also recognised my belated ability to focus on the task in hand had some merit. Who knows, but I just survived that one. Actually there was another student who did exactly the same to the same lecturer, but handed in hers an hour earlier. Anyway, I scraped through the second year, but it was damaging to the final degree outcome.

That would have made a difference if I was joining optometry now ... I wouldn't have been on a long list for a long list, let alone a short list for a position in the UK hospital eye service. But at the time, only a small number wanted to go along that route, and initially, I wasn't one of them. I had a pre-registration appointment with Andrew Field, one of the practitioners who sent some work to my father's business, and a top flight pre-reg post it turned out to be, I would say. However, in the middle of the final exams, an invitation to come along for a conducted tour of Moorfields Contact Lens Department appeared on the notice board in the students common room. I didn't see it, but a friend told me about it. I think my GA must have been behind it. Five of us responded, which by co-incidence, is the same number of days in the week. It turned out that there was a day on offer at the department, as a pre-reg, for each day. I was given Thursdays and started two weeks later. How could I apply for VSO when such a wonderful opportunity had just come my way, even if completely by accident.

My supervisor, Jennifer Chaston, had a different style to my private practice supervisor, but we all learned so much that year. The department was largely manned by dispensing opticians and a small number of ophthalmic opticians, Jennifer was full time, but most of the others were sessional. That year began a transformation in recruitment and from then on the department only took on ophthalmic opticians to the Contact Lens Department staff. There was another group of practitioners who were appointed at the inception of the CLD in 1951. These were not dispensers, or ophthalmic opticians, but state registered nurses, mostly male, who had achieved an ophthalmic diploma. I imagine that back in 1951, there would have been a brief meeting during which the then director pointed to one of them and said..." Trodd! You will make and fit contact lenses." I don't think there would have been any training or certainly no dissent, and so Troddy just got on with it. I joined when he was taking on the most difficult cases, working solely with PMMA impression sclerals, doing a wonderful job under very difficult circumstances.

The following year, the organisation of the contact lens department had moved along in leaps and bounds. Monty Ruben, the consultant director, and Jennifer recognised the growing need for research in contact lens practice. The single all week pre-reg appointee that year was Michel Guillon, a different type to the not so famous five in my year. He was able and driven to develop the research requirement, even as a pre-reg. None from the previous year were motivated in the same way, and some had already left or did so soon after. But I was going nowhere, and pleased that too much of an involvement in the research activities was not a pre-requisite. I did not have the same academic leaning, preferring to focus on the many and varied clinical challenges that came in on a regular basis. So if I had gone away on a far flung remote VSO destination four years earlier, I would not have seen the notice pinned up at City University, and my Thursdays at Moorfields in the pre-reg year would not have happened.

On qualifying, I immediately stepped up my days at Moorfields to two a week. Two or three years later, ophthalmic opticians became renamed and reborn as optometrists with the foundation of the British College of Optometrists. Jennifer moved on to pastures new, and Geoff Woodward replaced her as senior optometrist. The department continued to expand apace, he was soon appointed as the first principal Optometrist of the Contact Lens Department, and Michel replaced Geoff as senior. After a few years, Michel also moved on to Sydney to further his skills as a research optometrist, vacating his position as senior optometrist. Three or four people applied for the vacancy, including myself. I think it would be fair to say I had the most experience in the specific clinical skills required by the department, but the hospital administration had had plenty of time to assess my possible organisational skills, and came to a conclusion that "Couldn't organise a bunfight in a bakery" would fit well. Perhaps a bit unfair, but the person who was appointed did a better job than I would have done running the day to day matters.

Actually, it was my GA coming to my rescue again. I had made friends with Troddy when few others in the optometry group made any impact at all. He allowed me into what had been naughtily referred to as the Inner Sanctum and I was already sharing the impression PMMA scleral workload with him, and more to the point, learning the needful first hand at the sharp end. My second major interview followed soon after being turned down for the full time senior post. Geoff and I were having a corridor discussion. I pointed out that Troddy would be retiring in five years, and the department would need someone to replace him. Geoff said, "OK, start next week." I promised to be there five years, and that was over thirty five years ago, so I more than honoured my side of the agreement. Now, I would have had to have filled in a 20 page internet application form and there would have been a dozen other contenders. At the time, no-one was interested.

Troddy did retire five years later, and sadly died within a few months. I wish I could have shared with him the gas permeable development, but that was not to be. There was a fully functional contact lens manufacturing section within the department, and one or two heads had come and gone in the time I had been on the staff. One day, Lou, the head at the time, stunned me by declaring that he did not want to make any scleral lenses for me. I was already making all the PMMA fitted shells, but the powering procedures were awkward. I would have thought manufacturing, which involved ending up with oil and grease all over your hands, would be more appropriately separated from the clinical activities. However, the general consensus was that if I wanted to carry on with the project, I'd have to do it all myself. This was an amazing John McEnroe style "Are you being serious?" moment, but in reality was another divine intervention from my GA. I was forced to learn the manufacturing skills, but what an asset that turned out to be in the years to come. When Lou retired, I wrote on his leaving card to say that I now realise he always had my best interests at heart. We had a good laugh, and he took it in the spirit of friendship it was meant.

In the late 1980's and early 1990's high DK gas permeable materials replaced PMMA. The change was introduced at a late stage of material science development, so there was no need to find our feet with the early attempts which would have been ineffective with scleral lenses. In short, gas permeable materials simultaneously transformed scleral lens clinical practice and manufacturing. Moorfields was set up for RGP corneal lenses in the Contact Lens Service (recategorised from a Department), but would have needed a complete overhaul to take on RGP scleral lens production. We were looking at a massive task transferring most of our scleral lens wearers from PMMA to RGP, needing refitting in the reformed style, and lenses issued. Moorfields supported my establishment of Innovative Sclerals, and that became the preferred method for scleral lens delivery rather than on site. Where possible in that time, we transferred much of the production to Moorfields for the hospital's own internal use, ending up with a joint process for both preformed and impression scleral lenses.

We established an excellent working relationship for 20 years, until finally, my partners were all looking to retire, and it would have been impossible for me to carry on alone. This time, it was B&L, rather than my GA coming to the rescue and took over manufacture of the Innovative Sclerals range. And of course, at about the same time, every contact lens manufacturing company on the planet entered into what suddenly became the most exciting new development in contact lenses in recent times.

This is my 43rd year in specialised contact lens practice. If I was to be starting my career from the beginning, I'd do it all again. I have had massive help and support over the years from the establishment at Moorfields, Oxford Eye Hospital, my manufacturing partners, and I was able to learn so much from my colleagues at Moorfields. The British National Health Service allows health care practitioners in the UK to practise without having to offload the costs to the patients, so this has always been a major contribution when trying to develop clinical procedure. We can treat billionaires and people who do not have two pennies to rub together with equitability, so we are able to deliver a service where and when it is need most. And of course, who needs to be born with a silver spoon when you have a guardian angel looking after you at every step.

MELISSA BARNETT AND LYNETTE JOHNS

However your journey begins, whether it is from the guidance of an esteemed mentor, a unique patient that requires additional expertise, the opportunity to help people or your guardian angel nudging you, we hope that this text will help you along the way.

REFERENCES

[1] Ezekiel D. Gas permeable haptic lenses. J Br Contact Lens Assoc 1983; 6: 158-61. [http://dx.doi.org/10.1016/S0141-7037(83)80064-0]

[2] Visser R. Een nieuwe toekomst voor hoog-zuurstofdoorlatende scleralenzen bij verschillende pathologie. Visus 1990; 3: 11-6.

[3] Kok JH, Visser R. Treatment of ocular surface disorders and dry eyes with high gas-permeable scleral lenses. Cornea 1992; 11(6): 518-22. [http://dx.doi.org/10.1097/00003226-199211000-00006] [PMID: 1468214]

[4] Tan DT, Pullum KW, Buckley RJ. Medical applications of scleral contact lenses: 2. Gas-permeable scleral contact lenses. Cornea 1995; 14(2): 130-7. [http://dx.doi.org/10.1097/00003226-199503000-00001] [PMID: 7743793]

[5] Rosenthal P, Croteau A. Fluid-ventilated, gas-permeable scleral contact lens is an effective option for managing severe ocular surface disease and many corneal disorders that would otherwise require penetrating keratoplasty. Eye Contact Lens 2005; 31(3): 130-4. [http://dx.doi.org/10.1097/01.ICL.0000152492.98553.8D] [PMID: 15894881]

[6] Visser E-S. Advanced contact lens fitting. Part five: The scleral contact lens: clinical indications. Optician 1997; 214: 15-20.

[7] Visser E-S, Visser R, Van Lier HJ. Advantages of toric scleral lenses. Optom Vis Sci 2006; 83(4): 233-6. [http://dx.doi.org/10.1097/01.opx.0000214297.38421.15] [PMID: 16614579]

[8] Visser E-S, Visser R, van Lier HJ, Otten HM. Modern scleral lenses part I: clinical features. Eye Contact Lens 2007; 33(1): 13-20. [http://dx.doi.org/10.1097/01.icl.0000233217.68379.d5] [PMID: 17224674]

[9] Visser E-S, Visser R, van Lier HJ, Otten HM. Modern scleral lenses part II: patient satisfaction. Eye

Contact Lens 2007; 33(1): 21-5.
[http://dx.doi.org/10.1097/01.icl.0000228964.74647.25] [PMID: 17224675]

[10] Van der Worp E, Graf T, Caroline P. Exploring beyond the corneal borders. Contact Lens Spectr 2010; 6: 26-32.

[11] Tan B, Graham AD, Tsechpenakis G, Lin MC. A novel analytical method using OCT to describe the corneoscleral junction. Optom Vis Sci 2014; 91(6): 650-7.
[http://dx.doi.org/10.1097/OPX.0000000000000267] [PMID: 24830372]

[12] Visser E-S, Van der Linden BJ, Otten HM, Van der Lelij A, Visser R. Medical applications and outcomes of bitangential scleral lenses. Optom Vis Sci 2013; 90(10): 1078-85.
[http://dx.doi.org/10.1097/OPX.0000000000000018] [PMID: 23974663]

CHAPTER 1

History of Scleral Lenses

Timothy J. Bowden[1,†] and **Melissa Barnett**[2,*]

[1] *Bowden & Lowe, Kent, UK*

[2] *University of California, Davis, Sacramento, CA, USA*

Abstract: Scleral lenses have existed for centuries, longer than any other type of contact lens. They were first conceptualized by Leonardo DaVinci in the early 16th century and were first manufactured in Europe in the late 1800s. The first scleral lenses were blown glass scleral shells without power made in 1887 by Fredrich A. Müller and Albert C. Müller. The primary indication for these scleral lenses was to manage ocular surface disease. In 1889, Adolf Eugen Gaston Fick described the use of scleral lenses with optics added to correct vision. In 1889, Eugene Kalt described contact lenses as orthopedic appliances for the treatment of keratoconus. In that same year, August Müeller created a scleral lens for himself to correct his own 14D of high myopia. Modern advances of scleral lenses have overcome their previous shortcomings, including lens-induced corneal edema due to poor transmissibility of oxygen through the lens and poor reproducibility. Contemporary scleral lenses have re-emerged from a long history of contact lens successes and some failures. In recent years, there has been a burst of new designs and innovations worldwide. With modern materials, manufacturing, and advanced scanning equipment, scleral lenses are now very innovative and a million miles away from their early beginnings.

Keywords: Air bubble, Artificial eye, Blown glass contact lens, Cast, Clearance, Experiment, Fitting, Gas permeable, Glass, Glass mask, Impression, Keratoconus, Lens making, Material, Mold, Optician, PMMA, Refractive error, Scleral shell, Transitions.

INTRODUCTION

A question that is often asked is: when and by whom were contact lenses invented? Well, contact lenses were not so much invented as evolved. There have been many stages in this development, some theoretical, but in the main much more practical. Today, contact lenses are largely used for cosmetic reasons, but they originally were designed to deal with medical problems including keratoconus and symblepharon. Most of the early contact lenses were made by

* **Corresponding author Melissa Barnett:** University of California, Davis, Sacramento, CA, USA; Tel: 916-734-4641; Fax: 916-565-1640; E-mail: drbarnett@ucdavis.edu

† Deceased

Melissa Barnett & Lynette K. Johns (Eds.)

artificial eye makers. Who can be better to make something to fit onto the front surface of an eye and under the eyelids than a person who would already have the skills required?

Why were the first contact lenses designed as scleral lenses? This was a result of them being made by artificial eye makers. The first contact lenses were supported by the sclera, and the optic portion vaulted over the cornea. They could as easily have been made as corneal lenses. In fact, this happened in Japan when Kyoichi Tanaka designed his first contact lens. He had never seen a contact lens before, so what he designed was actually a corneal lens. This was the start of what was to become Menicon. It has now turned full circle. With new materials and new measuring, fitting, and manufacturing techniques, many eye care practitioners are turning to scleral lenses for improved vision and comfort for their visually compromised patients.

Artificial eye making originated in Egypt around 2000 BC to ensure that Egyptians could see in the afterlife, and it gradually spread throughout Europe, first through Venice and later through Germany, the UK and then the US (Fig. **1**). Artificial eye making was big business. Eye damage and eye loss were very common due to frequent, severe eye infections resulting from poor hygiene and no antibiotics, emerging industrial processes using lime and hot metals, and the non-availability of protective eyewear.

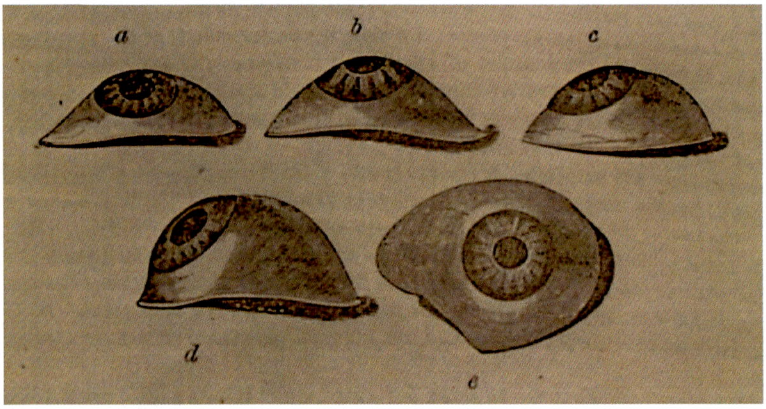

Fig. (1). Images of artificial eyes.

"The Optician" of 28th July 1898 reported that 2,000,000 artificial eyes were produced in the German Empire each year, and a single French firm was producing 300,000 per year. "The Optician" of 1st June 1899 reported a horse being fitted with an artificial eye made of vulcanite: "There is nothing a lover of horses dislikes more than a disfigured animal". It is no co-incidence that the earliest contact lenses from the Müller brothers of Wiesbaden, Germany, looked like artificial eyes, with the opaque scleral portion including representations of scleral and conjunctival blood vessels, but having a clear optic portion.

EARLY THEORISTS

It has previously been widely reported that the illustration in Leonardo da Vinci's Codex D, folio 3, of 1508 depicting a man with his head in a bowl of water somehow showed the invention of a contact lens (Fig. **2**). However, in the re-translation by Robert Heitz [1], this was not a prototype contact lens, but the beginning of understanding corneal neutralization. René Descartes, a French philosopher, mathematician, and scientist, described in his Discourse of La Dioptrique [2] in 1637 that a fluid-filled tube held against the eye enlarged the size of the retinal image. Philip de la Hire, a French mathematician, presented his dissertation in 1685 On the Neutralization of the Cornea [3]. He also speculated about whether the cause of myopia was either axial or refractive. Pierre Demours, a French physician, zoologist, and translator, and his father, a pharmacist, were the first to mention a conical cornea (keratoconus) in 1747 [4]. Pierre Demours also had a disagreement with Jean Descemet about a certain membrane in the cornea. Burchard Mauchart, 1748, John 'Chevalier' Taylor, 1766 [5], and Pickford [6], 1844, all made mention of keratoconus, but the first adequate description of keratoconus (Fig. **3**) was published by John Nottingham in 1854 [7]. A slit lamp view of keratoconus is shown in Fig. (**4**).

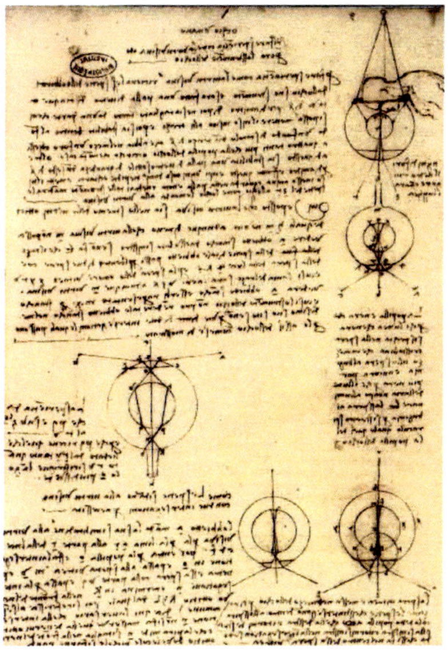

Fig. (2). The da Vinci Codex.

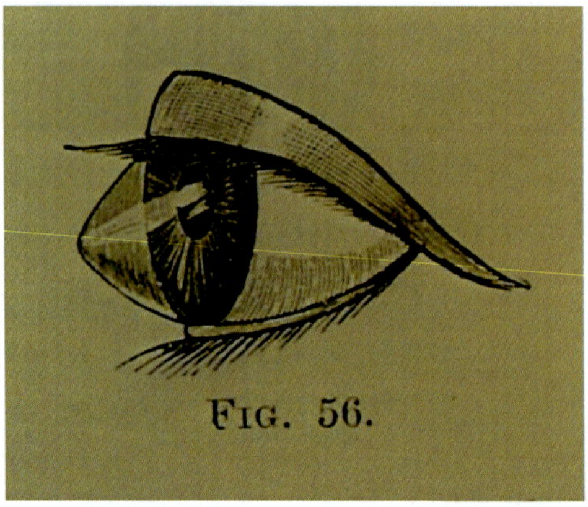

Fig. (3). Keratoconus described by Nottingham.

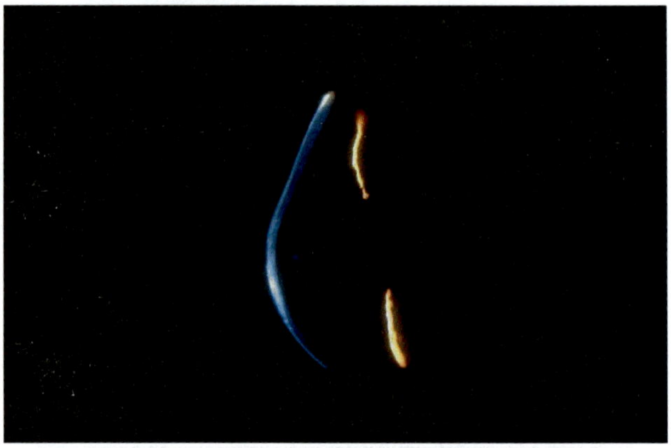

Fig. (4). Modern view of keratoconus.

In 1801, Thomas Young, an English physician and physicist, having studied medicine in London and Edinburgh and physics at Gottingen, identified the cause of astigmatism and published a three-color theory of perception. While a fellow at Cambridge University, he used a microscope lens with wax around the rim that was filled with water and held against the eye in an experiment on accommodation to neutralize the refractive effect of the cornea [8]. Inspired by Thomas Young, George Biddle Airy, British mathematician and astronomer, colluding and co-operating with John Herschel at Cambridge University, experimented with his own astigmatism. He described not only the optical theory of astigmatism, but also its correction with a theoretical back surface toric lens. He used the first few days of the moon's crescent (similar to a stenopaic slit) to distinguish the astigmatic axis of his own eye [9]. He was quoted in John Herschel's dissertation Light [10] regarding "the ingenious idea of a double concave lens, in which one surface should be spherical, the other cylindrical". The use of the spherical surface was to correct the general defect of an excessively convex cornea. "That of the cylindrical may be thus explained," he stated, and he went on to describe its application on the astigmatic cornea.

Sir John F. W. Herschel, son of Sir William Herschel (discoverer of Uranus), described the optical correction of malformed and distorted corneas using convex lenses applied to the eye in his dissertation previously mentioned. In a footnote, he suggested correcting "very bad cases of irregular cornea" by using "some transparent animal jelly contained in a spherical capsule of glass". He then went on to suggest whether "an actual mold of the cornea might be taken and impressed on some transparent medium" [10].

In 1859, William White Cooper [11], a London ophthalmologist, had glass masks made up by artificial eye makers Gray and Holford of Goswell Road, London, to separate the cornea from the lids in cases of symblepharon (Fig. **5**). These were clear glass shells, very similar to scleral lenses, but without an optic zone over the cornea.

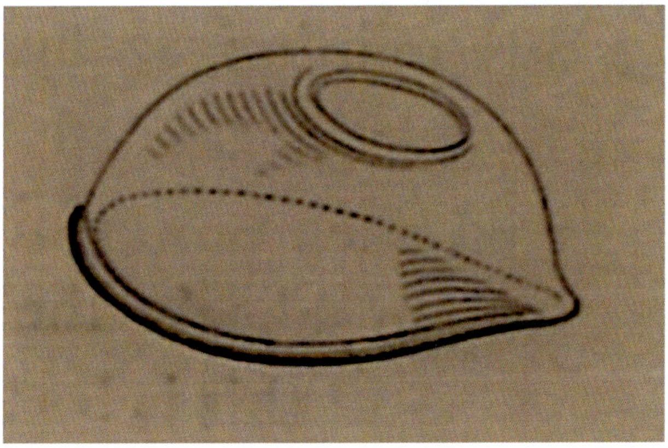

Fig. (5). Image of a glass mask, William White Cooper.

THE EVOLUTION OF THE SCLERAL LENS

The first scleral lenses—or perhaps more correctly, scleral shells, as they were not powered—were made in 1887 by Fredrich A. Müller and Albert C. Müller. The brothers were artificial eye makers working in their family business in Wiesbaden, Germany. They made and supplied a protective device for a patient of Dr. Theodore Saemisch. The patient had surgical damage to the lids of his right eye, leaving the cornea exposed, while sight in his left eye was very impaired due to myopia and cataract. By making a glass shell, which encased but did not touch the cornea, fluid was maintained around the cornea, preventing its further desiccation. The protective shell looked like an artificial eye, although the cornea was left clear [12]. The patient wrote a letter in 1908 (now lost) that since 1887 he had worn the lens continuously: day and night for 1½ –2 years at a time. Indeed, the lens was successfully worn with good tolerance and no apparent corneal damage for 21 years in total [13 - 15].

The Müller brothers continued to produce thin, lightweight, blown glass lenses with clear corneal regions and white scleral portions (Fig. **6**), which were well tolerated. Since the lenses were made of blown glass, the optic portion was variable and, as a result, the vision was also, but the tolerance of these glass lenses (and apparent avoidance of corneal edema) was good. This was probably due to the characteristic aspheric shape of their scleral zones, producing loose channels for the free passage of fresh tears carrying oxygen to the cornea and removing the waste products of corneal metabolism.

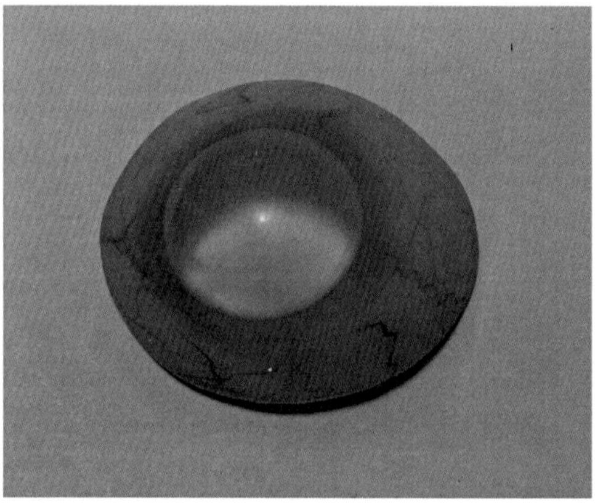

Fig. (6). Blown Glass Contact Lens.

Adolf Eugen Gaston Fick, a German ophthalmologist, began work in the Ophthalmic Clinic in Zurich under Professor Haab after returning from South Africa. He was interested in keratoconus and had been experimenting with rabbits' eyes, making molds of the cornea and constructing glass shells. He progressed to human cadaver eyes and had some glass scleral lenses made by Professor Ernst Abbe at Carl Zeiss in Jena in 1888. Professor Abbe had joined Carl Zeiss in Jena in 1866 as a research director. He was Professor of Physics and Mathematics at the University of Jena and a prolific inventor and writer of scientific papers on optics. Abbe developed the first Zeiss contact lenses from glass produced by Otto Schott, the son of a family of glass makers, who refined the chemistry of glass making. Previously, glass making was a cottage industry with very variable results from one batch to the next and from one family to another [17].

Fick described six patients on whom he had tried his lenses: one was keratoconic, and the other five had varying degrees of corneal opacities. In the keratoconic eye, vision improved from 2/60 to 6/36. However, at the time of publication, none of these patients were wearing the lenses for any length of time [16].

Fick was very observant, and from the plaster casts of human eyes, he noted in his article that the radius of curvature of the cornea was steeper than that of the sclera or globe of the eye, and that the conjunctiva flattened steadily away from the cornea. Fick observed clouding (corneal edema) in the epithelial layer, which was later called Fick's phenomenon or Sattler's veil. He recognized that an adaptation process enabled the wearer to become more tolerant to lens wear, and he found that air trapped behind the scleral lens on insertion retarded the onset of visual clouding. Additionally, inserting scleral lenses with boiled 2% grape sugar solution extended the wearing time for his rabbits to 8-10 hours before corneal clouding developed. He thought that cosmetic (prosthetic) contact lens shells could be used when corneal scarring precluded good vision.

For conical corneas, Fick suggested performing an iridectomy to produce an artificial pupil. A scleral lens, with an opaque iris and a black pupil, could then be fitted with a clear aperture positioned in line with the iridectomy. He suggested this option as an alternative to corneal tattooing and other such barbaric treatments, which often resulted in severe eye infections and potential eye loss.

Fick also observed that lenses could be used in aphakia for which "the high degree of hypermetropia could be diminished by increased curvature of the glass cornea" [16]. The lenses made for Fick by Professor Abbe had a back optic zone radius of 8 mm, optic zone diameter of 14 mm, a scleral band width of 3 mm, and a scleral zone radius of curvature of 15 mm.

Also in 1888, M. Straub introduced ophthalmic solutions of fluorescein for the investigation of corneal lesions. However, its fluorescent properties under blue light were not recognized for another 50 years [18, 19].

A year later in 1889, Eugene Kalt [20], an ophthalmologist in Paris, investigated contact lenses as "orthopedic appliances" in the treatment of keratoconus. He noticed that the contact lens changed the shape of the cornea, thus laying the groundwork that led to orthokeratology and to contact lenses being considered as a means of myopia control.

In the same year, August Müller, a final year medical student, presented his inaugural thesis at the University of Kiel for his doctorate in medicine. The dissertation entitled "Spectacle Lenses and Corneal Lenses" [21] included the correction of his own 14 diopters of myopia with contact lenses. It was the first time a reference had been made to a "corneal lens". The three lenses, made by Otto Himmler, a Berlin optician and instrument maker, measured 15-16 mm across and still exist in the Germanisch Museum in Munich. Due to his poor sight and his failure to achieve better vision with contact lenses, Müller did not pursue a career in ophthalmology, but instead went into orthopedics. However, he postulated that the various adverse signs and symptoms of lens wear could be ascribed to "... a disturbance of nourishment of corneal tissue..". However, this would not be validated for another 60-plus years, when it was demonstrated that the cornea requires atmospheric oxygen dissolved in tears to maintain a normal respiratory status [22].

Müller suggested that scleral lens discomfort arose from pressure on the conjunctiva from the scleral zone of the lens. His attempt to avoid air bubbles under the lenses by inserting the lenses underwater limited lens tolerance. The discomfort experienced by Müller due to this hypotonicity of the liquid behind the contact lens led him to use cocaine eye drops prior to lens insertion. However, the toxicity of cocaine to the cornea did not help much and added the risk of addiction.

To overcome some of the problems with solutions, Henri Dor, an ophthalmologist in Lyons, France, in 1892 recommended the use of physiological saline solution to insert contact lenses. This remained popular until the early 1940s [23].

In 1900, Dr. Louis de Wecker added another future use of scleral lenses when he used one as a splint to retain a corneal graft in position during healing [24]. A more detailed examination of the cornea was facilitated by the invention of the slit lamp in 1911 by Allvar Gullstrand of Sweden.

One year later, Zeiss produced its first scleral lens diagnostic fitting set for use by ophthalmologists. By this time, over 2,000 contact lenses had been made, mainly by Zeiss [25]. This was followed in 1916 by the first trial set especially for keratoconus [26].

Developments came along rapidly with Zeiss lenses made in 1918, with small lead pellets embedded in them to assist locating ophthalmic foreign bodies in conjunction with X-ray images (first discovered in 1896). That same year, Dr. Leonhard Koeppe described a contact lens for specialist observation of internal features of the eye using a slit-lamp biomicroscope. This type of short-term-use lens was termed a gonioscope [27].

In 1920, Zeiss manufactured a four-lens preformed fitting set for keratoconus. It was introduced and developed by Dr. W. Stock, who also suffered from keratoconus. The first lens had a 12 mm back scleral radius, but later a full range from 10.0 to 14.0 mm in 0.25 mm steps became available [28].

In the early 20th century, lens choice lay between the blown glass lenses produced by the firm of Müllers of Wiesbaden and the ground glass lenses such as those made by Carl Zeiss of Jena. The former lenses were inferior in consistency of optical quality, but superior in comfort and duration of wear. Zeiss lenses could correct reasonable amounts of ametropia, but their maximum wearing time was between 30 minutes and 2 hours. Poor wearing times did not preclude the use of these lenses for short-term application. In 1922, Zeiss was granted US and German patents for plastic (Cellon or Celluloid) scleral lenses. Appearance and discoloration stopped further development. Zeiss was also granted a patent for a lens formed between two lathe cut molds (Figs. **7a-c**).

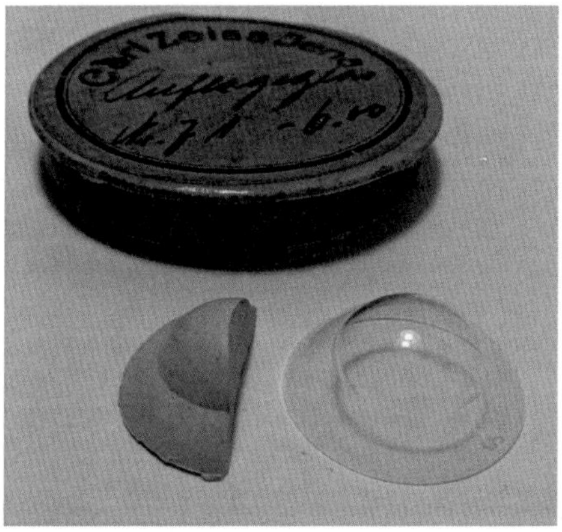

Fig. (7a). Zeiss back surface cast showing sharp transitions.

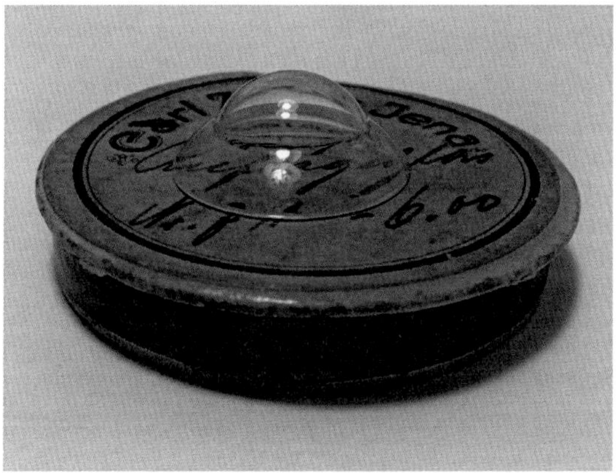

Fig. (7b). Zeiss lens profile.

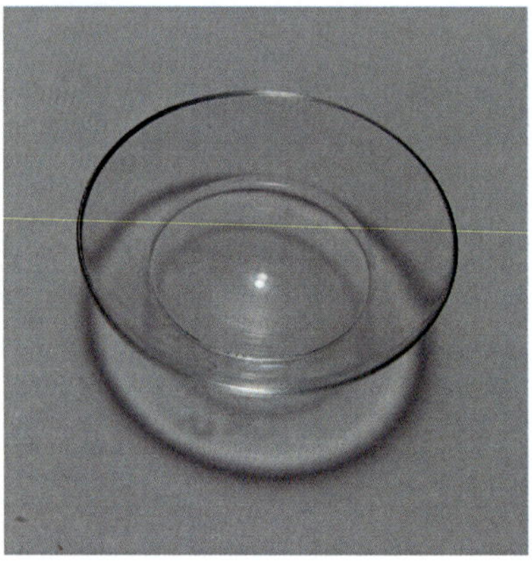

Fig. (7c). Zeiss lens showing sharp transitions.

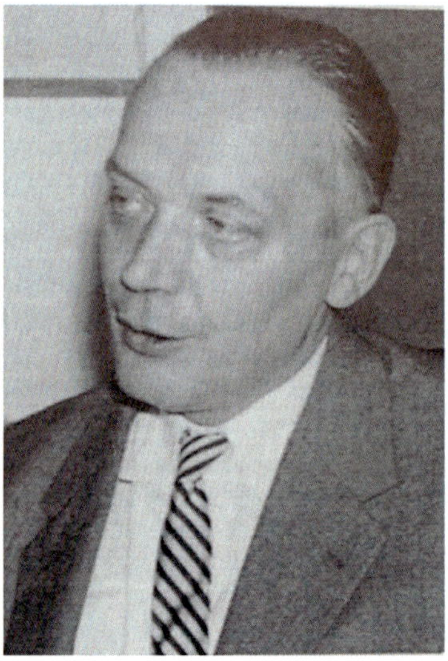

Fig. (8). Photograph of Adolf Müller Welt.

Adolf Wilhelm Müller-Welt of Stuttgart, Germany, descended from a family of glass artificial eye makers (Fig. **8**). In 1927, he started making scleral lenses, drawing from his experience in fitting artificial eyes. He described his lenses as having "a capillary tear layer over the cornea and retaining an air cushion beneath the scleral zone". The lenses, made from glass obtained from Schott of Jena, were blown over a series of preformed toric castings, which formed the scleral portion of the lens. These included areas of differing curvature to incorporate the insertions of the recti muscles [29]. The unfinished corneal portion was later ground and polished to the desired prescription. He was granted patent DRP. Nr. 553843 in 1932 and later introduced annealing to reduce the stresses produced in the glass during lens manufacture, thus improving the durability of the lenses (Fig. **5-7**).

Professor Leopold Heine, an ophthalmologist in Kiel, Germany, developed an "afocal" fitting set in 1929 for Zeiss (Fig. **9**) [30]. This utilized the increasing range of back optic zone radii to form a liquid lens of various powers under the lens to correct ametropia. The lens was fitted primarily to correct vision, so the physiological requirements of the eye were sacrificed for vision.

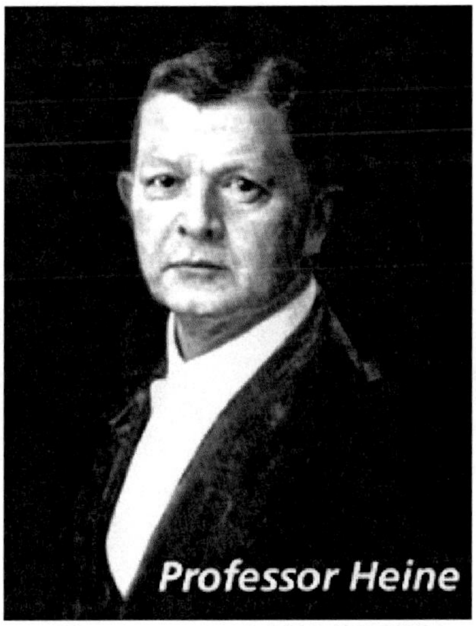

Fig. (9). Professor Leopold Heine.

In 1930, Josef Dallos, an ophthalmologist at the No. 1 Eye Clinic at the Royal Hungarian Peter Pazmany University at Budapest (Fig. **10**), developed an interest in the use of scleral lenses for the correction of visual defects. He felt that the best results would be obtained if he could closely follow the shape of the eye. Dallos investigated various impression materials and used Negocoll (derived from seaweed and described by Dr. Alphons Poller of Zurich) on the face of a cadaver. He prepared a positive cast of this impression in the wax-like substance Hominit, and the smooth appearance of the visible corneal segment convinced him that Negocoll would be a suitable medium for ophthalmic impressions [31]. Dallos used Müller lenses as impression trays [32] and filled the impression achieved with Homanit, making a positive cast. From this he made a negative cast with Plaster of Paris which was then converted into a brass die (Figs. **11a-d** and **12**) [33].

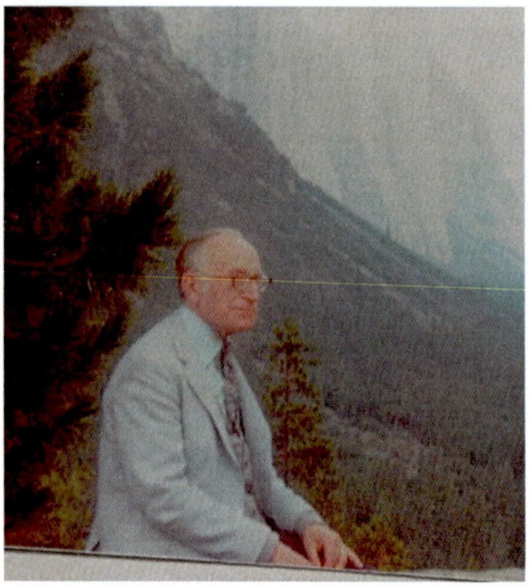

Fig. (10). Josef Dallos.

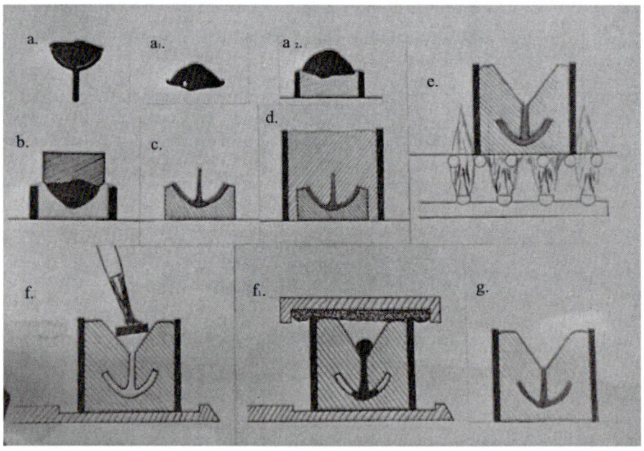

Fig. (11a). Sequence for lens making.

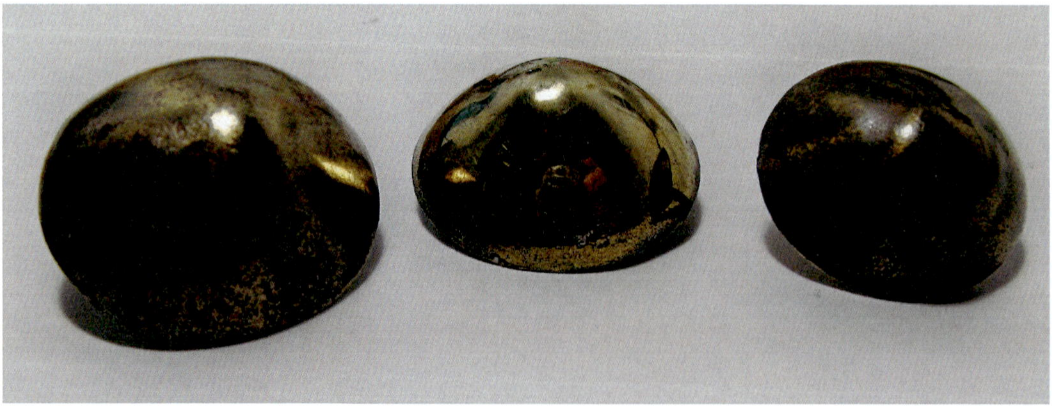

Fig. (11b). Dallos brass casts.

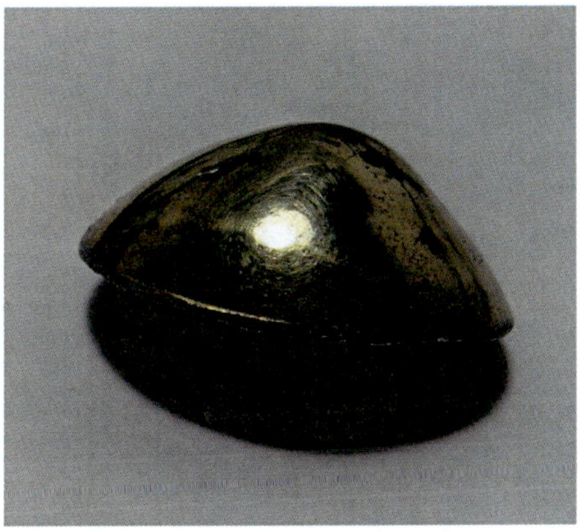

Fig. (11c). Profile view of Dallos brass cast.

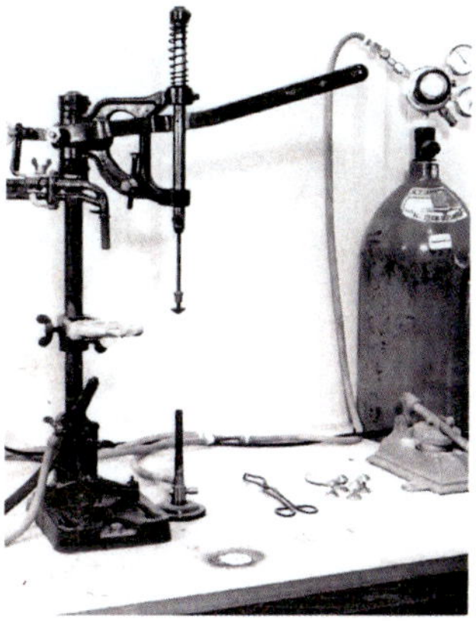

Fig. (11d). Dallos glass-making device. Image courtesy of Tony Sabell.

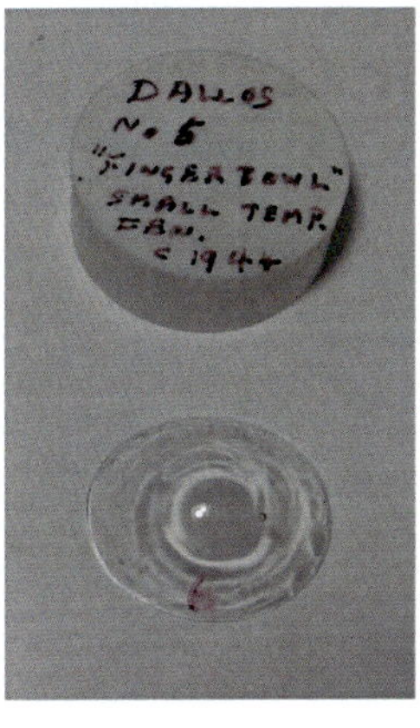

Fig. (12). Dallos lens.

The heated brass die was secured in the swinging arm of the press and pushed into the softened glass plate (thin glass photographic plates) at a suitable temperature, as judged by its color. The heat was then removed, and the glass solidified immediately. After ensuring a good fit of the lens, the central optical zone of the shell was then ground and polished. A similar technique was later used when PMMA materials were introduced. Working on the assumption that the natural body fluid offers the best chance of success, Dallos set out to conserve the tear reservoir to allow for its interchange by fresh tears, thus laying down the physiological principles for the successful fitting of scleral lenses.

In the 1930s, various plastics were being developed that would bring a great change to the development of contact lenses. A variety of materials were tried including cellulose nitrate (celluloid, highly flammable), cellulose acetate (used in spectacle frames), bakelite (made into multiple household objects), polyvinyl acetate (emulsion paint and adhesives), polyacrylates (developed by Otto Rohm and Otto Haas in their factory in Darmstadt and used in paint), and polystyrene (made by Imperial Chemical Industries [ICI]) into numerous household electrical items). In 1931, John Crawford and Rowland Hill, working separately for ICI in the UK, developed polymethylmethacrylate (PMMA), which had the registered trade name of "Perspex" but was also known as Lucite, Plexiglas, and Diakon. Rohm and Haas were licensed to use the ICI process to make Plexiglas sheets in Germany [34, 35]. However, the use of PMMA in Europe was held up due to a greater priority being given to military applications.

In 1933, Dallos suggested that if the front optic diameter was restricted to 8 mm (lenticulated), much higher optical values would be achievable without increasing the lens thickness and weight. At the same time, Professor Hans Hartinger of Zeiss suggested blending the sharp junction between the optic and scleral zones, and Zeiss trade literature offered the option of totally blended transition lenses [28]. This removed the "sharp edge" that touched the eye close to the limbal area. Using this same reasoning, Forknall, a UK optometrist, introduced the "offset scleral lens" in 1948 [36].

1935 saw Müller-Welt in Stuttgart introduce a fitting set of lenses with a toroidal scleral section for improved fitting and comfort, while Kohler and Danz, artificial eye makers of New York, US, made some blown glass lenses with ground optics; possibly the first contact lenses produced in the US.

In 1936, Theodore Obrig entered the contact lens arena (Fig. **13**). He had joined Gall & Lemke Optical Company (partially owned by his father) in 1914 as a graduate of Columbia University. As a medical student, he served in the US army as a bacteriologist and physiological chemist, returning to Gall & Lemke after the war. Around 1930, he became interested in contact lenses, fitting Zeiss ground glass lenses and later becoming an agent for Zeiss, fitting "on as many patients with high degrees of myopia, keratoconus and corneal scars as would submit to the ordeal [37]".

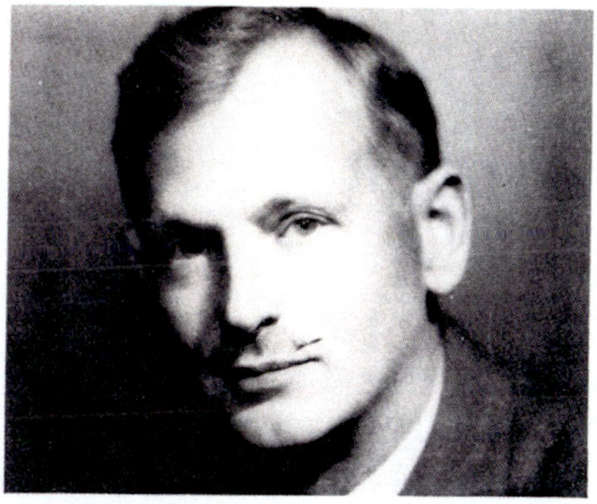

Fig. (13). Theodore Obrig.

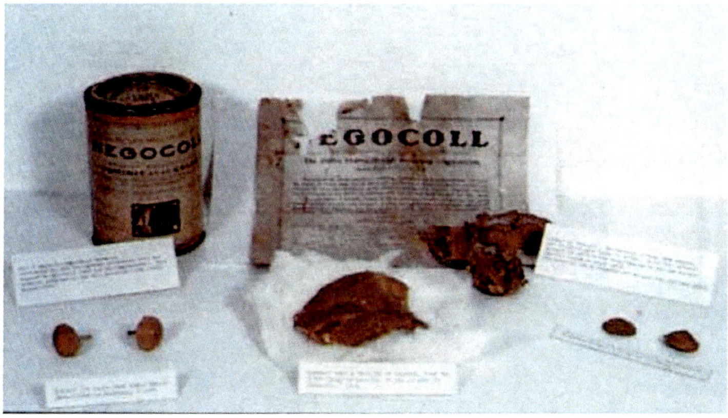

Fig. (14). Negocoll used by Dallos.

After a visit to Dallos in Budapest, Obrig started taking impressions of the eye and making lenses from the molds obtained. He used Negocoll, which was applied hot to the eye, to take the impressions using a funnel-shaped blown glass shell that was 22 mm in diameter, 7 mm deep, and had a 25 mm-long hollow handle plugged with cotton wool to retain the Negocoll (Fig. **14**). The shells were marked with colored spots or lines, red for right and light blue for left, which also indicated the position of the nasal canthus on the otherwise round shell. Some time later, he drilled perforations in the tray for the impression material to key onto as well as a variety of different sized, oval-shaped impression trays to conform to various eye shapes and sizes [38]. From the measurement of a number of impression casts, Obrig produced a table showing average corneal dimensions, which set the pattern of full corneal clearance fitting during the following decade.

Obrig encouraged Zeiss to make impression lenses, with the impressions being taken by the practitioner and sent to Zeiss in Jena. The finished lenses were relayed to US customers *via* the Zeiss office in New York. The lenses were made by blowing chemically resistant glass against a mold, with the optical portion being ground to prescription. Delivery took about four months. A pair of Zeiss lenses, en route to Leo Waldert, an optician in Rochester, New York, were on the Hindenburg (Fig. **15**) when it crashed and exploded at the Lakehurst Naval Base, New Jersey, on May 6, 1937 [39, 40].

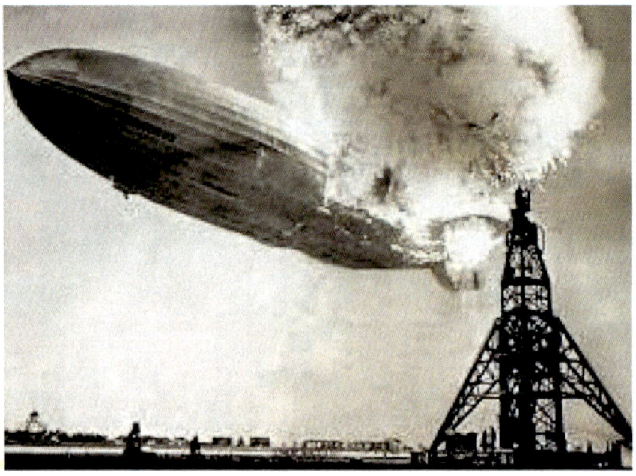

Fig. (15). Hindenburg in flames.

Cosmetically, the large optic zone of full corneal clearance was not acceptable, and the steep optic had to remain filled with fluid for the wearer to be able to see. A glove-like seal was required on the scleral zone, and any air seeping under the scleral portion resulted in an air bubble trapped in the steep apex of the lens in front of the pupil. Sattler's veil developed after about two hours of wear, visible to the wearer more readily indoors as a faint blue haze resembling tobacco smoke. Shortly after onset, the classic rainbow rings, resembling glaucoma halos, would be seen. Few patients could wear lenses for more than 30 minutes after the onset of these symptoms because the developing corneal edema produced photophobia, blepharospasm, and an unpleasant sensation of heat.

In the same year, Carl Hubert Sattler, an Austrian ophthalmologist working in Leipzig, investigated the corneal edema, which became known as Sattler's veil, induced by wearing ground spherical contact lenses [41]. By now, Joseph Dallos had accumulated so many glass shells from his earlier impressions that he was able to fit from his stock of "type shells". He demonstrated that the secret of fitting scleral lenses was not just the initial selection or the initial impression, but the careful tailoring of this first lens to the precise requirements of the individual eye to allow the exchange of tears beneath the lens. Because of his success, he continued to fit glass scleral lenses by this method until his death in 1979. He was never happy with PMMA lenses. He felt that by the time they were thin enough to be comfortable, they were not rigid enough to retain their shape. He later preferred to fit soft lenses.

Ida Mann was the first woman to become a consultant ophthalmologist at Moorfields Eye Hospital, London (1927), the first female professor of ophthalmology, and the first female professor at Oxford in 1945 (Fig. **16**). Together with Andrew Rugg-Gunn, an ophthalmologist from Western Eye Hospital, London, and Frederick Williamson-Noble, a consulting surgeon to St. Mary's, Paddington, Moorfields Eye Hospital, and later consultant to the Royal Navy, she visited Dallos in Budapest in 1936 to "learn the skills of making scleral lenses". They soon realized that the skills required were too complex to learn on a short trip and tried to persuade Dallos to move to the UK, but he refused. In the same year, William Feinbloom, a New York optometrist, introduced a scleral lens using a plastic material for the haptic portion that was bonded to a central glass optic zone (Fig. **17**) [42]. These were known as the U series from 1937 and as the T series from 1940 [25].

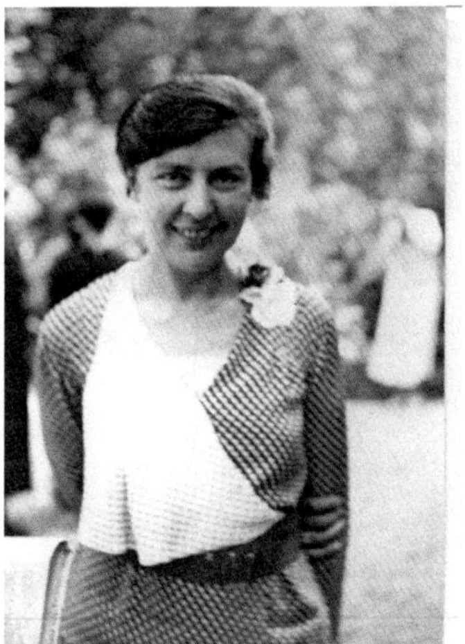

Fig. (16). Ida Mann.

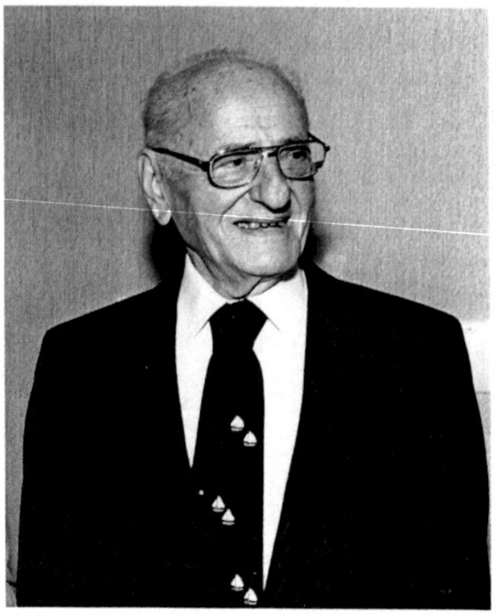

Fig. (17). William Feinbloom.

Preparations for war caused conditions to deteriorate in Hungary, and, as he was of Jewish descent, it was obvious that Dallos' work in Budapest could be destroyed. Ida Mann returned to Hungary on a rescue mission. Gerald Wingate, who owned the Theodore Hamblin Dispensing practices, had agreed to set up a contact lens clinic for Dallos at 18 Cavendish Square attached to their Wigmore Street premises. Josef Dallos and George Nissel, Dallos' brother-in-law, arrived in London in 1937. This was the first contact lens-only practice, and a commemorative plaque, unveiled by Dallos' widow, Vera Dallos-Pinter, in 2010, marks the spot (Fig. **18**). Dallos and Nissel commenced contact lens production and improvements in design.

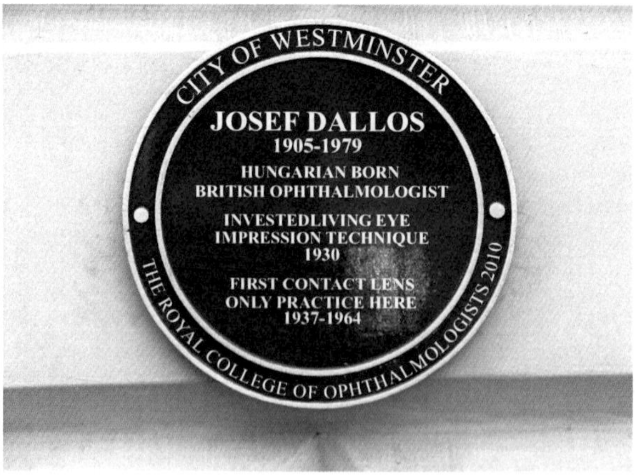

Fig. (18). The commemorative Dallos plaque at 18 Cavendish Square.

A major breakthrough occurred in 1938 when Theodore Obrig accidentally discovered that a blue filter introduced into a slit-lamp beam greatly enhanced the brightness of fluorescein solution. This made corneal abrasions and limbal pressure from contact lenses much more obvious [19]. In the same year, Obrig, together with engineer Ernest Mullen, made the first US all-plastic contact lens using the newly discovered "Plexiglas" (PMMA). The material was lightweight, optically clear, non-reactive, easily molded, ground, and polished, and inexpensive. He set up the Obrig Laboratories in the US, manufacturing an all-plastic, molded scleral lens.

Most fitters, except for Dallos and Müller Welt, concentrated on finding the right type of buffer solution to extend wearing time of lenses to reduce Sattler's veil. A 1% solution of sodium bicarbonate was used to fill the lens for insertion. At the start of symptoms, the lens was removed and refilled with a 2% solution. With the onset of additional symptoms, a 3% solution was used. This was called "stepping up" and gave a greater veil-free tolerance. Veiling also decreased with regular lens use [43].

Also in 1938, Dr. Istvan Györffy, a Hungarian ophthalmologist (Fig. **19**) working in the Maria Street Eye Clinic in Budapest (where Dallos had worked), was the first to use PMMA material for contact lenses in Europe. He came across the material during a visit to Germany in 1938 [44] and appreciated its potential. On his return to Budapest, he developed a technique for molding this sheet plastic and grinding the back and front optic surfaces. By late 1938, he had begun to fit acrylic scleral lenses and later went on to fit corneal lenses in this material [45 - 49]. Similar work was done that year by C. W. Dixey & Son Ltd., in London UK, who introduced lathe-turned, pre-formed acrylic scleral lenses, which were easier both to produce and to modify [50, 51]. Dixey's used a precision lathe to cut contact lenses from solid blocks of ICI Transpex material. The lathe was developed by dispensing optician Harry Birchall and engineer Cyril Winter. The process allowed greater variability in dimensions than was readily obtainable from the glass-grinding methods of Zeiss. The lenses could also be made thinner than Zeiss lenses without becoming excessively fragile, saving about 60% on the weight. A glass corneal lens made by Zeiss in 1932 measured 0.6 mm thick, whereas a 1948 acrylic lens measured 0.3 mm thick. The glass lens was at least four times the weight of the plastic one [52].

Although Zeiss had been at the very forefront of scleral lens design and manufacturing, the company suddenly stopped making lenses in the late 1930s to early 1940s, undoubtedly due to the other events that were happening in Europe at the time.

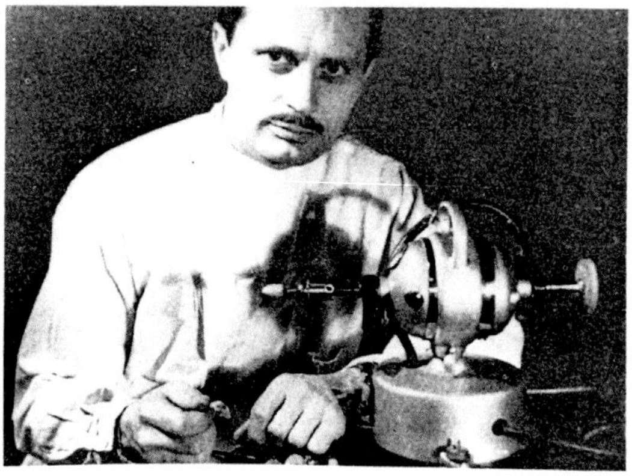

Fig. (19). Dr. Istvan Györffy.

In 1938, Dallos developed a telescopic combination of a contact lens and spectacle lens to enlarge the retinal image for cases of visual impairment. He also invented the Tholometer, a device modified from a Schiotz tonometer, to measure the sag, or vault, as he called it, of the cornea. This no longer exists, but a drawing survives (Fig. **20**).

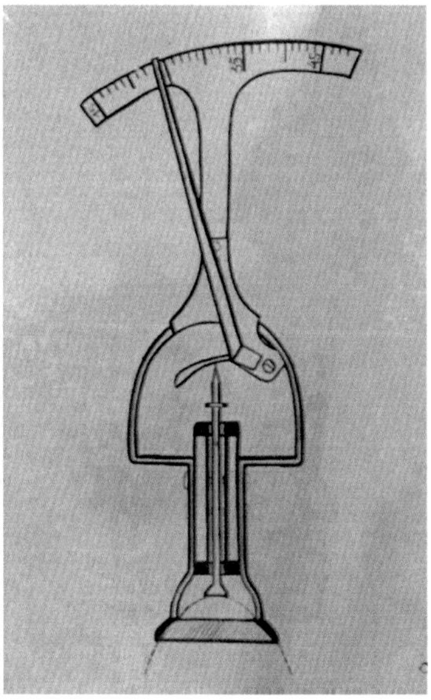

Fig. (20). Tholometer.

Around the same time, Dallos started the successful fitting of scleral lenses to 84 late-onset mustard gas keratitis casualties, their injuries dating from World War I [53]. Mustard gas was first used in trench warfare in Ypres, Belgium, in July

1917. The gas killed 4,086, but there were also 160,526 non-fatal mustard gas casualties from World War I [54]. Mustard gas is soluble in water, making it difficult to wash off. Hydrolysis, the splitting of a compound by water, is rapid, and the chemical causes blisters on contact with any damp skin or mucous membrane. The lungs and eyes are acutely targeted. Those surviving the lung effects endured loss of corneal epithelium, stromal opacification and thinning, followed by secondary infection and uveitis (Fig. **21**). Later, abnormalities of the limbal vascular bed, ischemia, and ulceration could occur [54]. Fitting scleral lenses helped restore optical function and made the eye more comfortable, but tolerance was still a problem.

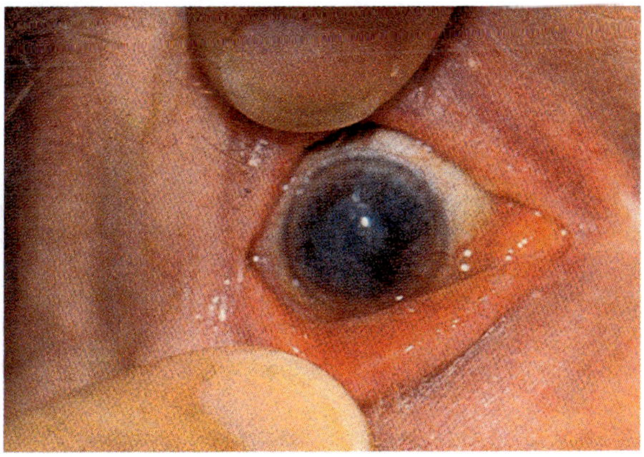

Fig. (21). Mustard Gas Keratitis.

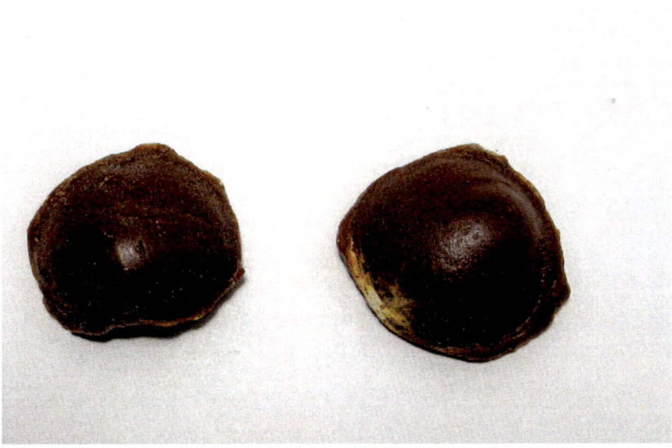

Fig. (22). Homonit casts used by Dallos.

In 1939, Dr. S. Maisler, a San Francisco doctor, described "a reversible hydrocolloid gel" introduced some months earlier by a San Francisco dental surgeon. This material – Kerr's hydrocolloid – was manufactured by the Detroit

Dental Manufacturing Company and was packaged in collapsible, toothpaste-type tubes. The tube was immersed in hot water and kneaded to soften the consistency. It was then applied onto the eye at 100–104°F (38–40°C) and set much quicker than previous impression materials (Fig. **22**). Maisler found that the blown glass impression trays as recommended by Obrig [38] were too fragile and described his own thin silver trays, which were sufficiently malleable to be adjusted for each eye (Fig. **23**) [55].

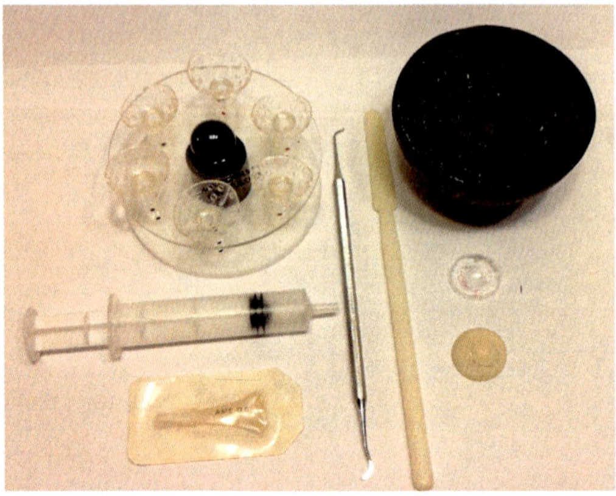

Fig. (23). Impression set from the 1980s.

Throughout WWII, Adolf Müller-Welt and his wife Ruth travelled all over Germany and occupied Europe fitting fluid-less glass scleral lenses to German officers who, at that time, were not allowed to wear spectacles while in uniform. They took with them cases of lens sets containing five to six thousand lenses in each and were thus able to fit almost all corrections [29]. Deteriorating conditions of war stopped such travel by 1944.

Theodore Obrig (Fig. **13**) introduced Ophthalmic Moldite, the first cold alginate impression material intended specifically for ophthalmic work, in 1943. This was a major breakthrough, as American optometrists were not allowed to use anesthesia without a physician being present due to drug laws. A cold injection method of molding avoided this requirement. Because the process was somewhat more comfortable, it helped the patient's eye remain stationary while the impression material was being applied, thus avoiding unseen interactions between the cornea and the impression shell [56]. By now, Obrig was using acrylic impression trays with hollow tubular handles and perforated bowls rather than his earlier blown glass ones [57]. This was followed in 1945 in the UK by Dental Zelex, a cold setting impression material, developed by Charles Keeler in Windsor, UK.

William Feinbloom in New York decided that minimal tangential touch on the sclera would not only evoke less sensation, but would enable an improved, balanced fit on the toroidally shaped sclera. He introduced the "Feincone lens" with an optic radius of 8.5 mm and cone angles of 43°, 46°, and 49°. Unfortunately, it was a full clearance lens and therefore did nothing to reduce the effects of Sattler's veil [58]. Meanwhile, in the UK, Norman Bier and Phillip Cole, both optometrists, introduced a small set of preformed fitting shells that supplemented the fitting sets of the Dixey lenses then in use. This was the "transcurve lens," and its originators claimed cosmetic superiority by virtue of a total diameter larger than that of the Dixey-type preformed lens. The most significant contribution associated with the transcurve lens was the introduction of the separate corneal measuring caps, later referred to as Fenestrated Lenses for Optic Measurement (FLOM) [59]. Around this time, Joseph Dallos and Norman Bier, working independently, formulated the fenestrated or "ventilated" scleral lens [60 - 62]. Earlier, Dallos had happened upon the idea by accident when he was forced to cut a 4mm hole in a glass scleral lens (Fig. **24**) to relieve the pressure on a "filtration scar" (trabeculectomy).

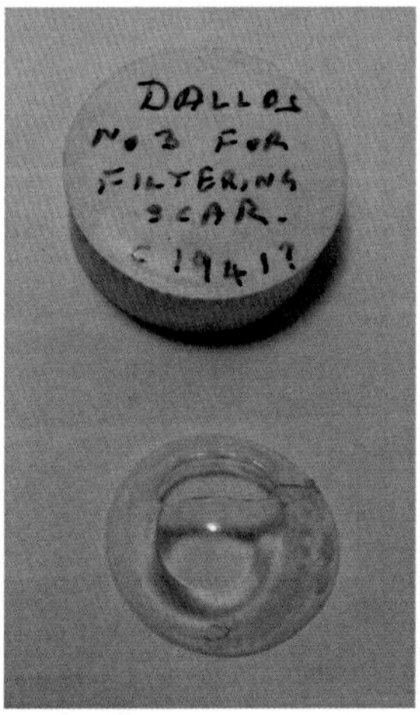

Fig. (24). Dallos lens to avoid a trabeculectomy scar.

Immediately, the comfortable wearing time of the lens doubled. He experimented with slots and holes (Fig. **25**) and found the most successful position for a small hole fenestration was on the temporal part of the lens close to the limbus, which had the effect of sucking in an air bubble on nasal gaze. Independently, Norman Bier (Fig. **26**) took out a patent, which was never enforced, for a series of slotted and fenestrated lenses to "permit lachrymal fluid and air to flow" through the lens. Tinted lenses also became available (Fig. **27**).

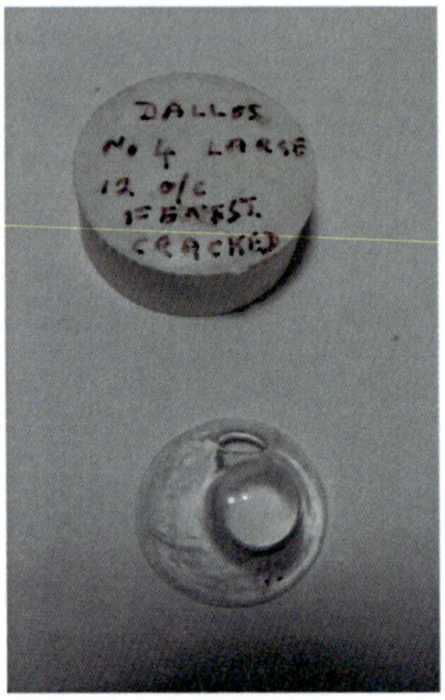

Fig. (25). Dallos lens with large fenestration at 12 o'clock.

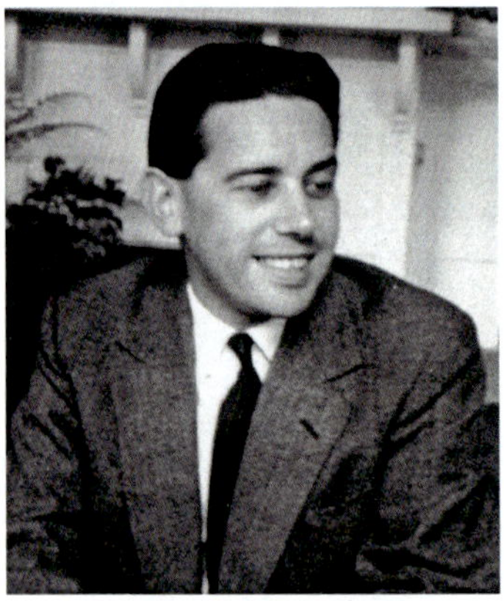

Fig. (26). Norman Bier.

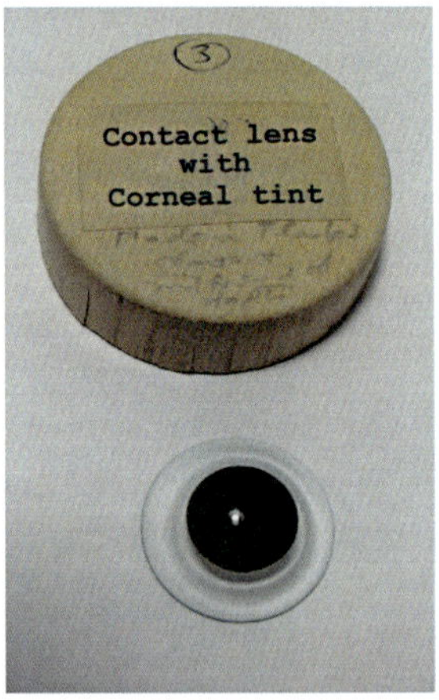

Fig. (27). Scleral lens with corneal tint.

It has often been queried as to how safe glass scleral lenses would be. In their book of 1946, Treissman and Plaice recount an apparently much-quoted case of a Zeppelin pilot who had fallen from his airship and was killed on hitting the ground [63]. Although his body and particularly his head were extremely damaged in the fall, the Zeiss lenses he was wearing were eventually recovered and found to be intact!

After the war, instead of scleral lenses being made by practitioners or in their own workshops, new contact lens laboratories appeared to supply independent practitioners. In the UK, George Nissel (Fig. **28**) was the first to set up his own lens manufacturing laboratory in Siddons Lane, London, in 1946 (a commemorative plaque was unveiled here in 2010 (Fig. **29**) just off Baker Street) and produced the "wide angle lens" based on the Feincone design. This was a scleral lens design with a spherical optic and scleral zone linked with a conical section. This design, together with the Feincone and Kelvin Conic lenses, aimed to reduce the vast numbers of permutations by standardizing the diameter of the optic zone. In 1947, Raymond Kelvin Watson (Fig. **30**), an optometrist in Manchester, UK, introduced his Kelvin Conic Lens [64], which was a scleral lens with a spherical optic zone and a conical scleral zone. It had an extra curve at the temporal side to provide a closer scleral fit [65]. Watson started the Kelvin Contact Lens company and developed methods of molding both scleral and corneal lenses [66]. In 1947, Obrig Laboratories opened a London branch in Park Lane, and Moldite became readily available in the UK. This lab would later be bought by Smith & Nephew in the early days of soft lenses.

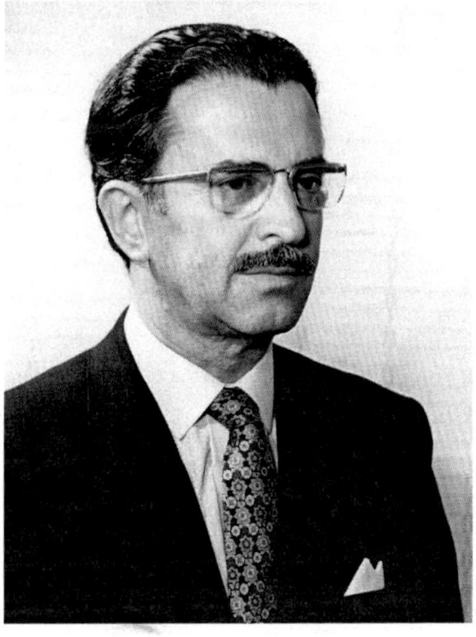

Fig. (28). George Nissel.

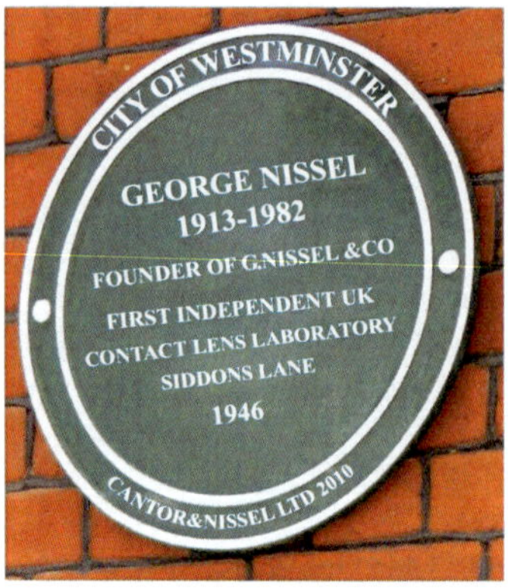

Fig. (29). George Nissel Plaque.

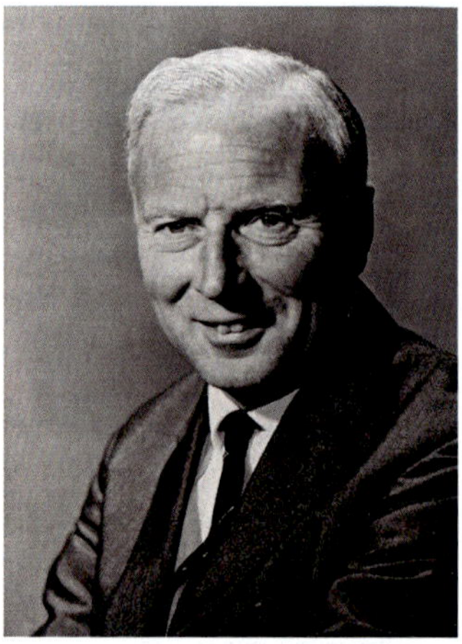

Fig. (30). Raymond Kelvin Watson.

Scleral lenses were also developed for covert operations. Norman Bier produced an underwater scleral lens (Fig. **31**) in 1951 that had a small "goggle" cemented to the front of each optic section, creating a small airspace to provide clear vision underwater without the risk of an alert sentry seeing the "flash" of the flat face plate of a diving mask. In the same year, Arthur Forknall, an optometrist from Wollaton in Nottingham, UK, designed the "offset lens" – again, a scleral lens with a spherical optic and an aspheric scleral zone that attempted to place even pressure on the sclera. It simplified fitting by eliminating the need to adjust the scleral zone radius when the total diameter was changed. As McKellen [67] pointed out, this design was neglected by most contact lens practitioners until it was later reintroduced by Montague Ruben as an offset corneal lens in 1966 [68].

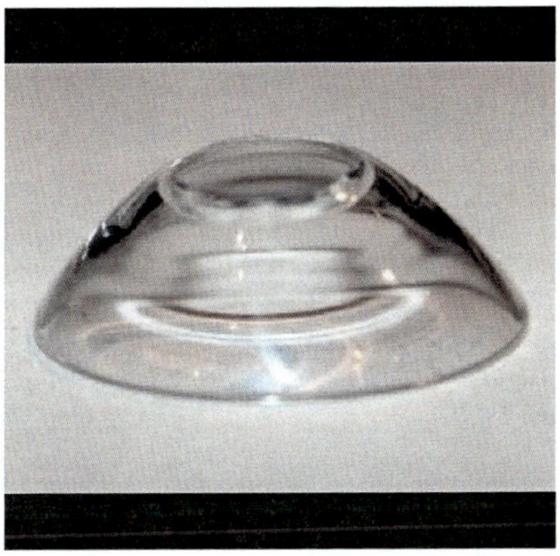

Fig. (31). Bier underwater lens courtesy of the Contact Lens Collection at the BOA Museum College of Optometrists, London.

In 1949, Alexander Cross, a London ophthalmologist, reported that there were at least 31 flying members of the RAF during WWII who wore contact lenses [69]. These were mainly to help experienced pilots back into the air following previous traumatic cataracts caused by shards of flying perspex from their aircraft canopies. It was those shards that gave Harold Ridely the idea for developing intraocular implants.

That year, Drs. Newton K. Wesley and George Jessen in Chicago produced yet another corneal molding technique called "concentric molding". It used a contact lens-like impression tray without a handle, and the inside surface was "scored or grooved" for good adhesion of the Moldite. The theory was provided that the impression tray had the same dimensions and proportions as the finished lens, it would center itself accurately with its optic zone corresponding to the patient's cornea, so that eye positioning was not critical [70]. Meanwhile, Frederick Burnett Hodd in London, UK, developed the method of using trays without handles, which, in certain circumstances, was superior to the use of trays with handles. In 1950, George Nissel packaged Ophthalmic Zelex into single-dose plastic tubes. More recently, dental alginates, such as Tissutex, Kromopan, and Orthoprint, have been used. Storey [71] published some observations on the possible use of polysulphide rubber impression materials, and silicone rubber impression materials became popular with some practitioners [72].

With the advent of the corneal lens by Tuohy in 1948 and the micro corneal lens by Frank Dickinson (UK), Jack Neill (US), and Wilhelm Söhnges (Germany), interest in scleral lenses started to wane. However, in 1957, Obrig Laboratories produced the Lacrilens, a molded PMMA scleral lens with a large perforation in the lower part of the lens, which connected to the corneal vault by means of two channels formed in a V shape [25]. In 1967, Fraser and Gordon (UK) designed the Apex lens specifically for the Hospital Service. The name Apex is derived from "aphakic experiment". The large semi-scleral design was quite thick and heavy in aphakic prescriptions, but it provided stable vision from its limbal locating characteristics [73]. However, its long-term use in PMMA material led to corneal neovascularization in many cases [74]. The design is still used in high-Dk materials for high prescriptions.

THE RE-EMERGENCE OF SCLERAL LENSES

John James Little in Edinburgh, UK, claims to have fitted the first gas permeable scleral lenses made from CAB material in the 1970s. Similarly, Arthur Irving claims that RGP scleral lenses were made by David Thomas contact lenses in Northampton, UK, around the same time. However, no records can be found for either of these events. Recorded at the BCLA conference in 1983, Don Ezekiel (Fig. **32**) from Perth, Australia, reported making scleral lenses using two different RGP materials. The design was later called the Gelflex Scleral and gained FDA clearance for use in the US. The following year, Brien Holden and George Mertz reported that the oxygen demand of the cornea was 70-75mm Hg, which helped to spur many manufacturers to create improved materials for contact lenses. Most of the major contact lens players had turned their attention away from any rigid lenses in favor of soft lenses, as this was where the big money lay. Because soft lenses did not make all of the distorted corneas go away, interest in scleral lenses continued.

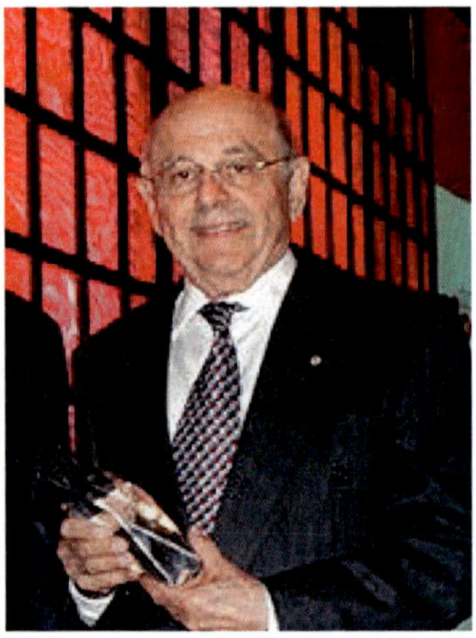

Fig. (32). Don Ezekiel.

In 1985, the spherical scleral lens was developed by Rients Visser of Visser Contactlenzen (The Netherlands), and production techniques were made possible by Ben Wanders from Procornea. Later improvements in this design included toric scleral lenses that were developed in a collaboration of Rients Visser and Ben Wanders. These scleral lenses are available in diameters ranging from 18.0-25.0 mm and are indicated for irregular corneal surfaces, dry eyes, mechanical protection, or to facilitate corneal healing. Front surface cylinders are available. The bitangential scleral lens designs were developed by Visser Contactlenzen in collaboration with Bart van der Linden from NKL Contactlenzen.

In 1987, the Panasil C impression material was developed by Kettenbach GmbH, although this was withdrawn in 1993. In 1992, Ken Pullum, a UK optometrist, founded Innovative Sclerals in Hertford, UK, to supply and fit RGP scleral lenses. As RGP materials could not be molded in the same way as glass or PMMA, he needed to find a different method of manufacturing. First, an impression was taken of the eye, then the cast was computer scanned, and the back surface of the lens was lathe cut using CAD/CAM technology. The front surface was finished by hand to keep the overall thickness down to an absolute minimum. This company was bought by Bausch + Lomb in 2015.

Robert L. Cotie and Alan Hirshberg of C&H Contact Lenses applied for a patent in 1994 on their Macrolens, a 14mm diameter rigid semi-scleral lens designed to provide the wearability and comfort of a soft lens. US Patent 5929968 was granted in 1999. It was renamed the SoClear lens, available from Dakota Sciences of Sioux Falls, South Dakota, US, and from Art Optical, Grand Rapids, Michigan, US, and is now available in four versions; SoClear Standard (STD), SoClear Keratoconus (Kera), SoClear Multifocal (MF), and SoClear Reverse Curve (RC). SO_2Clear scleral lenses are manufactured and available in the UK from No. 7 Contact Lenses. Distribution is also available throughout Australia, Europe, Hong Kong, Russia, Taiwan and Asia. Additionally, Con-lens in Denmark distributes So_2Clear lenses.

Also in 1994, the Boston Foundation for Sight, now known as BostonSight, of Needham, MA, US, gained FDA clearance for the Boston Scleral Lens and for lenses now used in prosthetic replacement of the ocular surface ecosystem (PROSE) treatment. PROSE lenses are available in the US, India, and Canada. The BostonSight SCLERAL is FDA approved and was launched in 2017. The BostonSight SCLERAL is the first scleral lens fitting system based on scleral anatomy and driven by clinical data. It offers right and left eye anatomical designs and front surface eccentricity options to improve both quantitative and qualitative vision. It is an evidence-based, data-driven fitting system that optimizes fitting efficiency in the 18.0mm, 18.5mm, and 19.0mm diameter category.

In 1995, a better impression material arrived in the shape of the Panasil Light Body. This was a polyvinyl siloxane impression material supplied in two cartridges that auto mixed in an application gun and was applied to the eye in an impression shell. It was thought to be accurate enough to identify fingerprints. This was surpassed in 2002 by the Tresident DH impression material.

Impressions or the use of preformed trial shells had always been the best way of fitting scleral lenses. Whereas keratometers and later topographers had been developed to measure the curvature and shape of the cornea, instruments were not available to measure the shape of the sclera. In 1938, Hembold designed a circular device made up of blunt pins. The device was pressed against the eye, and the pins would slide in and out so shape could then be reproduced at the opposite end of the eye. (Much like the Contour Gauge (Fig. **33**) that can be purchased in stores now to replicate the outline of architraves). For obvious reasons, this was not a great success. George Nissel turned to photographing the eye in various directions of gaze and then stitched the images together to get some idea of the shape of the cornea and sclera. He made a British Patent application 35161 / 38 on December 2, 1938 and US Patent 2279795 on April 14, 1942. An idea ahead of its time, it was limited by the technology of photography available.

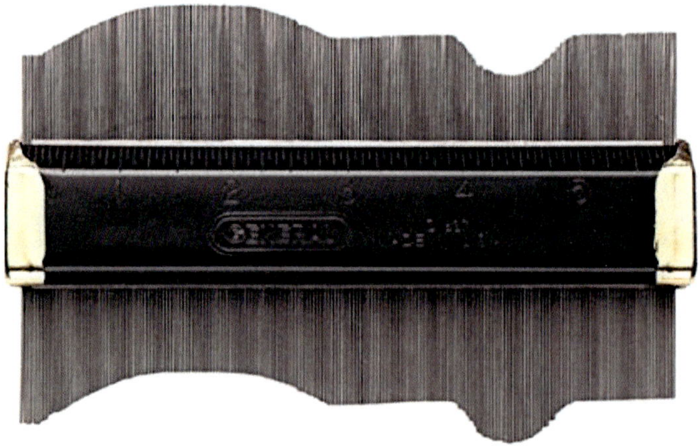

Fig. (33). Contour Gauge.

In 1997, the Falco mini-scleral lens from Switzerland was introduced, designed by Falco Linsen. The scleral lens designs SKV (aspheric scleral lens, limbal aspheric) and SKT (scleral-toric aspheric lens) were developed in collaboration with Eyeness A.G., Michael Wyss, and Michael Bärtschi and were introduced in 2009. The SKV, SKT (rotational symmetrical back surface), SMV (multicurve scleral lens), and SMT (limbal and scleral toric back surface, multicurve) are all 16.00 mm designs. The miniV (rotational symmetrical back surface) and miniT (limbal and scleral toric back surface) are both available in 14.80 mm diameters. The SKV, SKT, SMV, and SMT lenses are available in 15.0 and 17.50 mm diameters. Falco scleral lenses are available in multiple front surface designs including prism, prism and front toric, dynamic stabilization, front toric, and presbyopic (simultaneous bifocal and trifocal) designs. The Falco multifocal may be manufactured as either bifocal simultaneous or trifocal simultaneous designs. Distribution is available in Switzerland, Principality of Liechtenstein, Germany, Austria, Poland, Namibia, South Africa, UK, Italy, and Norway.

Dutch technical and scientific photographer Dr. Frans Jongsma invented the Eye Surface Profiler in 1998 based on the publication of his PhD thesis. Applications of the Eye Surface Prolifer design were first published in the PhD thesis of Dr. John de Brabander in 2002. In 2010, Dr. Ir Chris Velzel led the hardware re-design and miniaturization of the Profiler into its current shape. The Eye Surface Profiler measures the curvature of a 20 mm diameter of the front surface of the eye. It uses a technology called Fourier Transform Profilometry (Profilometry in short). Profilometry generates a dense 3D point cloud that describes the corneal and scleral shape. This 3D shape of the anterior surface of the eye enables practitioners to fit all types of lenses and to make new lens designs. However, it took another 15 years to bring this technology to market. The Eye Surface Profiler was launched in Europe in 2014 and the US in 2015. Distribution is available in all countries in Europe, the US, Australia, Canada, Malaysia, and Taiwan.

The Jupiter lens was designed by Dr. Robert Breece of MedLens Innovations in 2001 but is now made by Visionary Optics of Front Royal VA, US, following the untimely death of Dr. Breece in 2009. The Jupiter 15 mm and 18 mm come in three configurations to address different corneal geometries. First is the standard design in which the central corneal curve has a slightly steeper radius than the peripheral corneal curve. Most cases of corneal irregularity (keratoconus, post-surgical, *etc.*) can be fit with this design. In the advanced keratoconic design, the central curve is relatively steeper than the peripheral corneal curve. In the reverse geometry design, the central curve is relatively flatter than the peripheral corneal curve. The Jupiter lens was licensed to Essilor in 2006. The ProLOOK™ lens was introduced in 2016 by Essilor.

The MSD Corporation was established in 2006. The development of the corporation had started several years prior, when the company Unique Contact Lens was acquired in 1998 by Viscon. Viscon had a 13.5 mm thermal molded lens called the Epicon, which provided variable comfort. The 15.8 mm MSD lens was created with a unique patented hinge in the design. The name MSD, Mini Scleral Design, was created by MacDonald, Sturm, and Dootjes (MSD). Dr. Steve Byrnes helped with the further development and evolutionary process of the MSD scleral lens. The msd™ 15.8 mm and 18.0 mm as well as the msd™ 4FR 14mm and 14.5 mm are all available. With Blanchard as a distributor and manufacturer, msd™ is available in countries including Scandinavia, Mexico, and Serbia. The msd Select™ is also available with customizable parameters and an adjustable limbal zone and edge configuration, as are the multifocal msd Continu,™ a simultaneous vision design; msd TLZ™ torodial landing zone; msd™ front toric; and msd ULtra light™.

In 2006, Scot Brown of Scotlens developed the One8 design available in an 18.0 mm diameter. This design evolved into the 16.0 mm and 18.0 mm diameters and was renamed EasyScleral in 2012. EasyScleral is available as standard spherical, toric periphery, bi-toric, front surface toric, limbal zone alteration, and center thickness specification designs.

In 2007, William Masler, President of Acculens, Denver, US, designed the Maxim scleral lens. It since has had eight design updates and is licensed to Bausch + Lomb in the UK and to Mediphacos in Brazil. Masler designed the Comfort SL scleral lens in 2010 and the EasyFit scleral lens in 2013. In 2012, Troy Miller, the Vice President of Operations at Acculens, designed the Maxim Plus Multifocal scleral lens and the Comfort SL Plus Multifocal. The EasyFit Plus was designed in 2013, and the Maxim Plus Multifocal Center Progressive was designed in 2015. All Acculens designs are available with front toric, toric peripheral curves, and periscopic function. Outside of the US, Acculens products are manufactured and available under license in the UK, European Union, India, South America, Central America, Mexico, Canada, and the Middle East.

Valley Contax first introduced Valley scleral lenses in 2007. The Custom Stable™ (CS) generation was introduced in 2011. The Custom Stable is a complete family of scleral lenses designed by Josh Adams, NCLC, and his assistant Ryan Kulas. The CS family consists of lenses in diameters from 14.8 mm to 17.8 mm in both symmetrical landing zones (CS Prime) and toric landing zones (CS Elite). The reverse curve limbal clearance zone may be used to customize any fit. The CS Aurora multifocal is available on all types of scleral lenses with add powers from +1.25D to +3.50D. Custom Stable lenses are available in the US, and also distributed out of Italy and Singapore.

In 2008, Dr. Greg Gemoules (Fig. **34**) of Texas, US, published a paper on a novel method of fitting scleral lenses using high resolution optical coherence tomography (OCT) [75]. Since that time, he has developed his technique to include laser scanning of the anterior surface, which is downloaded into a computer program for 3D modeling to create a scleral lens called LaserFit®. The dimensions of the lenses and the radii of curvature of the various surfaces can be modified and cut on CNC lathes by TruForm Optics. Final powers feature wavefront-guided optics to control optical aberrations. Because the scleral lens is extremely stable, it allows the opportunity for aberration control.

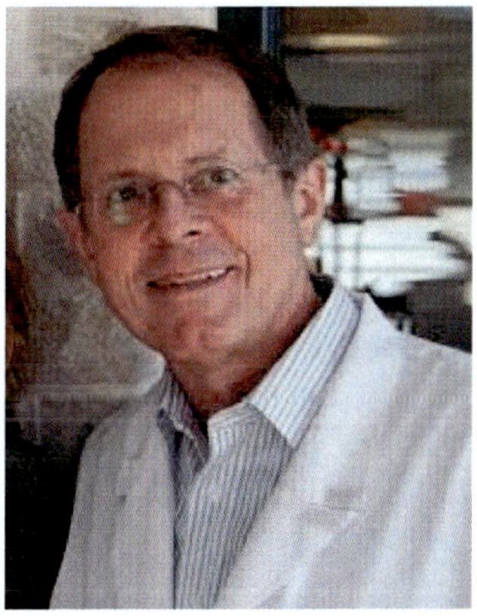

Fig. (34). Greg Gemoules.

The ICD family of scleral lenses was introduced in 2008 and designed by John Mountford (Australia), Don Noack (Australia), Patrick Caroline (US), Bob Heavyside (Canada), and Randy Kojima (Canada). The ICD is licensed and distributed by Paragon Vision Sciences through its global authorized manufacturer network. The initial diameter was 16.5 mm, and a diameter of 14.5 mm was introduced in 2015. Both diameters have tangent angle technology to allow a smooth transition from the limbus to the bulbar conjunctiva. Each has four zones that can be altered to achieve the required central and limbal clearance and allow proper landing on the sclera. Both lens diameters are available with a front surface toric option. This lens is distributed in the US, Australia, Mexico, UK, Sweden, Finland, Denmark, France, Algeria, Tunisia, Morocco, Spain, Portugal, Chile, Italy, San Marino, Vaticano, Israel, Hong Kong, Poland, Russia, Germany, South Africa, Canada, and Singapore.

In 2008, TruForm Optics introduced the DigiForm line of scleral lenses developed by TruForm's team of lens designers led by Jan Svochak. The 15.0 mm DigiForm came first, followed by the DigiForm 18.0 mm and 16.6 mm designs. All DigiForm lenses are template designs based upon a database of both oblate and prolate corneas acquired from a patented method of digital imaging. Fitting sets are supplied with laser marked base curve and sag values for cataloging. Toric and quadrant specific options are available. Multifocal options include near center and distance/near/distance. TruForm scleral lenses are available in the US, Australia, Brazil, Chile and Paraguay.

In October 2009, as a result of the increased interest in scleral lens fitting, the Scleral Lens Education Society was founded based on discussions between Dr. Rob Breece, Dr. Greg DeNaeyer, and Dr. Christine Sindt. The Scleral Lens Education Society "teaches contact lens practitioners the science and art of prescribing scleral contact lenses. The Scleral Lens Society supports public education that highlights the benefits and availability of scleral contact lenses". The founding board members were President: Dr. Greg DeNaeyer, Vice–President: Dr. Christine Sindt, Secretary: Dr. Bruce Baldwin, Treasurer: Dr. Jason Jedlicka, Public Education Committee Chair: Dr. Muriel Schornack, Fellowship Chair: Dr. Mindy Toabe, and International Chair: Dr. Eef van der Worp. The website, www.sclerallens.org, was launched in 2010 as the official website for the organization, containing information about scleral lens fitting, sponsors, scientific articles and publications, and videos on scleral lens handling as well as a forum for scleral lens practitioners to exchange information and advice.

In 2009, the Dyna Semi-Scleral® and Dyna Scleral® lenses were introduced by the R & D team at Lens Dynamics, Inc. under the direction of Al Vaske. The Dyna Semi-Scleral® is available from 13.5 mm to 16.0 mm, whereas the Dyna Scleral® has diameters from 16.1 mm to 21.0 mm. Both designs are available with reverse geometry, quad sym edge treatment, multifocal front, bitoric, and front toric options. Dyna scleral lenses are manufactured and distributed in the US, UK, Canada, Israel, Jamaica, Hungary, Mexico, Spain and Vietnam.

In 2009, Dr. Harvey Yamamoto designed and introduced the iSight™ Scleral lenses for GP Specialists. The iSight™ Scleral lens, with a standard diameter of 16.4 mm, is a uniquely designed scleral lens that utilizes multiple aspheric conical curves to achieve a more natural tangential fitting zone. The iSight™ Scleral lens can vault both the cornea and limbal zone while maintaining a minimal sagittal depth that promotes good tear exchange. Outside of the US, these lenses are distributed in Vietnam, Thailand, Cambodia, Laos, China, Japan, and Korea.

In 2010, Northern NLS scleral lenses introduced scleral lenses up to 18.0 mm. NLS lenses are designed by Dr. Jim Edwards *via* the WAVE software system. Two styles are offered: vaulting and alignment. Both are available in toric, bitoric, asymmetric, and multifocal (center near or center distance). Every lens is customizable with multiple parameters. Compound over-refraction is possible for compromised patients. Wave scleral lenses are available in the UK, Australia, Canada, Hong Kong, Kazakhstan, the Netherlands, Mexico, Spain, and Singapore.

Also in 2010, Walter Miller at Infinity Optical created the Infinity scleral lens. Infinity Optical was acquired by ABB Optical Group in March 2016. Lens diameters are available from 14.5 mm to 18mm. The Infinity lens allows a variable optic zone to control the central and limbal vault by changing a single curve.

EYEART Laboratories in Greece introduced the EPSILON scleral lens in 2010, designed by Lefteris Karageorgiadis, OD, Nikos Vasileiou, OD, and Nikos Karageorgiadis, MD. The Epsilon design is manufactured from 17.00 mm to 20.00 mm. Features include aspheric lens surfaces, toric landing zones with up to a 250 micron difference between the flat and steep meridians, front toric, and center near multifocal correction.

In 2011, the KERATOS ESCLERAL SG was introduced by Keratos in Colombia. Lens diameters of 15.0 mm to 17.0 mm are available in a tricurve design with three scleral landings. These lenses are distributed in Colombia, Ecuador, Argentina, Chile, Brazil, Panama and Curacao.

Paragon Vision Sciences launched NormalEyes in 2012, a 15.5 mm scleral lens design developed from the Paragon CRT lenses. Also in 2012, Onefit 14.9 mm diameter, aimed at failed soft toric lens wearers, was launched by Blanchard.

In 2012, Procornea (The Netherlands) developed Senso Sclera lenses designed by Mr. Ben Wanders. Senso semi scleral (14.4 mm), mini sclera (16.4 mm), and full scleral (20.0 mm) lens designs are also available. Senso full scleral lenses are indicated for extremely irregular corneas; these lenses have a toric periphery in the standard design. An ideal fit for Senso semi-scleral lenses is achieved by adjusting the combination of sagittal height, peri-factor of the periphery, and toricity. Lens weight is divided between the cornea and sclera, providing good comfort and clarity of vision.

In 2012, SLC Conica scleral lens was launched by MedLac. SLC Conica was designed by Dr. Marco Iovino (Avellino, Italy) and Dr. Riccardo Olent (Torino, Italy). SLC Conica is composed of four functional zones: the optical zone, compensator zone, limbal zone, and scleral zone. Standard scleral lens diameters are 16.8 mm and 18.5 mm. Custom diameters are available from 15.6 mm to 17.8 mm. Four different scleral lens designs are available: SLC Conica (symmetrical), SLC Conica Dual SAG (patented design in which two meridians have two different sag depths), SLC Conica front toric (patented design for cylindrical over-refraction correction with dynamic stabilization), and SLC Conica PK (oblate design for post-graft to obtain low limbal vaulting). Distribution is available in Italy and Greece.

The Atlantis scleral was launched at the end of 2013 by X-Cel Specialty Contacts. Design input was received from Buddy Russell, Craig Norman, Augusto Rosse, and Edgar Davilla. The standard diameter for Atlantis is 15.0 mm, but 16.0 mm to 17.5 mm diameters are also available. A unique edge design, based on a calculation process, aids in lens settling, deep sagittal depths, and flatter base curves. Scleral lens options include front toric, toric peripheral curves, lens notching, adjustable limbal sagittal depth, and multifocal. Outside of the US, Atlantis is distributed in Argentina, Bolivia, Colombia, Peru and Canada.

In 2013, Visionary Optics partnered with Dr. Greg DeNaeyer (Fig. **35**) to design a second-generation Jupiter lens. The final product became the Europa Scleral lens, which has three diameters of 16.0 mm, 18.0 mm, and 20.0 mm. Other lens parameters can be customized to suit any preferences and requirements. Scleral lens options include front toric, toric haptics, bitoric, lens notching, and front surface presbyopia correction. The company's Elara Scleral lens was introduced in 2015 as a mini-scleral lens that rests on the sclera and vaults over the cornea. The Elara Scleral design has a prolate geometry designed to fit regular corneas. Visionary Optics has a licensed manufacturer in Europe that manufactures Europa lenses and ships to accounts throughout Europe.

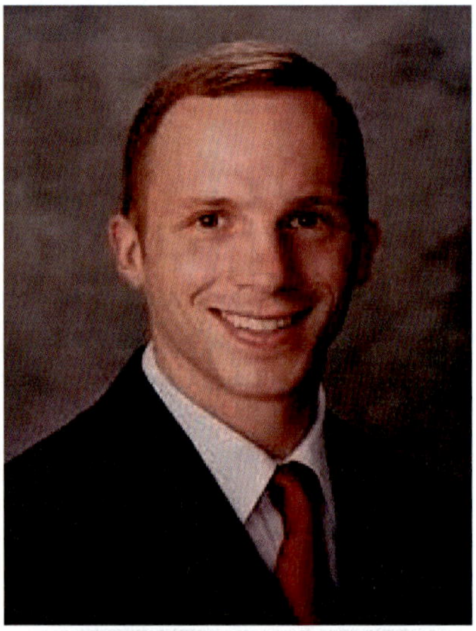

Fig. (35). Greg DeNaeyer.

Also in 2013, the AVT Scleral was designed by Keith Parker at Advanced Vision Technologies. In 2015, Sag Sight Technology (SST) was introduced to evaluate the size of the limbal zone where two identification marks (dots) indicate the 12 mm chord. The AVT scleral is available in sphere, toric, multifocal, toric peripheral curves, and any combination of the above. The Naturalens™ was introduced in 2017.

The same year, EyePrintPRO™ was developed by Christine Sindt, OD, and Keith Parker. EyePrintPRO™ is an impression-based transparent prosthetic scleral device. This device is designed to match the precise contours of the eye. An impression of the eye captures the curvatures of the entire ocular surface with 1-2 micron accuracy. EyePrintPRO™ lens options include toric, decentered optics, multifocal, prism, and higher-order aberration correction.

In 2013, the EyeSpace Scleral was designed by Lachlan Scott-Hoy. Lenses range in diameter from 16.0 mm to 20.0 mm. Larger lens diameters are available on request. The EyeSpace Scleral 2 was released in 2016. This latest offering accounts for spherical aberration and toricity by utilizing a fitting set, the EyeSpace software, and a topographer. OCT is useful, but not essential, to fit these lenses. They are distributed in New Zealand, Australia, South Africa, the US, and Singapore.

Rients Visser and his team (Visser Contactlenzen, Nijmegen, The Netherlands) collaborated with Bart van der Linden (NKL Contactlenzen, Emmen, the Netherlands, and a Menicon Group company) to realize the bitangential scleral lens design in 2013. The development of tangential scleral lenses resulted from a combination of a long history of tangential corneal lens designs and the fitting experience of Visser and his team. These scleral lenses are defined by a front optical zone, a spherical back optical zone, and a mid-peripheral zone that vaults the limbal area. These scleral lenses have two meridians with a different tangential angle to enable gentle application to the sclera. These two different meridians of the linear alignment zone are 90 degrees apart and make the back surface non-rotationally symmetrical, a so-called toric surface. A rotationally symmetric design is also available with the same tangential landing zone. Mini scleral lenses (14.0 mm to 17.5 mm) and large scleral lenses (18.0 mm to 24.0 mm) are available. Front surface cylinder is possible. These lenses are distributed within Europe by the Menicon Group Companies (names differ per location) and in the US and Canada by SynergEyes under the brand name SynergEyes VS and SynergEyes VS XL.

In 2014, Genesis was launched by Metro Optics for irregular corneas, including corneal abnormalities, and extreme dry eye. This lens is available in 15.6 mm and 18.2 mm diameters. In 2016, InSight Scleral® was developed by Drs. Neil Hodur and Jennifer Harthan in collaboration with the research and development team at Metro Optics. InSight Scleral® is a center distance design with the add power present in the mid-peripheral portion of the lens. Diameters range from 15.2 mm to 15.6 mm in the standard design and 13.5 mm to 20.0mm in the custom design. Peripheral curves range from flat 1 to steep 3. Toric peripheral curves are also available.

In 2014, Mini S was introduced by Soleko, Italy, designed by Carlo Tronti. This lens is available in 16.8 mm and 18.2 mm diameters and features multi-spherical geometry with aspheric transition curves. These lenses are also available outside of Italy.

Alden Optical, now part of Bausch + Lomb Specialty Vision Products, launched Zenlens in 2014, co-designed with Dr. Jason Jedlicka. Lens diameters of 16.0 mm and 17.0 mm are appropriate for a wide range of corneal prolate and oblate designs to fit an extensive range of corneal shapes. The lens utilizes a Smart Curve™, which allows modification of some parameters without altering others. The Zen RC for regular corneas was introduced in 2016. Distribution of these lenses outside of the US is available in Australia, Mexico, Canada, UK, Sweden, Finland, Denmark, France, Algeria, Tunisia, Morocco, Spain, Portugal, Chile, Italy, San Marino, Vaticano, Israel, Hong Kong, Poland, Russia, Germany, South Africa, Canada, and Singapore.

In 2015, Dr. Caroline Hodd, UK (Fig. **36**), No7 Contact Lenses, launched the Comfort 15. The lens has a 15.0 mm diameter, and the fit is all done by sag. The fitting set consists of lenses of different sag values from low to high, and the final lens is ordered by specifying sag and power. Keratoconus does not always mean that there is an increased sag. A little bump can have as great an effect as a big bump [76]. These lenses are distributed in Scandinavia, France, Germany, Italy, Israel, Cyprus, Middle East, South Africa, Portugal, Spain, Czech Republic, and Brazil.

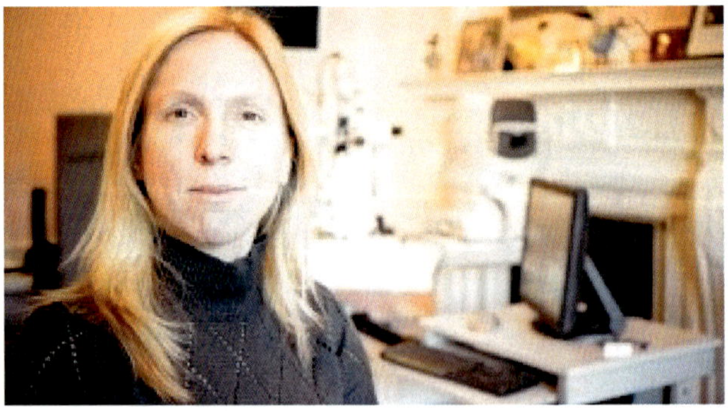

Fig. (36). Caroline Hodd.

Also in 2015, Visionary Lens, California, US, introduced Jeraly scleral lenses co-designed by Christa Brewster (Visionary Lens Consultant) and Jerry Crespo (Visionary Manufacturing Manager). Lens diameters from 14.5 mm to 22.00 mm are available to fit prolate or oblate corneas. The Jeraly lens is available with toric and multifocal features with reverse geometry corneal curves to optimize apical clearance. In the diagnostic fitting set, every diopter of base curve change is equal to 100 microns of sagittal depth change. Additional features include limbal and scleral landing zone adjustments and adjustable toric and quadrant haptic curves.

In 2016, Visionary Optics launched the sMAP3D designed by Precision Ocular Metrology, LLC, an associated company. The companies state that this was the first instrument to be able to measure the anterior curvature and elevation over a 22.00 mm area, 360 degrees. Readings taken in different angles of gaze are "stitched" together into one overall image. Software included can design a "virtual fit" with data sent directly to the lab for fabrication. Distribution outside of the US is available in Australia and New Zealand at the time of publication.

Also in 2016, Art Optical developed a spline-based 4-zone scleral lens called Ampleye. The diagnostic set includes prolate and oblate designs while integrating toric peripheries. Lens diameters of 16.0 mm, 16.5 mm, and 17.0 mm, as well as a wide variety of custom parameters including front toric, quadrant specific and multifocal designs, are available. These lenses are available in the US, Canada, Bermuda, Bolivia, Columbia, Korea, New Zealand, Sri Lanka, and Venezuela.

In 2017, the SynergEyes VS and SynergEyes VS XL were introduced by SynergEyes. This bitangential scleral lens design was created in a collaboration of Rients Visser and his team (Visser Contactlenzen, Nijmegen, The Netherlands) with Bart van der Linden (NKL Contactlenzen, Emmen, the Netherlands, a Menicon Group company) (see above). At the time of publication, lenses will be distributed in the US and Canada by SynergEyes.

Contemporary scleral lenses have re-emerged from a long history of contact lens successes and some failures. As can be seen in recent years, there is a burst of new designs and innovations worldwide. To the best of their ability, the authors sought to discover and describe every scleral lens at the time of publication, while new scleral lenses are currently in development. The authors attempted to reach every known scleral manufacturer. Manufacturers who responded to the outreach are included in this chapter. The authors apologize for any inadvertent omissions or oversight.

With modern materials, manufacturing and advanced scanning equipment, who knows how scleral lenses will evolve? Scleral lenses are now very innovative and a million miles away from their early beginnings.

Tim Bowden was a contact lens optician in Gillingham, Kent, UK, and has published Contact Lenses; The Story (www.contactlensesthestory.com) in 2009, charting the complete development of contact lenses from which he has drawn extensively for this chapter.

CONFLICT OF INTEREST

The authors declare no conflict of interest, financial or otherwise.

ACKNOWLEDGEMENTS

We are sincerely grateful for Tim Bowden's generosity, contributions, humor and insight for this chapter. His acknowledgment was "To my long-suffering wife Elisabeth, who still thinks I am sad." May he rest in peace. Melissa Barnett and Lynette Johns.

SCLERAL LENS TIMELINE

2000BC	Artificial eye making, Egypt
1508	Invention of a contact lens and understanding corneal neutralization, Leonardo da Vinci
1637	Fluid-filled tube against the eye enlarged the size of the retinal image, René Descartes
1685	Dissertation on the neutralization of the cornea, Philip de la Hire
1747	First mention of conical cornea (keratoconus), Pierre Demours
1748	Description of keratoconus, Burchard Mauchart, John 'Chevalier' Taylor (1766), Pickford (1844)
1801	Identified the cause of astigmatism, Thomas Young
1827	Described optical theory of astigmatism with a theoretical back surface toric lens, George Biddle Airy
1845	Described "an actual mold of the cornea might be taken and impressed on some transparent medium," Sir John F. W. Herschel
1854	First adequate description of keratoconus, John Nottingham
1859	Clear glass shells without an optic zone over the cornea (glass masks) made to separate the cornea from the lids in cases of symblepharon, William White Cooper
1866	Developed first Zeiss contact lenses from glass produced by Otto Schott, Abbe
1887	First scleral lenses, (scleral shells without power), Fredrich A. Müller and Albert C. Müller.
1888	Glass scleral lenses, Professor Ernst Abbe
1888	Fick, radius of curvature of the cornea and conjunctival shape
1888	Fick, corneal edema, later called Fick's phenomenon or Sattler's veil
1888	Ophthalmological solutions of fluorescein, M Straub
1889	Investigated contact lenses as 'orthopedic appliances' in the treatment of keratoconus, Eugene Kalt
1889	Correction of his own myopia (14D) with contact lenses. First reference to a corneal lens, August Müller.
1889	Three lenses made, 15-16 mm, Otto Himmler

1889	Cocaine eye drops prior to lens insertion. (did not help, added the risk of addiction), August Müller
1892	Use of physiological saline solution to insert contact lenses. (popular until the early 1940s), Henri Dor
1898	2,000,000 - Artificial eyes, German Empire
1898	300,000 - Artificial eyes per year, French firm
1899	Horse fit with an artificial eye made of vulcanite
1900	Contact lens used as a splint to retain a corneal graft in position during healing, Dr. Louis de Wecker
1911	Invention of slit lamp, Allvar Gullstrand, Sweden
1912	Zeiss produced first contact lens trial set for ophthalmologists
1916	First trial set especially for keratoconus
1918	Zeiss lenses made with small lead pellets embedded in them to assist locating ophthalmic foreign bodies in conjunction with X-ray images
1918	First gonioscope, Dr. Leonhard Koeppe
1920	Four-lens preformed fitting set for keratoconus by Zeiss, Dr. W Stock
1922	Zeiss granted US and German patents for plastic (Cellon or Celluloid) contact lenses
1927	Contact lenses described as having "a capillary tear layer over the cornea and retaining an air cushion beneath the scleral zone," Adolf Wilhelm Müller-Welt
1932	Granted patent DRP. Nr. 553843, Adolf Wilhelm Müller-Welt
1927	First woman ophthalmologist at Moorfields Eye Hospital, London, first female professor of ophthalmology, first female professor at Oxford, Ida Mann
1929	"Afocal" fitting set for Zeiss, Professor Leopold Heine
1930	Ophthalmic impressions, Josef Dallos
1930s	Development of various plastics
1931	Developed polymethylmethacrylate (PMMA), registered trade name "Perspex" also known as Lucite, Plexiglas and Diakon, John Crawford and Rowland Hill
1935	Fitting set of lenses with a toroidal scleral section, Müller-Welt
1935	Ground optics blown lenses, possibly the first contact lenses produced in the US, Kohler and Danz
1936	Table of average corneal dimensions, Theodore Obrig, US
1937	Pair of Zeiss lenses on Hindenburg when it crashed and exploded at the Lakehurst Naval Base, New Jersey
1936	Visited Dallos in Budapest to 'learn the skills of making scleral lenses,' Frederick Williamson-Noble
1936	Scleral lens using plastic material for the haptic portion and bonded to a central glass optic zone (Known as U series from 1937 and T series from 1940), William Feinbloom, New York
1937	First contact lens only practice, Josef Dallos and George Nissel

1938	Sattler (Sattler's veil)
1938	Fluorescein fluorescent properties under blue light, Theodore Obrig
1938	First US all-plastic contact lens using "Plexiglas", Theodore Obrig and Ernest Mullen
1938	First to use PMMA material for contact lenses, Dr. Istvan Györffy
1938	Fit acrylic scleral lenses, then fit acrylic corneal lenses, Dr. Istvan Györffy
1938	Developed lathe, Harry Birchall and Cyril Winter
1938	Lathe-turned preformed acrylic scleral lenses, C. W. Dixey & Son Ltd, UK
1938	Developed a telescopic combination of a contact lens and spectacle lens to enlarge the retinal image, Josef Dallos
1938	Invented the Tholometer to measure the sag, or vault, of the cornea, Josef Dallos
1938	Scleral lens fitting of 84 late-onset mustard gas keratitis casualties, Josef Dallos
1939	"A reversible hydrocolloid gel" set quicker than previous impression materials, Dr. S. Maisler
1939-1945	Fit fluid-less glass scleral lenses to German officers who were not allowed to wear spectacles while in uniform, Adolf Müller-Welt and his wife Ruth, Germany
1943	Ophthalmic Moldite, first cold alginate impression material, Theodore Obrig
1945	Dental Zelex, a cold setting impression material, Charles Keeler, UK
1945	"Feincone lens," William Feinbloom, New York
1945	Small set of preformed fitting shells "transcurve lens," Norman Bier and Phillip Cole, UK
1945	Introduction of separate corneal measuring caps, later referred to as Fenestrated Lenses for Optic Measurement (FLOM), Norman Bier and Phillip Cole, UK
1945	Fenestrated or "ventilated" scleral lens, Joseph Dallos and Norman Bier
1945	Patent for a series of slotted and fenestrated lenses to "permit lachrymal fluid and air to flow" through the lens, Norman Bier
1946	Zeiss lenses found to be intact of a Zeppelin pilot who fell from his airship and killed, Treissman and Plaice
1946	Produced the "wide angle lens" based on the Feincone design, George Nissel, UK
1947	"Kelvin Conic Lens," Raymond Kelvin Watson
1947	Kelvin Contact Lens company developed methods of molding both scleral and corneal lenses, Raymond Kelvin Watson
1947	Obrig Laboratories, UK Moldite readily available
1948	Underwater scleral lens
1948	Designed the "offset lens," Arthur Forknall, UK
1948	Corneal lens, Tuohy
1949	Fit at least 31 flying members of the RAF during WWII who wore contact lenses, Alexander Cross
1949	"Concentric molding," Drs. Newton K Wesley and George Jessen, US
1949	Method of using trays without handles, Frederick Burnett Hodd, UK

1950	Packaged Ophthalmic Zelex into single-dose plastic tubes, George Nissel
1957	Lacrilens, molded PMMA scleral lens with a large perforation in the lower part of the lenses which connected to the corneal vault by means of two channels formed in a V shape, Obrig Laboratories
1967	Apex lens, Fraser and Gordon, UK
1972	Possible use of polysulfide rubber impression materials, silicone rubber impression materials became popular, Storey
1970s	Fit the first gas permeable scleral lenses made from CAB material John James Little, Edinburgh, UK
1970s	RGP scleral lenses manufactured, David Thomas contact lenses in Northampton, UK
1983	Gelflex scleral lenses made using two different RGP materials, Don Ezekiel, Australia
1984	Oxygen demand of the cornea was 70-75mm Hg, Brien Holden and George Mertz
1986	Senso Sclera lenses Procornea, The Netherlands
1987	Panasil C impression material (Kettenbach GmbH), withdrawn in 1993.
1992	Innovative Sclerals (Ken Pullum, bought by Bausch + Lomb in 2015)
1994	Macrolens (C&H Contact Lenses), renamed SoClear lens (Dakota Sciences)
1994	Boston Scleral Lens receives FDA approval (Boston Foundation for Sight)
1995	Panasil Light Body impression material
1998	Eaglet Eye
1999	SoClear lens (Dakota Sciences)
1997	Falco mini-scleral lens (Falco Linsen)
2001	Jupiter lens (Medlens)
2006	Jupiter lens (Essilor)
2006	msdTM (MSD)
2006	One8 Scotlens
2007	Maxim scleral lens (Acculens)
2007	Valley lens (Valley Contax)
2008	LaserFit® (Dr. Greg Gemoules/TruFormOptics)
2008	ICD (Paragon Vision Sciences)
2008	DigiForm (TruForm Optics)
2009	Scleral Lens Education Society created (Founding board members Dr. Greg DeNaeyer, Dr. Christine Sindt, Dr. Bruce Baldwin, Dr. Jason Jedlicka, Dr. Muriel Schornack, Dr. Mindy Toabe, Dr. Eef VanderWorp)
2009	Dyna Semi-Scleral® and Dyna Scleral® (Lens Dynamics)
2009	iSight™ Scleral contact lenses (GP Specialists)
2010	Wave scleral lenses (Wave scleral lens)
2010	NLS semi-scleral lens (Northern contact lens)

2010	Infinity scleral lens (Infinity optical, acquired by ABB OPTICAL 2016)
2010	Comfort SL (Acculens)
2010	EPSILON scleral lens (EYEART Laboratories)
2011	Custom Stable™ (Valley Contax)
2011	KERATOS ESCLERAL SG (Keratos)
2012	NormalEyes (Paragon Vision Sciences)
2012	One Fit (Blanchard)
2012	SLC Conica (MedLac)
2012	EasyScleral (Scotlens)
2013	Atlantis scleral (Atlantis)
2013	EasyFit (Acculens)
2013	Europa Scleral lens (Visionary Optics)
2013	AVT Scleral (Advanced Vision Technologies)
2013	EyePrintPRO™ (EyePrintPro™)
2013	EyeSpace Scleral 2
2014	Genesis (Metro Optics)
2014	Eye Surface Profiler (Eaglet Eye)
2014	Zenlens (Alden Optical)
2015	Comfort 15 (No7 Contact Lenses)
2015	Jeraly scleral lenses (Visionary Lens)
2016	sMAP3D (Visionary Optics)
2016	InSight Scleral® (Metro Optics)
2016	Ampleye (Art Optical)
2016	Prolook (Essilor)
2016	Zen RC (Alden Optical)
2017	SynergEyes VS and SynergEyes VS XL (SynergEyes)
2017	Naturalens™ (AVT)

REFERENCES

[1] Heitz, R. The History of Contact Lenses. Vol 1. Early Neutralizations of Corneal Dioptric Power. J P Wayenborgh, Belgium, 2003.

[2] Descartes R. Discours de la Methode, Discours No 7. La Dioptrique 1637; p. 79.

[3] Historical Perspective Lecture, Nova South Eastern University, Fort Lauderdale, Fl, USA.

[4] Anthony T. An interrupted story: French translations from philosophical transactions in the seventeenth and eighteenth centuries

[5] Duke-Elder S. Ophthalmic Optics and Refraction. System of Ophthalmology 1970; 5: 713. [London: Kimpton].

[6] Pickford JH. Conical Cornea. Dublin: Hodges and Smith 1844.

[7] Nottingham J. Conical Cornea. London: John Churchill 1854.

[8] Young T. On the mechanism of the eye. Phil Trans R Soc 1801; 16: 23-88. [http://dx.doi.org/10.1098/rstl.1801.0004]

[9] Airy GB. On a peculiar defect in the eye, and a mode of correcting it. Trans Camb Phil Soc 1827; 2: 267-71.

[10] Herschel JF. 'Light' Section XII: 'Of the structure of the eye, and of vision'. Encyclopaedia Metropolitana 1845; 4: 396-404.

[11] Cooper WW. On Wounds and Injuries to the Eye. London: John Churchill 1859.

[12] Nissel G. The müllers of wiesbaden. Optician 1965; 150(3897): 591-4.

[13] Müller FA, Müller AC. Das Kunstliche auge. Wiesbaden: J. F. Bergmann 1910; pp. 68-75.

[14] Müller FE. Ueber die korrektion des keratokonus und anderer brechungsanomalien des auges mit müllers-chen kontaktschalen. Inaugural Dissertation University of Marburg 1920.

[15] Mann I. Contact lenses and Dr Josef Dallos. Contact Lens 1973; 4(4): 16.

[16] Fick AE. A Contact Lens (trans. C. H. May). Arch Ophthalmol 1888; 19: 215-26.

[17] Germany: Carl Zeiss International Available at: http://www.zeiss.com.

[18] Straub. Centralblatt f Augenheilk 1888.

[19] Obrig TE. A cobalt blue filter for observation of the fit of contact lenses. Arch Ophthalmol 1938; 20: 657-8. a [http://dx.doi.org/10.1001/archopht.1938.00850220129010]

[20] Pearson RM. Kalt, keratoconus, and the contact lens. Optom Vis Sci 1989; 66(9): 643-6. [http://dx.doi.org/10.1097/00006324-198909000-00011] [PMID: 2677884]

[21] Müller A. Brillengläser und hornhautlinsen. Inaugural Dissertation p 20 University of Kiel 1889; 20.

[22] Pearson RM. August müller's inaugural dissertation. J Br Contact Lens Assoc 1978; 1(2): 33-6.

[23] Dor H. Sur les verres de contact. Rev. Gén. Ophtalmol 1892; 11: 493-7.

[24] Mann I. The history of contact lenses. Trans Ophthalmol Soc U K 1938; 58: 129.

[25] Bowden TJ. Contact lenses; the story. Bower House Publications 2009.

[26] Rugg-Gunn A. Contact Glasses. Br. J Ophthalmol 1931; (Oct): 5.

[27] Koeppe L. Die mikroskopie des lebenden augenhintergrundes mit starken vergrösserungen im fokalen lichte der Gullstrandschen Nernstspaltlampe. Graefes Arch Ophthalmol 1918; 95: 282-306. [http://dx.doi.org/10.1007/BF01944342]

[28] Dallos J. Contact glasses, the 'invisible' spectacles. Arch Ophthalmol 1936; 15: 617-23. [http://dx.doi.org/10.1001/archopht.1936.00840160041003]

[29] Schiller F. Testimonial to Dr Adolf Wilhelm Mueller-Welt, DOS 1969. Available at: http://www.mueller-welt.com.

[30] Heine L. Die korrektur saemtlichr ametropien durch geschliffene kontaktschalen. Ber. 13′ Congr. Ophthal Amst 1929; 1: 232-4.

[31] Dallos J. Personal communication to Sabell 1977.

[32] (a). Sabell A G. An ophthalmic museum. Contact Lens J 1980; 9(2): 15-9. (b). Sabell A G. An ophthalmic museum. Contact Lens J 1980; 9(3): 16-9.

[33] Sabell AG. An ophthalmic museum. Contact Lens J 1980; 9(4): 10-8.

[34] Anderson JM. Contact lenses, clinical and other observations. Brighton: Courteney Press 1952; p. 11.

[35] London: Plastics Historical Society. http://www.plastiquarian.com

[36] Forknall AJ. Offset Contact lenses. Optician 1948; 116(3006): 419-21.

[37] Obrig T. Contact lenses. The Chilton Company 1942.

[38] Obrig TE. Molded contact lenses. Arch Ophthalmol 1938; 19: 735-58. b [http://dx.doi.org/10.1001/archopht.1938.00850170085006]

[39] Braff S. Contact lens Horizons. Max Shapero Lecture. Am J Optician & Phys Optician 1983; 60(10)

[40] Dickinson F, Hall KG. An Introduction to the Prescribing and Fitting of Contact Lenses. London: Hammond and Hammond. 1946.

[41] Sattler CH. Erfahrungen mit haftgläsern. Klin Mbl Augenheilk 1938; 100: 172-7.

[42] Feinbloom W. A plastic contact lens. Trans Am Acad Optom 1936; 10: 37-44.

[43] Bier N. Contact Lens Routine and Practice. 2nd ed. London: Butterworths 1957; pp. 141-5.

[44] Gyoerffy I. The history of the molded all-plastic lens. Br J Physiol Opt 1964; 21(4): 291-2. [PMID: 14266303]

[45] Györffy I. Kontaktschalen aus kunststoffen. Klin Mbl Augenheilk 1940; 104: 81-7.

[46] Györffy I. Therapeutic contact-lenses from plastic. Br J Ophthalmol 1950; 34(2): 115-8. [http://dx.doi.org/10.1136/bjo.34.2.115] [PMID: 15405355]

[47] Györffy I. The manufacture of haptic and corneal lenses in Budapest. Contact Lens 1968; 2(1): 9-15.

[48] Györffy I. Geschichte der Sklerallinsen aus PMMA. Contactologia 1980; 2: 143-9.

[49] Györffy I. Zur Geschichte der Korneallinsen aus PMMA. Contactologia 1981; 3: 106-9.

[50] Dixey, C. W. & Son Ltd. Dixey flexible contact lenses. Trade catalogue 1943.

[51] Ridley F. Recent developments in the manufacture, fitting and prescription of contact lenses of regular shape. Proc R Soc Med 1946; 39(12): 842-8. [PMID: 19993424]

[52] Graham R. The evolution of corneal contact lenses. Am J Optom 1959; 36: 55-72. [http://dx.doi.org/10.1097/00006324-195902000-00001]

[53] Tallet K. Mustard gas poisoning 1998. Availabel at: http://ourworld.compuserve.com/homepages/kylet1/gas.htm

[54] Department of Health. Treatment of poisoning by selected chemical compounds. London 2003.

[55] Maisler S. Casts of the human eye for contact lenses. Arch Ophthalmol 1939; 21: 359-61. [http://dx.doi.org/10.1001/archopht.1939.00860020163013]

[56] Steele E. American modifications of the contact lens molding technique. Optician 1948; 115(2968): 87.

[57] Obrig TE. A new ophthalmic impression material. Arch Ophthalmol 1943; 30: 626-30. [http://dx.doi.org/10.1001/archopht.1943.00880230058007]

[58] Feinbloom W. The tangent cone contact lens series. Optom Wkly 1945; 36: 1159-61.

[59] Bier N, Cole PJ. The transcurve contact lens fitting shell. Optician 1948; 115(2987): 605-6. [PMID: 18874359]

[60] Bier N. Application for British Patent No. 592055 Contact lens theory and practice. 2nd ed., London: Butterworths 1945.

[61] Bier N. The practice of ventilated contact lenses. Optician 1948; 116: 497-501.

[62] Dallos J. Sattler's veil. Br J Ophthalmol 1946; 30: 607-13. [http://dx.doi.org/10.1136/bjo.30.10.607]

[63] Treissman H, Plaice EA. Principle of the contact lens. London: Henry Kimpton 1946.

[64] Watson RK. The Kelvin contact lens. Optician 1947; 114(2948): 228-30. [PMID: 20265668]

[65] Sabell AG. An ophthalmic museum. Contact Lens J 1980; 9(6): 3-18. b

[66] McKellen GD. Conical contact lenses. Br J Ophthalmol 1949; 33(2): 120-7. [http://dx.doi.org/10.1136/bjo.33.2.120] [PMID: 18111354]

[67] McKellen GD. The 'offset' haptic lens. Optician 1963; 14: 105-7.

[68] Ruben M. Use of conoidal curves in corneal contact lenses. Br J Ophthalmol 1966; 50(11): 642-5. [http://dx.doi.org/10.1136/bjo.50.11.642] [PMID: 5926607]

[69] Cross A. Contact Lenses, An analysis of the results of use. BJO. 1949; 33: pp. 421-46.

[70] Jessen GN, Wesley NK. Concentric molding. Optom Wkly 1949; 40: 753.

[71] Storey JK. The possible use of polysulphide rubber impression material in contact lens work. Ophthal Opt 1972; 12: 1017-8.

[72] Silk A. Personal communication to Sabell 1982.

[73] Ruben M. The apex lens. Contact Lens 1967; 1(4): 14-28.

[74] Fraser J P, Gordon S P. The 'Apex' lens for uniocular aphakia. Ophthal Opt 1967; 7: 1190-253.

[75] Gemoules G. A novel method of fitting scleral lenses using high resolution optical coherence tomography. Eye Contact Lens 2008; 34(2): 80-3. [http://dx.doi.org/10.1097/ICL.0b013e318166394d] [PMID: 18327042]

[76] Hodd C. Personal communication 2015.

CHAPTER 2

Scleral Lens Anatomy

Lynette K. Johns[1,*] and **Melissa Barnett**[2]

[1] *The New England College of Optometry, Boston, Massachusetts, USA*

[2] *University of California, Davis, Sacramento, California, USA*

Abstract: Scleral lens terminology is vast and can be confusing. Since there are several designs with different parameters, manufacturers have created new terms for various aspects of scleral lenses. Not only do the parameters have a variety of names, but there are different names for large gas permeable lenses themselves. The Scleral Lens Education Society defined large diameter gas permeable lenses by their respective bearing patterns (corneal, corneo-scleral, and scleral) thereby reducing some confusion. The parameters, however, are more difficult to categorize. In this chapter, the anatomy of a scleral lens is described in four separate zones: optic zone, mid-peripheral zone, intermediate zone, and landing zone. The optic zone not only provides the optical correction but also can be manipulated to increase the clearance over the corneal surface. The mid-peripheral zone also can be manipulated to create more even clearance over the peripheral corneal surface. The intermediate zone is a critical junction between the mid-peripheral zone and scleral landing zone that bridges the limbus and can control the overall sagittal height of the lens. Lastly, the landing zone is the fitting zone of the scleral lens that aligns to the ocular surface and conjunctiva overlying the sclera and bears the weight of the entire lens. Due to the unique properties of the ocular surface shape, the landing zone can be rotationally symmetric or asymmetric to accommodate and facilitate proper alignment to the surface. All the terminology of the scleral lens anatomy is described in detail.

Keywords: Anatomy, Breaches, Bubble, Channels, Design, Diameter, Elevation, Fenestration, Intermediate zone, ISO, Landing zone, Measurement, Mid-peripheral, Optic zone, Radius, Sagittal depth, Sagittal height, Terminology, Toricity, Zone.

INTRODUCTION

Scleral lens terminology can be very confusing for not only novice practitioners, but experienced practitioners as well. Large diameter gas permeable lenses are labeled in a variety of ways. For example, mini-scleral, semi-scleral, full scleral, scleral contact lens, corneo-scleral, haptic lens, scleral prosthetic device, and

* **Corresponding author Lynette K. Johns:** The New England College of Optometry, Boston, Massachusetts, USA; Tel: 617-262-2020; Fax: 617-236-6323; E-mails: johnsl@neco.edu; lynettekjohns@gmail.com

prosthetic scleral lens device, naming just a few. In 2013, the Scleral Lens Education Society recommended internationally recognized nomenclature to describe scleral lenses based upon their fitting characteristics. Table **1** shows the recommended nomenclature.

Table 1. Scleral Lens Society recommended terminology for large diameter gas permeable lenses.

Lens Type	Description	Definition of Bearing Area
Corneal		Lens rests entirely on the cornea
Corneo-scleral		Lens rests partly on the cornea, partly on the sclera
Scleral	Mini-Scleral *Lens is up to 6mm larger than HVID*	Lens rests entirely on the sclera
	Large Scleral *Lens is more than 6mm larger than HVID*	

The reason that the Scleral Lens Education Society had made these recommendations was that the previous descriptions of large diameter gas permeable lenses was largely based on lens diameter. The problem with using diameters as defining large diameter lenses is that the fitting characteristics are dependent on fitting a relatively normal sized cornea. A 14.5 mm diameter was considered a semi-scleral lens, however, on a patient with a microcornea, the lens would likely not touch the cornea whatsoever and act as a full scleral lens. Conversely, if an 18.0 mm lens had difficulty clearing either the limbus or the apex of ectasia, the lens is acting as a corneo-scleral lens. This prompted the Scleral Lens Education Society to recommend terminology based on where the lens distributes its weight or bears on the ocular surface whether it is the cornea, conjunctiva overlying the sclera, or both.

The emphasis of this book is focused on scleral lenses, or lenses that completely clear the cornea and limbus and rest solely on the conjunctiva overlying the sclera. It is also theorized that the lens is supported by the tear fluid reservoir. Therefore, the attention is on scleral lenses. Scleral lenses have been widely adopted as the name for this category of large diameter gas permeable lenses. Unfortunately, scleral lens is a misnomer. The lens rests completely on the conjunctiva overlying the sclera and does not, in fact, have direct contact on the sclera. Since the conjunctiva is a loose connective tissue and conforms to the shape of the underlying sclera, it makes sense that the lens is referred to as a scleral lens since the rigid plastic conforms to the scleral shape.

Confusion continues to remain when referring to the different aspects of the lens design itself. There is no consensus regarding scleral lens terminology. The authors agree that there will be disagreement with proposed terminology provided herein; nevertheless, to maintain consistency throughout this book, some terminology will be suggested.

ISO TERMINOLOGY

The International Organization for Standardization (ISO) defined terminology for every type of contact lens and its associated parameters [1]. In the ISO text, scleral lenses are called "scleral contact lenses." Within the scleral lens community, there is a strong conviction that scleral lenses should not be termed scleral contact lenses as they do not contact the cornea. However, scleral "contact" lens is used in some circles, so the debate continues. Another problem with using the term contact lens is that within the realm of medically necessary contact lenses, to laypeople, contact lenses are considered an alternative to spectacles. This becomes a challenge for providers that require medical insurance pre-authorization and reimbursement.

In some situations, a scleral lens is referred to as a prosthetic device. A prosthesis replaces an organ or body part. For example, an ocular prosthesis replaces an absent or disfigured eye, whereas a prosthetic device replaces function. In this case, a scleral lens is replacing the function of an eye with visual rehabilitation, ocular surface lubrication and other functions. Occasionally, this decreases some of the challenges associated with medical insurance coverage and their definitions of contact lenses.

Scleral lenses are primarily in their adolescence. Previous scleral lenses were designed with polymethylmethacrylate (PMMA) materials and recently underwent a resurgence with gas permeable materials. While they are relatively young in the medical marketplace, there is a fair amount of agreement upon nomenclature in clinical practice. There are some similarities between the ISO vocabulary and words adopted in practice. In the ISO, impression scleral contact lenses are created by using a mold of the patient's eye. Currently, impression scleral lenses are being utilized with new lens design technology. The ISO also describes preformed scleral contact lenses. "Preformed" lenses that the ISO refers to are lenses that are created with a specified shape; however, these are commonly referred to as diagnostic or trial lenses. As an example, diagnostic or trial lenses are frequently used terms, and practitioners who fit scleral lenses will unlikely change their vernacular to the ISO term of preformed lenses and other recommended language.

Another problem when it comes to unifying the language of scleral lenses is that scleral lens designs have unique and varied properties. While the function of each of the various parameters is similar, the geometry varies between curves, tangents, angles and splines to name a few. To add to the confusion, scleral lens manufacturers also contribute to the multitude of terminology with their own proprietary features and language. Therefore, the purpose of this chapter is to encompass most of the terminology that is in the literature and known to the authors, and generalize it under functional categories.

The overall shape and anatomy of scleral lenses are divided into four categories in this chapter. For the sake of simplicity, they will be defined as the optic zone, mid-peripheral zone, intermediate zone and landing zone (Fig. **1** and **2**). The mid-peripheral zone is sometimes not considered an independent or fourth zone. See below.

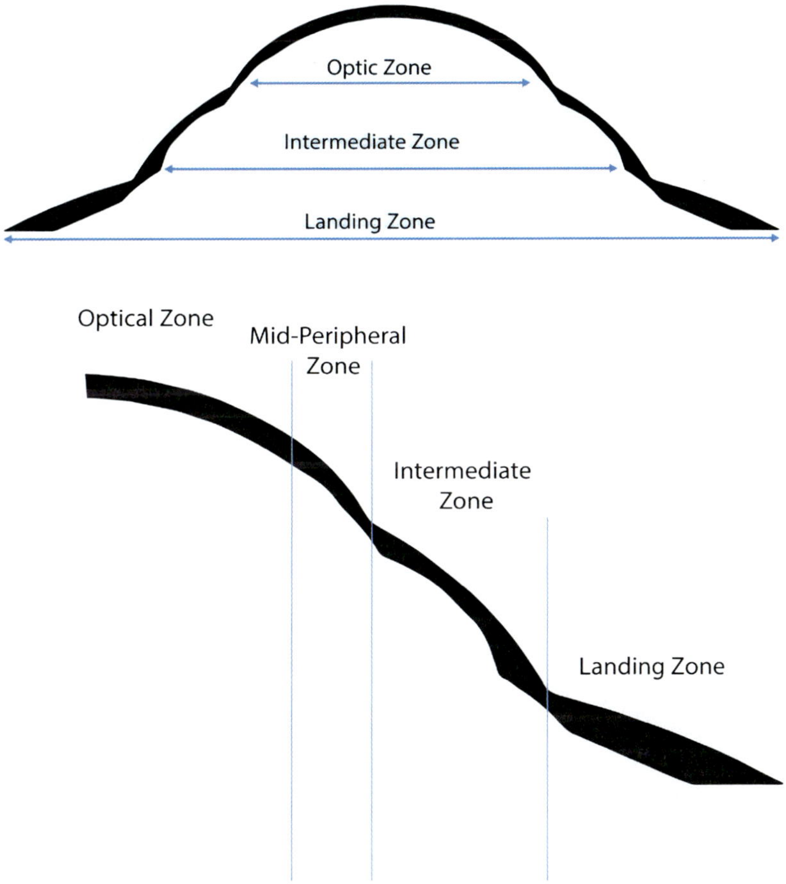

Fig. (1). Two views of the basic four zones of the anatomy of a scleral lens. The mid-peripheral zone overlies the cornea and is peripheral to the optic zone diameter of the lens.

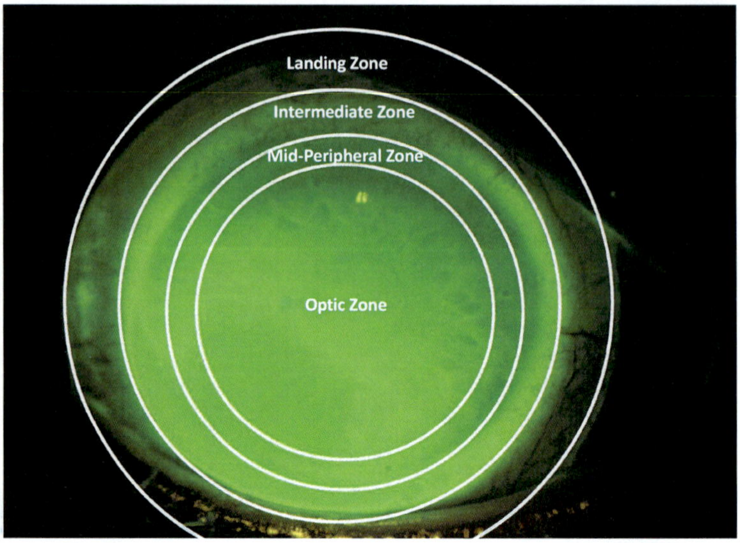

Fig. (2). This image depicts the four zones of a scleral lens on an eye with fluorescein.

THE OPTIC ZONE

The central portion of the lens will be referred to as the optic zone. The optic zone is used as a general term that encompasses the front optic zone radius, back optic zone radius or base curvature, front optic zone diameter, back optic zone diameter (Fig. **3**). These create the dioptric power, and are all traditional components of any contact lens. Some of these components are also defined in the ISO terminology.

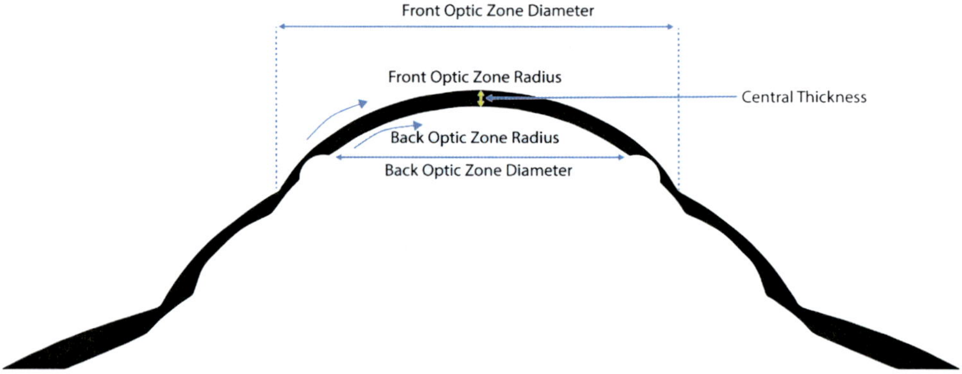

Fig. (3). Components of the optic zone.

Optic Zone Terminology

The characteristics of the optic zone of scleral lenses are labeled many ways by each manufacturer. They can be labeled in dioptric power of curvature, radius of curvature and in sagittal height or sagittal depth. As described earlier, the optic zone region consists of the back and front optic zone radii, the back and front optic zone diameters, as well as the overall power of the lens. An additional feature is the height or depth of the lens. The sagitta, sagittal depth or sagittal height is defined in the ISO as the, "maximum distance from a chord, which is perpendicular to the axis of rotation of a surface, to the curved surface [1]." The sagitta, sagittal height and sagittal depth all refer to the same measurement which can be confusing. To understand the difference, imagine a scleral lens on a countertop convex side up. The sagittal height of the lens is measured from a flat surface upward to the central curvature of the lens, whereas the sagittal depth starts the measurement from the central curvature downward to the flat surface (Fig. **4**). Since a scleral lens bridges over and does not touch the cornea, it is the authors' opinion to use the term height when referring to this measurement. However, the terms height and depth are used in practice interchangeably. There is further confusion, since the total sagittal height of the lens is measured using the chord of the lens from edge to edge. Not every manufacture labels their sagittal height as the total sagittal height of the lens. Some manufacturers use a pre-determined chord length, or the length of the plane where the landing zone begins. Keep in mind, that the sagittal height of the lens remains unchanged even on the eye. The sagittal height is acting as a labeled lens parameter. The clearance, or space between the cornea and the back surface of the lens that vaults over the cornea, is a different height measurement altogether.

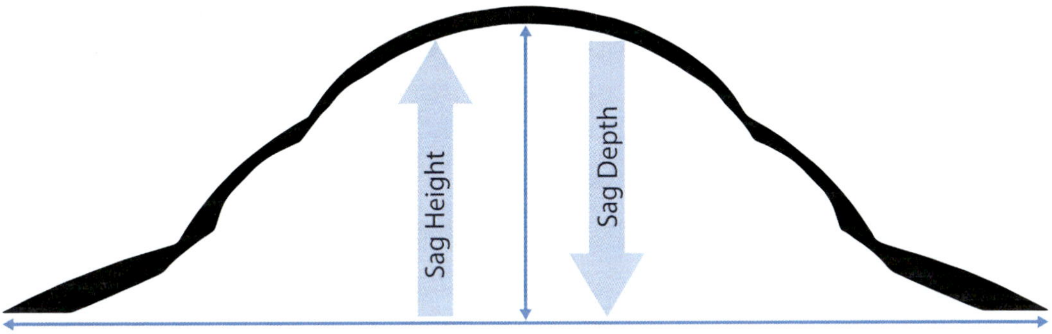

Fig. (4). Sagittal height and sagittal depth are the same measurement, but the differentiator is the direction from which it is measured.

Scleral lens manufacturers have begun to label the optic zone using all the terms of dioptric curvature, radii, and sagittal height. Central curvature and radii are consistent between manufacturers; however, the sagittal height, commonly called "sag height" or "sag," varies significantly among manufacturers. For example, if using one scleral lens brand to determine the patient's over-refraction and overall power, the practitioner needs to know both the curvature/radius and the power. It does not matter which brand is used and the information can be transferred across brands (7.9 radius with a -4.00 power will provide the exact same optical effect when using different brands). A 4500 μm sagittal height between brands will not necessarily provide the same clearance. Some practitioners have appealed to manufacturers to have the same sagittal heights among brands. Unfortunately, due to different proprietary curves and angles, this is not possible. If scleral lens laboratories were to define the sagittal height of their lenses as a total sagittal height (the reference chord being the edge to edge and the height determined from that plane to the central curvature of the lens), there will still be significant differences in the clearance effects of the scleral lenses on eyes (Fig. **5**).

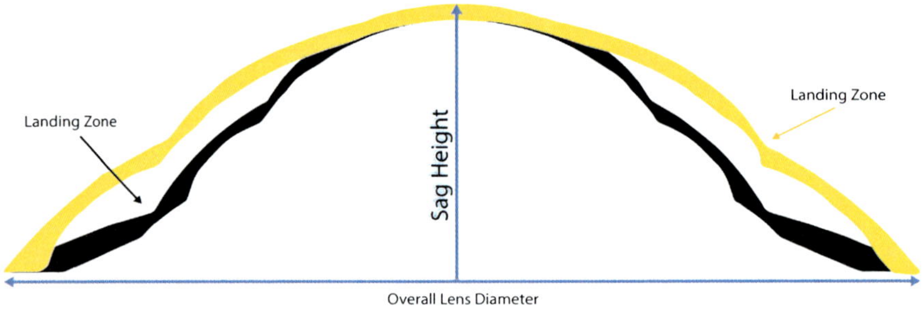

Fig. (5). Schematic of two lenses that would be labeled with the same overall sagittal height (vertical arrow) and the same overall diameter (horizontal arrow). The yellow curve may have a reduced central clearance since it may land more anterior to the cornea than the black lens as defined by the start of the landing zones (designated by arrows) on each lens.

When working with different designs, the nomenclature of this zone depends on the manufacturer. Examples of different names for the optic zone are clearance zone, clearance curve, central clearance zone, anterior clearance zone, apical clearance zone, corneal vault zone, corneal zone, base curve, base curve radius zone and other variations of these terms.

Optic Zone Functionality

One of the primary functions of a scleral lens is visual rehabilitation, and as with any contact lens, the optics are crucial. Due to the stability of scleral lenses, unique optical properties can be implemented in the optic zone. These include sphere, cylinder, asphericity, multifocality, optical decentration, and higher order aberration correction. When applying unique optics to the front surface of the scleral lens, it is important to stabilize the lens from rotation. Stabilizing features include prism ballast, double slab off prism, and truncation (although not widely used).

The optic zone also has associated fitting characteristics. The center thickness is a measurable parameter in all scleral lenses. Typically, the center thickness is measured at the geometric center of the lens, or within the center of the optic zone. The center thickness is very important for a variety of reasons. The center thickness needs to be thick enough to prevent breakage from typical handling and wear. With that in mind, it also needs to be thin enough to enhance oxygen permeability [2 - 4]. Often, diagnostic lenses are labeled with their center thicknesses. This is helpful for a practitioner determining the amount of clearance over the cornea. The clearance can be measured relative to the center thickness of the lens. This is covered in more detail in upcoming chapters. Keep in mind, the lens power can alter the thickness either at the center in high plus powered lenses or at the periphery of the optic zone in high minus powered lenses. If a diagnostic lens or an ordered lens is not labeled with the center thickness, the manufacturer can easily supply that information. Another problem that can affect the optic zone of the lens is flexure. The manufacturer can increase the center thickness to reduce or eliminate flexure (flexure can also be reduced with thickness changes of intermediate zone).

Unlike corneal lenses, the base curvature or back optic zone radius can be independent of the overall fitting characteristics of the scleral lens. However, manipulations to the back optic zone radius often impact the fitting relationship of the lens. In 2010, a study examining the fitting relationships of the flat and steep keratometric powers of patients with dry eye and keratoconus and the base curve of Jupiter™ scleral lenses demonstrated a loose association with these topographic parameters and the base curves. However, the topographic indices demonstrated a weak predictive association [5]. These findings are consistent in clinical practice with most designs; nevertheless, these fitting features have only been investigated with Jupiter lenses. Some manufacturers recommend keratometric values for initial lens selection. A potential advantage of matching optic zone curvature to keratometric values is the ability to create a more even clearance which can optimize oxygen availability and reduce conjunctival prolapse. Essentially, this creates a parallel curvature matching the curvature of the cornea with the back surface of the lens that generates a uniform clearance. Sometimes, the sagittal height is not labeled directly on the lenses. If a cornea requires more central clearance, the central sagittal height can be increased by steepening the back optic zone radius/base curve. Conversely, some manufactures do not label the curvature on their diagnostic lenses and only refer to the optic zone in sagittal depth. These designs can raise and lower the height to optimize clearance without changing the base curvature or back optic zone radius of the lens. At times, a combination of back optic zone radius/base curve and sagittal height changes is made to alter the scleral lens clearance.

MID-PERIPHERAL ZONE

It is debatable if the mid-peripheral zone is an independent zone or falls under the optic zone or intermediate zone category. This zone depends on the lens design. The mid-peripheral zone is located posterior to the optic zone and anterior to the intermediate zone, and is designed to clear the mid-peripheral cornea. Some designs have a zone dedicated to the mid-periphery, while other designs recommend changes in the back optic zone radius or base curvature to increase or reduce mid-peripheral clearance.

In designs that require changes in the base curvature to increase or reduce sagittal height, the optic zone diameter is fixed and likewise the clearance underneath the scleral lens. For example, if there is shallow clearance centrally and in the mid-periphery, changing the central base curvature will only increase the central clearance. The clearance under the edge of the optic zone diameter will not be altered. The curve posterior to the base curve can be elevated to lift over the mid-periphery. Next, the curve posterior to the mid-peripheral curve and in some cases the central base curve can be compensated to maintain central corneal clearance for this mid-peripheral change. This is where using steep and flat as terminology can be quite confusing. Additionally, not every lens design uses curvatures. Some designs use tangents and angles, wavelet theory and Fourier analysis, sigmoid functions or spline theory. The laboratory consultants are invaluable when troubleshooting all the aspects and zones of their designs. Even if the lens design is not based on curvature, the consultants understand the practitioner's use of steep and flat and can translate that into their designs. Also, the clearance over the mid-peripheral cornea can be measured either with OCT or an approximation of clearance compared to the central thickness of the lens. Since the measurement is in microns that, too can be communicated to the laboratory consultants and the appropriate increase or decrease can be ordered.

Other names for the mid-peripheral zone include peripheral corneal zone, peripheral clearance zone, peripheral curve 1 and mid peripheral/limbal zone. Again, this particular zone may be a part of the optic zone if the optic zone diameter is large or it may be integrated into an intermediate zone that clears the limbus as well.

Fenestrations

Fenestrations are small holes that can be applied either in the optic zone or in the mid-peripheral zone. They can be made by hand or are pre-made in the gas permeable button. Fenestrations are not commonly used in scleral lens practices; however, some designs and practitioners utilize fenestrated designs exclusively. The functions of fenestrations include reduction in lens suction and increased oxygenation to the cornea. Sometimes, these lenses are referred to as "air-ventilated." These holes inevitably create a bubble (Fig. **6**), but can be adjusted to reduce the bubble size and sometimes eliminate the bubble where tears are aspirated in and out with minimal air intrusion. The number and location of the fenestrations are variable and peripheral to the visual axis either in the peripheral optic zone or mid-peripheral zone. A circumferential channel can be created to allow motility of the bubble while preventing it from entering underneath the optic zone and obscuring vision. Bubble motility is important to prevent constant desiccation of the cornea underneath the bubble.

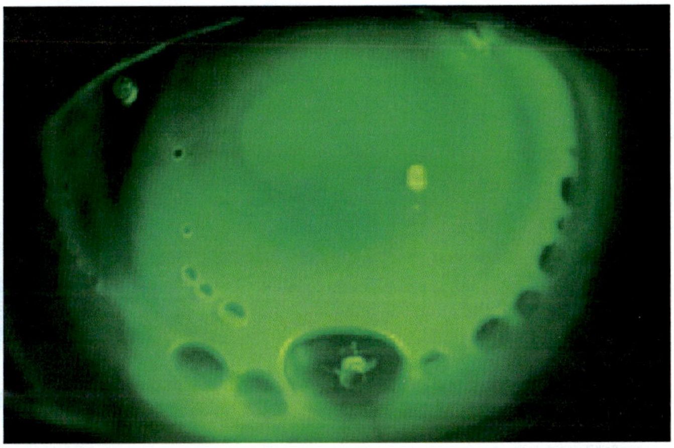

Fig. (6). Example of scleral lens with three fenestrations in the midperipheral zone with mid-peripheral bubbles. Image courtesy of Lynette Johns I-Site e-newsletter (July 2011).

To control the bubble from being too large or entering underneath the optic zone, modifications to the base curve can be incorporated into some designs. The base curve can be divided into quadrants where a steep base curve can be used inferiorly to more closely align to the cornea, while the superior, temporal and nasal quadrants can be modified independently. As long as power changes are made that correspond to the changes in base curve using the SAM-FAP method (steeper add minus-flatter add plus), the patient will not experience any visual fluctuation or disturbance while wearing a central base curve and powers divided in quadrants. Additionally, the clearance is lowered significantly while still preventing corneal contact to reduce bubble intrusion to the visual axis.

Since fenestrated lenses are air-ventilated, removal is quite easy. Typically, patients are educated not to remove the scleral lens by applying the removal plunger to the center of the lens. The exception is when the lens is fenestrated. The easiest way to remove a fenestrated lens is applying the plunger to the center of the lens, pulling it straight outward. It is not uncomfortable for the patient and there is no resistance or suction of the lens with this technique.

INTERMEDIATE ZONE

Clearing the limbus can be challenging when fitting scleral lenses. The intermediate zone connects the corneal zone (optic and midperipheral) to the scleral landing zone. Often, any manipulation to one zone can affect the other if the zones are not disengaged from one another. Therefore, the sagittal height of the lens can be further increased by increasing the height and/or length of this intermediate region.

Limbal clearance is largely impacted by the junction of the mid-peripheral zone and the intermediate zone; however, this is largely design dependent. The configuration of the zone can be considered reverse curvature or reverse geometry if this zone is a steeper curve or angle than the optic zone and mid-peripheral zone creating an oblate shape. Manipulating this zone is quite effective for managing challenging peripheral topographies or in conditions like post-penetrating keratoplasty, peripheral Salzmann's nodular degeneration, some cases of pellucid marginal degeneration and other irregularities.

The posterior junction of the intermediate zone is adjoined to the scleral lens landing zone. When the intermediate zone is quite steep and the landing zone is designed very flat, then a harsh junction can be created. This forms an "L" shape where the bend or elbow can compress into the conjunctiva. This can significantly impact scleral lens comfort and fitting characteristics. It is important to understand the location of the zones and the associated junctions when optimizing a scleral lens fit or troubleshooting a problematic lens design. The intermediate zone is sometimes called the limbal curve, limbal clearance curve, limbal zone, limbal clearance zone, transitional zone, limbal vault zone, peripheral curve 2 or limbal lift zone.

LANDING ZONE

The scleral lens landing zone is the most peripheral zone. This is arguably one of the most important regions of a scleral lens since it is the region where the lens first contacts or "lands" on the ocular surface. Scleral lenses actually land on the conjunctival surface; however, for an optimal fit, the shape of the landing zone should be very close to alignment with the overall scleral shape. Perfect scleral alignment may create a seal-off or suction event.

The landing zone of each scleral lens design can be quite complex and unique between manufacturers. As stated earlier, some designs use curvature, tangents and angles, wavelet theory and Fourier analysis, sigmoid functions, spline theory and probably other mathematical techniques. For this reason, a practitioner cannot empirically order a lens design from one manufacturer when using a different manufacturer's design. Additionally, some designs are impression molded lenses that most closely match the ocular surface shape. Unless the scleral lens was designed with impression molding, contemporary scleral lenses require diagnostic fitting and evaluation. In some instances, for regular/healthy corneas, the use of keratometry, corneal and/or scleral topography/profilometry, Scheimpflug tomography, and/or optical coherence tomography along with refraction are used to order a patient's first lens which can be evaluated like any diagnostic lens.

There can be multiple geometries for the scleral landing zone. Not only can this zone be comprised of multiple curves, tangents, *etc.*; the landing zone can be rotationally symmetric, toric, quadrant specific or divided in eight meridians or more around the total periphery of the lens. Unfortunately, eyeballs are not perfectly round, spherical globes. The burden lies with the practitioner to best design a scleral lens that gently aligns to each unique surface or meridian without compressing or impinging into the conjunctiva, while at the same time vaulting over the entire cornea and limbus. Instrumentation can be used to analyze the surface shape such as scleral topographers and optical coherence tomography. Some scleral lenses can be designed from scleral topographers. However, most contemporary scleral lenses are currently designed by observation and evaluation of diagnostic lenses. Understanding ocular surface shape, instrumentation and evaluation of scleral lenses will be extensively covered in upcoming chapters.

There are a variety of names used when referring to the landing zone and these include: scleral landing zone, scleral zone, scleral curve, peripheral curve 4, advanced peripheral system, peripheral zone, peripheral clearance zone, peripheral haptic or haptic.

Features of the Landing Zone

Toricity

The landing zone on all designs can be manipulated since one size does not fit all. The landing zone can be ordered flatter or raised from the ocular surface, or lowered and tighter depending on clinical observations. If there is disparity between landing zone in two meridians 90 degrees apart, then the lens can be designed with back surface toricity. The disparity can be too tight or too loose in one meridian, too loose or tight overall but looks different between the meridians, or too tight in one meridian and too loose in the other. Basically, the lens will be looser along one meridian and steeper or tighter 90 degrees apart. Fig. (**7**) demonstrates the disparity in a toric designed scleral lens. Studies have demonstrated improved centration, stability and comfort with toric landing zones [6, 7].

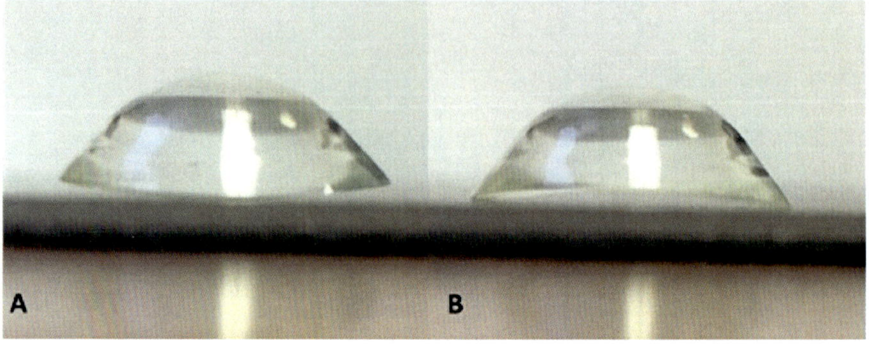

Fig. (7). Example of a toric lens from two perspectives. A. View along the steep meridian (centrally) with the flat meridian lifting off the table. B. View along the flat meridian (centrally) with the steep meridian edges touching the table. Image courtesy of Lynette Johns.

The ocular shape varies in many ways between eyes and patients: this will be discussed in the next chapter discussing ocular shape. Sometimes there is a difference in quadrants of the surface relative to the scleral lens. In this case, quadrant specific designs can be ordered depending on the lens design. In these instances, the landing zone and even zones more anteriorly can be altered independently using a quadrant specific design. In complex situations, the lens can be designed with eight meridians (Fig. **8**). Just as in quadrant specific designs, each meridian can be manipulated independently. Practitioners should always check with the manufacturer about the capabilities and features of each scleral lens design. If the patient has a unique and complicated ocular surface topography, impression molded lenses may be considered.

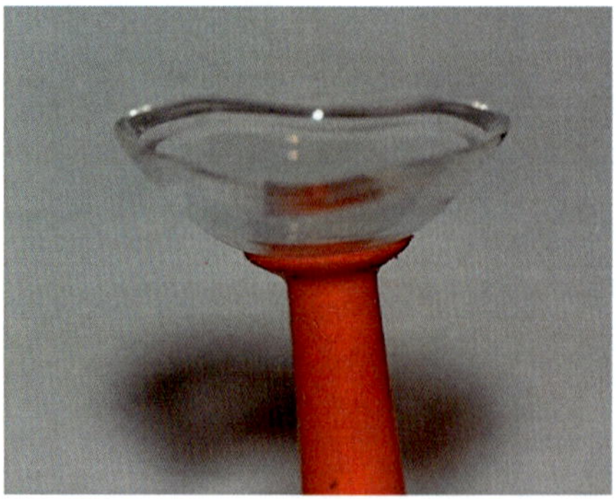

Fig. (8). An example of an eight-meridian lens. Image courtesy of Lynette Johns.

Back surface toricity should not be confused with front surface toricity. Front surface toricity is optical and incorporates the sphero-cylindrical optical properties of the lens. Front surface toricity of a scleral lens is similar to a soft toric lens. When residual astigmatism manifests in a sphero-cylindrical over-refraction, front surface toricity can be incorporated into the scleral lens design. Similar to a soft toric lens, the lens requires stabilization to ensure consistent vision. Stabilization is incorporated into rotationally symmetric (spherical) lenses by using either prism ballasting, dual thin zones, double slab-off prism and rarely truncation. These lenses typically have markings on the front surface to designate rotation. The practitioner should measure this rotation since it can have optical consequences when the cylindrical correction is not properly aligned. Just like soft toric lenses, when the rotation is clockwise or to the left, the amount/degrees of rotation are added to the front toric prescription. Conversely, when the rotation is counter-clockwise or to the right, then the amount/degrees or rotation are subtracted from the axis of the front toric prescription. This is commonly called LARS (left-add, right subtract). Practitioners should keep in mind when the lens is re-ordered with the optical axis compensation, the new lens will remain rotated to the same position since the compensation does not alter the fit or method of stabilization. If the scleral lens requires back surface toricity, quadrants or custom meridians, those modifications to the landing zone stabilize the lens effectively and can quickly return to the original orientation if the lens is applied rotated or the lens is rotated on the eye [6].

When both front surface toricity and back surface toricity are incorporated into the same lens, some practitioners refer to theses lenses as "bitoric." However, this is a misnomer, as the back optic zone radius is not toric. A true bitoric lens would have front surface toricity, and back optical zone surface toricity as well. Modifications to the back surface radii of the optic zone can be manufactured, and in some instances the back optic zone is manufactured in different meridional radii (fenestration cases). Therefore, terminology for a scleral lens with back surface (landing zone) toricity and optical front surface toricity needs to be established.

Breaches and Channels

In cases where scleral lenses seal-off and suction on the eye (Fig. **9**), breaches and channels can be incorporated to the lens design to improve tear exchange. Again, this depends on the manufacturer and the custom features of the design. A breach is an elongated radial excavation or tunneling of the back surface of the lens landing zone that may continue anteriorly (Fig. **10**). It may be quite subtle and not extend to the edge of the lens. The depth, number, and angular width of these breaches can vary based on customization requirements. They can be very wide and shallow (<100 μm), and not visible when viewing the lens.

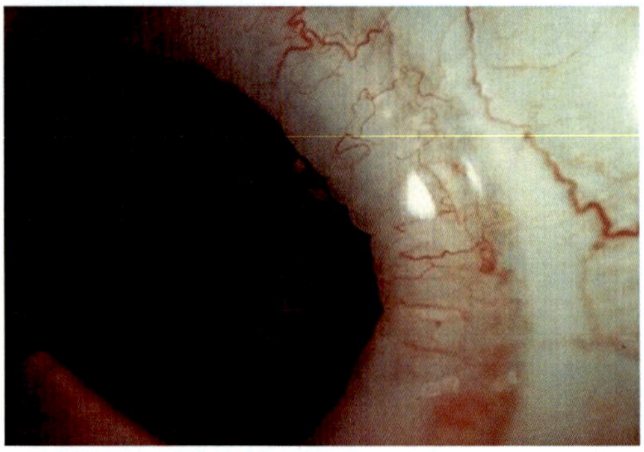

Fig. (9). Lens that is sealed-off and suctioned to the patients' eye. Note the limbal chemosis and hyperemia. Some patients who have an optimal fit with adequate tear exchange may experience exacerbations of chemosis and hyperemia due to their underlying ocular or systemic condition. These patients may be prone to seal-off and suction. If manipulations to the landing zone do not improve the occurrence of lens suction, breaches or channels can be incorporated into the lens design (depending on the manufacturer). Image courtesy of Lynette Johns and Optometry Times (July 2016).

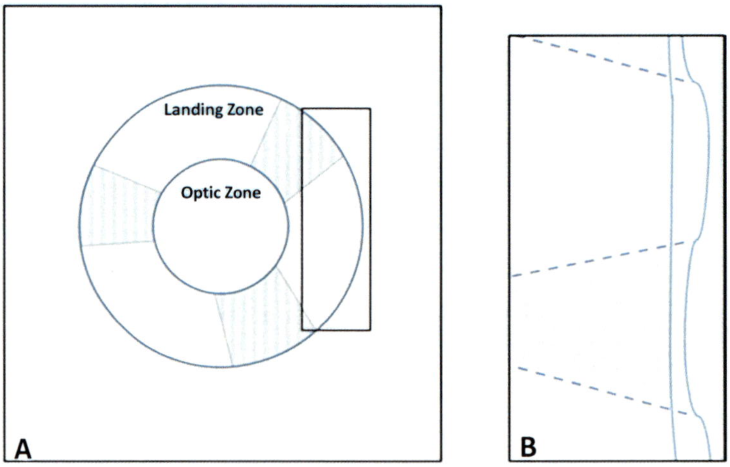

Fig. (10). (A) A diagram representing an example of radial breaches that extend from the edge of the lens on the back surface through the anterior zones. The boxed region (B) depicts the very edge of the lens showing the undulation of the back surface that can provide enhanced tear exchange to reduce or eliminate the occurrence of a suctioned or sealed-off lens.

Channels also can be employed to improve tear exchange (Fig. **11**). These channels can be milled into the back surface of the lens. These are distinct tunnels that can be visible when viewing the lens. Sometimes the edges of these channels are sharp and require post-processing polishing. Both channels and breaches can be made by hand (Fig. **12**).

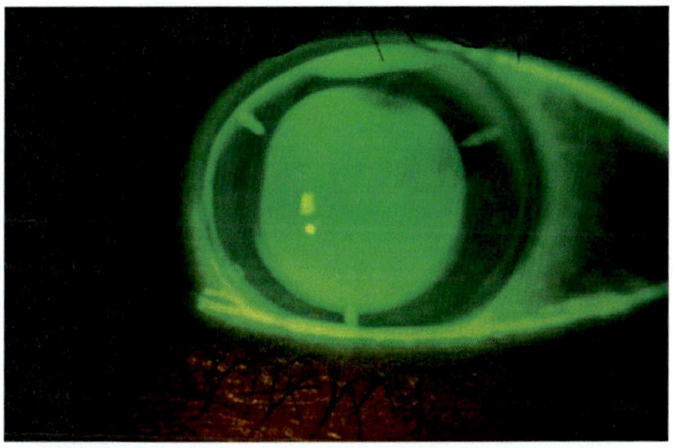

Fig. (11). Example of lathe milled channels enhancing tear exchange on an intralimbal corneal lens. Image courtesy of Lynette Johns.

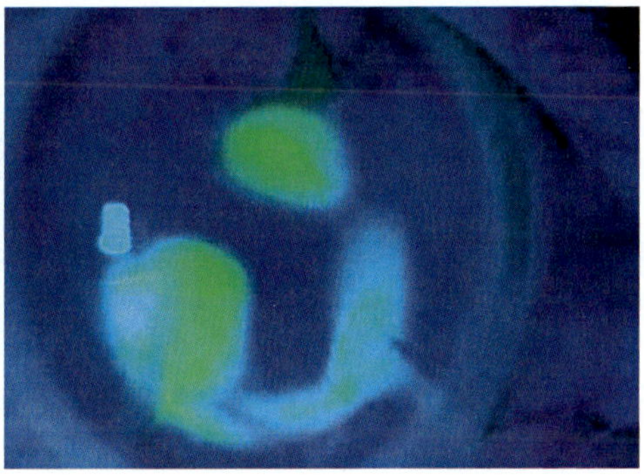

Fig. (12). Example of handmade breaches on a corneo-scleral lens. Image courtesy of Lynette Johns.

Notch / Microvault / Edge Vault

With scleral lenses, it is possible to go around any conjunctival elevation or abnormality such as an elevated pinguecula, pterygium or conjunctival cyst with a notch. Some manufacturers can incorporate a notch in a scleral lens. In cases of conjunctival elevations due to glaucoma surgical procedures (Fig. **13**), it is beneficial to avoid the abnormality altogether and create a notch in the scleral lens. Putting a notch in a scleral lens is quite straightforward. The first step is to measure the size (both length and width) of the conjunctival abnormality with a slit beam of the slit lamp or using scleral topography/profilometry. Next, measure the height and width of the conjunctival abnormality with the scleral lens on the eye. Then, mark the scleral lens with a sharpie or dry erase marker with the lens on the eye. (Inform the patient that the lens is being marked, not the eye). Then, measure the tracing on the lens after removing the scleral lens from the eye. Finally, call the laboratory consultant to discuss the plan and send the lens to the laboratory. It is important to note that this is a manual manipulation and is not exactly reproducible. If the notch is made too anteriorly, a bubble may form under the lens, and if the notch is too short, the lens may still impede on the elevation.

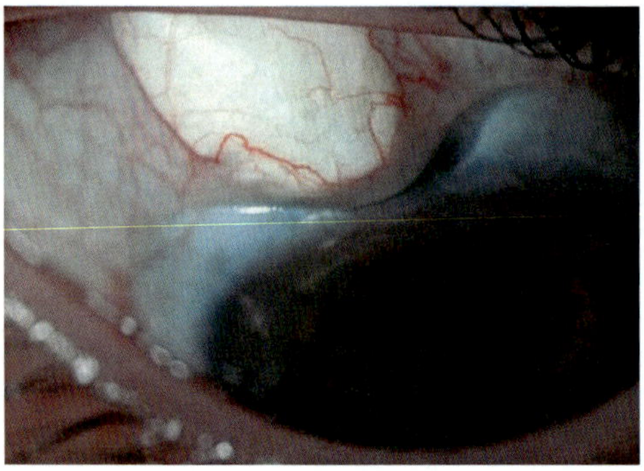

Fig. (13). Example of a scleral lens notch to accommodate a glaucoma drainage device with an overlying scleral patch. Image courtesy of Lynette Johns.

When inserting the lens on the eye, it is important to orient the lens on the eye with the correct orientation. In addition, it is beneficial to inform the patient and the staff person training the patient on scleral lens application and removal.

Some manufacturers create a focal vaulting feature within the lens or located at the edge. This feature creates a spherical elevation if located centrally inside the lens and a hemispherical ripple at the lens landing zone (Fig. **14**) while still maintaining the circular shape of the lens edge (Fig. **15**). Essentially, this feature vaults over a peripheral corneal or conjunctival elevation. The vaulting feature is specified by first determining the axis of the elevation relative to the center of the lens. Next, the distance from the center of the lens is determined by measuring the extent of the elevation from the edge. Finally, the width of the microvault or edge vault depends on the length of the lesion and depth of the feature is quantified.

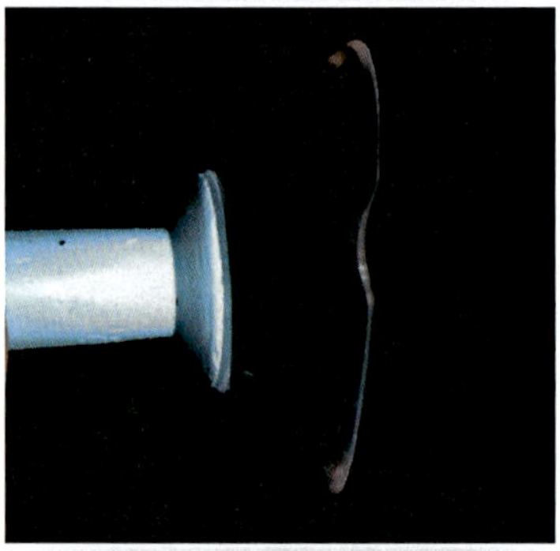

Fig. (14). An example of a focal elevation/vault at the edge of the lens manufactured for a patient with a pinguecula. Image courtesy of Lynette Johns I-Site e-newsletter (November 2016).

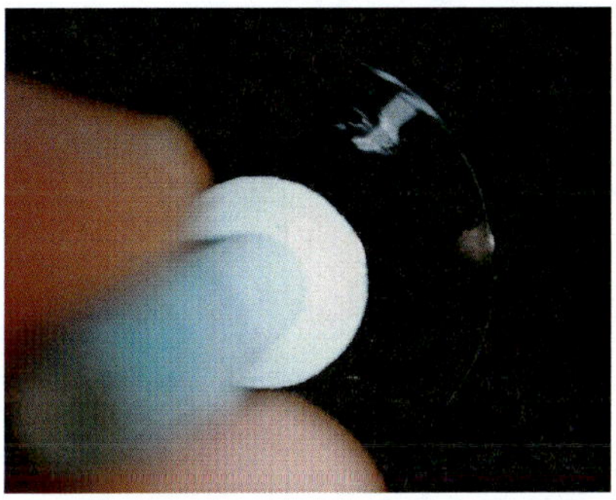

Fig. (15). This is the same lens shown in Fig. (**14**). Note the circular shape of the scleral lens edge is maintained with the focal vaulting feature located at 3 o'clock. Image courtesy of Lynette Johns I-Site e-newsletter (November 2016).

Lens Dots and Laser Markings

Often right lenses are labeled with one dot and the left lenses have either no dots, two dots or one dot of a different color. Dots not only indicate right versus left lenses, they also may indicate the orientation of stabilization in cases of back surface toricity, prism ballasting, dual thin zones, double slab-off prisms, quadrant or asymmetric landing zone peripheries. If the lens always rotates to a specific location, the patient should be instructed to systematically apply the lens being mindful of the location of the dot.

Lenses can be manufactured with laser markings on the anterior surface. The purposes of these markings on diagnostic lenses include labeling the diagnostic lens to prevent mixing them up, marking the zones of the lens, toric rotational markings, as well as labeling patient order numbers (Fig. **16**). Sometimes patients can be aware of the markings if they have sharp edges interacting with their eyelids. To determine if laser marking is causing symptoms, the lens can be rotated to see if the symptom is resolved.

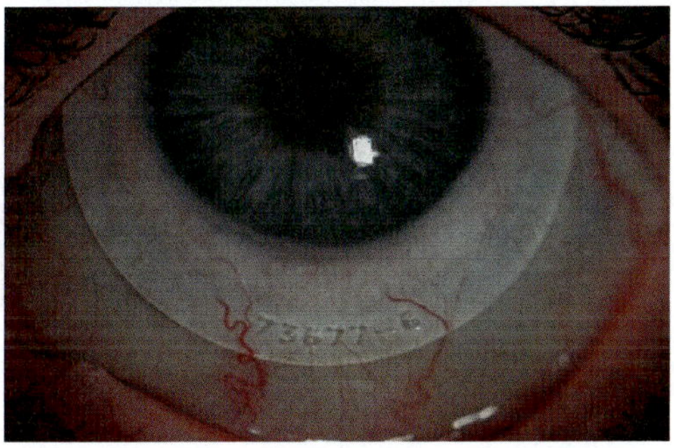

Fig. (16). Example of the laser mark on the anterior surface of the lens. This represents the reference identifier on a patient's lens.

SUMMARY

There are a multitude of terms for all aspects of scleral lenses. Unfortunately, with multiple designs and manufacturers, uniform labeling and terminology may be unlikely, which is unfortunate. It is important for practitioners to develop a relationship with their scleral lens manufacturers to understand the unique and specific aspects of their designs, as well as the customizable features and capabilities.

There are many scleral lens features that can be employed to troubleshoot complicated cases. Understanding the basic anatomy of a lens and all possible modifications that can be made to each zone can improve initial success and reduce the number of lens remakes. While contemporary scleral lenses are still young in the field of medical devices, manufacturers are actively researching and innovating their designs for the expanding role of these lenses.

CONFLICT OF INTEREST

The authors declare no conflict of interest, financial or otherwise.

ACKNOWLEDGEMENTS

We would like to thank Gloria Chiu, Karen Lee, Michael Lipson, Langis Michaud, Sheila Morrison, Florencia Yeh and Debbie Yeung for their edits of this chapter.

REFERENCES

[1] ISO 18369-1: 2006 +A1: 2009 Ophthalmic optics – Contact lenses – Part 1: Vocabulary, classification system and recommendations for labeling specifications. Geneva: International Organization for Standardization; 2009.

[2] Michaud L, van der Worp E, Brazeau D, Warde R, Giasson CJ. Predicting estimates of oxygen transmissibility for scleral lenses. Cont Lens Anterior Eye 2012; 35(6): 266-71. [http://dx.doi.org/10.1016/j.clae.2012.07.004] [PMID: 22878418]

[3] Jaynes JM, Edrington TB, Weissman BA. Predicting scleral GP lens entrapped tear layer oxygen tensions. Cont Lens Anterior Eye 2015; 38(1): 44-7. [http://dx.doi.org/10.1016/j.clae.2014.09.008] [PMID: 25447853]

[4] Compañ V, Oliveira C, Aguilella-Arzo M, Mollá S, Peixoto-de-Matos SC, González-Méijome JM. Oxygen diffusion and edema with modern scleral rigid gas permeable contact lenses. Invest Ophthalmol Vis Sci 2014; 55(10): 6421-9. [http://dx.doi.org/10.1167/iovs.14-14038] [PMID: 25190661]

[5] Schornack MM, Patel SV. Relationship between corneal topographic indices and scleral lens base curve. Eye Contact Lens 2010; 36(6): 330-3. [http://dx.doi.org/10.1097/ICL.0b013e3181eb8418] [PMID: 20631627]

[6] Visser ES, Visser R, Van Lier HJ. Advantages of toric scleral lenses. Optom Vis Sci 2006; 83(4): 233-6. [http://dx.doi.org/10.1097/01.opx.0000214297.38421.15] [PMID: 16614579]

[7] Visser E-S, Van der Linden BJ, Otten HM, Van der Lelij A, Visser R. Medical applications and outcomes of bitangential scleral lenses. Optom Vis Sci 2013; 90(10): 1078-85. [http://dx.doi.org/10.1097/OPX.0000000000000018] [PMID: 23974663]

CHAPTER 3

Understanding Anterior Ocular Surface Shape

Eef van der Worp[1,2,*], **Gregory DeNaeyer**[3] and **Patrick Caroline**[2]

[1] *University of Maastricht, Maastricht, The Netherlands*

[2] *Pacific College of Optometry, Forest Grove, OR, USA*

[3] *Arena Eye Surgeons, Columbus, OH, USA*

Abstract: Historically, there was little emphasis placed on the anterior shape of the eye, apart from the corneal shape, but with the resurgence of scleral lenses, recent interest in the anterior corneo-scleral junction has been examined, measured and quantified. Interestingly, the corneo-scleral junction had been found to be predominantly tangential. A variety of technology can be utilized to analyze the anterior ocular surface shape. Instrumentation includes keratometry, Placido-based topography, Scheimpflug topography, optical coherence tomography, and scleral topography. Curvature and elevation data, symmetry or asymmetry are critical in deciding whether a small diameter scleral lens, a large diameter scleral lens – or maybe a toric scleral lens is indicated when fitting a patient. Different metrics and indices define ocular surface shape. Consequences of inappropriate curvatures and parameters of lenses placed on the ocular surface can result in lens misalignment, excessive compression, impingement and/or edge lift that result in patient symptomatology. As with any contact lens, the overall goal is to provide optimal vision, fit and comfort. Therefore, it is crucial to understand the ocular surface shape to improve alignment and centration of the optics for optimal vision. Improvements in alignment reduce ocular signs and discomfort. A general understanding of ocular surface shape can lead to enhanced designs and improved patient outcomes.

Keywords: Anatomy, Anterior scleral shape, Conjunctival structures, Corneal shape, Corneal structures, Corneo-Scleral Profile, Decentration, Episcleral, Eye Dimensions, Eye muscle, OCT, Placido disc, Scheimpflug, Scleral Angles, Scleral shape, Sectorial, Spiral of Tillaux, Tangential Shape, Tenon's capsule, Toricity.

INTRODUCTION

Up until recently, little was known about the shape of the anterior eye outside of the cornea. That has changed quite dramatically in recent years. This chapter reviews what technology can be best used to analyze the anterior ocular surface

* **Corresponding author Eef van der Worp:** Pacific University College of Optometry, Forest Grove, OR, USA; Tel: +1 503 3522768; Fax: +1 503 3522929; E-mails: eefvanderworp@netherlens.com

Melissa Barnett & Lynette K. Johns (Eds.)

shape. This information is critical in deciding whether a small diameter scleral lens, a large diameter scleral lens – or maybe a toric scleral lens is indicated when fitting a patient. This chapter explores the metrics that define ocular surface shape and contains a consensus on terminology.

TOPOGRAPHY

Keratometry & Corneal Topography

The practical use of the use of central keratometry measurements to fit scleral lenses is very questionable. It is universally agreed that obtaining central keratometry values should be performed to obtain baseline measurements used to follow up and manage potential topographical changes. But otherwise, it seems that that central keratometry is not very useful in scleral lens practice.

What is the best method to analyze ocular surface shape when fitting and managing scleral lens patients? Corneal topography in contact lens practice is a large step forward from keratometry, and it is a very powerful tool if used correctly. Most of the corneal topographers in contact lens practices are reflection systems and typically based on Placido disc, after the Portuguese oculist who first described reflected images from the cornea [1]. Contemporary corneal topographers project a series of concentric rings or colored dots on the cornea, and the distances between the reflections of these are measured and analyzed. A practical limitation of this method is found in the peripheral cornea where the values either become less reliable and/or the instrument is unable to measure this area entirely, although systems that utilize this method have been used in experimental settings [2, 3]. The colored dot reflection systems have an advantage to ring reflection systems because they do not suffer (by definition) from "ring jam" since no reflected rings overlap. Some topographers utilize composite maps, in which five images are taken of a given eye (one central, four peripheral) and merged together into one image, providing coverage of the cornea.

Although Placido based corneal topography is limited to the cornea, there are ways to extrapolate the corneal data peripherally, which then could be used as an indicator for limbal and even anterior scleral shape. Potentially, some predictions can be made regarding the ocular shape beyond the corneal borders.

Corneal topography can be useful for monitoring corneal changes secondary to scleral lens wear. The landing zone of modern scleral lenses is on the sclera and its overlying tissues, leaving the cornea clear from mechanical pressure by the lens. In 2015, Soeters *et al.* found a number of corneal parameters to be significantly different (flatter) compared to 1 week or more after scleral lens removal in 20 eyes of 14 patients [4]. The average steep keratometry value was about 0.7 diopter (D) lower, the average flat keratometry value was 0.5 D lower and average maximum simulated keratometry value was 1.1 D lower. The duration of these changes is unknown.

In 2016, statistically significant corrneal flattening up to 0.08 mm +/- 0.04 mm was demonstrated while a scleral lens was worn for 8 hours and corneal clearance was maintained [5]. The superior mid-peripheral cornea was primarily involved in the flattening, which caused a slight increase in against-the-rule corneal astigmatism.

Higher-order aberrations (horizontal coma, vertical coma and spherical aberration) were found to undergo significant changes as well in scleral lens wear. Corneal clearance was statistically significantly reduced in East Asian participants, and greater superior-nasal corneal flattening was found compared to Caucasians.

Based on these observations, it seems that practitioners should be aware that corneal measurements following mini-scleral lens removal could potentially mask underlying corneal steepening. There is still a lot to learn about what is happening with scleral lens wear. Further discussion is beyond the scope of this chapter, which focuses on understanding scleral shape in order to better fit scleral lenses. Bearing in mind, corneal topographical changes underneath scleral lenses occur and should be monitored with the current evaluation techniques that are available.

Elevation Data

Relatively newer instruments, such as Scheimpflug systems, typically cover a larger corneal area, but are still limited to the corneal surface. A software update was recently developed for one of the Scheimpflug systems to make corneo-scleral section images in addition to the corneal data (Fig. **1**).

Scheimpflug corneal topographers scan optical sections of the cornea, similar to a slit lamp; as a result, by scanning across the cornea a full elevation map is created of both the anterior and the posterior cornea. These instruments can detect keratoconus at a very early stage, as early topographical changes occur with keratoconus appear in the posterior corneal surface [6].

The significance of height maps is that they represent shape compared to curve (radius) or power maps. In contact lens practice, it is 'shape' that is paramount to practitioners regarding the ocular surface. It is difficult to achieve an understanding of that shape, based on colored maps that represent curvature. When using a topographic map, red signifies a steep curvature but not directionality whether the curve is protruding or receding. As a result, the elevation difference and direction is not known based on the topographic map. A height or elevation map solves some of these problems and can be used in conjunction with a topographical map to determine millimeters of radius and microns of elevation. Hence, using microns to describe ocular surface shape and ocular surface differences makes much more sense, as stated in a position paper by Van der Worp, Hall and Caroline [7]. Placido disc systems, as described earlier in this section, can easily and quite accurately derive height information from their measured curvature data to create an elevation map.

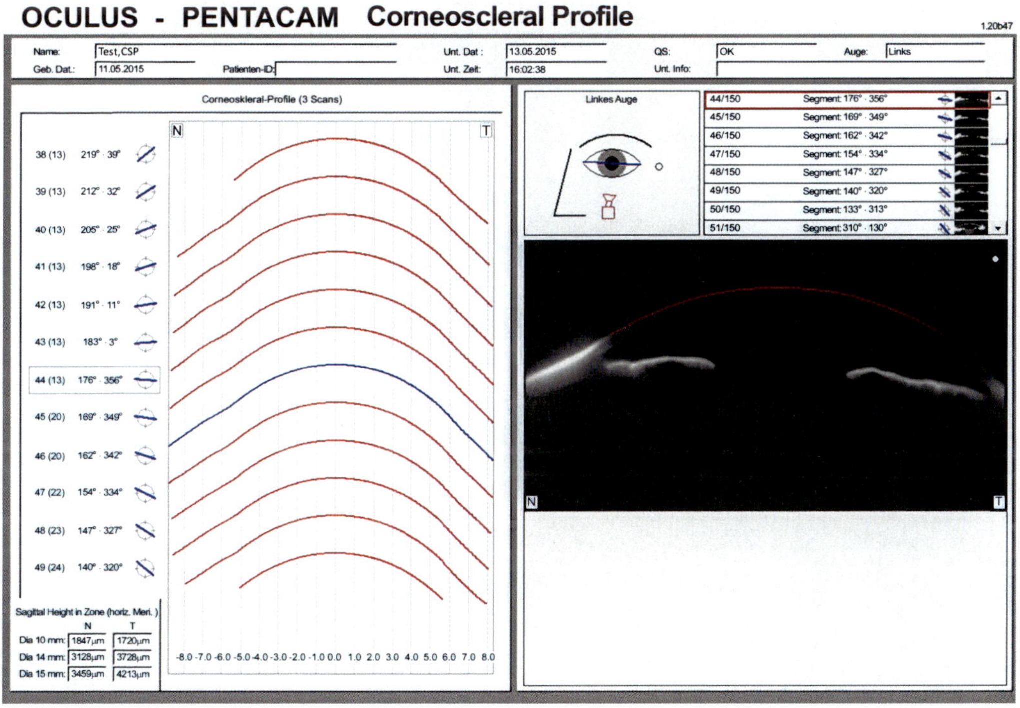

Fig. (1). Oculus Pentacam showing corneo-scleral profiles in different meridians.

Beyond the Corneal Borders

Height maps are generated by optical coherence tomography (OCT), some Scheimpflug devices and some recently introduced profilometry instruments, but, notably, they can also measure beyond the corneal borders. This can create information of the corneo-scleral profile, the limbal area, and the anterior scleral shape (Fig. **2**).

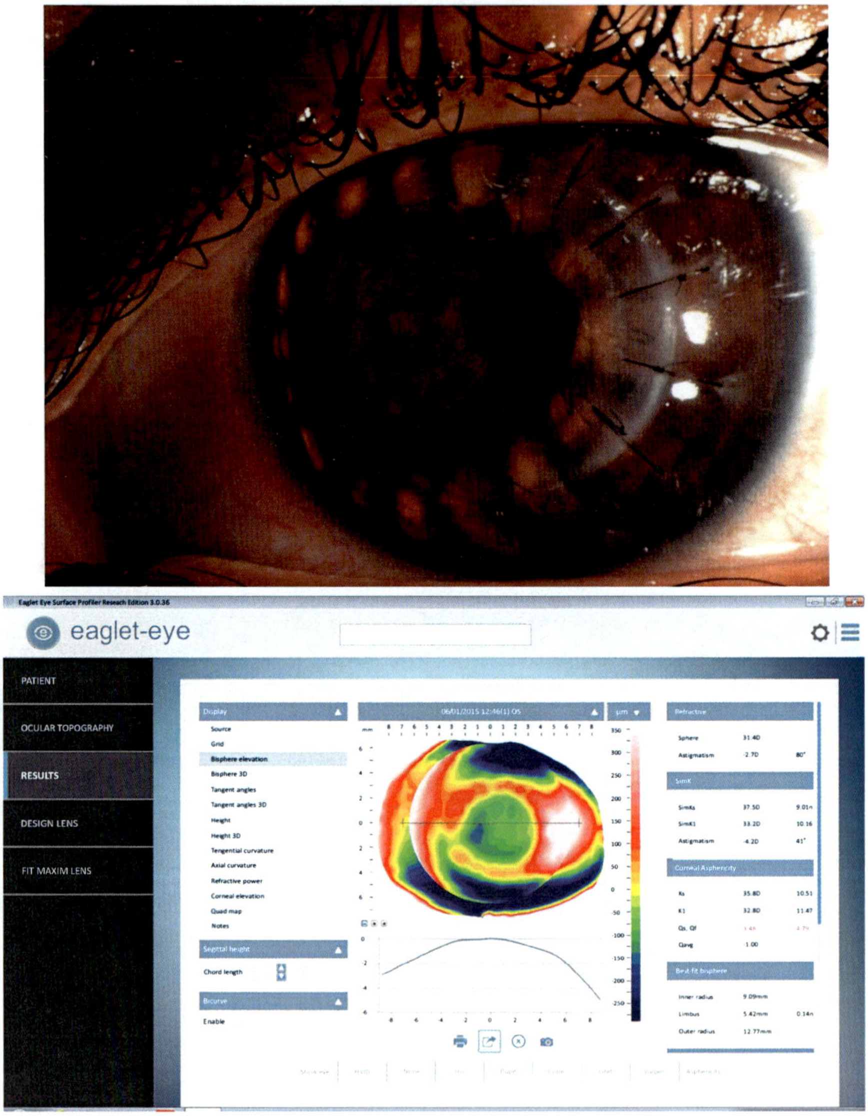

Fig. (2). (Top) Left eye with a corneal transplant. (Bottom) Elevation map (ESP, Eaglet Eye) of the same eye above. The red dots in the elevation map indicate localized elevation of the stitches. Images of courtesy of Brian Tompkins.

The first question is: over which area does the practitioner need shape information when fitting scleral lenses?

According to textbooks, when looking at the anterior ocular surface, there is about 7.0 mm between the limbus of the cornea and the insertion of the ocular rectus muscles (7.0 mm, 7.5 mm and 6.5 mm, respectively) in the temporal, superior and inferior direction. However, on the nasal side, there is only about 5.5 mm. This phenomenon is called 'the spiral of Tillaux', after the French physician who first described this phenomenon. If the average corneal diameter is about 12 mm for a normal eye, then the maximum diameter horizontally of a scleral lens before it interferes with the location of the eye muscle insertion is about 24 mm, assuming limited or no lens movement [8].

What do we know about the about the corneo-scleral junction profile and anterior scleral shape? In the German contact lens journal Die Kontaktlinse in 1992, Meier - a Swiss eyecare practitioner - defined in a publication different transitions from cornea to sclera [9]. Five different models are described:

Profile 1: a gradual transition from cornea to sclera in which the scleral portion is convex

Profile 2: a gradual transition from cornea to sclera in which the scleral portion is tangential

Profile 3: a marked transition in which the scleral portion convex

Profile 4: a marked transition in which the scleral portion is tangential

Profile 5: a convex corneal shape with a concave scleral shape

The profiles in the Meier scale are decreasing in sagittal height, in which the first profile has the highest sagittal height and profile number five has the lowest sagittal height. This is an important parameter for fitting scleral lenses. Other studies published in die Kontaktlinse tried to identify how often the different profiles were observed in the general population [10]. Profile 2 (gradual-tangential) followed by profile 3 (marked-convex) respectively were the first and second most commonly observed, the number one and two observed, followed by profile 1 (gradual-convex). Profile 4 (marked-tangential) was minimally observed and profile 5, (convex-concave), was almost nonexistent.

The question of how accurately these profiles can be subjectively rated by practitioners was also addressed in a study by Bokern *et al.* [11]. They found with 73 investigators a repeatability of only 54 percent. For some profiles, the repeatability was much lower.

Tangential Shape

When considering the corneo-scleral junction, one would expected this to be concave in shape, assumedly the cornea should have a steeper curve than the curve of the sclera. In fact, early generation scleral lenses were based on that idea (a marked corneo-scleral junction, and a radius of the sclera representing the overall radius of the globe).

Nevertheless, that appears not to be the case. Studies at Pacific University demonstrate that the shape of the corneoscleral junction appears to be straight in many cases based on OCT measurements [12, 13]. The scleral shape study at Pacific University evaluated 96 eyes of 48 normal subjects. The ocular shape was measured in eight different directions: nasal, nasal-inferior, inferior, inferior-temporal, temporal, temporal-superior, superior and superior-nasal. Most the junctions were tangential: only one quarter exhibited concave shapes, and few exhibited convex shapes. Moreover: within one eye, different profiles were measured in different meridians. Of note, the information found on the ocular surface with instruments such as the OCT is purely surface based. In other words, anatomically, there does seem to be a marked transition from cornea to sclera, but this is masked and filled by other tissue such as conjunctiva, Tenon's capsule and episclera [14, 15].

Nasal Flattening

What do the results from the previously described Pacific University scleral shape study mean, from a practical standpoint? First, it appears that practitioners should not assume the corneo-scleral junction to necessarily have the concave/convex shapes that would be expected based on theoretical consideration when fitting and designing a scleral lens [13]. It is suggested that using tangent angles rather than using curves (or very flat curves) may be appropriate in many cases when fitting scleral lenses. However, there are large differences in the various meridians even within the same eye.

It also appears from the Pacific shape studies that for the normal eye, the nasal portion on average is typically flatter compared to the other sections on the ocular surface (Fig. **3**). This could have a relatively small, but potentially significant effect on scleral lens centration [16]. In normal eyes and standard optical lenses, this would most likely not be bothersome. However, in eyes with large differences between nasal and temporal eye shape, and lenses with complex optics like multifocal and myopia-control lenses, this may become clinically relevant.

Ocular Sagittal Height (OC-SAG)

What is the ideal diameter or chord when it comes to scleral lens fitting? Fifteen millimeters seems to be a realistic baseline diameter, or chord, to work with as most instruments that go beyond the corneal borders provide a realistic measurement over that chord. Going larger than 15 mm can also make measurements in other meridians, like the vertical meridian, more difficult to measure.

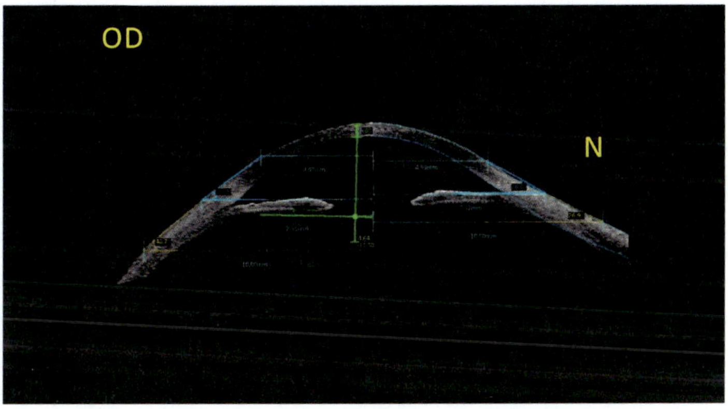

Fig. (3). Image of a right eye with a flatter nasal sclera(N) (limbal angle 28.8° scleral angle 26.9° from a horizontal axis) *versus* temporal sclera with a steeper appearance (limbal angle 36.9°, scleral angle 40.7°).

What does the anterior ocular surface area over a 15 mm chord look like? The central cornea is typically spherical, followed by a gradual flattening from the central cornea towards the periphery, usually described with a value called eccentricity. Next is the corneal-scleral junction shape which is usually unknown, followed by the shape of the anterior scleral surface. The latter two vary between individuals and even vary within the same eye. For the sake of simplicity, the ocular surface and sagittal height can be defined which is an average of all of the previous variables.

The OCT, while limited to single meridians, allows measurement for the first time of the sagittal height. Studies at Pacific University demonstrated the mean OC-SAG over 15mm in the horizontal meridian (n=55) to be 3735 sd ± 186 µm, with a range of 3290 – 4170 µm from the flattest (or shallowest) eye to the steepest (or highest) anterior ocular surface [17]. Meanwhile, studies at Waterloo University in Canada (n=40) over the exact same chord and direction established the OC-SAG to be 3740 sd ± 200 µm, with a range of 3140 – 4040 µm [18]. A study by Hall *et al.* at Visioncare Research LTD in the UK (n=50) found the OC-SAG to be 3740 sd ± 160 µm, ranging between 3290 – 4100 µm [19]. This experiment was repeated with the Eye Surface Profiler (Eaglet Eye) ESP in a study in the Netherlands [20 - 22]. In this Groenhof Study, only normal eyes (n=86) were measured. The OC-SAG over 15mm in the horizontal meridian was found to be 3755 sd ± 207 µm, with a range of 3290 – 4280 µm [21].

Terminology

Not every practitioner has an instrument available at this point to measure the total ocular surface area. Using current equipment can roughly estimate the overall ocular surface beyond the corneal borders. Corneal topographers, as described earlier in this chapter, can capture the corneal shape. The peripheral cornea can be captured or described as an angle rather than a curve. This peripheral angle can then be extrapolated onto the corneo-scleral zone. Thus, an estimate can be predicted about the overall ocular shape in that region. This way, an idea of the ocular surface shape can be approximated without direct measurement.

Based on this information, specific terminology needs to be defined so that practitioners are referencing the same measurements. First and foremost, ocular surface elevation can be defined either as a baseline chord to the top of the curve (height), or from the top of the curve to a baseline chord (depth). To be consistent, height has been proposed as the dominant terminology to describe the elevation of a given curve. This also applies to "sagittal height," rather than "sagittal depth." Some prefer "sagittal height" to describe ocular surface shape and "sagittal depth" to describe the sagitta of a contact lens. The consensus paper suggests using the term "sagittal height" for both the ocular surface and a contact lens [7]. When applying this terminology to the ocular surface, a baseline chord over a given diameter is first determined. Next, the height from that chord to the top of the curve (the cornea) is measured as the sagittal height. When referring to contact lens sagittal height, it describes the height from a base chord (typically the diameter of the lens) to the back surface curve of the contact lens, preferably in microns; however, millimeters are sometimes used.

The Model Eye

Based on the literature to date, the OC-SAG of the normal eye (without disease or irregularity) is roughly in the 3750 μm range with a maximum range of 1000 μm between the flattest and the steepest eye in this population [22, 23]. Therefore, these measurements provide baseline height information for a normal population so practitioners have perspective about scleral lens sagittal height.

Keratoconus is a main indication for scleral lens wear, and the overall sagittal height is typically higher as expected in corneal ectasias. When examining the differences between normal eyes and keratoconus eyes with OCT, Achong-Coan *et al.* found keratoconic eyes to be 205 μm higher on average than normal eyes (3940 *versus* 3735 μm) [24]. Interestingly, the study found that keratoconic eyes do not differ from normal eyes except in the central cornea.

Additional studies at Pacific University consistently demonstrate that the nasal area of the anterior sclera is more elevated than the temporal side (and other quadrants as well) from a baseline chord [12, 25]. Hall *et al.* evaluated this as well. They published a number of papers on the corneo-scleral junction (CSJ) in normal eyes and found similar results [19, 26]. The mean CSJ tended to be sharpest at the nasal side and became progressively flatter at the inferior, temporal and superior junctions. They reported that the CSJ angles were consistent with tangential extensions of the peripheral cornea to the sclera in many cases. Tan *et al.* confirmed these findings, stating that the squared orthogonalized residuals (SSRo) were significantly greater in the nasal quadrant [27]. The temporal quadrant demonstrated the flattest and smoothest topography. In the same study, whites demonstrated statistically significantly higher SSRo than Asians and Latinos.

In the context of contact lens terminology, it is stated that the nasal scleral portion is "flatter" than the rest according to the shape studies. In order to remain consistent with the elevation terminology used and proposed here, it may be best to refrain from using "flat" or "steep" terminology altogether and use "higher" and "lower" areas instead.

Using height terminology, the nasal side of the anterior sclera is therefore "more elevated" as seen from a reference baseline chord (Fig. **4**). The confusing part, to some degree, may be that the sagittal height (OC-SAG) on the nasal side actually has a lower value than the sagittal height on the temporal side.

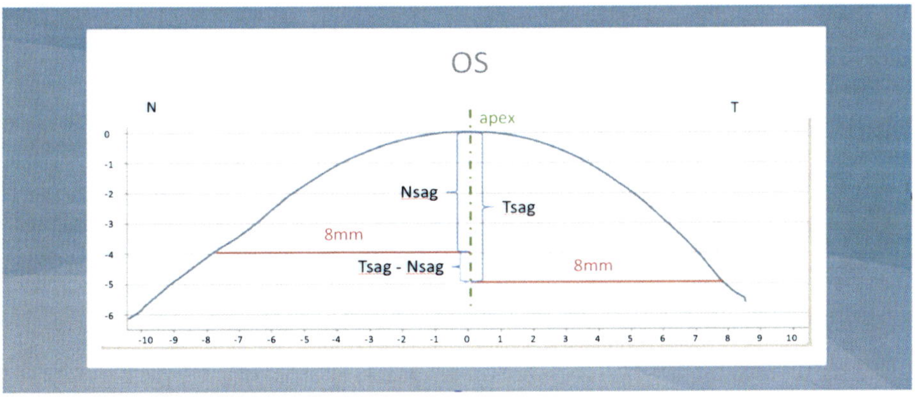

Fig. (4). This example shows there is a difference in the nasal sagittal height (Nsag) *versus* temporal sagittal height (Tsag) with the Eye Surface Profiler (Eaglet Eye).

Generally, in terms of elevation maps, the differences in height can be best displayed as absolute height differences (*e.g.*, the nasal side is 100 μm higher than the temporal side) from a horizontal plane. Even small differences in height (between two opposite meridians, as in corneal astigmatism) can be displayed.

In addition, a recent study at Pacific University by Kinoshita *et al.* evaluated corneal toricity and scleral asymmetry [28]. Of the ten subjects with a low amount of with-the-rule (WTR) corneal astigmatism, only one maintained a (WTR) orientation of scleral toricity at a 15.0 mm chord. None of the subjects demonstrated (WTR) scleral toricity at a 17.0 mm chord. Of the ten subjects with a high amount of corneal WTR astigmatism, three subjects maintained WTR scleral toricity at chords of 15.0 and 17.0 mm.

In summary, after reviewing the data presented in the aforementioned scleral shape and sagittal height studies, scleral shape is highly asymmetric. The presence of scleral toricity is often not in the same orientation and magnitude as the corneal toricity. The implications of this data may influence future scleral lens designs to improve lens positioning and optics. As future lens designs increase in diameter, practitioners may want to image both the cornea and sclera and utilize lens designs that take into account the highly asymmetric shape of the sclera.

Comparing Instruments

Ritzman *et al.* used three different instruments to measure large diameter chords on the corneal surface: the Visante by Zeiss, the Eye Surface Profiler by Eaglet Eye and the sMap3D™ by Visionary Optics, manufactured by Precision Ocular Metrology, LLC [29]. The sagittal height measurements of 30 eyes were taken in the 8 primary meridians at chords of 12.8 and 15.0 mm of 15 subjects. Additional sagittal height measurements were taken with the Eaglet ESP and sMap3D™ at a chord of 17.0 mm. The data from all three measurement techniques at all three chords lengths in 30 eyes was found to be consistent (Fig. **5**).

LENS FITTING

Clinically, what does all this mean and how can information about the anterior scleral shape be useful in scleral lens fitting? First of all, it can assist in making the right decision for a corneal GP lens *versus* a scleral lens, but also for starting with a rotationally symmetric scleral lens *versus* a toric scleral lens. It can additionally help the practitioner better understand, and alleviate common scleral lens problems such as localized conjunctival blanching and compression, air bubble formation behind the lens and conjunctival prolapse.

Corneal GP or Scleral GP?

Initial lens selection can be challenging for practitioners especially when deciding between corneal and scleral lenses. Investigators at Pacific University proposed a system based on height differences of the corneal elevation to aid practitioners with initial lens selection [30]. In their experience, a patient demonstrating less than 350 µm of corneal height differential was successful with a corneal GP lens 88.2% of the time. Therefore, they propose fitting a scleral lens if the patient demonstrates more than 350 µm difference in corneal height when evaluating the topography elevation map (Fig. **6**).

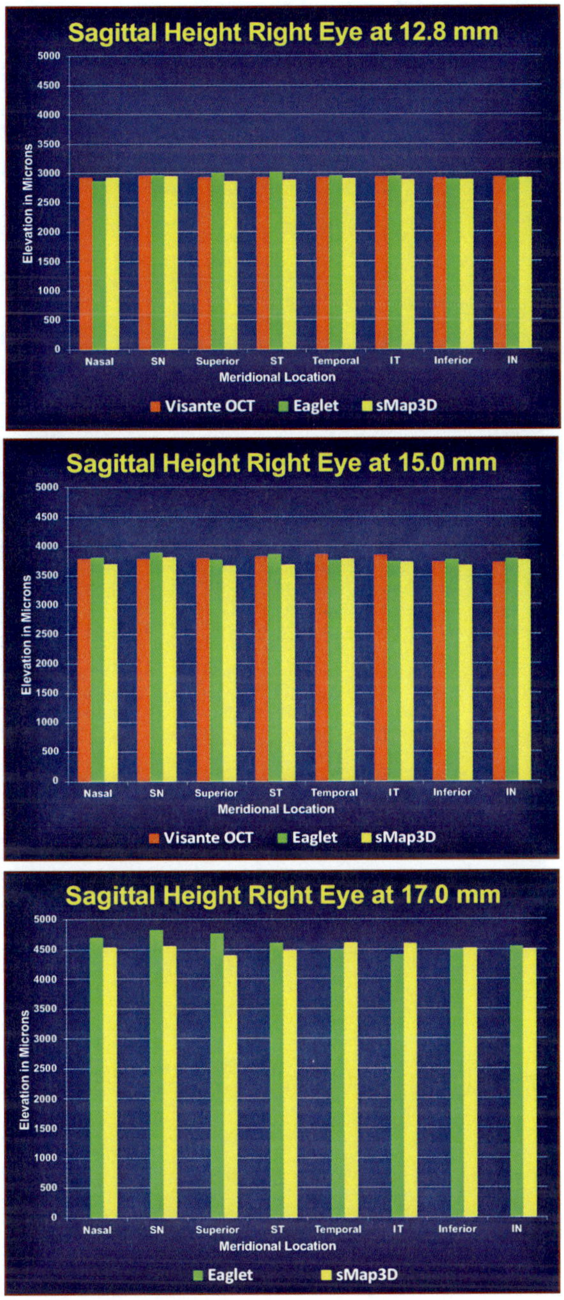

Fig. (5). Pacific University Scleral Shape Study measuring sagittal height over 12.8, 15 and 17mm using the Visante OCT (Zeiss) ESP (Eaglet Eye) and sMap3D™ (Visionary Optics). Image courtesy of Pat Caroline and Randy Kojima.

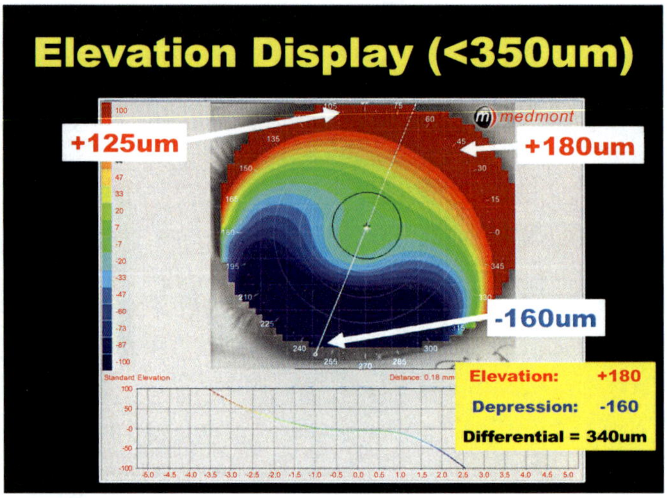

Fig. (6). Corneal elevation display, Medmont Topographer.

Scleral Lens Fitting & Anterior Ocular Surface Shape

Ritzman *et al.* evaluated 39 normal subjects (78 eyes) [29]. The sagittal height was measured in all eight meridians of the cornea, limbus and sclera at chords of 10.0, 12.8 and 15.0 mm. At the 10.0 mm (corneal) chord the average sagittal height difference between the two principle meridians was 45µm on the right eyes and 40 µm on the left eyes. This is approximately equivalent to -1.00 D of corneal astigmatism. At the 12.8 mm (limbal) chord they found no meaningful sagittal height differential between principle meridians; therefore, at the 12.8 mm chord the ocular surface can be best described as spherical (rotationally symmetric).

At the 15.0 mm (scleral) chord, the sclera shows a small amount of asymmetry in the 8 meridians with the nasal meridians being the highest and the temporal being the lowest. Scleral toricity (height differential) was approximately 105 µm between two opposing meridians of maximal difference. As described by Kinoshita *et al.*, a correlation between corneal and scleral toricity seems very unlikely [28].

This data seems to indicate that scleral asymmetry starts at the more symmetrical limbus and increases in asymmetry towards the extraocular muscles, possibly in line with the earlier described "Spiral of Tillaux." Based on the theoretical consideration of muscle insertion, this may explain nasal flattening in scleral shape studies [8].

Therefore, scleral lens designs of 14.5 mm or less are often rotationally symmetric; however, due to scleral asymmetry, scleral lens designs larger than

14.5 mm may often benefit from a toric periphery and/or a quadrant specific design.

Optics

A back surface toric or quadrant specific design is beneficial for comfort, and presents optimal alignment to the anterior surface shape. Secondly, there may be benefits for optics as well. Visser *et al.*, investigated toric scleral lenses on eye; it took on average five seconds for back toric scleral lenses to return to their initial position after the lenses were manually rotated to a different position [31] - showing the incredible stability of these lenses on eye. This was duplicated in another study by Visser *et al.* using a different toric scleral lens design, with similar results [32]. The median stability meridian in the right eyes was 140° (range 0-180°) compared to 137° (range 30-180°) in the earlier study; in the left eyes, this was 60° (range 0-180°) compared to 47° (range 0-170°) in the previous study [31, 32].

Due to the toric scleral lens stability, additional optical corrections to standard spherical or aspheric front optics designs [33] can be applied to the front surface of the lens such as a cylindrical correction, multifocality, and correction of higher order aberrations. This application can help further improve visual performance in these patients. However, an adaptive period may be needed where the patient has to acclimate to the "new optics." In other words, the human brain may not immediately and subjectively appreciate the superb optical quality provided by these lenses [34].

Scleral Lens Blanching & Compression

The topic of scleral lens blanching and compression is extensively discussed elsewhere in this book. Once the diagnostic lens is optimized for corneal clearance, the landing zone of the lens is assessed with respect to the ocular surface.

Conjunctival blanching is a phenomenon that occurs when localized areas of the conjunctival tissue around the limbus can be "whitened" because compression of the lens. This causes a restriction of blood flow. A ring of bearing on the inner part of the landing zone means the landing zone is too flat. Air bubbles underneath the peripheral edge of the lens also indicate a flat landing zone. Frothing may also be present underneath the peripheral edge. Fluorescein can be helpful in evaluating the landing zone.

For a steep lens periphery, the bearing would be on the outer part of the landing zone. Fluorescein pooling may be visible extending beyond the limbus over the adjacent scleral surface. A steep landing zone can increase the total lens clearance by lifting the entire lens off the corneal surface.

As noted earlier in this chapter, from clinical experience and studies on corneal shape, the anterior ocular surface is asymmetrical in shape. When a scleral lens is placed on this eye, one or more segments of the conjunctiva could be compressed, resulting in localized blanching. This can be a challenge; some companies truncate the lens or "grind" the back surface of the scleral lens where the blanching occurs to alleviate pressure in that specific area. Toric and/or quadrant specific scleral lens peripheries can be designed to overcome blanching or impingement as well, in a more structured and controlled way.

Conjunctival Prolapse

In some cases, loose conjunctival tissue (like in cases of conjunctivochalasis) can be drawn underneath the lens. This is typically caused by the negative pressure under the lens (Fig. 7). "Conjunctival prolapse" is also used to describe this. It appears to be more prominent in elderly patients. Loose conjunctiva is sometimes drawn underneath the transition/limbal zone of the lens, and may even appear underneath the optical zone. Excessive conjunctival tissue can be removed surgically, but it may recur. Neovascularization under the conjunctival flap has been noted clinically. In some patients with inflammatory conditions, the flap may adhere to the underlying cornea. Anterior ocular surface shape may be partly responsible for where the conjunctival tissue is drawn beneath the lens [35]. If the peripheral cornea and/or sclera is depressed infero-temporally, then the conjunctival prolapse would likely occur in this space. Fitting asymmetrical back surface scleral peripheries may help alleviate the problem.

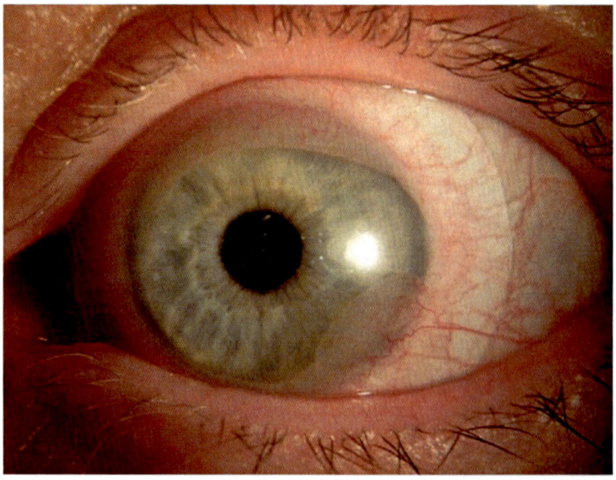

Fig. (7). Superior and infero-temporal conjunctival prolapse. Image courtesy of Greg DeNaeyer.

CLINICAL CASES

Case #1

Corneo-scleral measurement is critical to determine back surface haptic toricity of a scleral lens. Figs. (**8** and **9**) show a toric back surface haptic scleral lens on a toric sclera. At the time of the fitting, measurement of the sclera was unavailable and a clinical estimate of the amount of toricity needed to fit this highly with-th--rule toric sclera. The amount of toricity was underestimated and resulted in superior and inferior edge lift that caused bubble formation, as well as horizontal impingement.

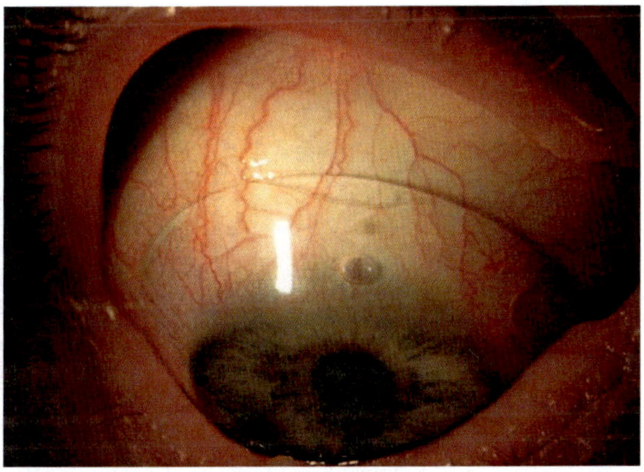

Fig. (8). A toric back surface haptic scleral lens with inadequate toricity that results in superior edge lift and bubble formation. Image courtesy of Greg DeNaeyer.

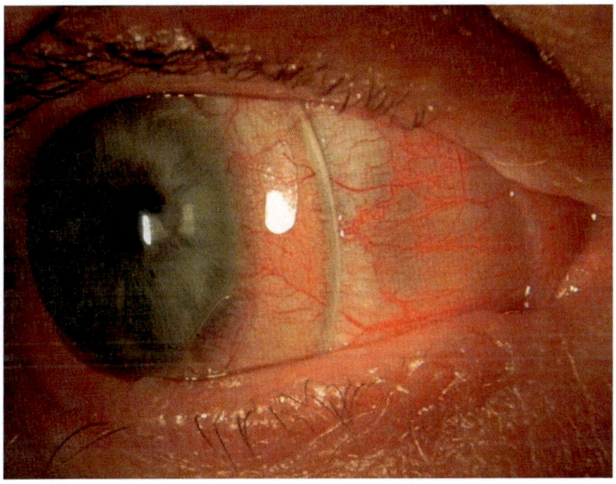

Fig. (9). Horizontal impingement secondary to uneven scleral haptic landing. Image courtesy of Greg DeNaeyer.

Case #2

A keratoconus patient with intrastromal ring segments was fit using sMap3D™ corneo-scleral topographer. Elevation maps measure 3.5 diopters of with-the-rule scleral toricity (Fig. **10**). A Europa Scleral™ 16.5 with a spherical back surface haptic was applied for the purposes of over-refraction (Fig. **11**). The mismatch of the back surface scleral lens on the toric sclera causes the inferior edge of the lens to slightly rest on the lower lid producing an immediate air bubble within the fluid reservoir. A Europa Scleral™ was ordered with 3 diopters of back surface toricity (Fig. **12**). Customized back surface peripheral toricity of the scleral lens resulted in 360 of scleral alignment.

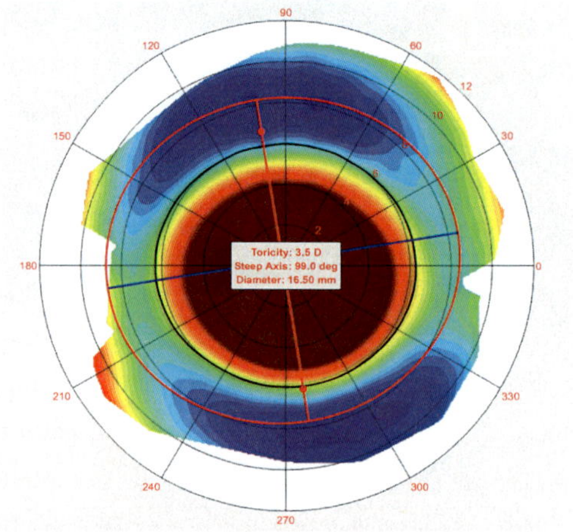

Fig. (10). 3.5 D WTR scleral toricity mapped with sMap3D™.

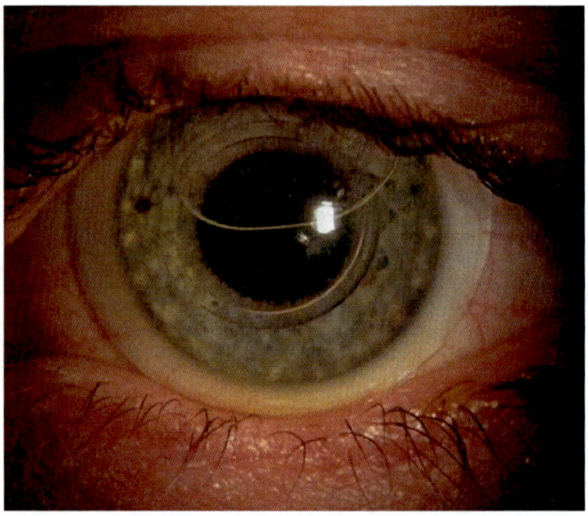

Fig. (11). Spherical back surface haptic scleral lens on a sclera with 3.5 diopters of toricity that results in edge lift and bubble formation. Image courtesy of Greg DeNaeyer.

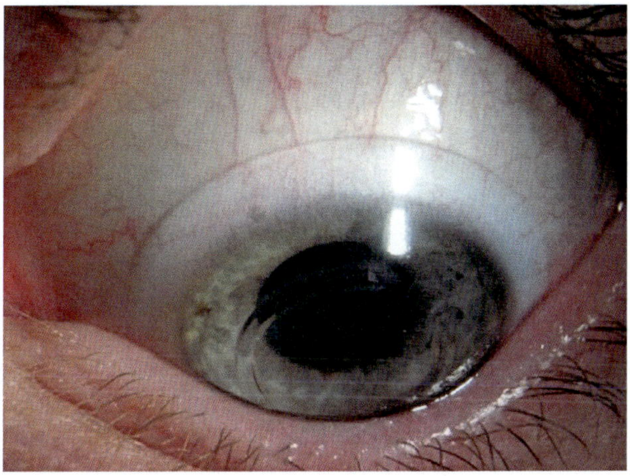

Fig. (12). Customized back surface scleral lens. Image courtesy of Greg DeNaeyer.

CONFLICT OF INTEREST

The authors declare no conflict of interest, financial or otherwise.

ACKNOWLEDGEMENTS

Declared none.

REFERENCES

[1] Bowden T. Contact lenses – the story. Bower House Publications 2009.

[2] Reddy T, Szczotka LB, Roberts C. Peripheral corneal contour measured by topography influences soft toric contact lens fitting success. CLAO J 2000; 26(4): 180-5. [PMID: 11071341]

[3] Szczotka LB, Roberts C, Herderick EE, Mahmoud A. Quantitative descriptors of corneal topography that influence soft toric contact lens fitting. Cornea 2002; 21(3): 249-55. [http://dx.doi.org/10.1097/00003226-200204000-00003] [PMID: 11917171]

[4] Soeters N, Visser ES, Imhof SM, Tahzib NG. Scleral lens influence on corneal curvature and pachymetry in keratoconus patients. Cont Lens Anterior Eye 2015; 38(4): 294-7. [http://dx.doi.org/10.1016/j.clae.2015.03.006] [PMID: 25865408]

[5] Alonso-Caneiro D, Vincent SJ, Collins MJ. Miniscleral lens wear influences corneal curvature and optics. Ophthalmic Physiol Opt 2016; 36(2): 100-11. [http://dx.doi.org/10.1111/opo.12270] [PMID: 26690831]

[6] de Sanctis U, Aragno V, Dalmasso P, Brusasco L, Grignolo F. Diagnosis of subclinical keratoconus using posterior elevation measured with 2 different methods. Cornea 2013; 32(7): 911-5. [http://dx.doi.org/10.1097/ICO.0b013e3182854774] [PMID: 23572130]

[7] Van der Worp E, Caroline P, Hall L. On a higher level – position paper on terminology regarding anterior ocular surface topography. Global Contact 2015; 68(2): 22-4.

[8] Van der Worp E. A guide to scleral lens fitting (English) Version 20 Book 2015. Available at: http://commons.pacificu.edu/mono/4/

[9] Meier D. Das cornea-skleral-profil – ein kriterium individueller kontaktlinsenanpassung. Die

Kontaktlinse 1992; 10: 4-11.

[10] Rott-Muff D, Keller U, Hausler M, Spinell M. Das cornea-skleral-profil und seine auswirkingen auf die form von weichlinsen. Die Kontaktlinse 2001; 5: 26-34.

[11] Bokern S, Hoppe M, Bandlitz S. Genauigkeit und wiederholbarkeit bei der klassifizierung des corneo-skleral profils. Die Kontaktlinse 2007; 26-8.

[12] Van der Worp E, Graf T, Caroline PJ. Exploring beyond the corneal borders. Contact Lens Spectr 2010; 6: 26-32.

[13] van der Worp E, Bornman D, Ferreira DL, Faria-Ribeiro M, Garcia-Porta N, González-Meijome JM. Modern scleral contact lenses: A review. Cont Lens Anterior Eye 2014; 37(4): 240-50. [http://dx.doi.org/10.1016/j.clae.2014.02.002] [PMID: 24631015]

[14] Caroline PJ, Andre MP. Scleral lens settling. Contact Lens Spectr 2012; 5: 60.

[15] Leach NE, van der Worp E, Bergmanson JP. Corneal and scleral topograpic anatomy.Clinical Ocular Anatomy and Physiology. 22nd ed., Houston: Texas eye research and technology center 2015.

[16] Sonsino J. Schornack, M. Troubleshooting Scleral Lenses. A successful fit can be life-changing, but practitioners must address the challenges of this lens type. Contact Lens Spectr 2013.

[17] Harkness B, Caroline P, Ritzmann M, Kojima R, Hayes JR. Comparison of sagittal height measurement methods and predicting central clearance of scleral contact lenses. Poster American Academy Optometry 2015.

[18] Sorbara L, Maram J, Fonn D, Woods C, Simpson T. Metrics of the normal cornea: anterior segment imaging with the Visante OCT. Clin Exp Optom 2010; 93(3): 150-6. [http://dx.doi.org/10.1111/j.1444-0938.2010.00472.x] [PMID: 20557556]

[19] Hall LA, Young G, Wolffsohn JS, Riley C. The influence of corneoscleral topography on soft contact lens fit. Invest Ophthalmol Vis Sci 2011; 52(9): 6801-6. [http://dx.doi.org/10.1167/iovs.11-7177] [PMID: 21685339]

[20] Jongsma FH, de Brabander J, Hendrikse F, Stultiens BA. Development of a wide field height eye topographer: validation on models of the anterior eye surface. Optom Vis Sci 1998; 75(1): 69-77. [http://dx.doi.org/10.1097/00006324-199801000-00027] [PMID: 9460789]

[21] Iskander D. The clinical utility of the Eye Surface Profiler. ARVO meeting, poster 533 2013.

[22] Van der Worp E. Hulscher. Speed Date – CL-SAG meets OC-SAG: part I. Global Contact 2015; (2): 34-5.

[23] Van der Worp E. What about the SAG? Global Contact 2013; 65(1): 22-7.

[24] Achong-Coan R, Caroline PJ, Kinoshita B, *et al.* How do normal and keratoconic eyes differ in shape? Poster Global Specialty Lens Symposium (GSLS). Las Vegas, USA 2012.

[25] Kojima R, Caroline PJ, Graff T, *et al.* Eye shape and scleral lenses. Contact Lens Spectr 2013; 4: 38-43.

[26] Hall LA, Hunt C, Young G, Wolffsohn J. Factors affecting corneoscleral topography. Invest Ophthalmol Vis Sci 2013; 54(5): 3691-701. [http://dx.doi.org/10.1167/iovs.13-11657] [PMID: 23548617]

[27] Tan B, Graham AD, Tsechpenakis G, Lin MC. A novel analytical method using OCT to describe the corneoscleral junction. Optom Vis Sci 2014; 91(6): 650-7. [http://dx.doi.org/10.1097/OPX.0000000000000267] [PMID: 24830372]

[28] Kinoshita B, Caroline P, Morrison S, Lampa M, Kojima R, Andre M. Corneal Toricity and Scleral Asymmetry - Are They Related? Poster Global Specialty Lens Symposium. Las Vegas. 2016.

[29] Ritzmann M. Scleral shape study - A study of the anterior scleral shape and its role in scleral lens fitting. Master Thesis - Faculty of Aalen University, Germany 2015.

[30] Caroline PJ, Andre MP. Selection of corneal *versus* scleral GP lens. Contact Lens Spectr 2015; 4: 64.

[31] Visser ES, Visser R, Van Lier HJ. Advantages of toric scleral lenses. Optom Vis Sci 2006; 83(4): 233-6.
[http://dx.doi.org/10.1097/01.opx.0000214297.38421.15] [PMID: 16614579]

[32] Visser ES, Van der Linden BJ, Otten HM, Van der Lelij A, Visser R. Medical applications and outcomes of bitangential scleral lenses. Optom Vis Sci 2013; 90(10): 1078-85.
[http://dx.doi.org/10.1097/OPX.0000000000000018] [PMID: 23974663]

[33] Hussoin T, Le HG, Carrasquillo KG, Johns L, Rosenthal P, Jacobs DS. The effect of optic asphericity on visual rehabilitation of corneal ectasia with a prosthetic device. Eye Contact Lens 2012; 38(5): 300-5.
[http://dx.doi.org/10.1097/ICL.0b013e3182657da5] [PMID: 22929305]

[34] Sabesan R, Johns L, Tomashevskaya O, Jacobs DS, Rosenthal P, Yoon G. Wavefront-guided scleral lens prosthetic device for keratoconus. Optom Vis Sci 2013; 90(4): 314-23.
[http://dx.doi.org/10.1097/OPX.0b013e318288d19c] [PMID: 23478630]

[35] Walker MK. A Proposed mechanism for scleral lens induced conjunctival prolapse. Poster Global Specialty Lens Symposium. Las Vegas. 2014.

CHAPTER 4

Scleral Lens Optics

Muriel Schornack*

Department of Ophthalmology, The Mayo Clinic College of Medicine, Rochester, Minnesota, USA

Abstract: Contact lens optics are crucial for patient's success and scleral lenses are not an exception. Scleral lenses provide an optimal and stable platform for housing standard and custom optics. Scleral lens optics are similar to corneal rigid gas permeable lens optics; however, there are additional variables of the post-lens tear film, decentration and tilt that are associated with scleral lenses. Unique fitting characteristics of scleral lenses may complicate empirical determination of lens power at this time. Practitioners may still need to use a diagnostic scleral lens and over-refract. Nevertheless, current scleral lenses can provide optical correction that rivals spectacles or other modes of contact lens correction. Furthermore, incorporation of higher order aberration correction on a rotationally and translationally stable scleral lens platform may eventually allow patients to achieve better visual acuity than other modes of correction. Looking ahead, the use of a scleral lens as a platform for magnification aids patients with low vision.

Keywords: Aberration, Bitangential, Centration, Correction, Decenter, Higher order, HOA, Optical system, Optics, Power, Prism, Prismatic, Refractive, Rotational, Spectacle, Stabilization, Tear lens, Telescope, Translational, Visual acuity.

INTRODUCTION

According to several large retrospective studies [1 - 3], the primary indications for scleral lens prescription have been corneal irregularity and ocular surface disease. Corneal irregularity most certainly causes distortion or aberration of vision, and potential optical benefits of scleral lenses are obvious in these cases. However, disruption of the corneal epithelium in ocular surface disease can also be responsible for a reduction in visual acuity. Improvements in visual acuity following scleral lens treatment for ocular surface disease have been reported [4].

Scleral lenses are defined by a set of unique fitting characteristics. Unlike all other lens designs, they do not rest upon the cornea. Rather, they land on the

* **Corresponding author Muriel Schornack:** Department of Ophthalmology, The Mayo Clinic College of Medicine, Rochester, Minnesota, USA; Tel: 507-284-3614; Fax: 507-284-4612; E-mail: Schornack.muriel@mayo.edu

Melissa Barnett & Lynette K. Johns (Eds.)

conjunctival tissue which overlies the sclera while completely vaulting the cornea and limbus. This creates a space between the posterior surface of the lens and the anterior surface of the eye, which serves as a fluid reservoir during lens wear. This fluid reservoir can vary widely in depth [5], and accumulation of debris in the post-lens fluid reservoir has been observed. Decentration, particularly in the inferotemporal direction, is another commonly observed phenomenon. This decentration may be accompanied by some lens tilt. Any or all of these factors could potentially impact optical performance of scleral lenses. Despite these variables, Salam has claimed that scleral lenses are not optically inferior to corneal lenses [6].

Tear Lens Power

When fitting corneal rigid gas permeable lenses, the tear film is generally assumed to be of negligible thickness when calculating the power of the contact lens/tear lens refractive system. Furthermore, reasonably close alignment between corneal contour and base curve of the optic zone of a corneal rigid gas permeable lens is generally necessary in order to achieve an appropriate lens fit. Negligible tear film thickness and general alignment between the lens and cornea in the optic zone of a corneal lens facilitates simple calculation or prediction of the lens power needed in order to produce the desired optical results.

Successful scleral lens wear can be achieved with a wide range of fluid reservoir depths (also described as "vault"). Sonsino *et al.* reported on a series of patients who were fit with scleral lenses for the management of keratoconjunctivitis sicca associated with chronic graft versus host disease. They found that the mean reservoir depth was 380 microns, with a standard deviation of 110 microns. Optimal visual acuity could be achieved with reservoir depths ranging from 220 to 600 microns of vault [5].

Because scleral lenses do not actually rest upon the cornea, the relationship between lens base curve and keratometry values need not be closely correlated. In a 2010 study, Schornack *et al.* reported only weak correlations between scleral lens base curve and steep or flat keratometric values derived from topography in patients with either a normal or abnormal corneal contour. The relationship between scleral lens base curve and reference sphere was similarly weak. None of the correlations were deemed sufficiently strong as to be predictive of base curve. The authors suggested that the measurement of sagittal depth needed to clear the cornea may actually be more useful than topography or keratometry in scleral lens fitting [7]. Since then, our understanding of scleral shape has expanded considerably. Emerging evidence suggests that corneal curvature is, in fact, of less importance than sagittal depth in fitting not just scleral lenses, but, possibly, a variety of lens designs.

Both fluid reservoir depth and potential disparity between scleral lens base curve and anterior corneal surface curvature could potentially affect the refractive power of the scleral lens/fluid reservoir complex. Given the depth of the fluid reservoir in some scleral lens fits, the tear film cannot be considered to be of insignificant thickness. As light leaves the back of the scleral lens and travels through the fluid reservoir, its vergence may change sufficiently to significantly contribute to the total refractive power of the optical system. Schornack *et al.* calculated this power change for a wide array of variables, including central keratometry readings, fluid reservoir depth, scleral lens power, and relationship between base curve and central keratometry readings [8]. To summarize their calculations, clinically significant changes in vergence were found to be theoretically possible, particularly in cases in which there is a high amount of convergence in various components of the optical system (high plus power lenses, steeper-than-K fits, increased fluid reservoir depth). Changes in vergence were less likely to be clinically significant when scleral lens power was relatively negative, scleral lens base curve was flatter than central K's, and fluid reservoir depth was relatively shallow. Even if spherical keratometry values were assumed, they concluded that the complexity of interactions between all variables made it impractical to attempt to calculate the scleral lens power necessary to achieve optimal visual acuity as one might do when fitting corneal rigid gas permeable lenses. Instead, they recommended that scleral lens power be determined by spherocylindrical over-refraction over diagnostic lenses. As of yet, there are no studies which confirm their calculations with on-eye assessments of scleral lens/fluid reservoir refractive systems.

Scleral lenses are known to "settle" on the eye over time. Although the exact mechanism or mechanisms by which this phenomenon occurs are not known, it does result in reduced central fluid reservoir depth. One could speculate that this change in fluid reservoir depth may affect the total refractive power of the lens/reservoir system. Britton *et al.* studied this phenomenon in 16 patients, and found that settling appeared to have a relatively small impact (0.25 D) on lens power needed to provide optimal visual acuity in this group of patients [9]. However, not all variables that could potentially contribute to change in vergence through the fluid reservoir were reported in this study. Furthermore, given variability in reported amounts of settling that can occur during scleral lens wear, one cannot yet conclude that changes in lens position over time will not have an effect on refractive power of the optical system. Additional studies in this area are necessary.

In addition to potential refractive contribution of the fluid reservoir, prismatic effects may also be created by any decentration of the lens (Fig. **1**). As noted previously, scleral lenses may have a tendency to decenter in an infero-temporal direction. Such decentration in a patient who requires a scleral lens in only one eye may create vertical diplopia. Alterations in lens design may improve centration. However, in cases in which the vergence system is very brittle, diplopia may persist despite optimization of lens design. Prismatic correction can be provided in the form of spectacles worn over the scleral lens. Incorporation of prismatic correction may also be possible with some scleral lens designs.

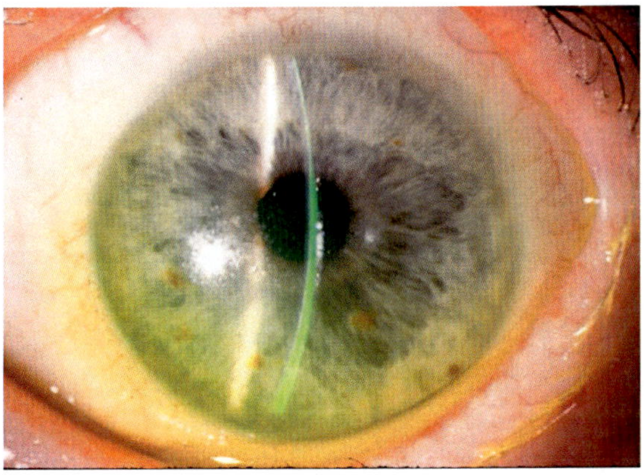

Fig. (1). Inferiorly decentered scleral lens demonstrating a base down post-lens tear prism. Image courtesy of Mayo Clinic.

Further Optical Considerations

In addition to induced prismatic effects, lens decentration could potentially reduce the quality of vision through the scleral lens displacing the optical center of the scleral lens from the visual axis of the eye. Neither precise quantification of scleral lens decentration nor assessment of the alignment of the optical center of the lens with the visual axis of the eye has been reported.

When considering the optics of refractive correction with either spectacles or contact lenses, we generally assume that light is incident normally along the optical axis. If light enters the lens at an oblique angle, astigmatism is induced. Differences in the relative elevation of the sclera in various quadrants of the eye may also lead to lens tilt. Scleral elevation varies between superior, inferior, nasal and temporal quadrants [10]. This could potentially cause lens tilt which could cause light to enter the lens at an oblique axis. Scleral lens tilt has not yet been calculated or measured, but it is likely to be relatively small in most eyes. In cases in which differences between elevations of the sclera in various quadrants are more pronounced, astigmatism may be induced along the axis of rotation. For plus power lenses, plus cylinder would be induced; for minus power lenses, induced cylinder would be minus in power. Thus, if a plus power lens rotated temporally along a vertical axis, plus cylinder axis 090 would be induced.

Future Possibilities

Improved Lens Stabilization/Centration

Early scleral lens designs that were commercially available in the United States featured spherical haptics. However, as early as 2006, Visser *et al.* suggested that lenses with toric haptics may provide better performance and comfort [11]. In 2013, Visser *et al.* further quantified lens design, visual outcomes, and patient satisfaction with bitangential peripheries. The second study confirmed the findings of the original work; lenses with bitangential peripheries provided good fitting characteristics (lens movement and position), visual acuity, and patient satisfaction [12]. Commercially available lenses now offer the option of toric, quadrant-specific, or custom haptics. Non-rotationally symmetric peripheral curves provide better alignment between the conjunctival tissue overlying the sclera and the landing zone of the lens. A more precise match between the posterior surface of the lens haptic and anterior ocular surface could improve lens stability, centration and optical performance in addition to reducing irritation or injection due to edge lift or impingement. The best means of achieving that match have yet to be determined. A recent study by Ticak *et al.* [13] showed that lenses stabilized using three different posterior surface peripheral curve designs all provided better stability that lenses with spherical haptics.

Correction of Higher Order Aberrations

As our ability to measure and quantify both scleral contour and higher order optical aberrations expands and our understanding of advantages and disadvantages of various methods of lens stabilization increases, scleral lenses may become a delivery platform for accurate and stable correction of higher order aberrations. Corneal irregularity is a common indication for scleral lens wear. In these eyes, both corneal and scleral rigid gas permeable lenses can neutralize the irregularity of the front surface of the cornea; stroma and inferior corneal surfaces are also often irregular. However, aberrations that arise from irregularities in the corneal stroma or posterior surface are not addressed in lenses with standard optics. Rotational and translational instability of corneal rigid gas permeable or soft lenses limits the utility of these lens designs as a platform for delivery of correction for higher order aberration. Several studies explored possibilities for achieving better visual performance using scleral lenses. In 2007, Gemoules and Morris reported combined higher order aberration reduction of 65% with corneoscleral lenses in patients with severe post-surgical irregularity [14]. Gumus *et al.* reported a greater reduction in spherical aberration in lenses which incorporated front surface optical eccentricity (86%) compared to lenses without an eccentricity adjustment (66%) [15]. Hussoin *et al.* reported on the optical impact of increasing front surface optical eccentricity on high contrast visual acuity, low contrast visual acuity, spherical aberration, horizontal coma, and vertical coma in 5 patients with keratoconus. These authors suggested that the amount of eccentricity that provided the best low contrast visual acuity appeared to correspond to the lens that provided best visual acuity [16]. Sabesan *et al.* reported successful correction of higher order aberrations in 6 patients (11 eyes) with advanced keratoconus using a custom scleral lens with wavefront-guided optics. Mean visual acuity also improved by an average of 1.9 lines with these lenses, and contrast sensitivity was also significantly improved. Of note, despite the fact that custom wavefront-guided scleral lenses effectively reduced higher order aberrations in these eyes to a magnitude that was comparable to those of a normal eye, logMAR acuity was 0.21, substantially worse than that of a normal eye [17]. More recently, Marsack *et al.* reported on the use of wavefront-guided scleral lenses in 7 subjects with moderate to severe keratoconus. Average gain of 1.5 lines of high-contrast visual acuity was reported, and higher order root mean square was reduced to within 1 SD or less than age-matched normals. However, as was the case in Sabesan's study, visual acuity in keratoconus patients with wavefront-guided scleral lens correction remained lower than that of normal eyes [18]. Clearly, this is an area in which additional research is needed.

Incorporation of Scleral Lenses into Telescope Systems

Several recent studies have described the design and fabrication of a wearable low vision aid that provides both 1x and 2.8x magnified visual paths incorporated into a 1.6 mm thick scleral lens [19, 20]. Still in the development stage, these telescopes may eventually provide an alternative to both external and implantable telescopes that may be used for patients with severe vision loss due to bilateral age-related macular degeneration or other macular conditions. Scleral lens-based telescopes could potentially have several advantages over other options. Placement of the telescope on the ocular surface would reduce the head movement required when using an external telescope to scan an entire visual scene. Placement of scleral lens-based telescopes would be considerably less invasive than an implantable telescope, and could easily be reversed if the patient was unable to adapt to the device.

Several prototypes of this device are described by Arianpour [20], and limitations of each design are identified. Possible methods of overcoming these limitations are discussed. Schuster *et al.* describes a scleral lens-based telescope (Fig. **2**) that is designed to be worn in combination with a pair of external glasses (Fig. **3**) [19].

Sensors within the glasses detect changes in reflection between closed and open eyes. The sensors then facilitate switching in between full-field view and magnified view through the telescope by detecting right-eye or left-eye blinks (monocular eye closures). The technology requires further refinement before practical application is possible, but testing has provided proof of concept for the lens design.

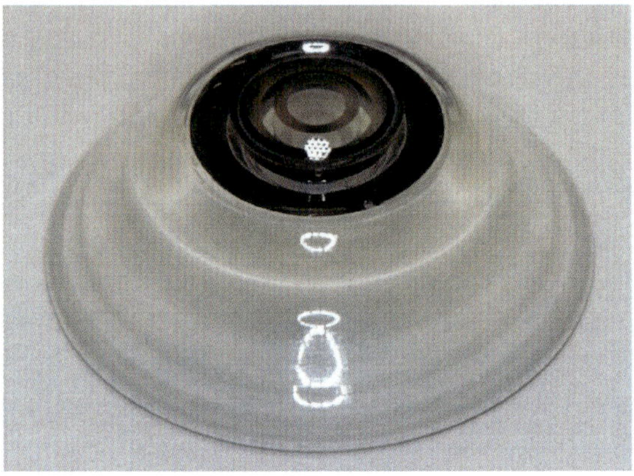

Fig. (2). Scleral lens-based telescope. Image courtesy of Glenn Schuster.

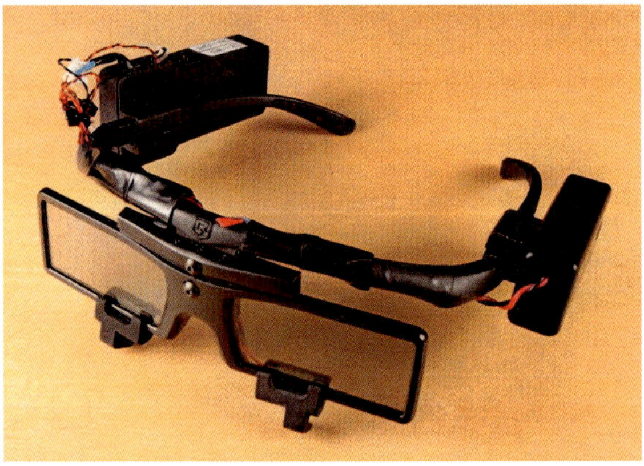

Fig. (3). Glasses used in conjunction with scleral lens-based telescope. Image courtesy of Glenn Schuster.

CONCLUSION

Unique fitting characteristics of scleral lenses may complicate empirical determination of lens power at this time. Practitioners may still need to use a diagnostic scleral lens and over-refract. Nevertheless, current scleral lenses can provide optical correction that rivals spectacles or other modes of contact lens correction. Furthermore, incorporation of higher order aberration correction on a rotationally and translationally stable scleral lens platform may eventually allow patients to achieve better visual acuity than other modes of correction. Looking ahead, the use of a scleral lens as a platform for magnification aids patients with low vision. This allows an alternative to external or implantable telescopes.

CONFLICT OF INTEREST

The author declares no conflict of interest, financial or otherwise.

ACKNOWLEDGEMENTS

Declared none.

REFERENCES

[1] Pullum KW, Buckley RJ. A study of 530 patients referred for rigid gas permeable scleral contact lens assessment. Cornea 1997; 16(6): 612-22. [http://dx.doi.org/10.1097/00003226-199711000-00003] [PMID: 9395869]

[2] Rosenthal P, Croteau A. Fluid-ventilated, gas-permeable scleral contact lens is an effective option for managing severe ocular surface disease and many corneal disorders that would otherwise require penetrating keratoplasty. Eye Contact Lens 2005; 31(3): 130-4. [http://dx.doi.org/10.1097/01.ICL.0000152492.98553.8D] [PMID: 15894881]

[3] Visser ES, Visser R, van Lier HJ, Otten HM. Modern scleral lenses part I: clinical features. Eye Contact Lens 2007; 33(1): 13-20. [http://dx.doi.org/10.1097/01.icl.0000233217.68379.d5] [PMID: 17224674]

[4] Schornack MM, Pyle J, Patel SV. Scleral lenses in the management of ocular surface disease. Ophthalmology 2014; 121(7): 1398-405. [http://dx.doi.org/10.1016/j.ophtha.2014.01.028] [PMID: 24630687]

[5] Sonsino J, Mathe DS. Central vault in dry eye patients successfully wearing scleral lens. Optometry and vision science: official publication of the American Academy of Optometry 2013.

[6] Salam A, Melia B, Singh AJ. Scleral contact lenses are not optically inferior to corneal lenses. Br J Ophthalmol 2005; 89(12): 1662-3. [http://dx.doi.org/10.1136/bjo.2005.074377] [PMID: 16299153]

[7] Schornack MM, Patel SV. Relationship between corneal topographic indices and scleral lens base curve. Eye Contact Lens 2010; 36(6): 330-3. [http://dx.doi.org/10.1097/ICL.0b013e3181eb8418] [PMID: 20631627]

[8] Schornack M, Nau C, Brown W. Estimation of refractive power of scleral lens/fluid reservoir optical systems in non-parallel scleral lens fits. Poster Global Specialty Lens Symposium. Las Vegas NV. 2014.

[9] Britton S, Bray C, Yeung D, Haines L, Sorbara L. Changes in over-refraction after scleral lens settling. Global Specialty Lens Symposium. Las Vegas NV. 2016.

[10] Van der Worp E, Graf T, Caroline PJ. Exploring beyond the corneal borders. Contact Lens Spectr 2010; 25(6): 26-32.

[11] Visser ES, Visser R, Van Lier HJ. Advantages of toric scleral lenses. Optom Vis Sci 2006; 83(4): 233-6. [http://dx.doi.org/10.1097/01.opx.0000214297.38421.15] [PMID: 16614579]

[12] Visser ES, Van der Linden BJ, Otten HM, *et al.* Medical applications and outcomes of bitangential scleral lenses. Optometry and vision science: official publication of the American Academy of Optometry 2013.

[13] Ticak A, Marsack JD, Koenig DE, *et al.* A comparison of three methods to increase scleral contact lens on-eye stability. Eye Contact Lens 2015; 41(6): 386-90.
[http://dx.doi.org/10.1097/ICL.0000000000000145] [PMID: 25943050]

[14] Gemoules G, Morris KM. Rigid gas-permeable contact lenses and severe higher-order aberrations in postsurgical corneas. Eye Contact Lens 2007; 33(6 Pt 1): 304-7.
[http://dx.doi.org/10.1097/ICL.0b013e318033edde] [PMID: 17993826]

[15] Gumus K, Gire A, Pflugfelder SC. The impact of the Boston ocular surface prosthesis on wavefront higher-order aberrations. Am J Ophthalmol 2011; 151(4): 682-90 e2.
[http://dx.doi.org/10.1016/j.ajo.2010.10.027]

[16] Hussoin T, Le HG, Carrasquillo KG, Johns L, Rosenthal P, Jacobs DS. The effect of optic asphericity on visual rehabilitation of corneal ectasia with a prosthetic device. Eye Contact Lens 2012; 38(5): 300-5.
[http://dx.doi.org/10.1097/ICL.0b013e3182657da5] [PMID: 22929305]

[17] Sabesan R, Johns L, Tomashevskaya O, *et al.* Wavefront-guided scleral lens prosthetic device for keratoconus. Optometry and vision science: official publication of the American Academy of Optometry 2013; 90(4): 314-23.

[18] Marsack JD, Ravikumar A, Nguyen C, *et al.* Wavefront-guided scleral lens correction in keratoconus. Optometry and vision science: official publication of the American Academy of Optometry 2014.

[19] Schuster GM, Arianpour A, Cookson S, *et al.* Wink-controlled polarization-switched telescopic contact lenses. Appl Opt 2015; 54(32): 9597-605.
[http://dx.doi.org/10.1364/AO.54.009597] [PMID: 26560792]

[20] Arianpour A, Schuster GM, Tremblay EJ, *et al.* Wearable telescopic contact lens. Appl Opt 2015; 54(24): 7195-204.
[http://dx.doi.org/10.1364/AO.54.007195] [PMID: 26368753]

CHAPTER 5

Medical Indications for Scleral Lens Use

Muriel Schornack*

Department of Ophthalmology, The Mayo Clinic College of Medicine, Rochester, Minnesota, USA

Abstract: Scleral lens indications are well established in published literature, beginning with descriptions of blown glass shells that were the precursors of scleral lenses in the late 1800s. Fick and Kalt explored the potential for optical correction of corneal irregularity in keratoconus with their original lenses, while Mueller described the use of a blown glass shell to correct significant myopic refractive error. Publications predating the introduction of rigid gas permeable scleral lenses in 1983 described the use of molded scleral shells or lenses to improve vision in cases of significant corneal irregularity, to protect the ocular surface and to correct refractive error. The introduction of rigid gas permeable contact lens materials sparked renewed interest in the scleral lens modality. Since Ezekiel's description of the use of rigid gas permeable scleral lenses in the management of keratoconus, high ametropia, marked corneal scarring and corneal surface compromise in 1983, interest in scleral lenses has steadily grown.

Whenever a scleral lens is placed on a diseased eye, practitioners must be aware that it is a therapeutic medical device. Use of scleral lenses in the management of ocular disease requires an understanding of the disease process. The eye should be monitored carefully to see that the desired outcome is obtained, and the therapeutic approach should be adjusted if the expected outcome is not achieved or if unexpected complications arise. Cooperation and collaboration with other eye care providers and specialists within other areas of medicine will allow practitioners to maximize the benefit for our patients.

Keywords: Auto-immune diseases, Clinical populations, Corneal ectasia, Corneal scars, Cosmetic, Dryness, Indications, Irregular corneas, Keratoconus, Keratoglobus, Managing expectations, Ocular surface, Ocular surface protection, Optics, Pellucid marginal degeneration, Post-corneal transplant, Prosthetic, Risk/benefit, Secondary corneal ectasias, Trauma.

* **Corresponding author Muriel Schornack:** Department of Ophthalmology, The Mayo Clinic College of Medicine, Rochester, Minnesota, USA; Tel: 507-284-3614; Fax: 507-284-4612; E-mail: Schornack.muriel@mayo.edu

Melissa Barnett & Lynette K. Johns (Eds.)

INTRODUCTION

Indications for the use of scleral lenses are well-established in published literature, beginning with descriptions of blown glass shells that were the precursors of scleral lenses in the late 1800s [1 - 3]. Fick and Kalt explored the potential for optical correction of corneal irregularity in keratoconus with their original lenses [1, 2], while Mueller described the use of a blown glass shell to correct significant myopic refractive error [3]. The development of moldable materials and fabrication techniques kept interest in scleral lenses alive throughout the first half of the 20th century. Publications predating the introduction of rigid gas permeable scleral lenses in 1983 described the use of molded scleral shells or lenses to improve vision in cases of significant corneal irregularity [4 - 7], to protect the ocular surface [7 - 16] and to correct refractive error [4, 5, 17]. The introduction of rigid gas permeable contact lens materials reduced the amount of corneal hypoxia caused by polymethylmethacrylate. These new materials sparked renewed interest in the scleral lens modality. Since Ezekiel's description of the use of rigid gas permeable scleral lenses in the management of keratoconus, high ametropia, marked corneal scarring and corneal surface compromise in 1983 [18], interest in scleral lenses has steadily grown. Indications for scleral lens wear and outcomes of scleral lens management of particular conditions have been reported in numerous publications from the 1990s to the present. As with early scleral shells, primary indications for modern scleral lens fitting include optical correction for irregular corneas, ocular surface protection and correction of refractive error.

Visual Improvement

Scleral lenses provide a smooth anterior ocular surface, and neutralize irregularity of the corneal surface. Because the lenses do not actually land on the cornea, there is no need to attempt to align the posterior surface of the lens with the surface of the cornea. Eliminating contact between the posterior surface of the lens and the anterior corneal surface provides several potential benefits. Better lens centration and stability can be achieved with scleral lenses compared to corneal lenses on eyes with highly irregular corneal surfaces. Lack of contact between the lens and the highly-innervated cornea may reduce lens awareness and result in more comfortable lens wear and adaptation. Corneal epithelial integrity may be better preserved with scleral lenses than with corneal rigid gas permeable lenses. Finally, scleral lenses may be less likely to mechanically induce central corneal warpage or reshaping during wear, although some reports have suggested that changes in corneal curvature may still occur [19, 20]. This may reduce variability in spectacle correction that can be observed in patients with corneal irregularity who wear corneal rigid gas permeable lenses.

The use of a variety of scleral lens designs in the management of both primary and secondary corneal ectasias has been documented in case reports, case series, and large retrospective reviews. Primary corneal ectasia encompasses conditions such as keratoconus, keratoglobus, and pellucid marginal degeneration. Secondary corneal ectasia may occur following refractive surgery. Corneal transplantation or post-traumatic scarring can also cause corneal surface irregularity that can limit the quality of vision that can be obtained with spectacles or hydrogel lenses. Corneal rigid gas permeable lens awareness can be a significant issue in patients with corneal irregularity. Scleral lenses have demonstrated the ability to provide good vision and comfort for these patients, and may allow them to delay or even avoid surgical intervention. General outcomes of scleral lens prescription for all forms of corneal ectasia have been reported [21 - 24]. In these studies, failure to achieve adequate vision and comfort with other lens modalities was considered an indication for scleral lens fitting. Significant improvements in visual acuity [21, 23, 24], NEI VFQ-25 scores [22], and ocular surface disease index scores [23] have been reported.

Primary Corneal Ectasia

Primary corneal ectasia encompasses a group of non-inflammatory ocular conditions characterized by thinning of the cornea and resulting in corneal surface distortion. Conditions within this family of disorders can be differentiated by the region of cornea affected and by their distinctive clinical appearances [25]. Keratoconus is the most common of these conditions, and generally causes bilateral asymmetric thinning of the paracentral cornea (Fig. **1**). Keratoglobus is characterized by generalized thinning and forward protrusion of the entire cornea (Fig. **2**). Pellucid marginal degeneration typically causes a crescent-shaped band of thinning in the peripheral cornea several millimeters from the limbus, usually in the inferior quadrant (Fig. **3**). Terrien's marginal degeneration causes slowly progressive non-inflammatory peripheral corneal thinning associated with neovascularization, opacification, and lipid deposition (Fig. **4**). All of these conditions can result in significant irregular astigmatism, and functional vision may not be able to be achieved with spectacle correction. Corneal rigid gas permeable lenses have traditionally been prescribed for patients with these conditions, and can provide excellent vision. In some cases, however, the degree or location of corneal irregularity makes it impossible to achieve an adequate fit with these lenses. The lenses may also elicit considerable awareness; some patients find that lens awareness or discomfort limits their ability to successfully wear corneal lenses. Scleral lenses provide another non-surgical alternative for patients with primary corneal ectasia.

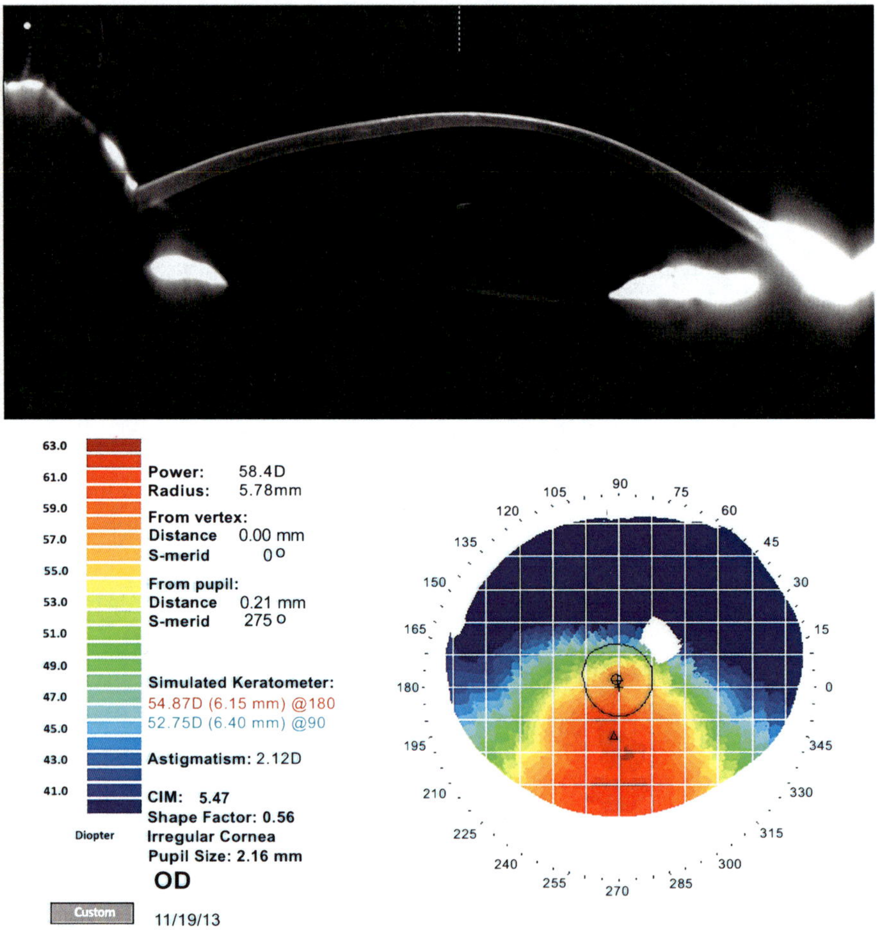

Fig. (1). (Top) Example of corneal topopgraphy in keratoconus. (Bottom) Corneal profile of keratoconus, note the corneal thinning at the apex of ectasia.

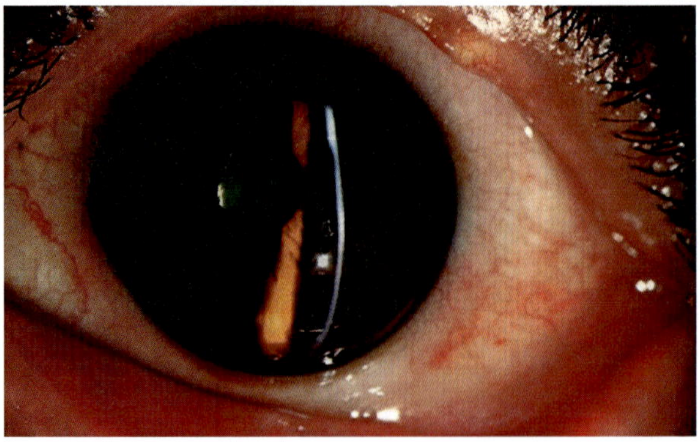

Fig. (2). Optic section demonstrating overall thinning of cornea with keratoglobus.

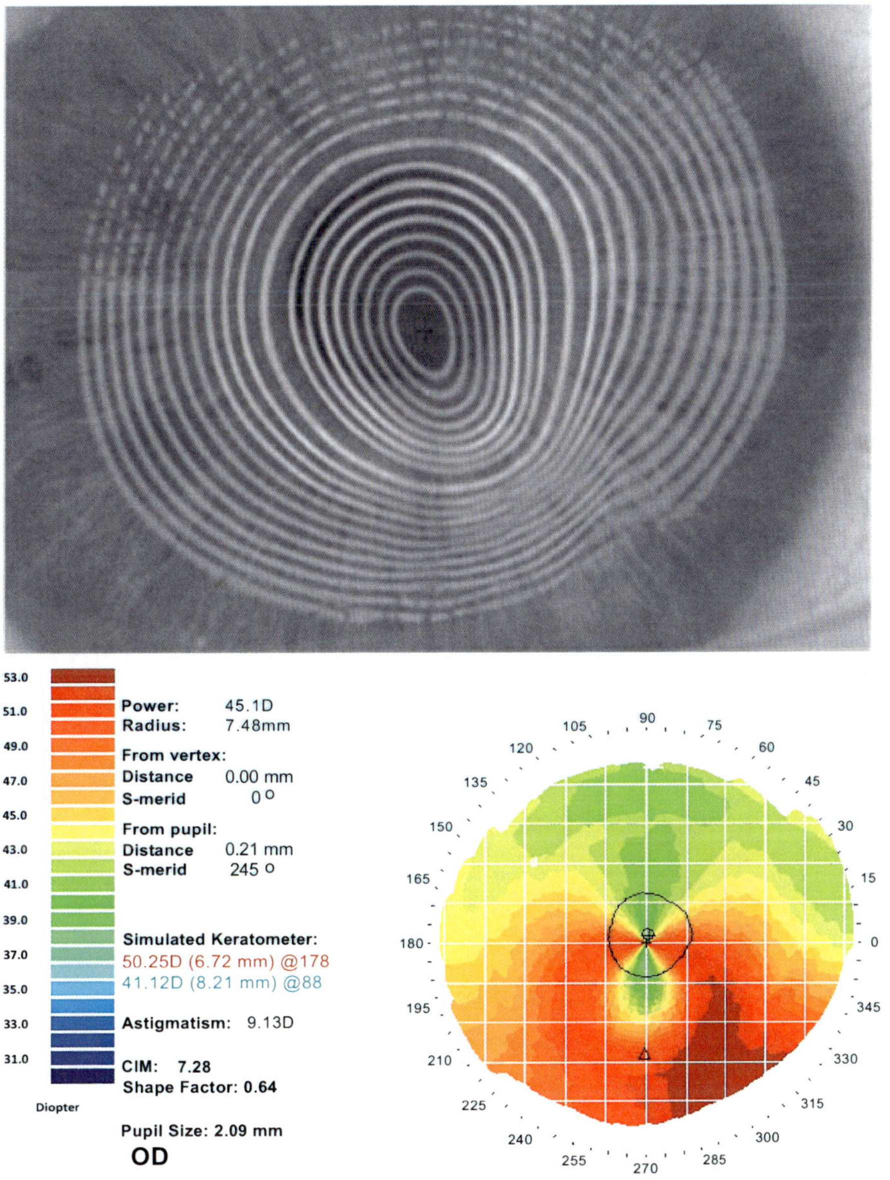

Fig. (3). (Top) Elongated and distorted topography mires on a cornea with pellucid marginal degeneration. The "ring jam" is associated with the area of ectasia. (Bottom) Topography of the same cornea demonstrating a classic pellucid topographical pattern known as either a crab claw or kissing doves.

A number of retrospective reviews pertaining to outcomes of scleral lens wear specifically identify keratoconus as a major indication for scleral lenses. In fact, keratoconus represents the largest single indication for scleral lens wear in published literature. In Schein's 1990 prospective study of 15 patients who were fit with early scleral lenses, 9 of the patients had keratoconus [26]. Tan reported on 343 scleral lens patients, of whom 38% were diagnosed with keratoconus [27]. Rosenthal's 2005 review of scleral lens outcomes included a total of 875 eyes, 262 of which were keratoconic [28]. Also in 2005, Pullum reviewed results of scleral lens fitting in 1003 patients (1560 eyes), and reported an indication of primary corneal ectasia in nearly 60% of these patients [29]. A large retrospective review of scleral lens outcomes by Visser *et al.* included 143 eyes with keratoconus (out of a total of 284 studied) [30]. Nearly 50% of eyes in Pecego's 2012 retrospective review were fit with scleral lenses for management of keratoconus [31]. Additional individual case reports and retrospective case series also include descriptions of scleral lenses for management of keratoconus [32 - 35], keratoglobus [36], pellucid marginal degeneration [28, 37] and Terrien's marginal degeneration [36].

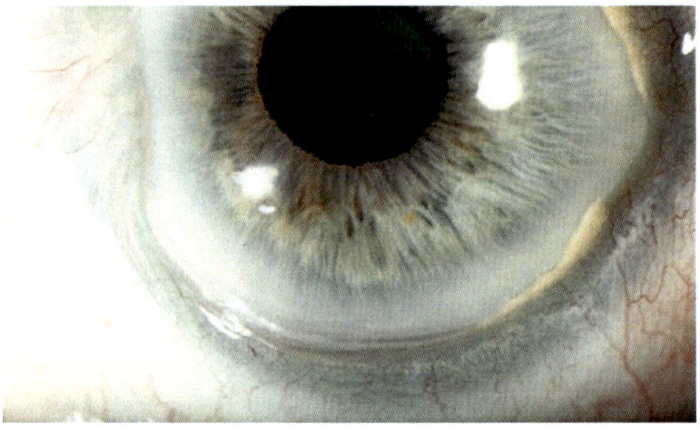

Fig. (4). Peripheral corneal degeneration with associated neovascularization and lipid deposition in a cornea with Terrien's marginal degeneration.

A study by DeLoss *et al.* [38] compared outcomes of scleral lens fitting to keratoplasty in patients with keratoconus. Results revealed that improvements in visual acuity are achieved more rapidly with scleral lens wear than with surgical intervention in patients with primary corneal ectasia. Furthermore, a statistically higher percentage of patients wearing scleral lenses achieved 20/25 visual acuity or better compared to those who underwent keratoplasty. Mean visual acuity was better in patients wearing scleral lenses compared to those who had undergone keratoplasty one year after intervention. More complications were observed in surgical patients compared to scleral lens wearers. This study suggests that scleral lenses should perhaps be considered for patients with keratoconus prior to surgical intervention for patients who cannot successfully wear other modes of correction.

Scleral lenses have also been prescribed to minimize visual distortion following corneal crosslinking for keratoconus. A prospective cohort study by Visser *et al.*

reported on the post-procedure use of scleral lenses in patients who had been wearing them prior to undergoing corneal crosslinking. No significant change was noted between pre-procedure distance visual acuity and acuity with scleral lenses one year after crosslinking. Wearing time and subjective tolerance for the lenses was also unchanged between pre- and post-procedure evaluation. However, over half (61%) of the eyes studied required adjustment of the scleral lens power or fit following crosslinking. This study demonstrates the utility of scleral lenses in the overall management of primary corneal ectasia, and shows that the lenses can be used in combination with other interventions [39].

While keratoconus comprises the largest collective number of cases described in the literature, prognosis for acceptable vision following surgical intervention for keratoconus is fairly positive, particularly if the area of ectasia is central and localized. However, in keratoglobus, pellucid marginal degeneration, and Terrien's marginal degeneration, the location and extent of ectatic cornea may complicate potential surgical approaches [37]. Furthermore, decentration (in pellucid and Terrien's marginal degeneration) and extent of the ectasia (in keratoglobus) can make it difficult to achieve an adequate fit with corneal rigid gas permeable lenses. The unique fitting characteristics of scleral lenses make this modality an ideal option for optical correction of these severe forms of primary corneal ectasia.

Acquired Corneal Ectasia

Although corneal transplants are among the most medically successful solid organ transplants, visual outcomes are not entirely predictable. Many patients who have undergone corneal transplantation need to continue to use contact lenses in order to achieve optimal visual acuity (Fig. **5**). Secondary corneal ectasia can also develop following any type of refractive surgery. Early refractive surgical procedures were not as precise as current techniques; many patients who had refractive surgery when the field was in its infancy may now be experiencing visual compromise due to corneal irregularity. Even in modern refractive surgery, optimal results cannot be guaranteed. Patients who have suboptimal outcomes may not be able to achieve adequate vision with spectacles or standard contact lenses. Ocular trauma can also cause considerable corneal irregularity, particularly following penetrating corneal laceration (Fig. **6**). Even severe corneal infection can lead to stromal loss that can result in an irregular corneal surface. Not only are scleral lenses useful in providing clear vision for patients with primary corneal ectatic conditions, but they can be used in visual rehabilitation for patients who have developed acquired corneal surface irregularity due to the conditions described above.

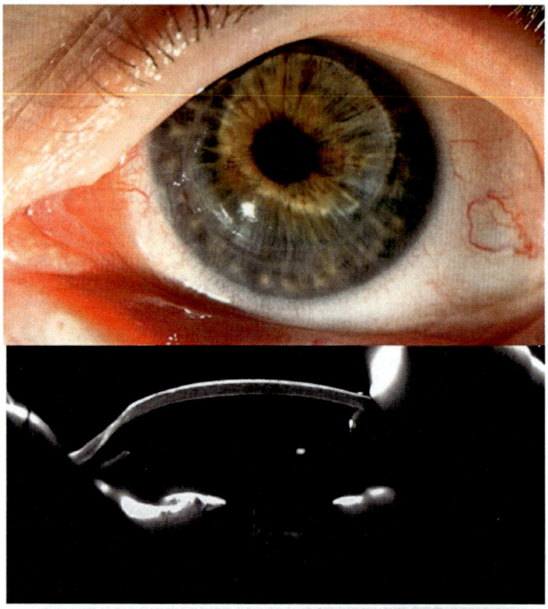

Fig. (5). (Top) Corneal transplant without sutures and irregular border of the graft-host junction. (Bottom) Corneal profile of corneal transplant.

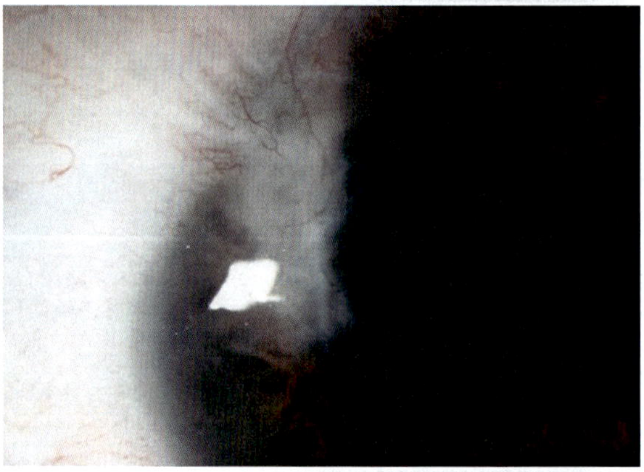

Fig. (6). Example of penetrating injury with fibrotic and vascularized scarring.

Corneal Transplant

Retrospective reviews have identified post-keratoplasty irregularity as an indication for scleral lens wear [28 - 30]. Irregular astigmatism and significant graft toricity are indications for post-keratoplasty scleral lens fitting. Long-term outcomes of scleral lens wear for visual rehabilitation following penetrating keratoplasty in 31 patients were reported by Severinsky *et al.* in 2014 [40]. Follow-up ranged from 0.5 to 8.8 years after successful completion of scleral lens fitting. Mean age of the corneal graft was 17.6 years, with a range of 4.3 to 42 years. In this population, 28 of 31 patients were successfully fit with scleral lenses. Scleral lenses provided significantly better visual acuity than spectacles in this population. Average wearing time was 11.9 hours daily, with the most successful wearers using their lenses for up to 13 hours daily. Graft complications occurred in 12 eyes; 10 eyes demonstrated graft rejection. Two cases of microbial keratitis were reported in this series. More recently, Barnett [41] and Alipour [42] published case series describing the use of scleral lenses following keratoplasty. Barnett *et al.* performed a retrospective review of visual results and patient-reported responses in a group of 34 patients (48 eyes) fit with scleral lenses between 0.9 and 49.5 years following transplantation. A mean gain of 2 lines of best-corrected visual acuity was reported; nearly 40% of eyes achieved 20/20 or better with scleral lenses, and 91.7% of eyes achieved visual acuity of 20/40 or better. Six eyes developed graft rejection, three of which were able to resume scleral lens wear following resolution of the rejection episode. No cases of microbial keratitis were reported in this study [41]. Alipour *et al.* prospectively evaluated 15.8 mm diameter scleral lenses in 45 patients (56 eyes) who had unacceptable vision following penetrating keratoplasty. While ideal or acceptable fit was achieved in all eyes, only 19 patients (23 eyes) actually ordered lenses. Barriers to completion of fit included cost, handling concerns and anticipated delays in receiving lenses. Of the patients who completed the fitting process, 11 (14 eyes) continued to wear lenses beyond the fitting period. No graft rejection episodes or cases of microbial keratitis were reported in this study [42].

These studies demonstrate the utility of scleral lenses in visual rehabilitation following keratoplasty, but also provide early insight into complications that may occur with scleral lenses used for this indication. Practitioners who choose to fit scleral lenses for this indication should have a thorough understanding of the possible complications that may occur in patients who have had corneal transplants. Practitioners should carefully monitor patients for early signs of these complications.

Post-refractive Surgery

Contact lens fitting following refractive surgery poses both physiological and psychological challenges. Alteration of normal corneal contour even in eyes that are defined as surgically successful may induce optical aberrations that can be quite visually debilitating to patients. Dry eye symptoms may become more pronounced following surgery. Post-surgical ectasia may cause progressive loss of clear vision (Fig. 7). Patients who have not achieved expected visual results may be disappointed or even angry. Patients who chose to undergo refractive surgery because they did not want to be dependent upon glasses or contact lenses, now may require specialty contact lenses in order to achieve functional vision. Some of these patients may be successful with standard hydrogel or corneal rigid gas permeable lens designs. In other patients, central corneal flattening may require the use of specialty hydrogel, hybrid, or reverse geometry rigid lens designs. When considering any type of contact lens fitting in a patient who has undergone refractive surgery, one must always be cognizant of the fact that the lens is being fit on a compromised cornea. Mechanical corneal warpage, corneal neovascularization, and flap dislocation are all possibilities when fitting contact lenses on eyes that have undergone refractive surgery.

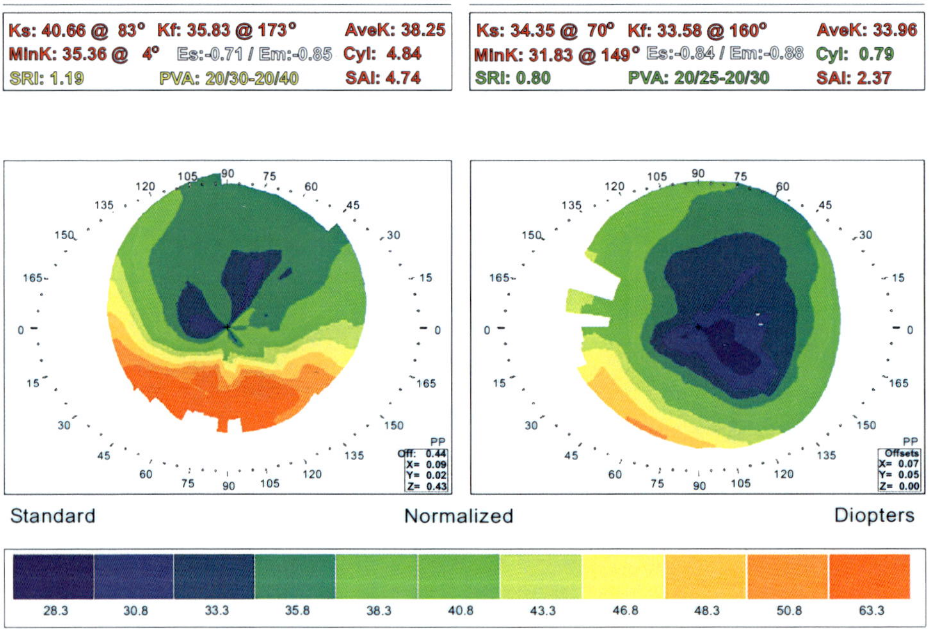

Fig. (7). Topographies of post-surgical corneas. Both eyes underwent radial keratotomy multiple times and LASIK. Image courtesy of Melissa Barnett.

Although scleral lenses do require specialized handling and care compared to other lens options, they represent a reasonable option for patients who have had disappointing results from refractive surgery. They do not contact the cornea, so the risk of flap dislocation or corneal warpage should theoretically be relatively low. Scleral lenses are available in reverse geometry designs, and can therefore be customized to provide any desired relationship between the posterior lens and anterior corneal surface. The post-lens fluid reservoir may provide relief from dry eye symptoms. However, decreased oxygen availability compared to a corneal lens may be more likely to lead to corneal neovascularization with scleral lenses compared to other designs. Literature regarding the use of scleral lenses following refractive surgery is relatively sparse. Rationale for the use of scleral lenses following refractive surgery is described by Parminder and Jacobs [43]. Scleral lenses are recognized as a possible contact lens option following LASIK [44]. Outcomes of scleral lens wear for management of dry eye symptoms following refractive surgery are reported in a retrospective review [45]. Two single case reports describe the use of a scleral lens following LASIK [46, 47].

Corneal Scarring/Ocular Trauma

Bacterial, fungal, or viral keratitis can cause extensive destruction of corneal stromal tissue. Upon resolution of the acute infection, corneal irregularity may persist, along with corneal opacity (Fig. **8**). If either irregularity or opacity is present along the visual axis, visual acuity and quality may be compromised. Scleral lenses can immediately provide some degree of visual improvement by creating a smooth anterior optical surface in such cases, although visual acuity may still be limited by a corneal opacity. An intriguing case report describes apparent corneal remodeling and restoration of corneal clarity with long-term use of a scleral lens [48]. This phenomenon warrants further investigation.

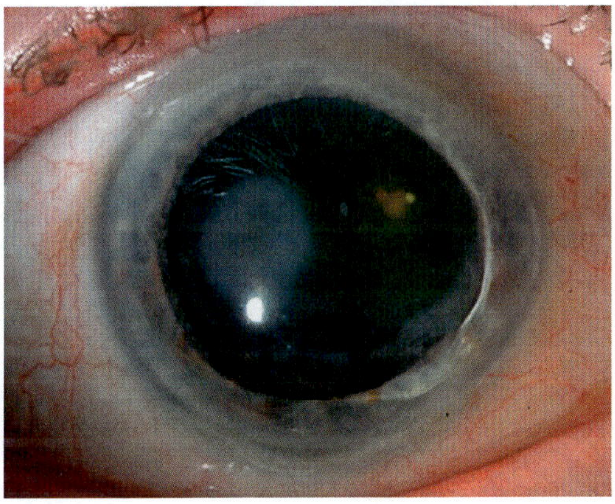

Fig. (8). Paracentral corneal opacity encroaching on the visual axis.

Penetrating corneal injury can result in poor vision due to corneal irregularity. As described above, scleral lenses can provide ocular surface protection in cases where orbital or periocular trauma causes disruption of normal lid function. In such cases, scleral lenses can not only provide improved vision, but may also help to maintain the integrity of the ocular surface.

Ocular Surface Protection and Restoration

Severe ocular surface disease can be defined as any condition which affects tear production, lid function, or epithelial integrity and results in compromise to the anterior surface of the eye. A broad constellation of conditions is associated with these clinical findings; systemic or ocular inflammatory disease, insults to neural pathways that supply motor or sensory innervation to the eye and adnexa, inherited corneal disorders, ocular or periocular trauma and undifferentiated dry eye syndrome can all contribute to ocular surface compromise. Symptoms of these conditions may include debilitating ocular pain, photophobia, or even vision loss due to corneal scarring. Clinical examination can reveal lid margin disease, decreased tear volume and/or stability, filamentary keratitis, corneal epithelial defects, or even stromal thinning or opacity. Traditional options for management of ocular surface disease all suffer from one or more inadequacies. Use of lubricant drops provide only a temporary increase in the volume of fluid that protects the cornea. Lid hygiene (warm compresses, lid massage, lid scrubs, manual and mechanical meibomian expression) cannot eliminate shear forces that may disrupt fragile corneal epithelium with every blink. Punctal occlusion decreases the rate of tear drainage, but does not distribute tears evenly over the ocular surface. Bandage hydrogel lenses require a relatively regular ocular surface and functional tear production in order to remain hydrated on the surface of the eye. While amniotic membrane placement may facilitate healing of an epithelial defect, it does not necessarily address underlying issues (such as exposure or neurotrophic keratopathy) responsible for the initial development of the defect, so its removal may lead to rapid relapse. Placement of a gold weight in the upper lid to reduce exposure still leaves a significant percentage of the corneal surface unprotected, and the weight is only effective when the patient is in an upright position. Protection of the cornea with either a conjunctival flap or tarsorrhaphy severely limits vision. Additional therapies include topical cyclosporine, topical lifitegrast, intense pulse light treatments, oral tetracycline derivatives and dietary supplementation.

Scleral lenses overcome many of the shortcomings of traditional management strategies for ocular surface disease. The post-lens fluid reservoir ensures continuous corneal lubrication, unlike artificial tears and punctal occlusion. Large diameter scleral lenses cover a majority of the surface of the eye, and provide protection for corneal and conjunctival tissue from potential aggravation due to friction between the ocular surface and the palpebral surface of the lids. Rigid lens materials do not absorb water, so patients who have been unable to use bandage hydrogel lenses due to dryness or corneal irregularity may find success with scleral lenses. Unlike conjunctival flap placement or tarsorrhaphy, scleral lenses not only allow for maintenance of the present level of vision, but may actually improve vision by providing a smooth anterior refractive surface and neutralizing aberrations caused by irregularities due to surface compromise. Rationale for the use of scleral lenses in the management of dry eye syndrome has been outlined in detail in a 2015 publication by Bavinger [49].

The utility of scleral lenses for ocular surface protection was recognized even before the introduction of rigid gas permeable scleral lenses [8, 9]. Retrospective reviews published since the advent of rigid gas permeable lenses have identified a number of ocular surface conditions that have been treated using scleral lenses, but all ocular surface conditions combined represent a minority of the total number of cases reported. Of 343 patients (517 eyes) described by Tan in 1995, ocular surface disease was identified as the indication for only 23 patients [27]. Rosenthal's 2005 review of 538 patients (875 eyes) included 374 eyes for which the primary indication was ocular surface disease [28]. Of the 1003 patients described by Pullum in 2005, an indication of ocular surface disease was recorded for just 11.3% of patients [29]. This suggests either that severe ocular surface disease is less common than corneal irregularity, or that the benefits of scleral lens wear for the management of severe ocular surface disease have yet to be fully appreciated. Several studies have specifically examined the outcomes of scleral lens management for ocular surface disease. In 2014, Schornack *et al.* reported on 115 patients with a variety of ocular surface conditions. Improvements in patient comfort, restoration and maintenance of ocular surface integrity, and statistically significant improvements in visual acuity were noted in this patient population [45]. Alipour also reported subject improvements in visual comfort and acuity in a small cohort of patients who were fit with mini-scleral lenses [50].

Inflammatory Ocular Surface Disease

As our understanding of tear film dysfunction and dry eye disease has evolved over the past several decades, there is emerging consensus that there is a significant inflammatory component within the etiology of the condition. It stands to reason that systemic or ocular conditions that can cause inflammation may lead to tear film dysfunction. Keratoconjunctivitis sicca is associated with both immune-complex mediated disease (for example, chronic graft versus host disease (GvHD) (Fig. **9**), Stevens-Johnson syndrome (SJS)), and systemic autoimmune disorders (rheumatoid arthritis, systemic lupus erythematosus, rosacea, ocular cicatricial pemphigoid (Fig. **10**), Sjögren's disease, and Graves' disease). Given the systemic nature of these conditions, an integrated therapeutic approach incorporating a variety of specialty areas of care is most appropriate for patients with these conditions. Depending upon the organ systems affected, cooperation between specialists in rheumatology, immunology, dermatology, hematology/ oncology, hepatology, neurology, gynecology, psychology/ psychiatry, orthopedics, dentistry, and optometry/ophthalmology is necessary to care for these patients. Scleral lenses can provide significant symptomatic relief and preservation of corneal epithelial integrity if keratoconjunctivitis sicca is present.

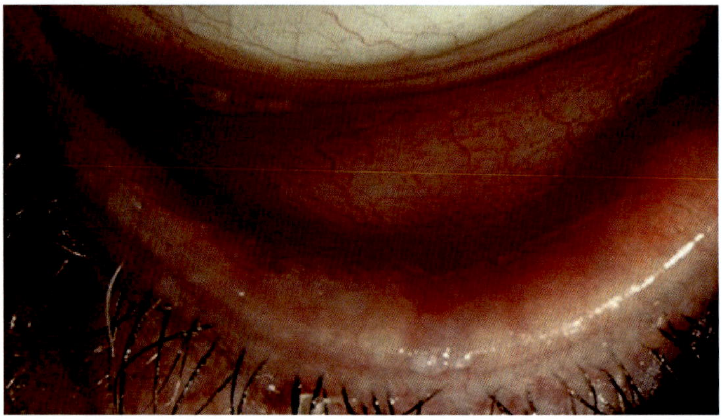

Fig. (9). Keratinization of the palpebral conjunctiva in a patient with graft versus host disease.

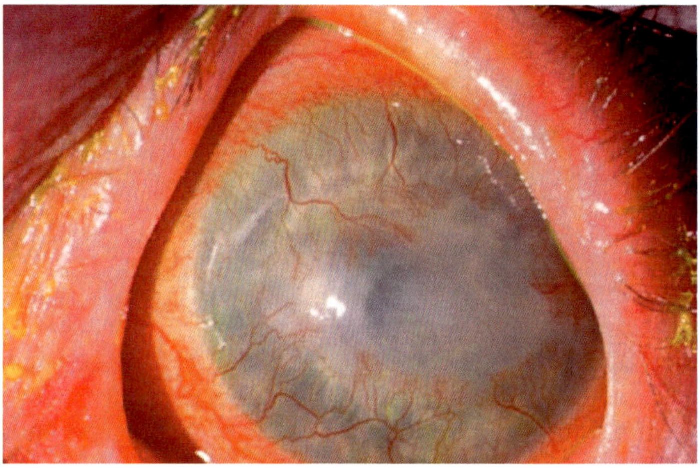

Fig. (10). Significant neovascularization and corneal opacity in a patient with ocular cicatricial pemphigoid.

Immune-Complex Mediated Ocular Surface Disease

The most robust literature supporting the use of scleral lenses in inflammatory ocular surface disease describes the management of immune-complex mediated disease. Large retrospective studies have specifically identified SJS [28 - 30, 45, 51, 52] as an indication for scleral lens wear. Outcomes of scleral lens therapy for SJS are described in several papers. Heur reported statistically significant improvements in both visual acuity and OSDI scores in a series of 19 patients [53]. Significant improvements in visual acuity and function (as assessed using the NEI VFQ-25) were reported by Papakostas [54]. In 2009, Tougeron-Brousseau reported statistically significant improvements in visual acuity, OSDI scores and VFQ-25 scores in 39 patients [54]. Perhaps even more compelling evidence of the efficacy of scleral lenses in the management of this condition is the fact that this form of therapy has been suggested in several overviews of current management strategies for ocular manifestations of the disease [55, 56].

The literature which supports the use of scleral lenses in the management of ocular manifestations of chronic GvHD is similarly compelling. The condition is specifically identified in several large reviews [31, 45, 51, 57]. The fact that the condition was not specifically identified as an indication in earlier studies could be due to the relatively recent expansion of the use of hematopoietic stem cell transplantation to treat systemic neoplastic disease. The earliest studies which reported improvements in both vision and comfort with scleral lens management of keratoconjunctivitis sicca associated with GvHD were published in 2007 and 2008 [58 - 60]. More recently, Theophanous reported not only visual improvements and reduced OSDI scores, but also reported improvements in clinical signs (decreased corneal staining, resolution of epithelial defects, resolution of filamentary keratitis) with scleral lens therapy [61]. Scleral lenses have been recognized as part of the therapeutic armamentarium for management of this condition in reviews of current management strategies for the condition [62, 63].

Scleral lenses were also reported to significantly improve visual acuity, decrease conjunctival hyperemia, and allow for resolution of corneal epithelial defects in a series of ten eyes with advanced atopic keratoconjunctivitis without primary corneal ectasia by Margolis *et al.* in 2007 [64]. Perhaps of even greater significance, primary corneal ectasia may be associated with atopic disease. Patients with keratoconus in addition to severe atopic disease may derive both optical and protective benefit from scleral lens wear. A 2012 case series described the use of scleral lenses in four patients with vernal keratoconjunctivitis, three of whom also had keratoconus. Improvements in visual acuity were noted in all patients, and no shield ulcers, infectious keratitis, or elevated intraocular pressure were noted in any of these patients during the follow-up period (mean 14.8 months) [65].

Autoimmune Disease-Associated Keratoconjunctivitis Sicca

Increased risk of keratoconjunctivitis sicca associated with a number of systemic autoimmune disorders is well established. In these conditions, antibodies circulating in the blood attack healthy tissue, and cause inflammation and destruction of normal tissue. If any component of the lacrimal system is targeted, disruption of the tear film can lead to discomfort, ocular surface tissue damage, or even vision loss. At present, there is no cure for these conditions; treatment is both palliative and supportive, preferably before irreversible tissue damage occurs. Supportive ocular management of these conditions is directed towards preserving the function of cells that produce components of the tear film, maintaining the integrity of the ocular surface, and reducing the severity of patient symptoms. Cooperation with other specialists who are managing other manifestations of the underlying condition is necessary in the care of these patients.

Ocular therapy tends to be additive; interventions of increasing complexity are added until therapeutic goals are met. Frequently, low-cost, low-risk interventions will be suggested initially. Smoking cessation, increasing environmental humidity and increasing water intake may be among the first recommendations. Regular use of supportive therapy such as lubricant drops, lid hygiene or nutritional supplements may be added if initial measures fail to achieve therapeutic goals. Punctal occlusion, topical medications (cyclosporine, lifitegrast, or steroid eyedrops), or oral medications (doxycycline) represent the next tier of treatment. If these measures fail to provide sufficient relief, moisture chamber glasses or scleral lenses may be prescribed.

Sjögren's disease often accompanies other systemic autoimmune disorders and is characterized by decreased production of tears and saliva. The condition has been frequently cited as an indication for scleral lens wear in large reviews [31, 45, 51, 52, 57]. At present, however, no studies specifically report the outcomes of scleral lens wear in patients with Sjögren's disease. Ocular cicatricial pemphigoid is an autoimmune disease that causes blistering and subsequent scarring of mucous membrane tissue, including conjunctival tissue in the eye. The condition is mentioned in several retrospective reviews [45, 52], and the use of scleral lenses in a single case has also been reported [66]. Graves' ophthalmopathy also arises from systemic autoimmune disease, but the etiology of its ocular symptoms is primarily exposure rather than lack of tear production. Successful treatment of Graves' ophthalmopathy with a scleral lens has been reported [67].

Neuropathic Ocular Surface Disorders

Neuropathy is defined as an abnormal or degenerative state of any part of the nervous system. The term can also refer to a physical condition resulting from this abnormality. Compromise sensory, motor or autonomic innervation to the eye and adnexa can lead to neuropathic ocular surface disorders. These disorders are most commonly associated with either the ophthalmic branch of the trigeminal nerve (CN V) or facial nerve (CN VII). Damage to the sensory component of the ophthalmic branch of the trigeminal nerve causes decreased corneal sensation and may lead to neurotrophic keratopathy. Compromise to the facial nerve may cause both brachial and visceral motor deficits. Brachial motor deficits can lead to exposure keratopathy if portions of the nerve that supply orbicularis muscles are affected. The visceral motor branch of the facial nerve innervates the lacrimal gland. Decreased tear production may result from damage to this branch of the nerve. Insult at any point along the pathway of the nerve may impair its function.

As was the case with inflammatory ocular surface disease, understanding of the pathophysiology underlying the ocular findings is of utmost importance when caring for patients with neuropathic ocular surface disease. One must understand cranial nerve structure, function, and anatomy in order to pinpoint the source of the insult. For example, particular combinations of neurologic deficits may suggest the presence of a specific intracranial lesion. While it is very important to maintain the health of the ocular surface, it may be even more critical to recognize potentially serious overall neurologic deficits and to refer the patient for further care when appropriate. Successful use of scleral lenses in the management of both isolated and combined neurotrophic and exposure keratopathy has been described in the literature in several individual case reports [68 - 70], as well as in reviews of scleral lens management of general ocular surface disease [45, 52].

Neurotrophic Keratopathy

Impaired corneal sensation disrupts feedback mechanisms that facilitate normal repair of corneal epithelium. Reduction or absence of corneal sensitivity can result in epithelial defects, ulceration, or even perforation of the cornea. The most common causes of neurotrophic keratopathy are herpes simplex and herpes zoster viral infections. Diabetes mellitus is also associated with an increased risk of this condition. Surgical insult to any part of the pathway of the fifth cranial nerve can also cause neurotrophic keratopathy, as can a space-occupying lesion along the nerve's pathway. Ocular trauma, such as a chemical burn or radiotherapy, may initiate a cycle of damage that can eventually result in loss of corneal sensation. In neurotrophic keratopathy, decreases in corneal epithelial vitality, metabolism, and mitosis eventually lead to loss of epithelial integrity. Once the epithelium has broken down, loss of normal feedback delays or prevents healing.

A patient with neurotrophic keratopathy may not report significant symptoms due to decreased corneal sensation. Early clinical signs may include reduced tear quality and break-up time, patchy or diffuse staining of the cornea or conjunctiva with sodium fluorescein or vital dye and neovascularization from the limbus extending towards the area of epithelial compromise. More advanced disease may present with a non-healing corneal epithelial defect. Stromal melting may ensue, as might opportunistic microbial infection.

Scleral lenses can provide a protected environment in which the corneal surface is continuously bathed in non-preserved fluid. The lens also protects potentially fragile epithelium from trauma induced by normal blinking. Ideally, scleral lens therapy should be initiated prior to the complete breakdown of the corneal epithelium and development of a non-healing epithelial defect. If introduced at an early stage of the disease, a scleral lens could significantly reduce morbidity. However, scleral lenses may also facilitate healing of epithelial defects when introduced at a later stage in the disease process.

Exposure Keratopathy

Disruption of normal blink function or lid integrity can result in corneal damage if the lids do not regularly and completely distribute tears over the entire ocular surface. Physiologic lagophthalmos, overly-aggressive blepharoplasty or ptosis repair, surgical or traumatic disruption of the lid margin, movement disorders (Parkinson's disease and progressive supranuclear palsy), and any insult to the facial nerve may result in corneal exposure. Patients with exposure keratopathy may experience symptoms characteristic of dry eye syndrome, including discomfort, a sandy or gritty sensation, photophobia, and fluctuating or blurred vision. Clinical findings characteristic of this condition may include lid margin irregularities, incomplete or weak blink on attempted eye closure or diffuse or coalesced corneal epithelial defects (Fig. **11**). Long-term exposure can lead to development of corneal scarring and neovascularization, and may increase the risk of microbial keratitis.

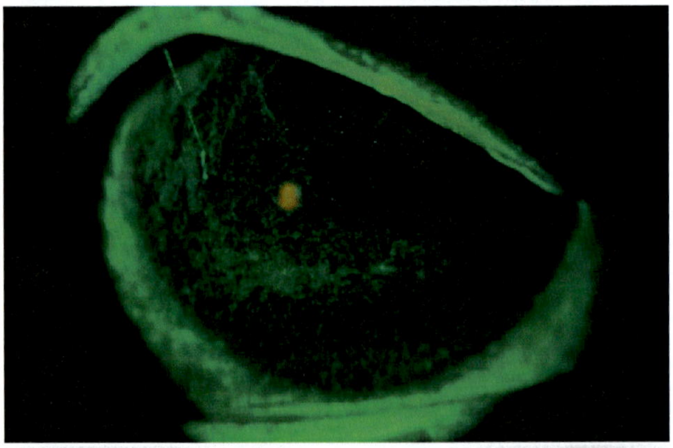

Fig. (11). Dense corneal punctate epithelial erosions associated with exposure keratopathy. Image courtesy of Lynette Johns.

If a patient exhibits clinical signs of exposure keratopathy in the absence of symptoms, clinicians should consider the possibility of damage to both the trigeminal and the facial nerves. When present, concurrent insult to both of these nerves creates a challenging clinical scenario. Compromised lid closure or blink function, along with reduced lacrimal gland stimulation, causes an insufficiency in tear quantity and distribution. Desiccation of epithelial cells leads to frank epithelial defects. Decreased corneal sensation disrupts the normal mechanism of epithelial cell replacement. The cascade culminates in the development of a non-healing corneal defect in a patient who may be asymptomatic, and therefore unaware of the cycle of destruction that has taken place.

As in neurotrophic keratopathy, scleral lenses can provide continuous protection and hydration of the ocular surface despite the lack of normal lid function. Corneal epithelial integrity can be maintained in the post-lens environment. Other therapeutic options certainly exist (moisture chamber goggles, tarsorrhaphy, placement of gold weight in the upper lid), but none of these options provide the level of ocular surface protection offered by scleral lenses. Furthermore, scleral lenses may be more cosmetically acceptable than other therapeutic modalities.

Ocular and Orbital Trauma

Damage to sensory or motor innervation to the eye or surrounding tissues can lead to ocular surface damage and subsequent vision loss. Likewise, direct trauma or insult to those tissues, either accidental or iatrogenic, can also cause corneal or conjunctival compromise. Descriptions of specific applications for scleral lenses following ocular trauma or insult suggest their utility may eventually expand well beyond commonly reported indications.

Treatment of malignancy of the eye, head or neck, requires a finely tuned balance between therapies that is aggressive enough to eradicate the neoplasm, but still preserves ocular and orbital tissues essential for maintenance of ocular health and vision. Surgical removal of the lesion can compromise ocular structures or their sources of innervation. Radiotherapy can cause collateral damage to all tissue in its path. Lin *et al.* described a case in which a scleral lens has been used to provide ocular surface protection in a patient with keratoconjunctivitis sicca secondary to GvHD who subsequently developed an undifferentiated sarcoma. Surgical excision of the lesion involved the lower eyelid, and the patient was subsequently treated with radiotherapy. Despite all of these challenges, the patient has maintained an intact corneal surface and excellent visual acuity [71]. Another case report described the use of a scleral lens following excision of papillary squamous cell carcinoma of the upper lid [72]. Both of these cases demonstrate that scleral lenses can provide excellent protection of the ocular surface, and can be used to reduce the risk of ocular morbidity associated with periorbital surgery or radiation.

Severe facial trauma may also result in secondary compromise to the ocular surface, particularly if eyelids are involved. Kalwerisky *et al.* described the use of scleral lenses to maintain corneal integrity in 10 patients (16 eyes) with severe periorbital thermal injuries. One eye required emergent keratoplasty, but the remainder of the eyes were successfully managed with scleral lenses. Six eyes developed infiltrates which resolved with addition of non-preserved fortified antibiotics to the fluid in the bowl of the lenses. All eyes of patients who recovered from their injuries maintained visual acuity of 20/70 or better, and four eyes achieved best-corrected vision of 20/20 [73]. Although periocular trauma is not commonly cited as an indication for scleral lens therapy, these results suggest that scleral lenses may help to limit functional vision loss in patients who experience such injuries.

Limbal Stem Cell Deficiencies

Limbal stem cells are believed to be responsible for maintaining corneal epithelial integrity. They also act as a barrier to prevent conjunctival epithelial cells from migrating onto the corneal surface. These cells reside in the palisades of Vogt, in the area of the corneo-scleral junction. If this cell population is absent or compromised, the corneal epithelium is not adequately renewed or repaired. Conjunctival epithelial cells migrate onto the surface of the cornea, and neovascularization develops (Fig. **12**). Resultant corneal scarring or inflammation may cause loss of vision.

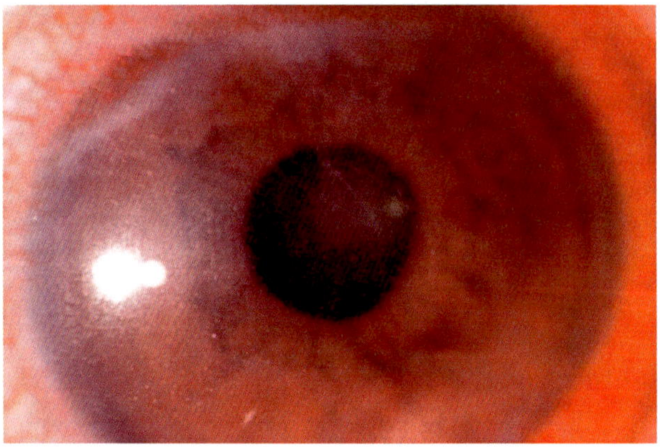

Fig. (12). Corneal limbal stem cell deficiency with limbal pannus.

Limbal stem cell deficiencies can be genetic or acquired. Aniridia and Peters' anomaly are associated with genetic forms of the disease. Acquired stem cell deficiency can result from inflammatory, infectious, traumatic, or neoplastic challenge to the ocular surface. Inflammatory conditions that can compromise limbal stem cell population include SJS, ocular cicatricial pemphigoid, GvHD, staph hypersensitivity or chronic ocular allergy. Fungal, viral or bacterial corneal infections can lead to stem cell deficiency. Traumatic causes of limbal stem cell deficiency include thermal or chemical burns, radiation or chemotherapy, ocular surgery involving the limbus, toxicity caused by preservatives in topical ocular medication, or even contact lens wear.

Standard medical therapy for the condition may include removal of the offending agent and any or all of the standard therapeutic interventions for dry eye syndrome. Surgical interventions include mechanical debridement of conjunctivalized corneal epithelium, amniotic membrane transplantation or limbal conjunctival autografts.

Scleral lenses may offer an additional non-surgical therapeutic alternative if standard medical therapy fails to achieve the desired effect. They provide a continuously hydrated, protected environment over the limbus. Scleral lenses have already been shown to be effective in specific conditions associated with acquired limbal stem cell deficiency [53, 54, 59, 60, 74]. Schornack described a case in which scleral lenses were specifically used to treat clinically diagnosed limbal stem cell deficiency. After resolution of symptoms, scleral lens wear was discontinued. The patient remained symptom-free even after discontinuation of scleral lens wear. This suggests that creation of a protective microenvironment beneath a scleral lens may have allowed for recovery of the regenerative potential of a challenged, but not obliterated, stem cell population [75].

Corneal Dystrophy/Degeneration

Scleral lenses have proven to be useful in correcting optical aberrations which arise from irregularities on the surface of the cornea, protecting and preserving corneal epithelial integrity, and improving ocular comfort. Given the success of scleral lenses in the management of both corneal irregularity and ocular surface compromise, one could predict that corneal dystrophy or degeneration could be treated effectively with this modality.

Corneal dystrophies (Fig. **13**) are hereditary conditions characterized by accumulation of abnormal tissue (Fig. **14**) in some layer of the cornea. The conditions are bilateral and usually progressive, and are classified based upon the layer of cornea affected. They are generally not associated with other ocular or systemic disease. Corneal degeneration causes tissue change that may lead to progressive deterioration and possible vision loss. Degeneration may be unilateral, and can also be associated with systemic disease or aging changes in the eye. In addition to causing optical aberrations due to surface irregularities, some corneal dystrophies and degenerations have been identified as risk factors for the development of recurrent corneal erosions. If the integrity of the corneal epithelium and its connections to deeper layers of the cornea are compromised by either dystrophy or degeneration, patients may experience delayed epithelialization, persistent sloughing of newly formed epithelium, and recurrent episodes of epithelial loss [76]. The use of scleral lenses in the management of recurrent corneal erosions associated with lattice and Avellino dystrophy [77], anterior basement membrane dystrophy [31, 45, 51], and Salzmann's nodular degeneration [78, 79] has been reported.

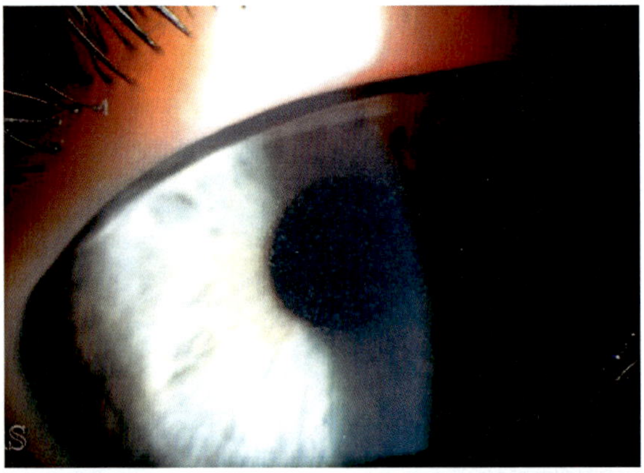

Fig. (13). Meesmann's corneal dystrophy.

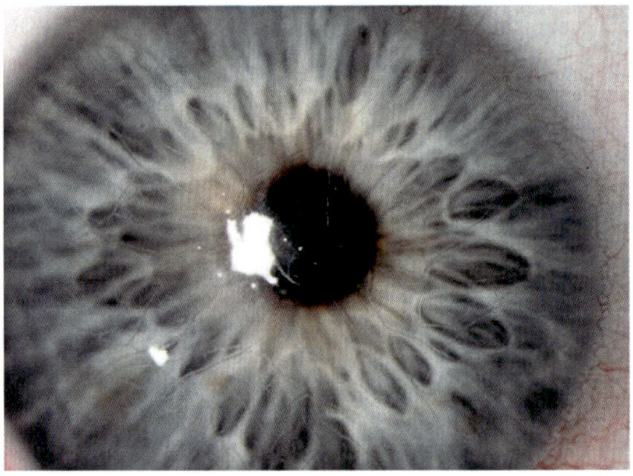

Fig. (14). Corneal amyloidosis with branching transparent lattice deposits.

Persistent Epithelial Defects

Persistent epithelial defects can be associated with a number of conditions described above. If there is a disruption in the intricate and interconnected epithelial system, then limbal stem cells are activated, new epithelial cells are directed to the site of the lesion, and robust connections between epithelial cells and underlying tissues are formed (Fig. **15**). Imbalance of this system can potentially result in an epithelial defect that does not heal well. Once again, understanding of the underlying disease process or deficit is essential in the overall management of the condition. For example, a persistent epithelial defect caused by prolonged exposure may have different characteristics and may require a different overall therapeutic approach compared to a defect that arises from limbal stem cell deficiency or an insult to the ophthalmic branch of the trigeminal nerve.

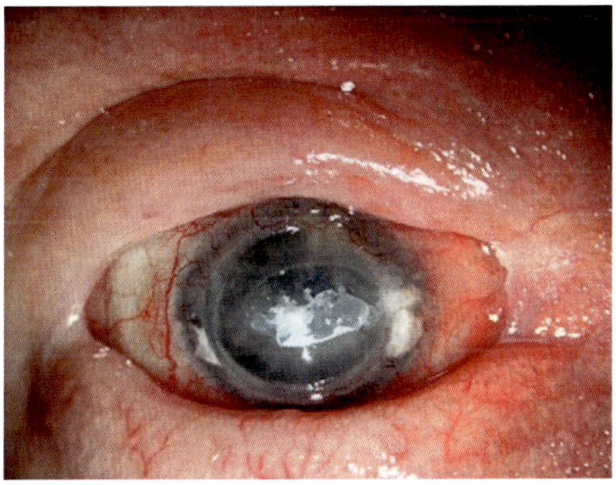

Fig. (15). Persistent non-healing epithelial defect.

However, regardless of etiology or specific treatment strategy for the underlying condition, re-epithelialization is a critical goal in the early management of persistent epithelial defects. Traditional medical intervention should certainly be attempted. In some cases, aggressive lubrication, discontinuation of medications that contain toxic preservatives, punctal occlusion, or placement of a bandage soft contact lens can promote resolution of the epithelial defect. Use of autologous serum or amniotic membrane grafting can be used if traditional medical management fails to provide adequate results. More aggressive surgical intervention (tarsorrhaphy, limbal stem cell transplantation) may also be considered [80].

Scleral lenses have demonstrated efficacy in the treatment of persistent epithelial defects. The post-lens fluid reservoir continuously hydrates the cornea. Interaction between the eyelid and a bandage soft contact lens is eliminated; this may facilitate the formation of intact hemidesmosomes between fragile new epithelial cells and Bowman's layer. Non-preserved medication or nutrient solution may be placed in the bowl of the lens, providing prolonged contact with the ocular surface. For this application, continuous wear of scleral lenses may be indicated.

The use of rigid gas permeable lenses in the management of persistent epithelial defects was first described by Tappin in 2001. In this study, seven cases of successful re-epithelialization of persistent epithelial defects were presented. Underlying pathology in these cases was varied, and included exposure keratopathy, neurotrophic keratopathy, SJS, and post-radiation keratopathy [81].

More recently, case reports and case series representing scleral lens management of 43 patients with persistent epithelial defects have been published [77, 82 - 85]. Resolution of persistent epithelial defects with scleral lenses was also described in 22 patients in Schornack's 2014 review [45]. Also in 2014, Katzman included scleral lens therapy in his overview of management strategies for persistent epithelial defects [80].

Usually, patients are instructed to remove scleral lenses prior to sleeping. However, in cases involving persistent epithelial defects, the protection provided by scleral lenses may also be necessary during sleeping as well as waking hours. The decision to recommend overnight wear of a lens must be carefully considered; persistent epithelial defects may permit opportunistic microbial infection of the cornea, and overnight wear of contact lenses is strongly associated with an increased risk of microbial keratitis. In 2014, Ciralsky *et al.* published a standardized protocol for continuous wear of scleral lenses for the management of persistent epithelial defects. Eight eyes which were managed using this protocol experienced uneventful resolution of their epithelial defects. Application of this protocol may minimize the risk of complications while providing full-time protection of the cornea during re-epithelialization of persistent epithelial defects. The protocol is described below [86]:

1. Wear of the scleral lens 24 hours a day until complete re-epithelialization was achieved.
2. Brief daily removal of the device for cleaning, disinfection with Clear Care (Alcon, Fort Worth, TX, USA) and Optimum CDS or ESC (Lobob Laboratories, San Jose, CA, USA), and rinsing with Unisol 4 Saline (Alcon, Fort Worth, TX, USA). Of note, Unisol 4 is no longer available. Alternative products include LaciPure (Menicon America, Inc., Waltham, MA, USA) or Purilens Plus (The Lifestyle Company, Inc., Freehold, NJ, USA).
3. Replacement of the reservoir fluid with one drop of moxifloxacin 0.5% (Vigamox™, Alcon, Fort Worth, TX, USA) followed by Unisol 4 saline (see above).
4. Prompt transition from continuous to long-term, daytime only scleral lens wear following epithelial defect resolution.

Undifferentiated Dry Eye Disease

In cases where ocular surface tissue damage is either already present or imminent due to compromise in ocular or periocular structures, scleral lenses have repeatedly been shown to be valuable. They protect and hydrate the ocular surface, and provide a barrier between the corneal epithelium and the lids. In the management of undifferentiated dry eye disease, literature on outcomes of scleral lens management is less clear. Schornack described a subset of patients with undifferentiated dry eye disease. Of 76 patients who presented for initial evaluation, 37 chose not to pursue scleral lenses following initial examination, and 5 did not complete the fitting process. Of the 34 patients who did complete the fitting process, 19 had minimal or no signs of ocular surface compromise that is normally associated with dry eye disease. All of the 34 patients who were fit with scleral lenses reported initial improvements in ocular comfort, but 71% of them eventually discontinued scleral lens wear. Average duration of lens wear was 10 months in those who discontinued wear (range 2-40 months). Those who discontinued lens wear cited lens handling difficulties, lack of symptomatic relief, lens sensation, and adequate relief with less aggressive intervention as their reasons for dropping out of scleral lens wear [45].

Some patients with undifferentiated dry eye disease achieved satisfactory symptomatic relief with the lenses, therefore management of this condition with scleral lenses is a reasonable option. However, patients with severe symptoms in the absence of clinical signs of disease may experience limited relief with this modality. It is possible that a more protracted office trial with diagnostic lenses may improve success rates by allowing patients to experience the sensation of wearing the lens for several hours or more prior to committing to the fitting process. Frank discussion on the chronic nature of dry eye disease, and the need for continual intervention to achieve symptomatic relief may also increase the chance of success with this modality. Emphasis on maximizing the benefits of less invasive or burdensome intervention prior to initiation of scleral lens wear may be prudent.

Weak associations between patient symptoms and clinical signs of primary dry eye disease confound prediction of successful or unsuccessful scleral lens wear. Patients with minimal clinical evidence of aqueous deficiency or meibomian gland dysfunction can be severely symptomatic. Rosenthal has postulated that the apparent disconnect between clinical signs and subjective patient symptoms may be due to increased sensitivity and responsiveness of pain receptors on the ocular surface to innocuous stimuli, and has termed the phenomenon "corneal evaporative hyperalgesia [87]." Scleral lenses may be useful in the diagnosis of this condition, because they instantly and completely block corneal surface evaporation, maintain continuous hydration of the corneal surface, and block the corneal surface from any lid sensation. If a patient's pain response persists despite scleral lens application, it is unlikely that scleral lenses will provide adequate symptomatic relief.

NOVEL APPLICATIONS

Several novel applications for scleral lenses have been suggested. Mechanical support of the upper lid in cases of complex ptosis can be provided by scleral lenses. While the solution may provide functional vision, patient satisfaction with cosmesis may be limited [88].

The use of scleral lenses as drug delivery devices has also been described. Kalwerisky placed topical fortified non-preserved antibiotics in the bowl of the lens to treat corneal infiltrates [73]. Ciralsky recommended placement of non-preserved antibiotics in the bowl of the lens prior to lens application in lenses that were being worn continuously to manage persistent epithelial defects [86]. Scleral lenses have also been used to deliver anti-VEGF agents to the cornea to treat neovascularization [89, 90]. A recent study reported the delivery of stem cells on a scleral lens carrier for management of a chemical burn in an animal model [91].

SUMMARY OF MEDICAL INDICATIONS

While it is generally acknowledged that scleral lenses can play an important role in the management of corneal irregularity and ocular surface disease, there is not yet consensus on placement of scleral lenses within the overall management of these conditions. Prior to developing evidence-based recommendations, many questions need to be answered. As of yet, complications of scleral lens wear have not been defined. The incidence of complications and risk factors for complications have yet to be identified. It cannot be safely assumed that the risk factors for complications of scleral lenses are identical to other types of contact lenses. There are significant differences in lens fitting parameters and the interaction between scleral lenses and ocular surface structures. One could argue that scleral lenses should be considered only after more traditional management strategies have failed. This approach would be logical when using scleral lenses to provide improved vision in cases of corneal irregularity. Well-established and well-studied lens options (hydrogel or silicone hydrogel lenses, hybrid lenses, corneal rigid gas permeable lenses) should perhaps be investigated prior to considering scleral lens fitting. However, if all other options have been exhausted, scleral lenses should certainly be considered prior to surgical intervention. In cases of ocular surface disease, placement of scleral lenses within a management strategy becomes somewhat unclear. Once again, it could be considered rational to employ traditional medical management prior to scleral lens therapy. In cases that require immediate and aggressive intervention, scleral lens use may be indicated before exhausting all other options. One could also argue for the use of scleral lenses prior to the development of severe epitheliopathy or ocular surface damage for eyes that are at high risk of severe corneal compromise. In these cases, prophylactic use of scleral lenses could actually reduce the risk of permanent damage to ocular structures, and may alleviate the need for more aggressive intervention. As literature in the area of scleral lenses matures, practitioners should be able to gain greater confidence in our ability to appropriately prescribe scleral lenses in a way that maximizes the benefits while minimizing the risks associated with their use.

Whenever a scleral lens is placed on a diseased eye, practitioners must be aware of the fact that it is not simply a contact lens; it is a therapeutic medical device. Use of scleral lenses in in the management of ocular disease requires an understanding of the disease process that is unfolding in the eye. The expected outcome of scleral lens therapy needs to be defined. The eye should be monitored carefully to see that the desired outcome is obtained, and the therapeutic approach should be adjusted if the expected outcome is not achieved or if unexpected complications arise. Cooperation and collaboration with other eye care providers and specialists within other areas of medicine will allow us to maximize the benefit for our patients.

CONFLICT OF INTEREST

The author declares no conflict of interest, financial or otherwise.

ACKNOWLEDGEMENTS

Declared none.

REFERENCES

[1] Efron N, Pearson RM. Centenary celebration of Fick's Eine Contactbrille. Arch Ophthalmol 1988; 106(10): 1370-7.
[http://dx.doi.org/10.1001/archopht.1988.01060140534019] [PMID: 3052382]

[2] Pearson RM. Kalt, keratoconus, and the contact lens. Optom Vis Sci 1989; 66(9): 643-6.
[http://dx.doi.org/10.1097/00006324-198909000-00011] [PMID: 2677884]

[3] Pearson RM, Efron N. Hundredth anniversary of August Muller's inaugural dissertation on contact lenses. Surv Ophthalmol 1989; 34(2): 133-41.

[4] Ridley F. Scleral Contact Lenses. Their Clinical Significance. Arch Ophthalmol 1963; 70(6): 740-5.
[http://dx.doi.org/10.1001/archopht.1963.00960050742004]

[5] Taub RG. Scleral contact lenses. Eye Ear Nose Throat Mon 1967; 46(1): 84.
[PMID: 6038409]

[6] Gould HL. Management of keratoconus with corneal and scleral lenses. Am J Ophthalmol 1970; 70(4): 624-9.
[http://dx.doi.org/10.1016/0002-9394(70)90899-8] [PMID: 5505480]

[7] Ruedemann AD Jr, Jardon F. Ten years experience with scleral lenses. Trans Am Ophthalmol Soc 1970; 68: 245-76.

[8] Klein M. Contact lens in cases of neuroparalytic keratitis. Br J Ophthalmol 1943; 27(5): 221-2.

[http://dx.doi.org/10.1136/bjo.27.5.221] [PMID: 18169923]

[9] Gould HL. Treatment of neurotrophic keratitis with scleral contact lenses. Eye Ear Nose Throat Mon 1967; 46(11): 1406-14.
[PMID: 6064085]

[10] Krachmer JH. The therapeutic and cosmetic indications for flush-fitting scleral contact lenses. J Iowa Med Soc 1968; 58(9): 944-6.
[PMID: 5683275]

[11] Constable JD, Carroll JM. The emergency treatment of the exposed cornea in thermal burns. Plast Reconstr Surg 1970; 46(3): 309-12.
[http://dx.doi.org/10.1097/00006534-197009000-00021] [PMID: 5448360]

[12] Goren SB, Shoch D. The use of the flush-fitting scleral contact shell after surgical intervention on acoustic neuroma. Trans Am Ophthalmol Soc 1970; 68: 277-91.

[13] Gould HL. The dry eye and scleral contact lenses. Am J Ophthalmol 1970; 70(1): 37-41.
[http://dx.doi.org/10.1016/0002-9394(70)90666-5] [PMID: 5421652]

[14] Gould HL. Management of the dry eye using scleral lenses (a report on 66 cases). Eye Ear Nose Throat Mon 1970; 49(3): 133-40.
[PMID: 5481594]

[15] Goren SB, Clemis JD. Care of the eye in facial paralysis. Arch Otolaryngol 1973; 97(2): 227-8.
[http://dx.doi.org/10.1001/archotol.1973.00780010233030] [PMID: 4568448]

[16] Burns CL, Chylack LT Jr. Thermal burns: the management of thermal burns of the lids and globes. Ann Ophthalmol 1979; 11(9): 1358-68.
[PMID: 400375]

[17] Mills PV, Lewis EM. Scleral contact lens wear in unilateral aphakia. Br J Ophthalmol 1971; 55(2): 116-24.
[http://dx.doi.org/10.1136/bjo.55.2.116] [PMID: 5550535]

[18] Ezekiel DF. Gas permeable haptic lenses. J Br Contact Lens Assoc 1983; 6: 158-61.

[19] Soeters N, Visser ES, Imhof SM, Tahzib NG. Scleral lens influence on corneal curvature and pachymetry in keratoconus patients. Cont Lens Anterior Eye 2015; 38(4): 294-7.
[http://dx.doi.org/10.1016/j.clae.2015.03.006] [PMID: 25865408]

[20] Vincent SJ, Alonso-Caneiro D, Collins MJ. Miniscleral lens wear influences corneal curvature and optics. Ophthalmic Physiol Opt 2016; 36(2): 100-11.
[http://dx.doi.org/10.1111/opo.12270] [PMID: 26690831]

[21] Arumugam AO, Rajan R, Subramanian M, Mahadevan R. PROSE for irregular corneas at a tertiary eye care center. Eye Contact Lens 2014; 40(2): 71-3.
[http://dx.doi.org/10.1097/ICL.0000000000000006] [PMID: 24418864]

[22] Baran I, Bradley JA, Alipour F, Rosenthal P, Le HG, Jacobs DS. PROSE treatment of corneal ectasia. Cont Lens Anterior Eye 2012; 35(5): 222-7.
[http://dx.doi.org/10.1016/j.clae.2012.04.003] [PMID: 22633003]

[23] Lee JC, Chiu GB, Bach D, Bababeygy SR, Irvine J, Heur M. Functional and visual improvement with prosthetic replacement of the ocular surface ecosystem scleral lenses for irregular corneas. Cornea 2013; 32(12): 1540-3.
[http://dx.doi.org/10.1097/ICO.0b013e3182a73802] [PMID: 24145631]

[24] Romero-Jiménez M, Flores-Rodríguez P. Utility of a semi-scleral contact lens design in the management of the irregular cornea. Cont Lens Anterior Eye 2013; 36(3): 146-50.
[http://dx.doi.org/10.1016/j.clae.2012.12.006] [PMID: 23291263]

[25] Krachmer JH, Feder RS, Belin MW. Keratoconus and related noninflammatory corneal thinning disorders. Surv Ophthalmol 1984; 28(4): 293-322.

[http://dx.doi.org/10.1016/0039-6257(84)90094-8] [PMID: 6230745]

[26] Schein OD, Rosenthal P, Ducharme C. A gas-permeable scleral contact lens for visual rehabilitation. Am J Ophthalmol 1990; 109(3): 318-22. [http://dx.doi.org/10.1016/S0002-9394(14)74558-1] [PMID: 2309865]

[27] Tan DT, Pullum KW, Buckley RJ. Medical applications of scleral contact lenses: 1. A retrospective analysis of 343 cases. Cornea 1995; 14(2): 121-9. [http://dx.doi.org/10.1097/00003226-199503000-00001] [PMID: 7743792]

[28] Rosenthal P, Croteau A. Fluid-ventilated, gas-permeable scleral contact lens is an effective option for managing severe ocular surface disease and many corneal disorders that would otherwise require penetrating keratoplasty. Eye Contact Lens 2005; 31(3): 130-4. [http://dx.doi.org/10.1097/01.ICL.0000152492.98553.8D] [PMID: 15894881]

[29] Pullum KW, Whiting MA, Buckley RJ. Scleral contact lenses: the expanding role. Cornea 2005; 24(3): 269-77. [http://dx.doi.org/10.1097/01.ico.0000148311.94180.6b] [PMID: 15778597]

[30] Visser ES, Visser R, van Lier HJ, Otten HM. Modern scleral lenses part I: clinical features. Eye Contact Lens 2007; 33(1): 13-20. [http://dx.doi.org/10.1097/01.icl.0000233217.68379.d5] [PMID: 17224674]

[31] Pecego M, Barnett M, Mannis MJ, Durbin-Johnson B. Jupiter Scleral Lenses: the UC Davis Eye Center experience. Eye Contact Lens 2012; 38(3): 179-82. [http://dx.doi.org/10.1097/ICL.0b013e31824daa5e] [PMID: 22543730]

[32] Cotter JM, Rosenthal P. Scleral contact lenses. J Am Optom Assoc 1998; 69(1): 33-40. [PMID: 9479934]

[33] Looi AL, Lim L, Tan DT. Visual rehabilitation with new-age rigid gas-permeable scleral contact lenses--a case series. Ann Acad Med Singapore 2002; 31(2): 234-7. [PMID: 11957565]

[34] Ye P, Sun A, Weissman BA. Role of mini-scleral gas-permeable lenses in the treatment of corneal disorders. Eye Contact Lens 2007; 33(2): 111-3. [http://dx.doi.org/10.1097/01.ICL.0000258593.20221.c6] [PMID: 17496707]

[35] Schornack M, Patel SV. Postsurgical applications for scleral lenses. *Optometry* -. J Am Optom Assoc 2010; 81(6): 272.

[36] Mahadevan R, Fathima A, Rajan R, *et al.* An ocular surface prosthesis for keratoglobus and Terrien's marginal degeneration. Optometry and vision science: official publication of the American Academy of Optometry 2014; 91(4 Suppl 1): S34-9.

[37] Biswas S, Brahma A, Tromans C, *et al.* Management of pellucid marginal corneal degeneration. Eye 2000; 14(Pt 4): 629-34. [http://dx.doi.org/10.1038/eye.2000.155]

[38] DeLoss KS, Fatteh NH, Hood CT. Prosthetic replacement of the ocular surface ecosystem (PROSE) scleral device compared to keratoplasty for the treatment of corneal ectasia. Am J Ophthalmol 2014; 158(5): 974-82. [http://dx.doi.org/10.1016/j.ajo.2014.07.016] [PMID: 25058902]

[39] Visser ES, Soeters N, Tahzib NG. Scleral lens tolerance after corneal cross-linking for keratoconus. Optometry and vision science: official publication of the American Academy of Optometry 2015.

[40] Severinsky B, Behrman S, Frucht-Pery J, Solomon A. Scleral contact lenses for visual rehabilitation after penetrating keratoplasty: long term outcomes. Cont Lens Anterior Eye 2014; 37(3): 196-202. [http://dx.doi.org/10.1016/j.clae.2013.11.001] [PMID: 24300196]

[41] Barnett M, Lien V, Li JY, *et al.* Use of scleral lenses and miniscleral lenses after penetrating keratoplasty. Eye Contact Lens 2015.

[PMID: 26214530]

[42] Alipour F, Behrouz MJ, Samet B. Mini-scleral lenses in the visual rehabilitation of patients after penetrating keratoplasty and deep lamellar anterior keratoplasty. Cont Lens Anterior Eye 2015; 38(1): 54-8.
[http://dx.doi.org/10.1016/j.clae.2014.10.001] [PMID: 25457628]

[43] Parminder A, Jacobs DS. Advances in scleral lenses for refractive surgery complications. Curr Opin Ophthalmol 2015; 26(4): 243-8.
[http://dx.doi.org/10.1097/ICU.0000000000000173] [PMID: 26058019]

[44] Steele C, Davidson J. Contact lens fitting post-laser-*in situ* keratomileusis (LASIK). Cont Lens Anterior Eye 2007; 30(2): 84-93.
[http://dx.doi.org/10.1016/j.clae.2006.12.005] [PMID: 17329148]

[45] Schornack MM, Pyle J, Patel SV. Scleral lenses in the management of ocular surface disease. Ophthalmology 2014; 121(7): 1398-405.
[http://dx.doi.org/10.1016/j.ophtha.2014.01.028] [PMID: 24630687]

[46] Mahadevan R, Jagadeesh D, Rajan R, *et al.* Unique Hard Scleral Lens Post-LASIK Ectasia Fitting. Optometry and vision science: official publication of the American Academy of Optometry 2014.

[47] Kramer EG, Boshnick EL. Scleral lenses in the treatment of post-LASIK ectasia and superficial neovascularization of intrastromal corneal ring segments. Cont Lens Anterior Eye 2015; 38(4): 298-303.
[http://dx.doi.org/10.1016/j.clae.2015.02.003] [PMID: 25746152]

[48] Cressey A, Jacobs DS, Carrasquillo KG. Management of vascularized limbal keratitis with prosthetic replacement of the ocular surface system. Eye Contact Lens 2012; 38(2): 137-40.
[http://dx.doi.org/10.1097/ICL.0b013e31823bafbc] [PMID: 22327201]

[49] Bavinger JC, DeLoss K, Mian SI. Scleral lens use in dry eye syndrome. Curr Opin Ophthalmol 2015; 26(4): 319-24.
[http://dx.doi.org/10.1097/ICU.0000000000000171] [PMID: 26058032]

[50] Alipour F, Kheirkhah A, Jabarvand Behrouz M. Use of mini scleral contact lenses in moderate to severe dry eye. Cont Lens Anterior Eye 2012; 35(6): 272-6.
[http://dx.doi.org/10.1016/j.clae.2012.07.006] [PMID: 22902924]

[51] Dimit R, Gire A, Pflugfelder SC, Bergmanson JP. Patient ocular conditions and clinical outcomes using a PROSE scleral device. Cont Lens Anterior Eye 2013; 36(4): 159-63.
[http://dx.doi.org/10.1016/j.clae.2013.02.004] [PMID: 23499361]

[52] Romero-Rangel T, Stavrou P, Cotter J, Rosenthal P, Baltatzis S, Foster CS. Gas-permeable scleral contact lens therapy in ocular surface disease. Am J Ophthalmol 2000; 130(1): 25-32.
[http://dx.doi.org/10.1016/S0002-9394(00)00378-0] [PMID: 11004256]

[53] Heur M, Bach D, Theophanous C, Chiu GB. Prosthetic replacement of the ocular surface ecosystem scleral lens therapy for patients with ocular symptoms of chronic Stevens-Johnson syndrome. Am J Ophthalmol 2014; 158(1): 49-54.
[http://dx.doi.org/10.1016/j.ajo.2014.03.012] [PMID: 24699156]

[54] Papakostas TD, Le HG, Chodosh J, Jacobs DS. Prosthetic replacement of the ocular surface ecosystem as treatment for ocular surface disease in patients with a history of Stevens-Johnson syndrome/toxic epidermal necrolysis. Ophthalmology 2015; 122(2): 248-53.
[http://dx.doi.org/10.1016/j.ophtha.2014.08.015] [PMID: 25282251]

[55] Ciralsky JB, Sippel KC, Gregory DG. Current ophthalmologic treatment strategies for acute and chronic Stevens-Johnson syndrome and toxic epidermal necrolysis. Curr Opin Ophthalmol 2013; 24(4): 321-8.
[http://dx.doi.org/10.1097/ICU.0b013e3283622718] [PMID: 23680755]

[56] Iyer G, Srinivasan B, Agarwal S, Kamala Muralidharan S, Arumugam S. Comprehensive approach to

ocular consequences of Stevens Johnson Syndrome - the aftermath of a systemic condition. Graefes Arch Clin Exp Ophthalmol 2014; 252(3): 457-67.
[http://dx.doi.org/10.1007/s00417-014-2568-8] [PMID: 24469247]

[57] Agranat JS, Kitos NR, Jacobs DS. Prosthetic replacement of the ocular surface ecosystem: impact at 5 years. Br J Ophthalmol 2015.
[PMID: 26644423]

[58] Jacobs DS, Rosenthal P. Boston scleral lens prosthetic device for treatment of severe dry eye in chronic graft-versus-host disease. Cornea 2007; 26(10): 1195-9.
[http://dx.doi.org/10.1097/ICO.0b013e318155743d] [PMID: 18043175]

[59] Takahide K, Parker PM, Wu M, *et al.* Use of fluid-ventilated, gas-permeable scleral lens for management of severe keratoconjunctivitis sicca secondary to chronic graft-versus-host disease. Biol Blood Marrow Transplant 2007; 13(9): 1016-21.
[http://dx.doi.org/10.1016/j.bbmt.2007.05.006] [PMID: 17697963]

[60] Schornack MM, Baratz KH, Patel SV, Maguire LJ. Jupiter scleral lenses in the management of chronic graft versus host disease. Eye Contact Lens 2008; 34(6): 302-5.
[http://dx.doi.org/10.1097/ICL.0b013e318188e205] [PMID: 18997537]

[61] Theophanous C, Irvine JA, Parker P, *et al.* Use of prosthetic replacement of the ocular surface ecosystem scleral lenses in patients with ocular chronic graft-versus-host disease. Biology of blood and marrow transplantation: J Am Soc Blood and Marrow Transplant 2015; 21(12): 2180-4.

[62] Espana EM, Shah S, Santhiago MR, Singh AD. Graft versus host disease: clinical evaluation, diagnosis and management. Graefes Arch Clin Exp Ophthalmol 2013; 251(5): 1257-66.
[http://dx.doi.org/10.1007/s00417-013-2301-z] [PMID: 23504086]

[63] Nassar A, Tabbara KF, Aljurf M. Ocular manifestations of graft-versus-host disease. Saudi J Ophthalmol 2013; 27(3): 215-22.
[http://dx.doi.org/10.1016/j.sjopt.2013.06.007] [PMID: 24227989]

[64] Margolis R, Thakrar V, Perez VL. Role of rigid gas-permeable scleral contact lenses in the management of advanced atopic keratoconjunctivitis. Cornea 2007; 26(9): 1032-4.
[http://dx.doi.org/10.1097/ICO.0b013e3181245172] [PMID: 17893528]

[65] Rathi VM, Sudharman Mandathara P, Vaddavalli PK, Dumpati S, Chakrabarti T, Sangwan VS. Fluid-filled scleral contact lenses in vernal keratoconjunctivitis. Eye Contact Lens 2012; 38(3): 203-6.
[http://dx.doi.org/10.1097/ICL.0b013e3182482eb5] [PMID: 22367220]

[66] Schornack MM, Baratz KH. Ocular cicatricial pemphigoid: the role of scleral lenses in disease management. Cornea 2009; 28(10): 1170-2.
[http://dx.doi.org/10.1097/ICO.0b013e318199fa56] [PMID: 19770718]

[67] Harthan JS. Therapeutic use of mini-scleral lenses in a patient with Graves' ophthalmopathy. J Optom 2014; 7(1): 62-6.
[http://dx.doi.org/10.1016/j.optom.2012.11.002] [PMID: 24646903]

[68] Grey F, Carley F, Biswas S, Tromans C. Scleral contact lens management of bilateral exposure and neurotrophic keratopathy. Cont Lens Anterior Eye 2012; 35(6): 288-91.
[http://dx.doi.org/10.1016/j.clae.2012.07.009] [PMID: 22902053]

[69] Schornack MM. Poster 9: Management of neurotrophic keratopathy with a scleral rigid gas permeable contact lens. *Optometry* -. J Am Optom Assoc 2007; 78(6): 273-4.

[70] Weyns M, Koppen C, Tassignon MJ. Scleral contact lenses as an alternative to tarsorrhaphy for the long-term management of combined exposure and neurotrophic keratopathy. Cornea 2013; 32(3): 359-61.
[http://dx.doi.org/10.1097/ICO.0b013e31825fed01] [PMID: 23073486]

[71] Lin SJ, Jacobs DS, Frankenthaler R, Rubin PA. An ocular surface prosthesis as an innovative adjunct in patients with head and neck malignancy. Otolaryngol Head Neck Surg 2008; 139(4): 589-91.

[http://dx.doi.org/10.1016/j.otohns.2008.06.032] [PMID: 18922350]

[72] Samimi DB, Chiu GB, Burnstine MA. PROSE scleral lens: A novel aid for staged eyelid reconstruction. Ophthal Plast Reconstr Surg 2013.
[PMID: 24317103]

[73] Kalwerisky K, Davies B, Mihora L, Czyz CN, Foster JA, DeMartelaere S. Use of the Boston Ocular Surface Prosthesis in the management of severe periorbital thermal injuries: a case series of 10 patients. Ophthalmology 2012; 119(3): 516-21.
[http://dx.doi.org/10.1016/j.ophtha.2011.08.027] [PMID: 22133791]

[74] Tougeron-Brousseau B, Delcampe A, Gueudry J, *et al.* Vision-related function after scleral lens fitting in ocular complications of Stevens-Johnson syndrome and toxic epidermal necrolysis. Am J Ophthalmol 2009; 148(6): 852-9 e2.
[http://dx.doi.org/10.1016/j.ajo.2009.07.006]

[75] Schornack MM. Limbal stem cell disease: management with scleral lenses. Clinical & experimental optometry: journal of the Australian Optometrical Association 2011; 94(6): 592-4.

[76] Ramamurthi S, Rahman MQ, Dutton GN, Ramaesh K. Pathogenesis, clinical features and management of recurrent corneal erosions. Eye (Lond) 2006; 20(6): 635-44.
[http://dx.doi.org/10.1038/sj.eye.6702005] [PMID: 16021185]

[77] Ling JD, Gire A, Pflugfelder SC. PROSE therapy used to minimize corneal trauma in patients with corneal epithelial defects. Am J Ophthalmol 2013; 155(4): 615-9.
[http://dx.doi.org/10.1016/j.ajo.2012.09.033]

[78] Chiu GB, Bach D, Theophanous C, *et al.* Prosthetic Replacement of the Ocular Surface Ecosystem (PROSE) scleral lens for Salzmann's nodular degeneration. Saudi J Ophthalmology: Official J Saudi Ophthalmol Soc 2014; 28(3): 203-6.

[79] Schornack M. Scleral lenses in the management of salzmann's nodular degeneration. *Optometry* -. J Am Optom Assoc 2009; 80(6): 293-4.

[80] Katzman LR, Jeng BH. SManagement strategies for persistent epithelial defects of the cornea. Saudi journal of ophthalmology: official journal of the Saudi Ophthalmological Society 2014; 28(3): 168-72.

[81] Tappin MJ, Pullum KW, Buckley RJ. Scleral contact lenses for overnight wear in the management of ocular surface disorders. Eye (Lond) 2001; 15(Pt 2): 168-72.
[http://dx.doi.org/10.1038/eye.2001.54] [PMID: 11339584]

[82] Rosenthal P, Cotter JM, Baum J. Treatment of persistent corneal epithelial defect with extended wear of a fluid-ventilated gas-permeable scleral contact lens. Am J Ophthalmol 2000; 130(1): 33-41.
[http://dx.doi.org/10.1016/S0002-9394(00)00379-2] [PMID: 11004257]

[83] Grover S, Jacobs DS, Colby KA. Boston Ocular Surface Prosthesis for persistent epitheliopathy after treatment of conjunctival melanoma. Cornea 2010; 29(4): 459-61.
[http://dx.doi.org/10.1097/ICO.0b013e3181b55b40] [PMID: 20164756]

[84] Gumus K, Gire A, Pflugfelder SC. The successful use of Boston ocular surface prosthesis in the treatment of persistent corneal epithelial defect after herpes zoster ophthalmicus. Cornea 2010; 29(12): 1465-8.
[http://dx.doi.org/10.1097/ICO.0b013e3181da58b9] [PMID: 20847682]

[85] Lim P, Ridges R, Jacobs DS, Rosenthal P. Treatment of persistent corneal epithelial defect with overnight wear of a prosthetic device for the ocular surface. Am J Ophthalmol 2013; 156(6): 1095-101.
[http://dx.doi.org/10.1016/j.ajo.2013.06.006] [PMID: 24075432]

[86] Ciralsky JB, Chapman KO, Rosenblatt MI, *et al.* Treatment of refractory persistent corneal epithelial defects: A standardized approach using continuous wear PROSE therapy. Ocul Immunol Inflamm 2014.
[PMID: 24654929]

[87] Rosenthal P, Borsook D. Ocular neuropathic pain. Br J Ophthalmol 2016; 100(1): 128-34. [http://dx.doi.org/10.1136/bjophthalmol-2014-306280] [PMID: 25943558]

[88] Shah-Desai SD, Aslam SA, Pullum K, Beaconsfield M, Rose GE. Scleral contact lens usage in patients with complex blepharoptosis. Ophthal Plast Reconstr Surg 2011; 27(2): 95-8. [http://dx.doi.org/10.1097/IOP.0b013e3181d07408] [PMID: 21057345]

[89] Keating AM, Jacobs DS. Anti-VEGF treatment of corneal neovascularization. Ocul Surf 2011; 9(4): 227-37. [http://dx.doi.org/10.1016/S1542-0124(11)70035-0] [PMID: 22023817]

[90] Lim M, Jacobs DS, Rosenthal P, Carrasquillo KG. The Boston Ocular Surface Prosthesis as a novel drug delivery system for bevacizumab. Semin Ophthalmol 2009; 24(3): 149-55. [http://dx.doi.org/10.1080/08820530902802013] [PMID: 19437350]

[91] Espandar L, Caldwell D, Watson R, Blanco-Mezquita T, Zhang S, Bunnell B. Application of adipose-derived stem cells on scleral contact lens carrier in an animal model of severe acute alkaline burn. Eye Contact Lens 2014; 40(4): 243-7. [http://dx.doi.org/10.1097/ICL.0000000000000045] [PMID: 24901976]

CHAPTER 6

Scleral Lenses for the Regular / Normal / Non-Diseased Cornea

Langis Michaud*

École d'Optométrie, de l'Université de Montréal, Québec, Canada

Abstract: A regular/normal/non-diseased cornea is characterized by a prolate surface, with no indices of irregularity, warpage or distortion. For consistency, the term regular cornea will be used in this text. Anterior corneal surface elevation and posterior corneal surface elevation of a regular cornea which do not exhibit ectasia or irregularities of either surface. These patients present with common refractive errors: myopia, regular astigmatism, hyperopia and presbyopia. Prescribing scleral lenses for patients with regular corneas or switching patients from other modalities to scleral lenses is very feasible. First, practitioners determine the need, which is improving vision and/or comfort. Scleral lenses can significantly enhance the lens wearing experience of regular cornea patients, especially in astigmatic, presbyopic or marginal dry eye patient populations. For regular cornea patients and the correction of common refractive errors, the risk-to-benefit ratio needs to be evaluated and an appropriate lens selected. In conclusion, scleral lenses are becoming part of practitioners' standard armamentarium to improve the contact lens experience of their patients.

Keywords: Astigmatism, Comfort, Convenience, Ease, Environment, Handling, Healthy, HOA, Multifocal, Non-distorted, Normal, Optics, Options, Physiological, Presbyopia, Prolate, Refractive surgery, Regular, Sports, Visual acuity.

INTRODUCTION

A regular/normal/non-diseased cornea is characterized by a prolate surface, with no indices of irregularity, warpage or distortion. For consistency, the term regular cornea will be used in this text. Anterior corneal surface elevation and posterior corneal surface elevation of a regular cornea which do not exhibit ectasia or irregularities of either surface (Fig. **1**). These patients who have normal corneas present with common refractive errors: myopia, regular astigmatism, hyperopia and presbyopia.

* **Corresponding author Langis Michaud:** École d'optométrie, de l'Université de Montréal, Montréal, QC, Canada; Tel: 514-343-6111 ext 8945; Fax: 514-343-6082; E-mail: langis.michaud@umontreal.ca

Melissa Barnett & Lynette K. Johns (Eds.)

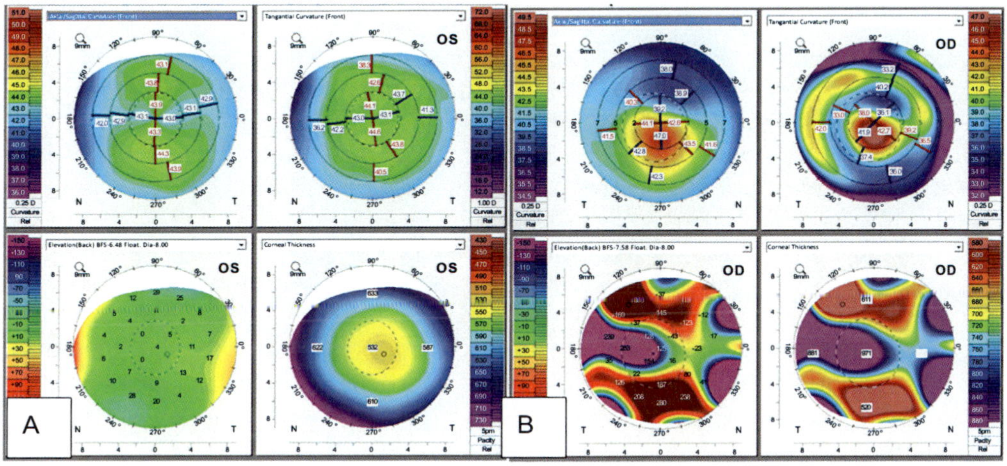

Fig. (1). A. Example of an Oculus Pentacam® analysis of a normal cornea. The posterior elevation is displayed in the bottom left map. B. Example of a cornea with keratoconus demonstrating anterior elevation in the top images as well as posterior elevation in the bottom left map. Images courtesy of Melissa Barnett.

Why Consider Scleral Lenses for Regular Corneas?

Traditionally, scleral lenses were prescribed to manage irregular corneas or ocular surface disease. The benefits from their usage are numerous and, in such circumstances, it is easy to assume that the risk/benefit ratio is low [1]. Despite the reported success of scleral lenses in diseased and irregular corneas, is the risk/benefit ratio still low if we consider fitting a 30-year-old computer worker or a 15-year-old baseball player while other contact lens options are available? To answer this question, a practitioner should balance the advantages and disadvantages of fitting scleral lenses appropriately. This chapter highlights considerations for fitting patients who have regular corneas with scleral lenses.

Conventional Contact Lens Dropout Rates

In 2014, there were an estimated 39.2 million contact lens wearers in the United States [2]. In 2010, the contact lens dropout rate was 15.9% annually [3]. Of the lapsed patients, 52.4% discontinued lens wear because of long-standing lens-related discomfort, and 14.2% discontinued because of reduced visual acuity. In addition, 4.5% of patients could not achieve adequate presbyopia correction with contact lenses [3]. Three out of four patients dropped out because of vision or comfort-related reasons. A patient who discontinues lens wear becomes a net loss for practitioners who dedicate effort and chair time to keep these patients in contact lenses. In the United States, the median value over the lifetime of a single patient dropping out of contact lens use is estimated to be between $19,947 and $24,556 [3].

Numerous strategies over the years have attempted to address contact lens dropout [4]. Options include modifications of the material, design and fitting of the lens; mode of lens wear, and care regimen. Despite more than 40 years of constant innovation and changing these variables, up to 51% of soft lens wearers still permanently discontinue contact lens wear [5]. The re-emergence of scleral lenses has become a recent option to correct common refractive errors.

Benefits of Scleral Lenses for Regular Corneas

Scleral lenses address the primary reasons why soft contact lens wearers drop out. Typically, visual acuity is the primary reason for contact lens dropout in astigmatic and presbyopic patients. Contact lens discomfort is another reason for dropout. Scleral lenses address both discomfort and visual acuity [3]. From a practitioner perspective, lens fitting behavior may also account for contact lens dropout.

Comfort

Contact lens discomfort is multifactorial in origin, and scleral lenses address most of these aspects. First, scleral lenses are made of gas permeable materials that do not dehydrate over time. Their physical and optical properties are maintained for the entire duration of wear. Second, if a scleral lens is fit optimally, there is a reservoir space between the back surface of the lens and the cornea. This reservoir is filled with a preservative-free fluid to keep the ocular surface continuously bathed. Consequently, scleral lenses can help patients with regular corneas that also have associated ocular dryness [6]. Third, due to the rigid polymers, scleral lenses are less likely to absorb biocides from lens care regimens and thereby prevent continuous exposure to an absorbed chemical compared to soft lenses. Uptake and release of preservative agents or buffers may trigger allergic and toxic reactions on the ocular surface. Some preservative agents are known to increase inflammatory reactions, which, in turn, can increase symptoms of discomfort [7].

The solution most commonly used to fill scleral lenses is preservative free and often non-buffered. According to the SCOPE study, 61.4% of practitioners recommend hydrogen peroxide as their regimen of choice, which is also preservative free [8]. Consequently, with the use of scleral lenses, interactions between care regimen solutions and ocular surface are minimized, which helps improve contact lens related comfort.

Visual Acuity/Optics

Visual acuity is improved with the use of scleral lenses because they are made of rigid gas permeable materials. Scleral lenses can offer larger optic zones compared to any other lenses including corneal gas permeable, soft spherical, soft toric and hybrid lenses. With a larger optic zone, haloes and glare are often reduced, with a corresponding improvement in vision – even under the most challenging conditions. For patients with large pupils who suffer from glare and haloes, scleral lenses may reduce their symptoms.

Higher-order aberrations (HOAs) can pollute visual performance (Fig. **2**) and are more prevalent in patients with irregular corneas or lenticular opacities [9]. For regular "normal" eyes, the presence of HOAs is often a result of the inherent optics of the corrective lenses. Soft lenses intrinsically induce HOAs if the lenses are not designed to optically compensate for HOAs [10].

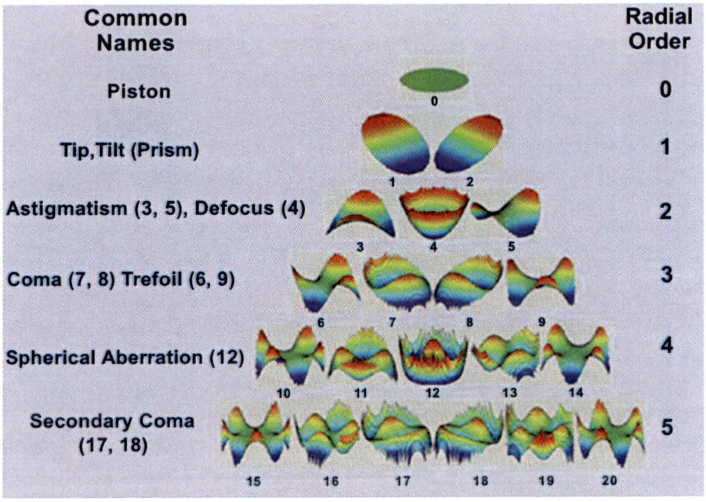

Fig. (2). Examples of higher-order aberrations. Image courtesy of Ken Lebow (Contact Lens Spectrum November 2008).

Despite controversial results in clinical studies, the increased level of HOAs may be associated with high myopia or moderate hyperopia [11]. With scleral lenses, the post-lens tear reservoir fluid and wavefront-guided optics help reduce HOAs [12] and compensate for any corneal distortion that may occur after several months or years of soft contact lens wear.

Scleral lenses make a difference for astigmatic and presbyopic patients. It has been shown that a small amount ($\geq$ 0.75D) of astigmatism should be properly corrected [13] to improve visual acuity by three to six letters [14]. Rigid gas permeable lenses are preferred to soft lenses to improve visual outcomes, especially in moderate to severe astigmatic patients [15]. The gas permeable material offers a stable optical surface and does not dehydrate during regular wear or under challenging conditions. Scleral lenses offer the full optical advantages of gas permeable lenses to compensate for refractive astigmatism and are more stable on the ocular surface than any other type of lens. Significant amounts of corneal astigmatism, for example 3.50D, can be corrected with a scleral lens with spherical optics. If the spherical design does not correct the full amount of astigmatism, then front surface optical toricity can be employed. Scleral lenses are known to be stable with many different mechanisms to enhance lens rotational stability.

Lens Behavior in Presbyopia

For presbyopia, many elements are crucial to reaching a satisfactory fit. First, lens centration is paramount [16]. Most soft lenses tend to decenter infero-temporally [17], leading to a misalignment of the lens optics and the visual axis. The lateral movement of the lens becomes significant when the patient converges and the eye moves in the opposite direction than the lens. This negatively alters the visual outcome with soft multifocal contact lenses [18]. This centration problem can be resolved with scleral lenses. For instance, mini-scleral lenses remain well-centered on the eye, while larger-diameter scleral lenses tend to decenter inferiorly and temporally [19]. Some manufacturers are able to design a multifocal lens with decentered optics to compensate for lens misalignment. In addition to centration, the second important factor is to fully correct any refractive astigmatism in presbyopic patients. As previously stated, scleral lenses can correct astigmatism with a spherical power; however, front toric optics can also be utilized to improve distance and near vision.

Dry eye is a very important consideration in the presbyopic population. With constant lubrication of the cornea and ocular surface, scleral lenses can help relieve dry eye symptoms while providing improved lens comfort over the duration of lens wearing time. This benefit of scleral lens wear can maintain presbyopic patients in comfortable contact lens wear and reduce the rate of contact lens dropout.

Scleral Lens Limitations

Physiological Issues

With the re-emergence of scleral lenses, there are few known facts, and many unanswered questions remain. One question in recent years has been the potential presence of chronic hypoxia related to scleral lens wear. A theoretical model of oxygen delivery to the cornea through a scleral lens system was published in 2012 [20]. Based on the principle that a scleral lens and its tear fluid layer act as oxygen barriers in series, the authors considered several lens thicknesses and clearance levels to estimate the effective Dk/t values of every possible combination. "Dk" refers to the permeability of the material or the fluid to oxygen, and "t" is the thickness of the element to diffuse through. The authors concluded that any combination in which the lens is thicker than 250 microns and the tear fluid is over 200 microns will lead to the development of corneal hypoxia. Different theoretical models found similar findings [21 - 23].

Clinically, practitioners did not see obvious signs of chronic corneal hypoxia. There were almost no reports of corneal hazing, microcysts or neovascularization. However, clinical studies have been published confirming that scleral lens wear can be associated with induced corneal swelling varying from 1% to 4% in regular corneas [24, 25], keratoconus [26] and especially in cases in which the endothelial cell layer is compromised [27, 28]. An interesting *in vivo* study confirmed a reduction in oxygen diffusion to the cornea if the tear fluid layer thickness increases [29]. In this study, instead of relying on optical pachymetry, the authors used the equivalent oxygen percentage (EOP) approach to evaluate oxygen consumption of the cornea directly with electrodes after exposure to several gases. A reference curve was developed after scleral lenses were fit with 200 and 400 microns of clearance. Their results stated that increased clearance reduced oxygen diffusion to the cornea by 30%. Considering an optimal EOP level of 9.9% to avoid corneal hypoxia [30], scleral lenses (18.0 mm in diameter, with an average lens thickness of 310 microns, fit with 200 microns of clearance), lead to an EOP value of 9.0%, while the same lens with 400 microns decreased EOP to 6.2% [29].

After examining theoretical and practical studies, it has been shown that scleral lenses induce corneal edema with variable lens thicknesses and corneal clearances. Some authors believe that this level of induced edema is benign because it is comparable to physiological corneal edema upon awakening. Physiological edema is eliminated within the first hour of exposure to the atmosphere after eye opening. In the case of scleral lenses, the induced 1–4% edema lasts the entire duration of wear. The long-term effect of such chronic exposure over time is unknown. In the case of a compromised corneal endothelial layer, corneal edema may appear very rapidly. However, hypoxia is not always clinically visible. Corneal edema manifests when hypoxia reaches 5% to 8%, and clinical signs correlate with the amount of edema [31]. Loss of corneal transparency occurs when edema reaches 15% [32]. Neovascularization occurs when hypoxia becomes chronic and affects the limbus as well as the central cornea. Corneal blebs are transient and are not easily assessed after a few minutes following awakening [33]. Epithelial microcysts are associated with overnight wear with lower-oxygen-permeable soft lenses. Microcysts have never been reported in patients wearing lenses during the day, even if oxygen permeability was below the Holden-Mertz criteria [34]. Overnight wear of scleral lenses is not recommended because it is linked to a high level of corneal hypoxia [35].

Scleral lens thickness varies among designs and manufacturers. For a given lens design, the thickness is typically the same across the entire surface. However, exceptions occur with front surface toricity, prism ballasting, slab off prism and back surface toricity in which the lens may be thicker in different regions. More convex lenses are usually thicker centrally compared to concave lenses. In contrast, if the lens is highly decentered inferiorly, then inferior clearance of the post-lens tear reservoir can be significantly increased. It should also be noted that the post lens tear reservoir varies considerably with time. The most recent studies on settling indicate that the average loss of fluid is 80 microns for large-diameter scleral lenses and 100 microns for mini-scleral lenses [36], with high inter-subject variation.

Handling

Two of the most significant reported barriers to scleral lens wear are scleral lens handling and economic concerns [37]. For irregular cornea patients, visual restoration is the primary goal of scleral lenses, and patients are quite motivated to succeed with scleral lens application, removal and handling. However, for patients with regular corneas (fit with scleral lenses to either compensate for refractive error or because they are lapsed soft lens wearers), handling can become a significant barrier.

Small-diameter scleral lenses may be easier to handle. Scleral lenses 15.0 mm in diameter are not much larger than standard soft toric contact lenses. They can even be favorable compared to average soft disposable contact lenses (14.2 mm diameter). Smaller-diameter scleral lenses may be perceived as less intimidating than large-diameter scleral lenses and may be easier to handle. Small-diameter scleral lenses may be a good alternative for patients with small palpebral apertures. Many manufacturers offer video training on their websites on how to handle scleral lenses. The Scleral Lens Education Society (http://www.sclerallens.org/how-use-scleral-lenses) also provides video training for all types of scleral lenses.

There are a variety of proposed methods for applying scleral lenses. The applicator method involves resting the lens upon either a soft lens applicator or DMV plunger. The tripod method involves resting the lens on three fingers without devices (Fig. **3**). Another way to balance a scleral lens is using an orthodontic ring (small round rubber band put on the tip of the finger to mimic soft lens insertion technique). Otherwise, two fingers and a stable arm can be used to balance the lens. Lastly, a scleral lens stand can balance the lens while the patient uses both hands to open the eyelids and lower their eye downward toward the lens.

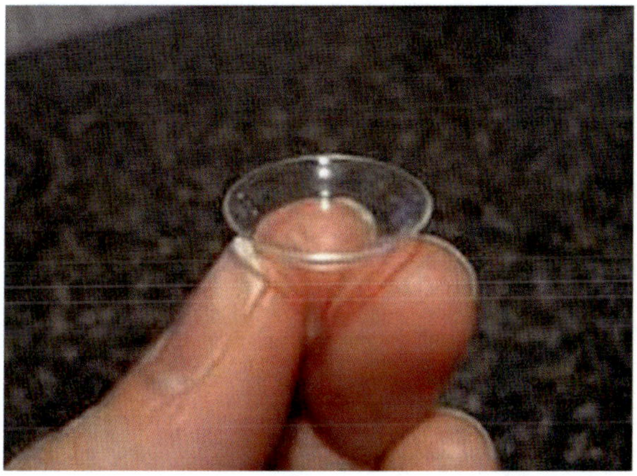

Fig. (3). Example of balancing a scleral lens with three fingers as a tripod. Image courtesy of Lynette Johns.

There are alternative scleral lens removal strategies. One method requires the use of a plunger that allows the patient to break the seal of the scleral lens and the ocular surface prior to removal. Another method involves using fingers to remove the lens, similar to removing a corneal gas permeable lens.

Scleral Lenses Compared to other Options, Including Refractive Surgery

For patients with regular corneas, the goal of contact lens fitting or refractive surgery is to correct refractive error including hyperopia, myopia, astigmatism and/or presbyopia. All of the options below can be considered to achieve an optimal result.

- Visual acuity: Overall, gas permeable lenses and hybrid lenses provide sharper and crisper visual acuity compared to soft lenses [38], especially when significant astigmatism is present. For higher refractive errors, contact lenses are preferable to refractive surgery because of the high rate of post-operative regression [39].
- Comfort: Daily disposable soft contact lenses can help patients improve their contact lens wearing experience since care regimens are no longer used [4]. However, not all daily disposable contact lenses perform equally well. The improvement of the contact lens wearing experience is based not only on material, but also on the severity of the initial symptoms [40]. As previously stated, scleral lenses can also improve end-of-day dryness [6].
- Pupil size/high-order aberrations: Contrary to general belief, pupil size does not influence post-surgical outcomes of refractive surgery [41]. Pre-operative

refractive error and post-operative uncorrected visual acuity are key elements that explain the presence of symptomatic glare or haloes post-operatively [42]. Soft contact lenses in patients with regular astigmatism can increase the amount of high -order aberrations [43]. Studies have demonstrated that scleral lenses are effective in reducing higher-order wavefront aberrations in patients with irregular astigmatism who did not achieve sufficient vision with conventional methods of optical correction [44, 45]. As of yet, no study has been published on the effect of scleral lenses for higher-order aberrations with regular astigmatism. Based on the author's clinical experience, scleral lenses can help reduce the amount of coma and trefoil as a result of the full compensation of corneal irregularity and the improved optical qualities including a larger optic zone and image quality.

- Convenience/handling: Soft contact lens handling and convenience are easier compared to scleral lenses. In general, patients preferred soft lenses for handling and convenience, but rigid corneal gas permeable lenses for visual acuity [38]. However, some patients find soft lenses too delicate to handle, and they appreciate the rigid nature of a scleral lens.
- Environmental conditions: Soft contact lenses tend to dehydrate [46]. The loss of water content during wearing hours affects soft lens stability, parameters and behavior. Visual acuity can also be compromised. Rigid corneal gas permeable and scleral lenses do not dehydrate and, consequently, maintain parameters over the lens wearing time.

Exposure to airborne allergens or challenging environments can trigger ocular discomfort, redness, tearing and immune system reactions. In such environmental conditions, contact lenses can help reduce the level and intensity of symptoms, especially when daily disposable contact lenses are worn [47]. Because scleral lenses are effective in managing severe allergies in patients with vernal keratoconjunctivitis and atopic keratoconjunctivitis, it is logical to consider scleral lenses as a valid option for reducing exposure to allergens in symptomatic patients with regular corneas [48, 49].

The tables below (Tables **1** and **2**) provide a theoretical approach to rationalizing the use of each modality based on this author's experience in regular cornea patients.

Table 1. Modalities of visual correction for specific patient needs.

	Glasses	Soft Contact Lenses	RGP Lenses	Scleral Lenses	Hybrid Lenses	Refractive Surgery
Refractive error correction	1	2	1	1	1	2
Higher-order aberrations	3	2	1	1	1	3

(Table 1) contd.....

	Glasses	Soft Contact Lenses	RGP Lenses	Scleral Lenses	Hybrid Lenses	Refractive Surgery
Comfort	1	3	4	2	2	2
Convenience	2	2	1	3	2	1
Environmental conditions	4	2	3	1	3	5
Adverse events	1	3	2	2	2	2
Cost	3	2	1	4	3	4
TOTAL	15	16	13	14	14	19

1: Optimal result 2: Good result 3: Average 4: Under expectation 5: Not to be considered.

Table 2. Main arguments/factors for the management of regular cornea patients based on the author's experience.

	Glasses	Soft Contact Lenses	RGP Lenses	Scleral Lenses	Hybrid Lenses	Refractive Surgery
Does not tolerate something in the eye	O	X	X	?	X	O
Wants a "permanent" option	X	X	X	X	X	?
Handling issues	O	O	O	O Mini-scleral	?	O
Vision is not optimal	O	X	O	O	O	X
Dry eye / discomfort	X	?Daily disposable	X	O	X	X
Symptomatic of haloes, glare, night driving issues	X	X	X	O	X	X
Convenient option / ease of wear	O	O	O	?	?	O
Affordability / cost	O	O	O	X	X	X
High refractive errors	X	X	O	O	X	X
Presbyopia	O	?	O	O	O	X
Ocular surface disease – risk factor for infections / inflammations	O	X	O	O	?	X
Sport activities	X	O	X	O	O	O
Allergy / challenging environment	X	O Daily disposable	X	O	?	X
Chair time involved, including follow-ups	O	O Except presbyopia	?	X	?	X

X: Not recommended
O: Valid option
?: Individualized determination, some lens designs may be indicated.

There is no single, easy, simple, convenient and affordable solution for optimal results in every patient. For each patient, the practitioner should evaluate the advantages and disadvantages of each procedure/device, discuss each option with the patient and determine the ideal option for each individual. Many times, scleral lenses will help improve the patient's contact lens experience. Skilled practitioners will recognize scleral lens limitations and when other options are preferred.

Specific Populations with Regular Corneas

Children can wear contact lenses safely and can take care of their lenses on their own by the age of 8–10 [50]. Many types of contact lenses have been studied and fit in young patients. Between 0–2 years of age, contact lenses are mostly used to correct aphakia or very high refractive errors, with silicone lenses preferred over other modalities. By the age of 18–24 months, the cornea increases in size and the tear film evolves, making the silicone soft contact lenses challenging to fit and difficult to tolerate for the patient. Customized silicone hydrogel and rigid gas permeable lenses can then be considered, the latter being the exception and not the rule.

Hyperopia is relatively frequent at a younger age: 8.4% of children are hyperopic at age 6, 2–3% from 9 to 14 years of age, and approximately 1% at age 15 [51]. Hyperopia is more prevalent in Caucasian and rural populations.

The pattern is different for myopia, with differences found between age groups, ethnicities and ocular and social backgrounds. A recent analysis in North America estimates the prevalence of myopia in children aged 6 to 72 months: Caucasians 1.2%, Hispanics 3.7%, Asians 3.98%, and African Americans 6.6% [52]. A greater difference was found in older children of different ethnicities. This prevalence evolves with age: at age 12, myopia affects 42.7% of Asian teenagers, while 8.3% of Caucasian Europeans demonstrate nearsightedness. At age 17, these numbers increase to 59.1% and 17.7%, respectively.

Astigmatism (>1.0D) is found in 22.9% of Caucasian children aged 6 to 7, and its prevalence decreases to 17.1% at 10 years of age. Even though the overall prevalence remains in the range of 17–22% during adolescence, astigmatism decreases in some children, while other children acquire it. It is difficult to estimate who will evolve and who will regress [53]. Ethnic origins also play a role; astigmatism is found at a higher degree and prevalence in native and aboriginal people.

In some patients, corneal astigmatism can be compensated partially, or entirely, by internal lenticular astigmatism. Most of the time, these patients do not present with refractive astigmatism. However, if a scleral lens is applied, the post-lens fluid reservoir will compensate for the corneal cylinder. Lenticular astigmatism, typically against-the-rule astigmatism, will manifest on refraction. Very rarely, the posterior cornea shows a high level of astigmatism, which is usually counterbalanced by anterior corneal astigmatism. Front surface toric scleral lenses are the only way to compensate for this lenticular or posterior corneal induced astigmatism. A front toric scleral lens can be stabilized by a prism ballast system, dual thin zone, double slab off, or by back surface toric peripheral curve designs.

For common refractive errors, daily disposable soft lenses are the most commonly prescribed types of contact lenses fit in children [54] if myopia control is not considered. Additionally, scleral lenses are not a preferred option for a pediatric population. In this population, scleral lenses are reserved for the treatment of ocular surface disorders (Stevens-Johnson syndrome, vernal keratoconjunctivitis, familial dysautonomia, *etc.*) and/or when all other options have failed to correct common refractive errors [55].

High convex powered scleral lenses are sometimes used in aphakic children. Since convex lenses have higher center thicknesses, the cornea may be deprived of oxygen, thus inducing physiological issues. In these cases, patients should be followed more closely.

Scleral lens handling can be a major challenge; thus, close parental supervision is necessary. Compliance is another concern that should be addressed on regular follow -up appointments.

For teenagers, the scenario can be different. Some practitioners fit young athletes with scleral lenses as a protective device against a challenging environment. Scleral lenses may be a better option for patients requiring corneal rigid gas permeable lenses. For example, baseball or football players can be exposed to dusty environments. When biking, the eyes are exposed to wind and dehydration of the ocular surface. If visual correction is needed, soft contact lenses will usually perform well. However, performance can be altered by environmental conditions. Scleral lenses can offer a better alternative, especially if the patient has irregular corneal astigmatism [56]. Scleral lenses are more stable, do not dehydrate and protect the ocular surface from exposure to dust, foreign particles and wind. Scleral lenses even protect the cornea in the event of severe contact or a traumatic incident while a patient is active [57].

Presbyopia is a highly prevalent condition and will affect 2.1 billion people in the world by the year 2020 [58]. Many of these patients require correction of vision with glasses and/or contact lenses. However, contact lens dropout rates among presbyopic patients remain high because of problems with vision and comfort [59]. In addition, presbyopic patients are often unaware of the multitude of contact lens options. Consequently, there is a gap between the high demand from presbyopic patients, the multifocal contact lens industry and eye care practitioners. Many features of scleral lenses can help improve visual and physiological outcomes when fitting presbyopic patients and can thereby help prevent contact lens dropout.

Because of the vast number of patients entering presbyopia, there has been a multitude of scleral multifocal designs introduced over the past few years [58]. Each manufacturer has its own proprietary design for multifocal lenses. The table below illustrates several designs for regular and irregular corneas. Detailed information about each multifocal scleral lens can be found on the website and in the fitting guide of each manufacturer. It is crucial to follow the fitting guide and manufacturer's recommendations for enhanced success. Every scleral lens design is different and requires unique and specific approaches for troubleshooting.

Just like soft multifocal lenses, it is recommended to have two or three different options with different designs for presbyopic patients. Designs may include near-centered, distance-centered and aspheric (Table **3**). At the time of publication, most manufacturers do not offer specific diagnostic multifocal fitting sets. Most scleral multifocal lens fits are based on the monofocal fitting set accompanied by manufacturer laboratory consultation.

Table 3. A summary of the wide range of multifocal scleral lenses that are available.

Type	Designs	Power Range	Add Range	Diameter	Base Curve
Acculens: Maxim, Comfort SL, Easy Fit	Center near	+20.00 to -20.00D cylinder to -6.00D	+1.00 to +3.50D	14.5 to 20.5 mm	Custom
Art Optical: Ampleye	Center near	Custom	+1.00 to +3.50D	16.5mm, 16.0mm, 17.0mm	6.04 to 8.44mm
Art Optical/Dakota Sciences: SO_2 Clear	Center near	+20.00 to -20.00D in 0.25D steps	+1.00 to +3.50D in 0.25D steps	13-15mm	5.83-9.00mm
Advanced Vision Technologies: SST	Center distance	Custom	+1.00 to +3.00D	Custom	Custom
Blanchard: Onefit 2.0	Center near	+20.00 to -20.00D in 0.25D steps	Standard add of +2.25D	14.6-15.2mm	6.80-9.00mm
Essilor: Jupiter Plus	Center distance	+20.00 to -20.00D	Up to +1.75D	15-18.2mm	Custom
EyePrint Prosthetic	Center distance	Custom	Custom	Custom	Custom

(Table 3) contd.....

Type	Designs	Power Range	Add Range	Diameter	Base Curve
Falco	Simultaneous or alternating	Custom	+0.12 to +5.00D	15-17.5mm	Custom
GP Specialists: iSight	Center near or center distance	+20.00 to -20.00D in 0.25D steps	+0.50 to +5.00D	14.2-24mm	Custom
Lens Dynamics: Dyna semi-scleral	Front aspheric	+12.00 to -20.00D	Up to +2.75D	13-16mm	5.50-8.50mm
Lens Dynamics: Dyna scleral	Front aspheric	+12.00 to -20.00D	Up to +2.75D	16.1-19mm	7.00-9.50mm
Metro Optics: InSight scleral	Center distance	Custom Cyl to 8.00D	Custom	15.2-20mm	Custom
Northern: semi-scleral	Center near for hyperopes and center distance for myopes	Custom	Up to +5.00D	14mm – 18mm	Custom
Procornea: Senso	Semi-scleral Center near or center distance	+20.00 to -25.00 in 0.25D steps	+1.00 to +2.50D in 0.50D steps	13-15mm in 0.2mm steps	6.50-9.80mm in 0.05mm steps
TruForm Optics: DigiForm	Center near	+30.00 to -30.00D	Up to +3.50D in 0.25D steps	15.0 – 18mm	Custom
Valley Contax: Custom Stable Aurora	Center near	+30.00 to -30.00D	+1.00 to +3.50D	14.8-17.8mm	Custom
Visionary Optics: Europa for Presbyopia	Center near	Custom	+1.00 to +3.50D	16.0-20.0 mm	Custom
Wave: Multifocal	Center near and center distance	+30.00 to -30.00D	Up to +5.00D	12.5-18.0mm	Custom
X-Cel Specialty Contacts: Atlantis Multifocal	Center distance	+20.00 to -20.00D	+0.75 to +4.00D	15.0 to 17.5mm	6.5 to 9.12mm

Higher-Order Aberration Control

Common refractive errors are classified as defocus, which are lower-order aberrations. Higher-order aberrations (HOAs) are considered optical aberrations of the ocular refractive media and are mainly composed of coma, trefoil and spherical aberrations. Significant HOAs can reduce visual acuity by dispersing light (Fig. **4**). This is perceived as haloes and glare around a light source. Chromatic and other aberrations are also part of the human optical refractive system. However, these can improve visual acuity, and their correction does not contribute to enhanced visual acuity [60].

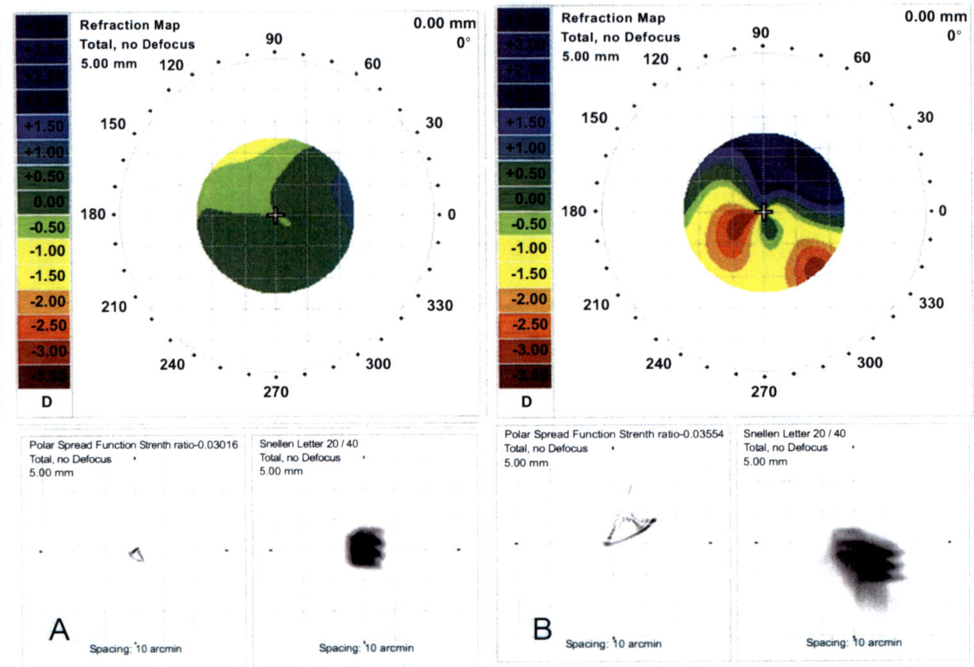

Fig. (4). (A) Example of refractive map (top), point spread function (bottom left) and simulated Snellen 20/40 letter (bottom right) of a normal eye using iTrace™, Tracey Technologies. (B) The same maps imaged of an eye with keratoconus. Images courtesy of Langis Michaud.

During the eye's natural aging process, the extent and significance of HOAs vary over time [61]. There is also a high level of inter- and intra-subject variability. As a reference, aberrations are measured in microns and are considered clinically significant at 300 microns. Rigid gas permeable lenses were found to be effective in significantly reducing HOA levels in post-surgical corneas [62] and keratoconus [63].

Scleral lenses provide good compensation for corneal irregularities with the post lens fluid reservoir. In addition, scleral lenses have limited movement and rotation when properly stabilized, optimizing aberration control. Customized scleral lenses specifically designed to compensate for HOAs can further improve the reduction of HOAs [12]. Customized HOA correction in scleral lenses is an area of new development and is not widely available.

Risk/Benefit Ratio

The risk/benefit ratio should be considered for each individual scleral lens fitting. Although scleral lenses have many positive attributes, there are also many unanswered questions. Thus, a cautious approach should be taken when fitting scleral lenses.

The risk/benefit assessment is necessary when fitting scleral lenses on regular corneas. These patients have many other contact lens options available. Regular cornea patients can be fit with scleral lenses in numerous situations. In fact, there are clear benefits of wearing scleral lenses in the following conditions:

- A visual need that is not fully compensated for by the current mode of correction.

  This patient is already wearing glasses or another type of contact lenses and encounters problems such as suboptimal visual acuity, fluctuating vision, the presence of halos and glare and/or discomfort.

  Benefits: Since scleral lenses are comprised of gas permeable material, they typically provide optimal visual acuity. The lens is stable and does not dehydrate, which reduces visual fluctuations. Scleral lens designs enable the largest possible optic zones, and the post-lens fluid reservoir compensates for surface irregularities. Scleral lenses improve symptoms of dry eye because they retain fluid on the ocular surface for the entire duration of wear.

- A visual need that is not compensated for by other means.

  An example is a patient with astigmatism who is becoming presbyopic and suffers from dry eye. Very few contact lens options can fully and adequately correct both astigmatism and presbyopia. Scleral lenses, along with hybrid lenses, can be very effective for these patients.

  Benefits: Scleral lenses provide astigmatic presbyopic patients true multifocal optics rather than relying on other options that may reduce visual acuity. These patients do not lose tridimensional visual acuity with monovision correction. Spherical scleral lenses can compensate for a significant amount of corneal astigmatism.

- Environmental challenges

  Scleral lenses can help patients suffering from chronic allergies such as pollens, airborne allergens, or dusty, windy and challenging environments.

  Benefits: Scleral lenses act as a shield to dramatically reduce exposure to allergens and other environmental challenges.

- Sports, specific activities, targeted populations

Improving vision and comfort is important when considering scleral lenses for sports activities, particularly those activities in challenging environments. Off-label, scleral lenses can act as an ocular shield in an industrial environment [64]. Scleral lenses can also be used to treat ocular surface disorders in children or for other specific reasons in a case-by-case approach if indicated.

Benefits: To help patients who have specific needs under challenging circumstances.

To counterbalance these benefits, there are potential risks associated with scleral lens wear.

- Physiological Issues

Thick scleral lenses, fitted with clearance > 250 microns, may trigger hypoxia to the cornea, on a chronic basis, with no studies on its long-term impact.

- Troubleshooting Issues

Tight lens syndrome, conjunctival prolapse, accumulation of debris in the reservoir, epithelial bogging, conjunctival misalignment and lens decentration are a few of the issues that may be encountered with scleral lenses. Optically, lens-induced astigmatism may occur. Most of these problems are considered benign, but practitioners would prefer to avoid them if possible. Options are available to minimize these issues, and methods are covered in chapter 12.

If there is a high prevalence of debris accumulation in the reservoir, lens wear can be negatively impacted. Debris accumulates and remains trapped in the post-lens fluid reservoir. This debris may force patients to discontinue scleral lens wear, especially if they have alternative corrective options. Debris in the reservoir is mainly lipid based and mucoid in nature [65].

- Giant Papillary Conjunctivitis

Giant papillary conjunctivitis is the most frequent gas permeable lens-related complication with corneal gas permeable lens wearers [66] and is rarely reported in scleral lens wearers. Here again, few clinical studies have ever reported the incidence or prevalence of papillary reactions secondary to scleral lens wear. Tan *et al.* rated this occurrence at 1.7% of eyes fit with scleral lenses [67], which is far lower than the results (25%) published on the use of first-generation hybrid lenses [68]. A practitioner must consider the specific scleral lens design versus another type of lens to reduce the risk of inducing a papillary reaction.

Scleral lenses have minimal movement and, in most cases, are fit large enough that the entire blinking process is done on its surface. Consequently, there is limited lens edge-to-lid interaction, which is probably the most important factor triggering mechanical stress on the fragile, non-keratinized conjunctival cells.

Mechanical insult can be increased if lens wettability is not optimal [69]. Some materials (Boston materials from Polymer Technology, Rochester, NY) are associated with a higher wetting angle than others, such as Optimum (Contamac, Essex, UK) or Tyro (Menicon, Japan). The selection of material for scleral lenses can have an impact on potential adverse events and patient comfort [66]. However, recent data found no differences in comfort provided by two types of materials with different wetting angles [70].

- Handling

In some cases, a patient may be required to remove scleral lenses once or twice a day to replenish the fluid reservoir if there are no other options to restore vision and comfort. Although not convenient, it could be acceptable. It is a different scenario for the computer worker who is unlikely to remove and reapply scleral lenses during work hours.

- Infections

Fortunately, there are few reports of microbial keratitis associated with scleral lens wear.

- Adverse Events

Corneal compromise is mostly limited to reactions to preserved solutions to fill the lens or to other non-compliant behavior, such as overnight lens wear. Use of scleral lenses has less reported risks than any other type of lenses. This is a benefit, especially for patients prone to infections or presenting with multiple risk factors.

- Convenience/Handling

While many new patients may be intimidated by the size of scleral lenses, the diameters of some mini-scleral lenses are not much larger than a soft lens. Practitioner confidence and proper education can overcome much of the intimidation with applying and handling scleral lenses. If a scleral lens is misaligned when applied, corneal abrasions may occur. If bubbles are trapped in the liquid reservoir, patients may experience discomfort from focal corneal desiccation or a temporary dellen. Patients may experience extreme discomfort if the plunger is applied to the center of the lens for removal.

Lens-Induced Astigmatism

Performing keratometry or topography over a scleral lens may demonstrate residual or induced astigmatism, which is considered a sign of lens flexure [71]. Flexure is well documented in corneal gas permeable lenses. When there is a misalignment of the lens to the corneal surface, the lens, although rigid, may bend. This bend will produce a change in lens surface keratometry and induce astigmatism. It is speculated that the blink expresses the post-lens tear fluid, and the lack of fluid cannot resist against the bend in the lens [72]. While this has been reported in corneal gas permeable lenses with a variety of materials, the phenomenon has also been observed with scleral lenses. However, this phenomenon of induced astigmatism and change in over-keratometry of the lens surface has not been thoroughly investigated with scleral lenses as it has with corneal lenses. In clinical experience, increasing the lens center thickness reduces this occurrence, but oxygen permeability may be affected. Just as the cornea demonstrates toricity, the sclera has asymmetry and toricity as well [73]. Flexure with scleral lenses may be caused by the lens misalignment with the toric sclera. Incorporating back surface toricity with corneal lenses reduces flexure [74, 75]. Similarly, adding back surface toric peripheral curves to the scleral landing zone improves overall scleral alignment and has been observed to reduce presumed lens flexure and induced astigmatism [76].

Considering these elements, scleral lenses have many benefits. It is possible to duplicate the very positive experience of fitting irregular cornea and diseased eye patients with these lenses. However, when considering scleral lenses for regular cornea patients, it is important to weigh the potential risks associated with this modality.

Design/Fit and Wear

Soft lens design and fit could be one of the factors to consider for improving contact lens discomfort (CLD) [77]. These findings suggest that improved comfort comes from less lens movement, enhanced tear exchange, and a diameter that exceeds the visible cornea in every quadrant and every gaze. Edge designs also influence the overall comfort of patients fit with soft lenses.

It is conceivable that scleral lens design may improve CLD in symptomatic wearers. Scleral lenses have a large diameter, exceed the visible cornea in every quadrant, and vault over the cornea. If aligned properly, the edges minimize interaction with the palpebral and bulbar conjunctiva. Toric peripheries help improve comfort in larger-diameter scleral lenses [78]. Furthermore, due to minimal scleral lens movement, there is limited tear exchange: 0.2% per minute of wear [79].

Lens Care

The potential negative interaction between lens care products and the ocular surface has been well recognized. In fact, multipurpose preserved solutions may cause irreversible tissue sensitivity reactions and reduced cell integrity as well as delay cell healing by reducing cellular metabolic rates [80]. The same findings were observed in solutions used with gas permeable lenses [81]. This type of reaction may not directly influence patient comfort. However, eliminating contact lens solutions is a good way to reduce the frequency and intensity of CLD [82].

Soft lenses absorb biocides, preservatives and buffer agents; however, gas permeable materials are less likely to absorb solution additives. Consequently, the uptake and release of chemicals during overnight soaking is different, and chemical exposure is usually reduced with gas permeable lenses. In his annual report, Bennett indicated that 13% of practitioners recommend the use of hydrogen peroxide systems as their preferred care regimen for gas permeable lenses [83]. Hydrogen peroxide systems do not contain preservatives and are perceived as a safer option. The newest products also contain moisturizers and surfactants to improve the lens surface, making it more wettable and resistant to deposits [84]. Lens surface conditioning optimizes wettability and tear film stability.

Soft and gas permeable lenses disrupt the natural equilibrium of the tear film on the ocular surface and contribute to its destabilization [85]. With plasma treatment, the surfaces of gas permeable lenses undergo radiofrequency ionized oxygen that make the hydrophobic surfaces more hydrophilic. As a result, the wetting angle and surface tension are improved along with reduced deposition of lipids, proteins and bacteria [86]. If the material can be plasma treated and conditioned during overnight soaking, tear film stability may improve once the lens is worn and, consequently, reduce the occurrence of CLD. Hydrogen peroxide, which does not require rubbing, contributes to maintaining the wetting angle for a longer time compared to a multipurpose care regimen [87].

Environmental Factors

When considering inherent patient factors, scleral lenses should not be regarded differently from any other type of contact lens. It is of prime importance to treat any ocular surface condition prior to contact lens fitting. Anterior and posterior blepharitis, Demodex or any current inflammatory or infectious condition should be managed and treated appropriately. Dry eye disease should be managed according to known clinical algorithms. Treatments such as Omega-3 oral supplementation, oral doxycycline, and long-term use of topical cyclosporine or lifitegrast can be utilized if needed. Chronic use of topical medications should be addressed when fitting scleral lenses on patients with regular corneas. Contact lens wear may be contraindicated in the presence of some chronic topical medications.

Tear exchange is minimal and occurs at a reduced rate with scleral lenses. Topical drugs that are applied once the lens is worn do not accumulate at a high rate in the fluid reservoir. On the contrary, drugs placed in the reservoir prior to lens insertion should remain for most of the scleral lens wearing time. However, little is known about the dosage and concentration of medications in a scleral lens.

Although scleral lenses prevent the possibility of a toxic reaction, other complications can occur. Topical medications are formulated to penetrate the cornea and possibly even deeper, depending on the nature of the disease to be treated. With soft or scleral lens wear, the medication is not able to reach the ocular surface, and the cornea may not be able to effectively achieve the concentration needed for physiological impact. At the very least, the medication effect is reduced. Topical medications should be applied without the scleral lens on the eye. Patients can remove their lenses, apply the medication, wait 5–10 minutes and then resume scleral lens wear. It is also important to recommend non-preserved artificial tears/comfort drops and care products due to the possibility of crossed-effects or a toxic reaction between preserved agents from medications or solutions in contact with the ocular surface.

From an environmental perspective, scleral lenses compare favorably to other types of contact lenses. Any contact lens will reduce exposure to allergens and pollens. Dust or particles may get under small-diameter gas permeable lenses and potentially dislodge the lenses. This does not occur with scleral lenses due to minimal tear exchange once the lens is stabilized. Some soft lenses may dehydrate and become uncomfortable if worn in challenging environments. Scleral lens material is not influenced by external conditions such as desiccation. Scleral lenses can be a valid option to benefit patients with regular corneas in challenging, dusty or allergenic environments.

CONCLUSION

Prescribing scleral lenses for patients with regular corneas or switching patients from other modalities to scleral lenses is feasible. First, practitioners identify a patient's need, which is likely to improve vision and/or comfort. Scleral lenses can significantly enhance the lens wearing experience of patients with regular corneas, especially in astigmatic, presbyopic or marginal dry eye patient populations. For patients with regular corneas and common refractive errors, the risk-to-benefit ratio needs to be evaluated, and an appropriate lens selected. In conclusion, scleral lenses are becoming part of a practitioner's standard armamentarium to improve the contact lens experience of their patients.

CONFLICT OF INTEREST

The author declares no conflict of interest, financial or otherwise.

ACKNOWLEDGEMENTS

Declared none.

REFERENCES

[1] van der Worp E, Bornman D, Ferreira DL, Faria-Ribeiro M, Garcia-Porta N, González-Meijome JM. Modern scleral contact lenses: A review. Cont Lens Anterior Eye 2014; 37(4): 240-50. [http://dx.doi.org/10.1016/j.clae.2014.02.002] [PMID: 24631015]

[2] Nichols JJ. 2014 Annual Report. Contact Lenses 2014. *C. L.* Spectrum 2015; 30(January): 22-7.

[3] Rumpakis J. New Data on Contact Lens Dropouts: An International Perspective. Rev Optom 2010; 147(1): 37-42.

[4] Nichols JJ, Willcox MD, Bron AJ, *et al.* The TFOS International Workshop on Contact Lens Discomfort: Executive Summary. Invest Ophthalmol Vis Sci. 54: TFOS7-TFOS13.

[5] Dumbleton K, Caffery B, Dogru M, *et al.* The TFOS International Workshop on Contact Lens Discomfort: report of the subcommittee on epidemiology. Invest Ophthalmol Vis Sci 2013; 54(11): TFOS20-36. [http://dx.doi.org/10.1167/iovs.13-13125] [PMID: 24058130]

[6] Alipour F, Kheirkhah A, Jabarvand Behrouz M. Use of mini scleral contact lenses in moderate to severe dry eye. Cont Lens Anterior Eye 2012; 35(6): 272-6. [http://dx.doi.org/10.1016/j.clae.2012.07.006] [PMID: 22902924]

[7] Kalsow CM, Reindel WT, Merchea MM, Bateman KM, Barr JT. Tear cytokine response to multipurpose solutions for contact lenses. Clin Ophthalmol 2013; 7: 1291-302. [http://dx.doi.org/10.2147/OPTH.S44642] [PMID: 23847409]

[8] Ellen S. SCOPE Study: Current consensus of prescribers' scleral lens wear and care recommendations. American Academy of Optometry meeting New Orleans.

[9] Maeda N. Evaluation of optical quality of corneas using corneal topographers. Cornea 2002; 21(7) (Suppl.): S75-8. [http://dx.doi.org/10.1097/01.ico.0000263123.53521.4d] [PMID: 12484703]

[10] Roberts B, Athappilly G, Tinio B, Naikoo H, Asbell P. Higher order aberrations induced by soft

contact lenses in normal eyes with myopia. Eye Contact Lens 2006; 32(3): 138-42. [http://dx.doi.org/10.1097/01.icl.0000195570.73454.a5] [PMID: 16702868]

[11] Khan MS, Humayun S, Fawad A, Ishaq M, Arzoo S, Mashhadi F. Comparison of higher order aberrations in patients with various refractive errors. Pak J Med Sci 2015; 31(4): 812-5. [PMID: 26430409]

[12] Sabesan R, Johns L, Tomashevskaya O, Jacobs DS, Rosenthal P, Yoon G. Wavefront-guided scleral lens prosthetic device for keratoconus. Optom Vis Sci 2013; 90(4): 314-23. [http://dx.doi.org/10.1097/OPX.0b013e318288d19c] [PMID: 23478630]

[13] Holden BA. The principles and practice of correcting astigmatism with soft contact lenses. Aust J Optom 1975; 58: 279-99.

[14] Richdale K, Berntsen DA, Mack CJ, Merchea MM, Barr JT. Visual acuity with spherical and toric soft contact lenses in low- to moderate-astigmatic eyes. Optom Vis Sci 2007; 84(10): 969-75. [http://dx.doi.org/10.1097/OPX.0b013e318157c6dc] [PMID: 18049362]

[15] Michaud L, Barriault C, Dionne A, Karwatsky P. Empirical fitting of soft or rigid gas-permeable contact lenses for the correction of moderate to severe refractive astigmatism: a comparative study. Optometry 2009; 80(7): 375-83. [http://dx.doi.org/10.1016/j.optm.2008.11.008] [PMID: 19545851]

[16] Plainis S, Atchison DA, Charman WN. Power profiles of multifocal contact lenses and their interpretation. Optom Vis Sci 2013; 90(10): 1066-77. [http://dx.doi.org/10.1097/OPX.0000000000000030] [PMID: 23995515]

[17] Belda-Salmerón L, Drew T, Hall L, Wolffsohn JS. Objective analysis of contact lens fit. Cont Lens Anterior Eye 2015; 38(3): 163-7. [http://dx.doi.org/10.1016/j.clae.2015.01.006] [PMID: 25726510]

[18] Young C, Kading DL, Brujic M. Strategies for Success with Specialty Multifocal Contact Lenses. Go beyond the rack to customize lenses to meet the needs of your presbyopic patients. Review of Cornea and Contact Lenses 2013.

[19] DeNaeyer G. Scleral lens decentration 2014.http://www.pentavisionevents.com/ckfinder/userfiles/files/DeNaeyer-Scleral%20Lens%20Decentration.pdf

[20] Michaud L, van der Worp E, Brazeau D, Warde R, Giasson CJ. Predicting estimates of oxygen transmissibility for scleral lenses. Cont Lens Anterior Eye 2012; 35(6): 266-71. [http://dx.doi.org/10.1016/j.clae.2012.07.004] [PMID: 22878418]

[21] Jaynes JM, Edrington TB, Weissman BA. Predicting scleral GP lens entrapped tear layer oxygen tensions. Cont Lens Anterior Eye 2015; 38(1): 44-7. [http://dx.doi.org/10.1016/j.clae.2014.09.008] [PMID: 25447853]

[22] Compañ V, Oliveira C, Aguilella-Arzo M, Mollá S, Peixoto-de-Matos SC, González-Méijome JM. Oxygen diffusion and edema with modern scleral rigid gas permeable contact lenses. Invest Ophthalmol Vis Sci 2014; 55(10): 6421-9. [http://dx.doi.org/10.1167/iovs.14-14038] [PMID: 25190661]

[23] Compañ V, Oliveira C, Aguilella-Arzo M, Edgrington T, Weissman B. Modeling Corneal Oxygen with Scleral Gas Permeable Lens Wear. Opt Vis Sci 2016. Epub ahead of print

[24] Ng LH, Wang Z. Chan C-Y. Yueng W-N. Corneal physiological changes after short-term scleral lens wear. BCLA meeting. Liverpool, UK. 2015.

[25] Miller WL, Vance K, Johnson L, Bergmanson JP. Scleral contact lens effect on central and peripheral corneal thickness. Invest Ophthalmol Vis Sci 2015; 56: 6103 .http://iovs.arvojournals.org/article.aspx?articleid=2336208&resultClick=1

[26] Soeters N, Visser ES, Imhof SM, Tahzib NG. Scleral lens influence on corneal curvature and pachymetry in keratoconus patients. Cont Lens Anterior Eye 2015; 38(4): 294-7.

[http://dx.doi.org/10.1016/j.clae.2015.03.006]

[27] Lau J, Reeder R. Localized corneal graft rejection from scleral lens wear with excessive limbal clearance 2015.http://www.pentavisionevents.com/ckfinder/userfiles/files/Lau%20-%20Scleral%20 Contact%20Lens%20Complications%20with%20Excessive%20Limbal%20Clearance.pdf

[28] Ryff B, Lasby A, Pack L. Corneal decompensation after scleral lens wear in a compromised cornea 2015.http://www.pentavisionevents.com/ckfinder/userfiles/files/Ryff%20-%20Corneal%20 Decompensation%20after%20Scleral%20Wear%20in%20a%20Compromised%20Cornea.pdf

[29] Giasson CJ, Morency J, Michaud L. Measuring oxygen levels under scleral lenses of different clearances. Invest Ophthalmol Vis Sci 2015; 56: 6074.http://iovs.arvojournals.org/article.aspx?articleid=2336175&resultClick=1

[30] Benjamin WJ, Hill RM. Human cornea: individual responses to hypoxic environments. Graefes Arch Clin Exp Ophthalmol 1988; 226(1): 45-8.
[http://dx.doi.org/10.1007/BF02172717] [PMID: 3342975]

[31] Efron N, Ed. Stromal edema Contact Lens Complications. 2nd ed. Edinburgh: Butterworth-Heinemann 2004; pp. 132-40.

[32] Efron N. Contact lens-induced changes in the anterior eye as observed *in vivo* with the confocal microscope. Prog Retin Eye Res 2007; 26(4): 398-436.
[http://dx.doi.org/10.1016/j.preteyeres.2007.03.003] [PMID: 17498998]

[33] Holden BA, Williams L, Zantos SG. The etiology of transient endothelial changes in the human cornea. Invest Ophthalmol Vis Sci 1985; 26(10): 1354-9.
[PMID: 3930418]

[34] Holden BA, Sweeney DF. The significance of the microcyst response: a review. Optom Vis Sci 1991; 68(9): 703-7.
[http://dx.doi.org/10.1097/00006324-199109000-00005] [PMID: 1745495]

[35] Smith GT, Mireskandari K, Pullum KW. Corneal swelling with overnight wear of scleral contact lenses. Cornea 2004; 23(1): 29-34.
[http://dx.doi.org/10.1097/00003226-200401000-00005] [PMID: 14701954]

[36] Kauffman MJ, Gilmartin CA, Bennett ES, Bassi CJ. A comparison of the short-term settling of three scleral lens designs. Optom Vis Sci 2014; 91(12): 1462-6.
[http://dx.doi.org/10.1097/OPX.0000000000000409] [PMID: 25279781]

[37] Alipour F, Behrouz MJ, Samet B. Mini-scleral lenses in the visual rehabilitation of patients after penetrating keratoplasty and deep lamellar anterior keratoplasty. Cont Lens Anterior Eye 2015; 38(1): 54-8.
[http://dx.doi.org/10.1016/j.clae.2014.10.001] [PMID: 25457628]

[38] Fonn D, Gauthier CA, Pritchard N. Patient preferences and comparative ocular responses to rigid and soft contact lenses. Optom Vis Sci 1995; 72(12): 857-63.
[http://dx.doi.org/10.1097/00006324-199512000-00003] [PMID: 8749332]

[39] Alió JL, Soria F, Abbouda A, Peña-García P. Laser *in situ* keratomileusis for -6.00 to -18.00 diopters of myopia and up to -5.00 diopters of astigmatism: 15-year follow-up. J Cataract Refract Surg 2015; 41(1): 33-40.
[http://dx.doi.org/10.1016/j.jcrs.2014.08.029] [PMID: 25465210]

[40] Michaud L, Forcier P. Comparing two different daily disposable lenses for improving discomfort related to contact lens wear. Cont Lens Anterior Eye 2015. S1367-0484(15)30034-5

[41] Chan A, Manche EE. Effect of preoperative pupil size on quality of vision after wavefront-guided LASIK. Ophthalmology 2011; 118(4): 736-41.
[http://dx.doi.org/10.1016/j.ophtha.2010.07.030] [PMID: 21093922]

[42] Schallhorn S, Brown M, Venter J, Hettinger K, Hannan S. The role of the mesopic pupil on patient-

reported outcomes in young patients with myopia 1 month after wavefront-guided LASIK. J Refract Surg 2014; 30(3): 159-65.
[http://dx.doi.org/10.3928/1081597X-20140217-02] [PMID: 24763720]

[43] Gatti RF, Lipener C. Optical performance of different soft contact lenses based on wavefront analysis. Arq Bras Oftalmol 2008; 71(6) (Suppl.): 42-6.
[http://dx.doi.org/10.1590/S0004-27492008000700009] [PMID: 19274410]

[44] Gumus K, Gire A, Pflugfelder SC. The impact of the Boston ocular surface prosthesis on wavefront higher-order aberrations. Am J Ophthalmol 2011; 151(4): 682-690.e2.
[http://dx.doi.org/10.1016/j.ajo.2010.10.027] [PMID: 21269603]

[45] Hussoin T, Le HG, Carrasquillo KG, Johns L, Rosenthal P, Jacobs DS. The effect of optic asphericity on visual rehabilitation of corneal ectasia with a prosthetic device. Eye Contact Lens 2012; 38(5): 300-5.
[http://dx.doi.org/10.1097/ICL.0b013e3182657da5] [PMID: 22929305]

[46] Pritchard N, Fonn D. Dehydration, lens movement and dryness ratings of hydrogel contact lenses. Ophthalmic Physiol Opt 1995; 15(4): 281-6.
[http://dx.doi.org/10.1016/0275-5408(95)00004-W] [PMID: 7667020]

[47] Wolffsohn JS, Emberlin JC. Role of contact lenses in relieving ocular allergy. Cont Lens Anterior Eye 2011; 34(4): 169-72.
[http://dx.doi.org/10.1016/j.clae.2011.03.004] [PMID: 21530362]

[48] Rathi VM, Sudharman Mandathara P, Vaddavalli PK, Dumpati S, Chakrabarti T, Sangwan VS. Fluid-filled scleral contact lenses in vernal keratoconjunctivitis. Eye Contact Lens 2012; 38(3): 203-6.
[http://dx.doi.org/10.1097/ICL.0b013e3182482eb5] [PMID: 22367220]

[49] Margolis R, Thakrar V, Perez VL. Role of rigid gas-permeable scleral contact lenses in the management of advanced atopic keratoconjunctivitis. Cornea 2007; 26(9): 1032-4.
[http://dx.doi.org/10.1097/ICO.0b013e3181245172] [PMID: 17893528]

[50] Walline JJ, Jones LA, Rah MJ, *et al.* Contact Lenses in Pediatrics (CLIP) Study: chair time and ocular health. Optom Vis Sci 2007; 84(9): 896-902.
[http://dx.doi.org/10.1097/OPX.0b013e3181559c3c] [PMID: 17873776]

[51] Castagno VD, Fassa AG, Carret ML, Vilela MA, Meucci RD. Hyperopia: a meta-analysis of prevalence and a review of associated factors among school-aged children. BMC Ophthalmol 2014; 14: 163.
[http://dx.doi.org/10.1186/1471-2415-14-163] [PMID: 25539893]

[52] Foster PJ, Jiang Y. Epidemiology of myopia. Eye (Lond) 2014; 28(2): 202-8.
[http://dx.doi.org/10.1038/eye.2013.280] [PMID: 24406412]

[53] O'Donoghue L, Breslin KM, Saunders KJ. The changing profile of astigmatism in childhood: the NICER study. Invest Ophthalmol Vis Sci 2015; 56(5): 2917-25.
[http://dx.doi.org/10.1167/iovs.14-16151] [PMID: 26024077]

[54] Efron N, Morgan PB, Woods CA. Survey of contact lens prescribing to infants, children, and teenagers. Optom Vis Sci 2011; 88(4): 461-8.
[http://dx.doi.org/10.1097/OPX.0b013e31820efa0f] [PMID: 21336226]

[55] Gungor I, Schor K, Rosenthal P, Jacobs DS. The Boston Scleral Lens in the treatment of pediatric patients. J AAPOS 2008; 12(3): 263-7.
[http://dx.doi.org/10.1016/j.jaapos.2007.11.008] [PMID: 18258469]

[56] Booras K. 2014. http://www.aaopt.org/scleral-contact-lenses-applications-sports-vision

[57] Altman B. Injury of a mini-scleral contact lens wearer. Contact Lens Today 2013.

[58] Barnett M. Multifocal scleral lenses 2015. http://www.clspectrum.com/articleviewer.aspx?articleID=113639

[59] Brujic M, Miller J. 2011. http://www.reviewofcontactlenses.com/content/d/dry_eye/c/27244/

[60] Charman WN, Chateau N. The prospects for super-acuity: limits to visual performance after correction of monochromatic ocular aberration. Ophthalmic Physiol Opt 2003; 23(6): 479-93. [http://dx.doi.org/10.1046/j.1475-1313.2003.00132.x] [PMID: 14622350]

[61] Athaide HV, Campos M, Costa C. Study of ocular aberrations with age. Arq Bras Oftalmol 2009; 72(5): 617-21. [http://dx.doi.org/10.1590/S0004-27492009000500003] [PMID: 20027396]

[62] Gemoules G, Morris KM. Rigid gas-permeable contact lenses and severe higher-order aberrations in postsurgical corneas. Eye Contact Lens 2007; 33(6 Pt 1): 304-7. [http://dx.doi.org/10.1097/ICL.0b013e318033edde] [PMID: 17993826]

[63] Jinabhai A, Radhakrishnan H, O'Donnell C. Visual acuity and ocular aberrations with different rigid gas permeable lens fittings in keratoconus. Eye Contact Lens 2010; 36(4): 233-7. [http://dx.doi.org/10.1097/ICL.0b013e3181e52dd1] [PMID: 20543704]

[64] Walker M, Caroline P, Kinoshita B, *et al.* The protective advantage of scleral contact lenses. Global Specialty Lens Symposium. Las Vegas. 2015.

[65] Caroline P. McMahon J. Lotoczky, J. Rosen C. Michaud L. Scleral lenses: new opportunities, new challenges. Global Specialty Lens Symposium.

[66] Forister JF, Forister EF, Yeung KK, *et al.* Prevalence of contact lens-related complications: UCLA contact lens study. Eye Contact Lens 2009; 35(4): 176-80. [http://dx.doi.org/10.1097/ICL.0b013e3181a7bda1] [PMID: 19474751]

[67] Tan DT, Pullum KW, Buckley RJ. Medical applications of scleral contact lenses: 1. A retrospective analysis of 343 cases. Cornea 1995; 14(2): 121-9. [http://dx.doi.org/10.1097/00003226-199503000-00001] [PMID: 7743792]

[68] Ozkurt Y, Oral Y, Karaman A, Ozgür O, Doğan OK. A retrospective case series: use of SoftPerm contact lenses in patients with keratoconus. Eye Contact Lens 2007; 33(2): 103-5. [http://dx.doi.org/10.1097/01.ICL.0000258592.12598.28] [PMID: 17496704]

[69] Bourassa S, Benjamin WJ. Clinical findings correlated with contact angles on rigid gas permeable contact lens surfaces *in vivo*. J Am Optom Assoc 1989; 60(8): 584-90. [PMID: 2794327]

[70] Fortuin MF, Schilperoort J, Evans BJ, Edgar DF, Manon HM, Kiers H. Randomised controlled study comparing comfort-related outcomes between two rigid gas permeable (RGP) lenses with different sessile drop contact angles. Ophthalmic Physiol Opt 2011; 31(2): 190-9. [http://dx.doi.org/10.1111/j.1475-1313.2010.00812.x] [PMID: 21309806]

[71] Barnett M. 2012. http://www.reviewofcontactlenses.com/content/c/37103/

[72] Corzine JC, Klein SA. Factors determining rigid contact lens flexure. Opt Vis Sci 74(8): 639-45. [http://dx.doi.org/10.1097/00006324-199708000-00025]

[73] Van der Worp E, Graf T, Caroline PJ. Exploring beyond the corneal borders. Contact Lens Spectr 2010; 6: 26-32.

[74] Meyler J G, Ruston D. Toric RGP Contact Lenses made easy. Optician 1996; 209(5504): 30-5.

[75] Meyler J, Morgan P. Advanced contact lens fitting. Part 2. Toric rigid lens fitting. Optician 1997; 5604(213): 18-23.

[76] Messer B. The developing role of scleral lenses in today's society. Contact Lens Spectrum 2013; 28(10): 40-55.

[77] Van der Worp E. Reviving the art of soft lens fitting. Contact Lens Spectrum 2013; 28(9): 44-55.

[78] Visser ES, Visser R, Van Lier HJ. Advantages of toric scleral lenses. Optom Vis Sci 2006; 83(4): 233-

6.
[http://dx.doi.org/10.1097/01.opx.0000214297.38421.15] [PMID: 16614579]

[79] Vance KD, Miller W, Bermangson J. Measurement of tear flow in scleral contact lens wearers. American Academy of Optometry meeting.

[80] Choy CK, Cho P, Boost MV. Cytotoxicity and effects on metabolism of contact lens care solutions on human corneal epithelium cells. Clin Exp Optom 2012; 95(2): 198-206.
[http://dx.doi.org/10.1111/j.1444-0938.2011.00687.x] [PMID: 22233282]

[81] Choy CK, Cho P, Boost MV. Cytotoxicity of rigid gas-permeable lens care solutions. Clin Exp Optom 2013; 96(5): 467-71.
[http://dx.doi.org/10.1111/cxo.12039] [PMID: 23638722]

[82] Lazon de la Jara P, Papas E, Diec J, Naduvilath T, Willcox MD, Holden BA. Effect of lens care systems on the clinical performance of a contact lens. Optom Vis Sci 2013; 90(4): 344-50.
[http://dx.doi.org/10.1097/OPX.0b013e318288e10c] [PMID: 23478632]

[83] Bennett ES. GP annual report 2015. C.L. Spectrum 2015; 1(October)http://www.clspectrum.com/articleviewer.aspx?articleID=113321

[84] Schafer J, Steffen R, Rah MJ. Patient satisfaction with a novel one-step hydrogen peroxide solution. Clin Ophthalmol 2014; 8: 2035-40.
[PMID: 25336902]

[85] Tyagi G, Alonso-Caneiro D, Collins M, Read S. Tear film surface quality with rigid and soft contact lenses. Eye Contact Lens 2012; 38(3): 171-8.
[http://dx.doi.org/10.1097/ICL.0b013e31824da99c] [PMID: 22510586]

[86] Huang , *et al.* The application of low-temperature plasma technology on the surface modification of biomaterials. Mater Rev 2004; 18: 72-4.

[87] Samaha D. 2011. http://www.aaopt.org/hydrogen-peroxyde-better-alternative-care- regiment-rgp-a-d-rigid-contact-lenses

CHAPTER 7

Instrumentation

Jeffrey Sonsino[1], **S. Barry Eiden**[2,*] and **Randy Kojima**[3]

[1] *Optique, PLLC, Nashville, TN, USA*

[2] *North Suburban Vision Consultants, Ltd., Keratoconus Specialists of Illinois, Deerfield, IL, USA*

[3] *Pacific University College of Optometry, Forest Grove, OR, USA*

Abstract: When modern scleral lenses became popular, the instruments used to help evaluate the health of the cornea and conjunctiva in the presence of the lenses were somewhat rudimentary. Practitioners observed the cornea and conjunctiva with the biomicroscope, used manual keratometry or Placido topography to map the corneal curvature, and relied on sodium fluorescein to judge the depth of the post-lens tear reservoir. The instrumentation industry quickly fills unmet needs, and the scleral lens market is no exception. In fact, the pace of innovation of instrumentation that is used to evaluate these relatively complex medical devices has been, and will continue to be, dramatic for years beyond the publication of this textbook. At the time of publication, currently available instrumentation is reviewed and may likely change with innovation and technology. Innovations and advances in modern imaging technology have enhanced traditional methods of scleral lens fitting. While not every piece of equipment is required for fitting scleral lenses, any additional information provided by unique instrumentation aids the practitioner to achieve fitting success.

Keywords: Clearance, Confocal, Documentation, Endothelial cell, Frequency domain, Lens thickness, OCT, Oxygen, Pachymetry, Pentacam, Photography, Sagittal depth, Scan, Scheimpflug, Scleral topographers, Technology, Time domain, Topography, Ultrasound, Vault.

INTRODUCTION

When modern scleral lenses became popular, the instruments used to help evaluate the health of the cornea and conjunctiva in the presence of scleral lenses were somewhat rudimentary. Practitioners observed the cornea and conjunctiva with the biomicroscope, used manual keratometry or Placido topography to map the corneal curvature, and relied on sodium fluorescein to judge the depth of the post-lens tear reservoir. The instrumentation industry quickly fills unmet needs, and the scleral lens market is no exception. In fact, the pace of innovation of

* **Corresponding author S. Barry Eiden:** North Suburban Vision Consultants, Ltd, Keratoconus Specialists of Illinois, Deerfield, IL, USA; Tel: 847 412 0311; Fax: 847 412 0316; E-mail: sbeiden@nsvc.com

instrumentation that is used to evaluate these relatively complex medical devices has been, and will continue to be, dramatic for years beyond the publication of this textbook. Currently available instrumentation is reviewed in this publication and may likely change with future innovation and technology.

Anterior Segment Optical Coherance Tomography

Optical Coherance Tomography (OCT) provides real time, *in vivo*, cross sectional imaging of scleral lenses on eyes. Gemoulis first used OCT to aid in the fitting of scleral lenses shortly after OCT was adapted for use in the anterior segment [1]. Although the technology to empirically fabricate scleral lenses from OCT data has not been developed, practitioners have used OCT to aid in many aspects of scleral lens design [2].

What is OCT?

OCT is an interferometry technique used to image semi-transparent structures. Interferometry is a class of techniques used in other sciences in which electromagnetic radiation is superimposed onto itself to detect certain information about the waves. In the case of OCT, near-infrared light emitted by a superluminescent light-emitting diode (LED) is split into two beams using a beam splitter. The two beams travel different paths within the device and then further onto the target. The beams recombine and hit a detector. Whatever stands in the way of the beams creates a phase shift and interference. The images viewed are due to a change in refractive index or opacity.

First-generation OCT relied on time domain mechanics. Time domain OCT contained mechanical moving parts that performed rapid A-scans. Therefore, there was a physical limit to the speed of image acquisition, resulting in a lower resolution image (8-10 μm). The next-generation OCT is spectral domain. In spectral domain OCT, all wavelengths of light are recorded simultaneously by a spectrometer. This results in 50 to 1,000 times faster acquisition speed and higher resolution (3-5 μm).

The basic types of scans on the commercially available OCT units are cross line scans, line scans, and pachymetry measurements. Cross line scans take a near-simultaneous vertical and horizontal scan and present the data on a single page (Fig. **1**). Line scans usually take the horizontal slice, although the axis of the line scan can be controlled by the examiner. Rotating the line scan allows the examiner to image an area of concern in an exact plane (Fig. **2**). Pachymetry mapping is the third type of anterior segment imaging applicable to scleral lenses. In this application, the pachymetry map is not used to determine corneal thickness as the name implies. Pachymetry measurements allow the examiner to image eight axes near-simultaneously in a radial pattern (Fig. **3**). Subsequently, the examiner can select the type of scan desired based on the number of scans required for the given application.

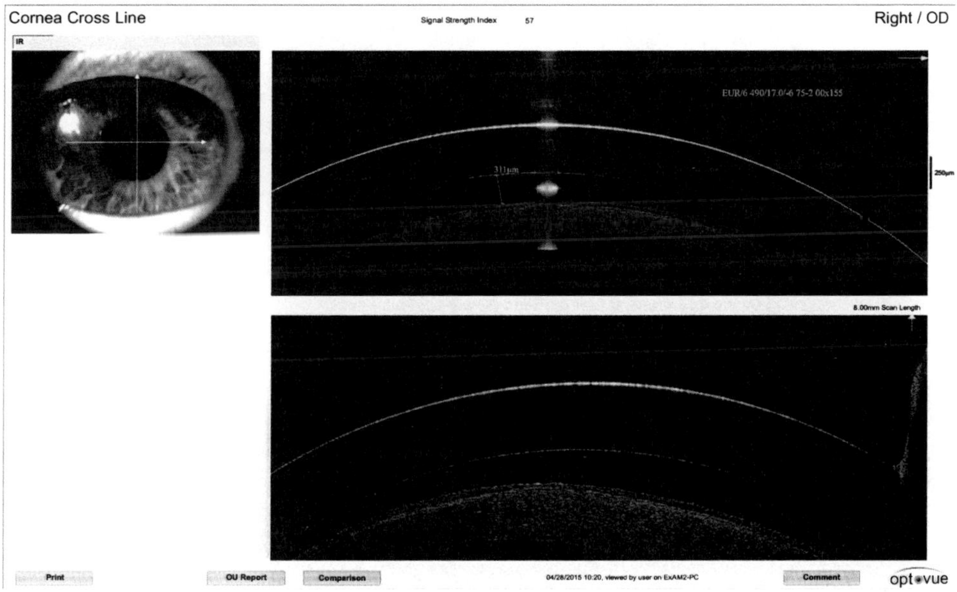

Fig. (1). Anterior segment OCT cross line scan (Optovue, Fremont, CA) of a keratoconic eye with a scleral lens. There are three images presented with this scan: en face image (top left), horizontal line scan (top right), and vertical line scan (bottom right). The horizontal line scan is labelled with vault measurement and lens parameters entered manually by the examiner.

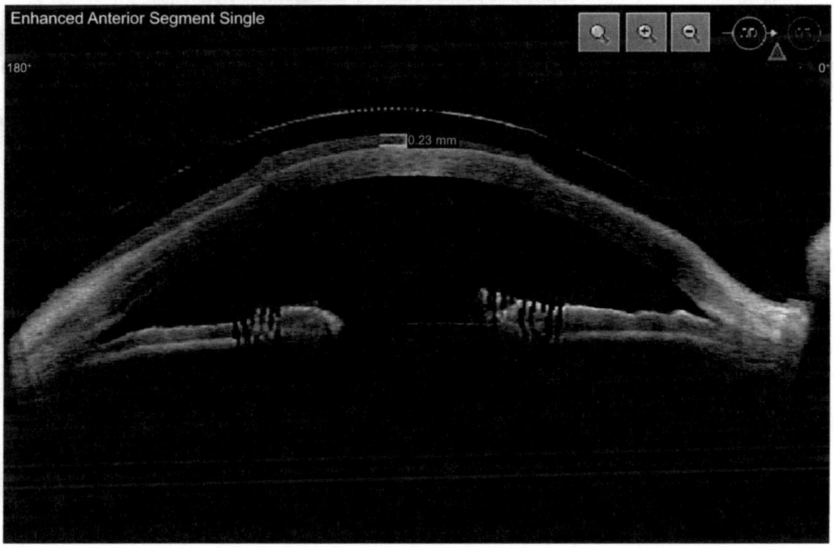

a

Fig. 2 contd.....

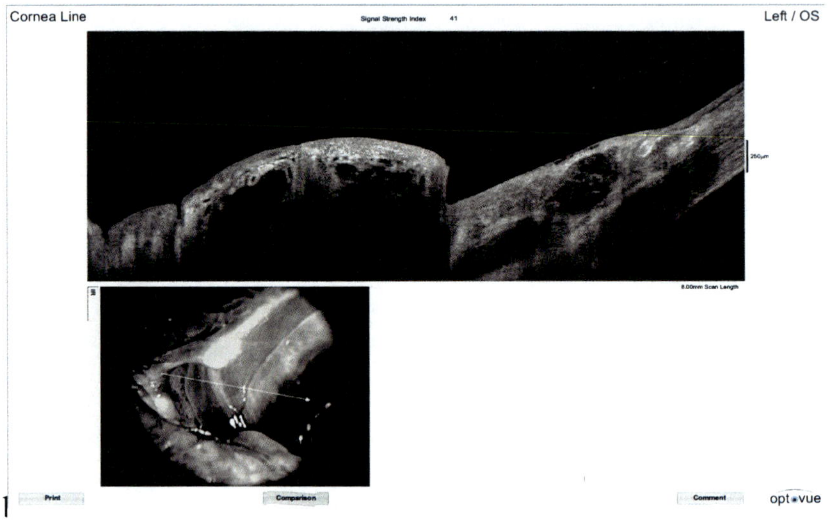

Fig. (2). (a) Anterior segment OCT line scan (Carl Zeiss Meditec, Dublin, CA) of a left eye on a patient with ocular graft-*versus*-host disease. In this limbus-to-limbus view, the entire scleral lens is visible. This time domain system has lower resolution than current spectral domain OCTs. (b) Anterior segment OCT line scan rotated by the operator (Optovue, Fremont, CA). The line scan was rotated to show the edge of a scleral lens impinging a trabeculectomy with poor bleb morphology. The axis of the line scan is shown in the en face image (white arrow below).

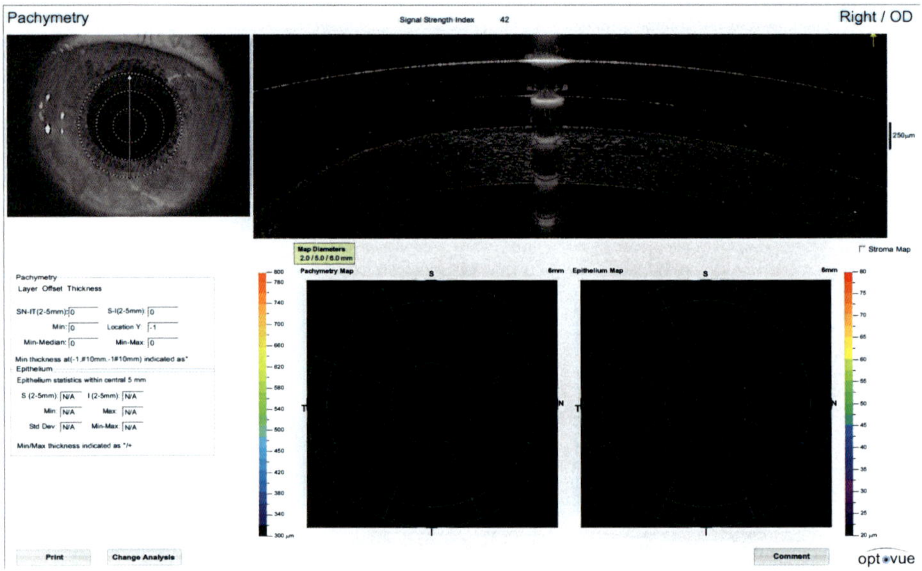

Fig. (3). Anterior segment pachymetry image (Optovue, Fremont, CA) of a patient wearing a scleral lens. Five axes are imaged near-simultaneously in one scan and can be accessed by hovering a mouse over different axes.

One of the key reasons to use anterior segment OCT in the evaluation of scleral lenses is to measure the distance between two surfaces using a caliper tool. The most common measurement taken is vault, or clearance, between the posterior surface of the lens and the cornea and sclera. Using the caliper tool to measure vault allows the examiner to make decisions about the fit in relationship to the ocular structures with a level of precision not found with sodium fluorescein evaluation (Fig. **4**) [1, 3]. One limitation when measuring the vault of scleral lenses on anterior segment OCT images is that the caliper tools were not designed to read through a scleral lens. Therefore, the difference in index of refraction between tears and the lens material makes the absolute value of the measurement somewhat inaccurate. If the lens material is kept consistent, the vault measurement will be repeatable and consistent between measurements.

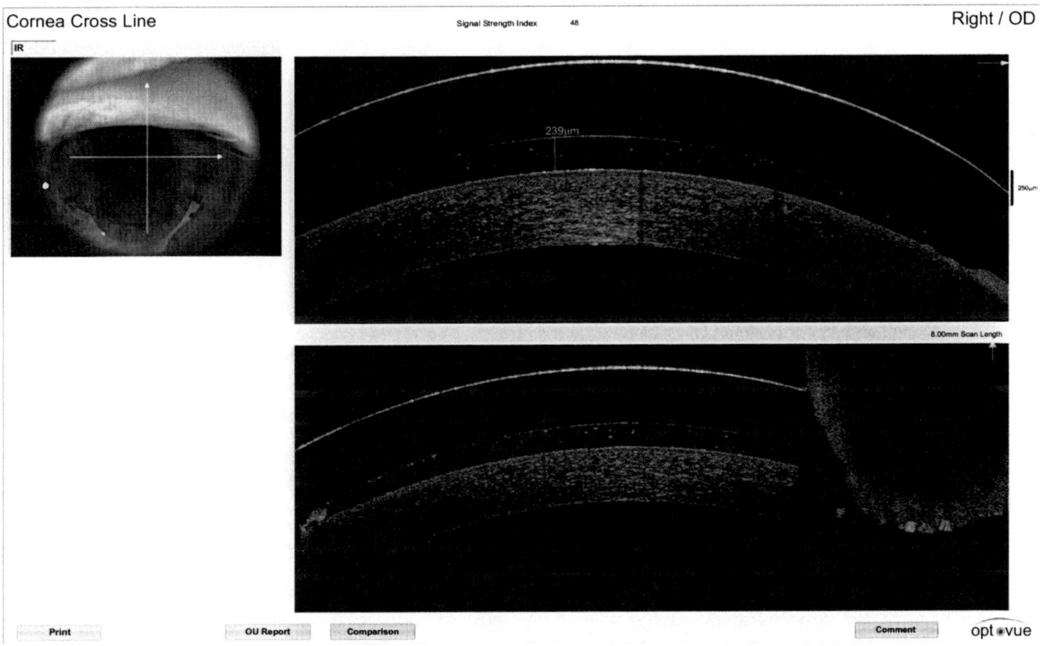

Fig. (4). Vault measurement on an anterior segment OCT image (Optovue, Fremont, CA) in a patient with ocular cicatricial pemphigoid. Since the diagnosis dictates a relatively normal corneal shape, the caliper tool can be used in the horizontal line scan.

Proper placement of the caliper tool to measure vault depends on the underlying diagnosis. For example, in a patient with severe dry eye in ocular graft-*versus*-host disease, measuring the vault can be accomplished in the horizontal cross line scan at the closest or furthest points between the posterior lens surface and the cornea. However, if the underlying diagnosis is keratoconus, the caliper should be placed near the apex of the cone (cross-referencing the corneal topography for location) (Fig. **5**). With this location, the examiner can ensure that the apex of the cone is truly vaulted, even with the expectation of lens settling throughout the day.

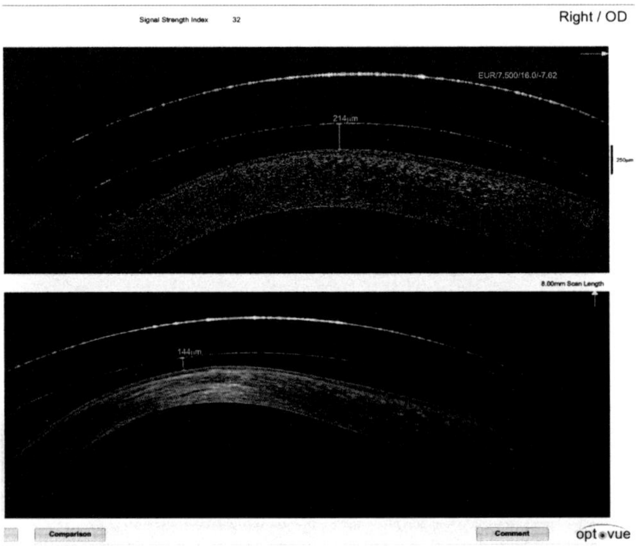

Fig. (5). Vault measurement on anterior segment OCT (Optovue, Fremont, CA) of a patient with keratoconus wearing a scleral lens. The caliper tool is placed near the apex of the cone. Although there is no way to pinpoint the exact location of the apex of the cone using anterior segment OCT, this point can be estimated when comparing to corneal topography.

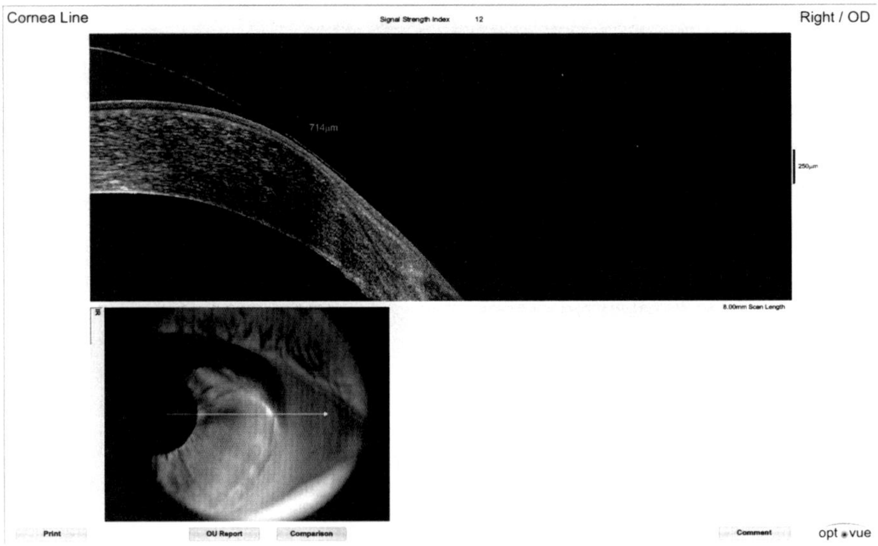

a.

Fig. (6a). Measurement of corneal touch initially.

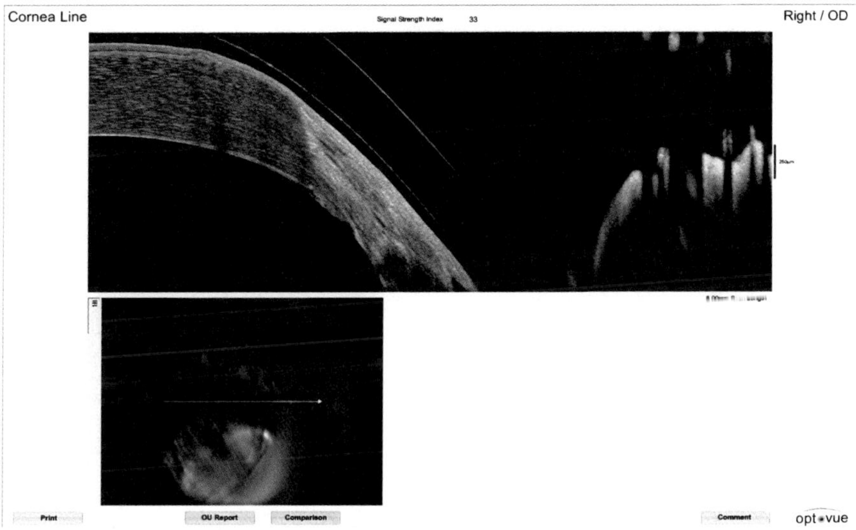

b.

Fig. (6b). Measurement of corneal touch improved with subsequent parameter changes.

A second function of the caliper tool is to measure areas of concern. For example, areas of touch between the posterior lens surface and the cornea can be measured and compared between subsequent lens redesign and imaging to determine whether the proper parameters were changed (Fig. **6a and b**). The significance of edge bearing into an elevated area of the conjunctiva can be assessed to aid in clinical decision making (Fig. **2**).

With the advent of scleral lens designs that incorporate novel intermediate curves or tangential mid-peripheral zones, it is important to assess the peripheral cornea and its relationship to the scleral lens. Lenses that accommodate oblate corneas, such as post-RK or post-LASIK, or that have oblate shapes themselves to accommodate conditions such as pellucid marginal degeneration or Salzmann's nodular degeneration can be precisely evaluated for risk of bearing on underlying decentered treatment zones or corneal and conjunctival elevations. The technique for obtaining a mid-peripheral scan is slightly different from obtaining a central scan. The best images are obtained when the examiner uses a fixation target to move the patient's gaze rather than moving the machine to accommodate primary gaze. The reason is that in primary gaze, computer software must de-warp the image, so the image is not as pure. When manipulating the patient's gaze (to the left or right) and using a line scan, the cornea and sclera appear flat (Fig. **7**).

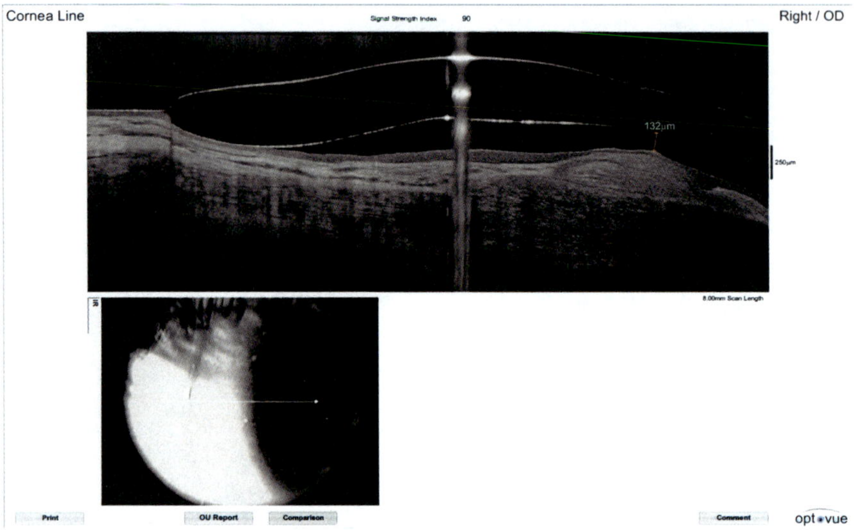

Fig. (7). Imaging of the mid-periphery of a patient with Salzmann's nodular degeneration using anterior segment OCT (Optovue, Fremont, CA). The patient was fit with a scleral lens with a tangential mid-periphery that nicely vaulted and accommodated the elevated peripheral nodules.

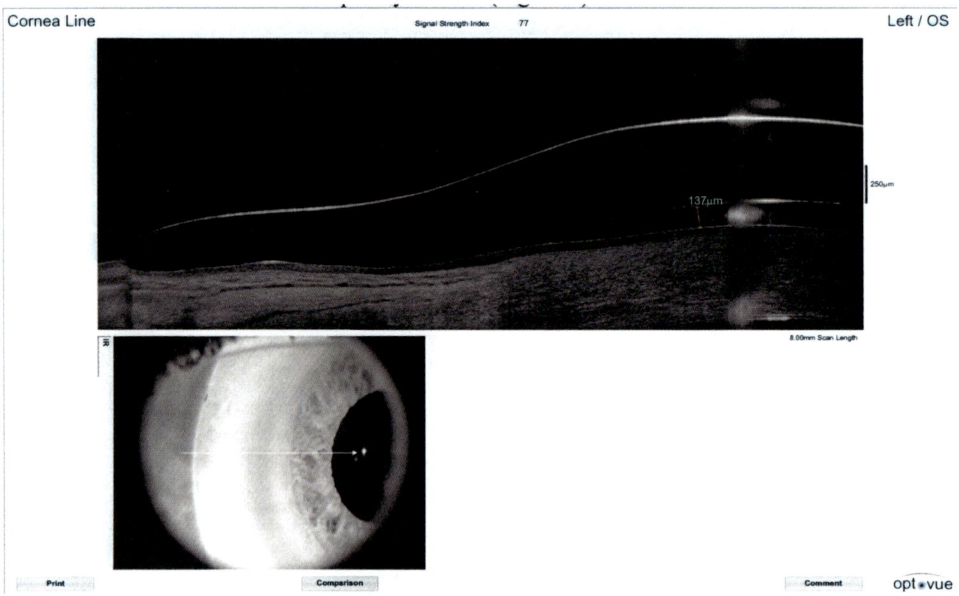

Fig. (8). Imaging the periphery of a lens with anterior segment OCT to determine whether a pinguecula is adequately cleared. When other scleral lens designs failed due to impingement on a nasal pinguecula, an impression-based lens was fit to vault the exact area. After 9 months of wear, the patient experienced symptom-free wear.

Finally, OCT can be used to assess the edge alignment of scleral lenses on the conjunctiva and underlying sclera. This is most useful when there are anatomic variants on the conjunctiva such as pingueculae, glaucoma blebs, or scleral patch grafts. Some scleral lens designs are capable of sectorally vaulting specific areas. OCT of the lens periphery allows the practitioner to determine whether anatomic variants are adequately cleared (Fig. **8**).

Pachymetry

Pachymetry is the measurement of corneal thickness. Corneal thickness can be a tool for indicating whether scleral lenses are contraindicated, establishing a baseline prior to scleral lens fitting, monitoring corneal physiology, and determining whether a scleral lens should be modified.

Baseline corneal thickness may demonstrate a very thin cornea due to keratoconus, suggesting the relative severity of disease progression. Conversely, a post-penetrating keratoplasty eye that has a very thick graft (and low endothelial cell count) may be contraindicated for scleral lenses due to impending graft failure.

Some scleral lenses may need to be modified when there is an increase in measured corneal thickness, suggesting corneal edema. Therefore, it is always a good idea prior to initiation of scleral lens wear to take baseline pachymetry measurements. After baseline is established and scleral lens wear commences, subsequent pachymetry measurements can help determine whether there is subclinical corneal edema necessitating re-evaluation.

Michaud *et al.* demonstrated key criteria for fitting scleral lenses by which the risk for corneal edema can be minimized [4]. If corneal edema is detected with pachymetry after long-term wear, the fit can be modified to satisfy the criteria of highest Dk material, a center thickness of no greater than 250 µm, and vault of no greater than 200 µm [4].

Pachymetry may be measured using either optical or ultrasound methods. The gold standard method of measuring pachymetry has most commonly been ultrasound, although there are shortcomings with this technique [5, 6]. For instance, repeat measurements are not precise because a probe tip must be held to the cornea by an examiner. Similarly, if the probe tip is tilted, an oblique measurement will yield a falsely high thickness.

Newer methods of optical measurement are less operator-dependent and more computer-driven. Contrary to ultrasound pachymetry, optical techniques are non-contact. Optical measurements may be taken by different methods including

Scheimpflug, OCT, specular microscopy, and intra-operatively using low coherence reflectometry [5, 7].

Scleral Topography

Scleral topographers are the most recent devices available to aid the evaluation of scleral lenses. Unlike corneal topographers, they can image out to a diameter of 22.00 mm, rather than a standard corneal diameter of 12.0 mm.

There are currently two models available in the market: the Eye Surface Profiler (ESP) (Eaglet Eye, Netherlands) and the sMap3D (Precision Ocular Metrology, New Mexico, USA, distributed by Visionary Optics, Virginia, USA). The ESP measures 350,000 points to derive height data of the cornea and sclera. The measurement with ESP is taken with the patient in primary gaze. The measurement with sMap3D is based on direct triangulation, which is performed by using a uniquely coded projected pattern to identify matching points across multiple views. The sMap3D combines topographic measurement of primary, superior, and inferior gaze directions. Software then stitches the images together to generate superior and inferior scleral data in addition to nasal and temporal data. Both scleral topographers are fluorescein based, project patterns on the ocular surface, and use two offset cameras to triangulate height data.

The ESP uses software to fit various commercially available scleral lens designs based on sagittal height and curvature data. The sMap3D has functionality to either have the practitioner design every lens parameter or download the scleral topography directly to Visionary Optics' consultative service to produce a best-fit Europa Scleral Lens (Visionary Optics, Virginia, USA).

Scheimpflug Tomography

Tomography is the process of generating a "tomogram," or a two-dimensional image of a slice or section through a three-dimensional object. One method to achieve this is using Scheimpflug imaging. The Scheimpflug principle was first introduced by Theodor Scheimpflug [8], a cartographer of the Austrian navy, over 100 years ago. The result is the ability to image with extended depth of focus. The Scheimpflug principle has been applied in ophthalmic instrumentation to obtain optical sections of the entire anterior segment of the eye, from the anterior surface of the cornea to the posterior surface of the lens. This technology is used by instruments such as Pentacam (Oculus) and Galilei (Zeimer) to measure the anterior and posterior corneal surfaces as well as other anterior segment structures. *via* the use of a rotating Scheimpflug camera (single camera in Pentacam or dual cameras in Galilei), a 360-degree representation of the anterior segment is achieved (Fig. **9**).

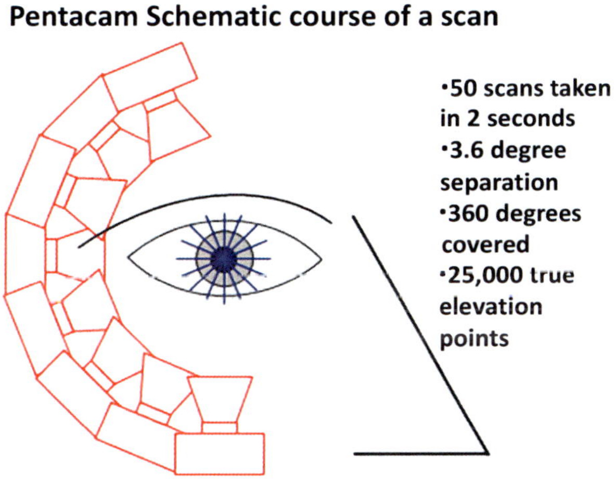

Fig. (9). Rotating Scheimpflug camera scan used with Pentacam standard tomography (Oculus) demonstrating 360-degree anterior segment coverage.

Scheimpflug tomography of the anterior segment provides true elevation-based data that enables measurements of anterior corneal elevation, posterior corneal elevation, and full corneal thickness (also known as global pachymetry) as well as high quality imaging and structural measurements of the anterior segment (Figs. **10** and **11**). Elevation data can also be used to derive corneal curvature measurements analogous to curvature data obtained by Placido-based corneal topography. True elevation corneal measurements and data of both the anterior and posterior cornea, along with global pachymetry data, allow for highly accurate detection of corneal ectatic diseases such as keratoconus. Specifically, posterior corneal elevation anomalies will precede, and be more advanced, than anterior corneal elevation and curvature anomalies in keratoconus [9]. There are many cases in which the anterior corneal surface, both in terms of curvature and elevation, are normal, but a posterior corneal elevation anomaly exists (Figs. **12a and b**). This can result in a false negative for keratoconus detection if only the anterior corneal surface was analyzed (such as with Placido-based corneal topography). Conversely, some conditions or situations exist that appear to be suggestive of keratoconus, when in fact the cornea is quite normal. Displaced corneal apices and large deviations of the visual axis (large angle kappa) are two examples in which Placido topography, or any representation of anterior corneal surface curvature, would suggest keratoconus, and elevation-based Scheimpflug tomography would reveal an otherwise normal cornea [10]. Additionally, anomalies of global pachymetry are also highly diagnostic of keratoconus (Fig. **13**). Although in many cases of keratoconus the thinnest point of the cornea is below the normal range of minimum corneal thickness, the rate of change of corneal thickness from the thinnest point peripherally is most sensitively diagnostic of ectatic corneal disease. This is true even in cases in which the thickness of all points of the cornea is statistically normal [11]. Another example of the benefits of Scheimpflug tomography is for the differential diagnosis of pellucid marginal corneal degeneration (PMD). Traditionally, the classic "kissing dove" or "crab claw" pattern seen on curvature topography maps has been considered pathognomonic of PMD. However, it is established that in PMD, there is localized peripheral corneal thinning found inferiorly about one millimeter from the limbus. When examining global pachymetry maps and corneal elevation maps in the vast majority of cases with traditionally classic topography curvature maps thought to be PMD, the thinnest point of the cornea is significantly more central than previously determined. In fact, the global pachymetry maps, and both the anterior and posterior corneal elevation maps, are quite typical of keratoconus [12]. Typical PMD patterns are observed only in a very small percentage of cases.

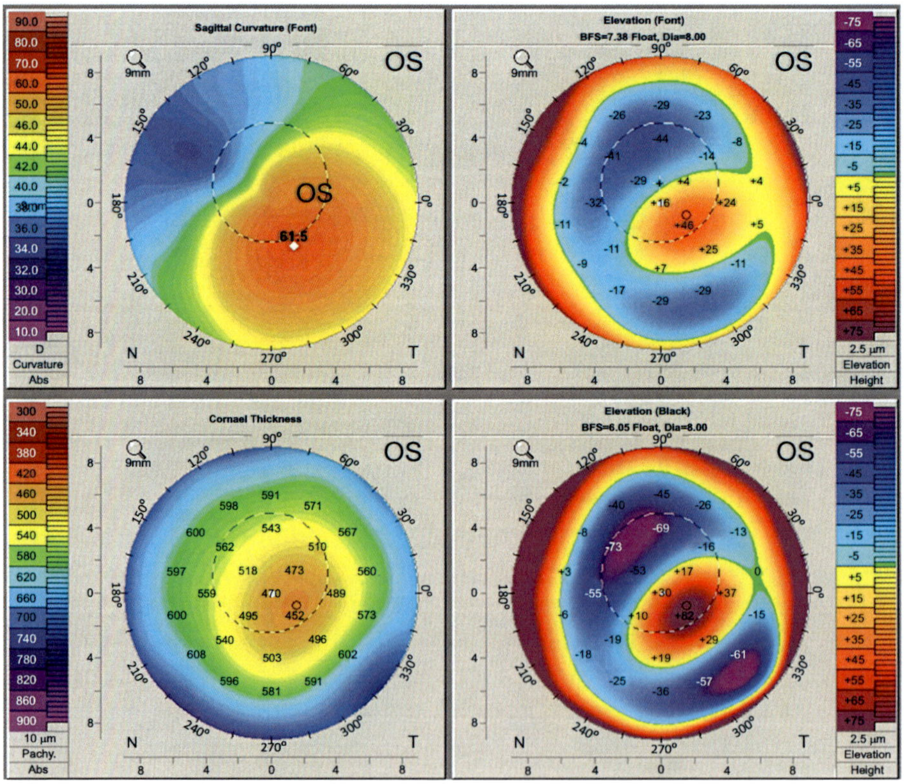

Fig. (10). The 4-Map Refractive display of Pentacam corneal tomography for a case of keratoconus. Upper left is anterior corneal curvature, upper right is anterior corneal elevation, lower right is posterior corneal elevation, and lower left is global corneal thickness (pachymetry).

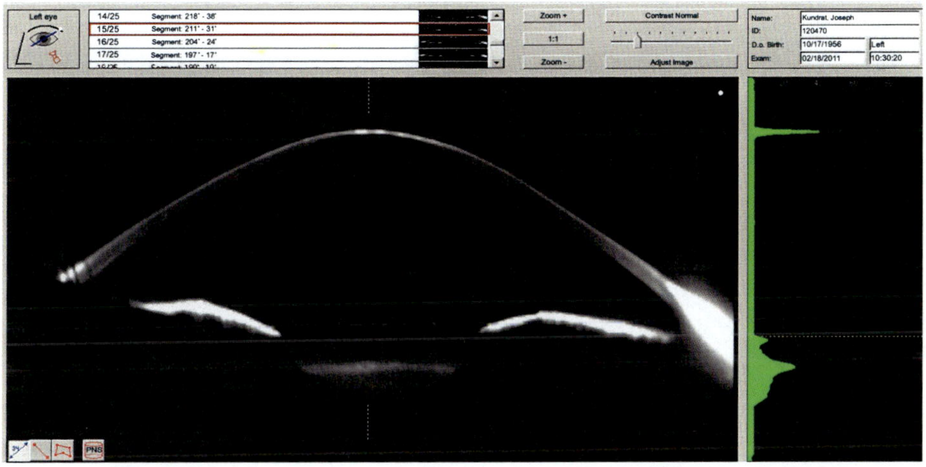

Fig. (11). Scheimpflug image of a case of advanced keratoconus along an oblique meridian.

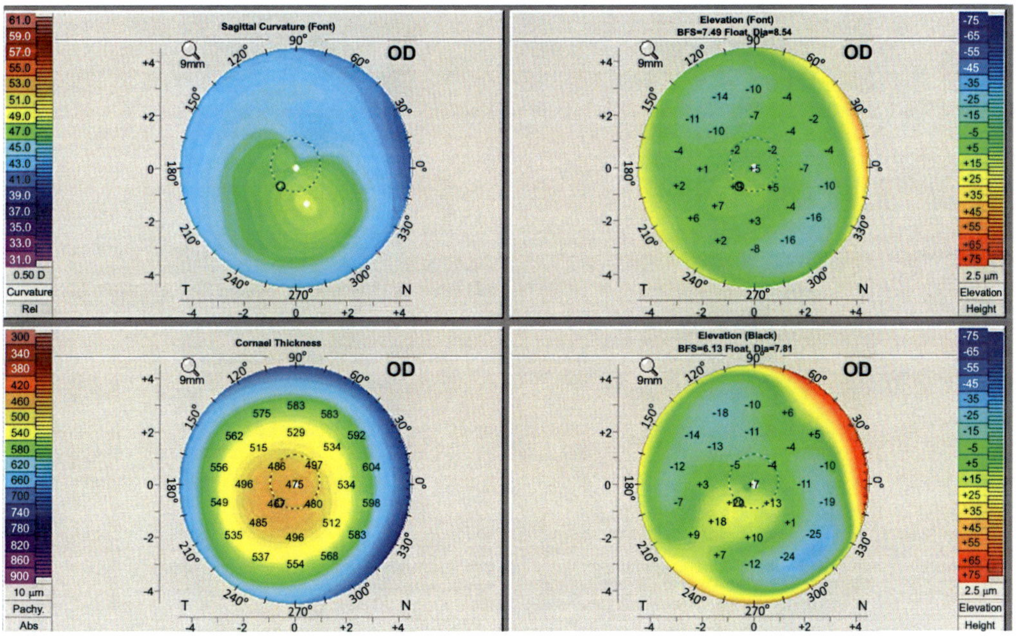

Fig. (12a). Pentacam 4-Map display right eye of a patient with normal anterior curvature and elevation but with abnormality of the posterior elevation and global pachymetry.

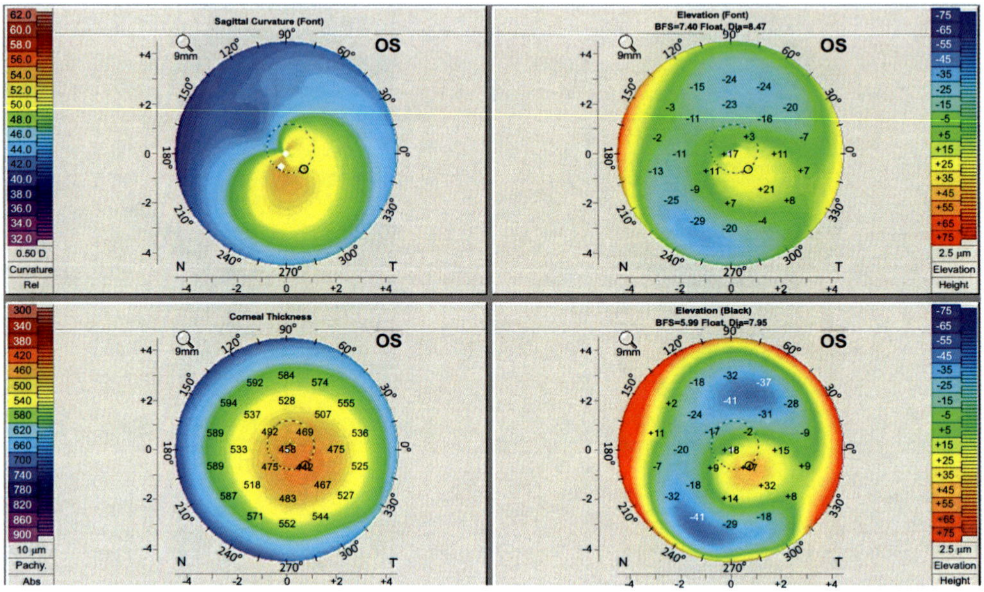

Fig. (12b). Pentacam 4-Map display of left eye of same patient as in Fig. (**3a**). This shows classic abnormalities of both the anterior and posterior cornea as well as global pachymetry.

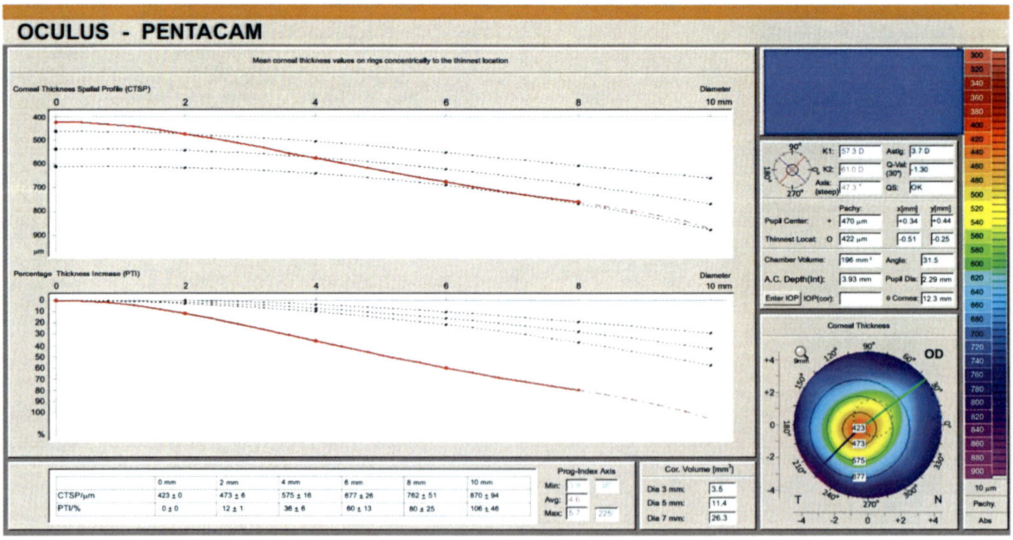

Fig. (13). Pentacam display of absolute corneal thickness with the corneal thickness spatial profile (CTSP) chart and the rate of change of corneal thickness from the thinnest point out to the periphery with the percentage thickness increase (PTI) chart.

Anterior segment imaging and associated structural measurements are also quite useful information acquired from Scheimpflug tomography. Corneal, iris surface, anterior chamber angle, and crystalline lens imaging are used in disease documentation and to assess change over time. Measurements of the anterior chamber angle, anterior chamber depth, and volume in 360 degrees are very useful in assessing patients potentially at risk for angle closure glaucoma. Quantification of lens opacities via a method termed densitometry can be used to document and monitor for the progression of cataracts. Finally, the various measurements obtained from Scheimpflug tomography have been shown to be highly valuable in IOL calculations, especially for patients with keratoconus or those who have undergone refractive surgical corneal procedures [13].

One of the newest developments in Scheimpflug tomography is its ability to image and measure corneo-scleral profiles. These measurements can be used to detect and quantify asymmetries of scleral shape when measured in 360 degrees. Software is being developed to enable this data to be used in the virtual design of both corneal and scleral lenses (Fig. **14**).

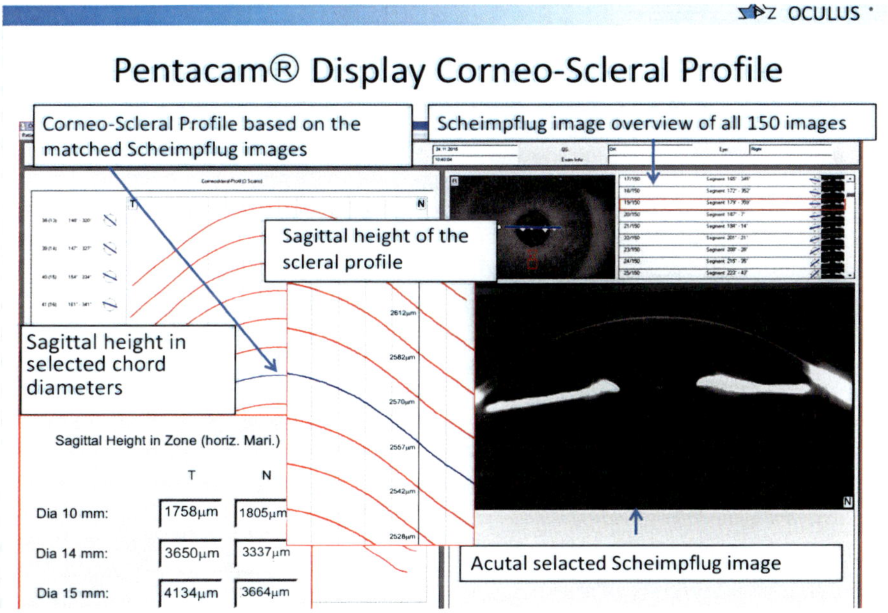

Fig. (14). Pentacam scleral profile software display.

Specular Microscopy

Specular microscopy is a non-invasive imaging technology that allows the practitioner to visualize, analyze, and document corneal endothelial cells. Utilizing contemporary computerized specular microscopy systems, practitioners can determine endothelial cell size, shape and concentration of cells within a square millimeter area (cell count) and image intracellular and extracellular anomalies. Specular microscopic systems work by projecting light onto the cornea and capturing the image that is reflected from the optical interface between the corneal endothelium and the aqueous. The software can then compute the cell count, the percentage of normally shaped cells (typically hexagonal) and the uniformity of the cell sizes within the analyzed area (Fig. **15**). The corneal endothelium is a single cell layer with the primary physiological function to maintain corneal thickness and transparency. The cornea naturally imbibes aqueous from the anterior chamber, which is required to provide various nutrients to the cornea. However, without the proper functioning of endothelial cells to actively pump fluid out of the stroma via active transport mechanisms, the cornea would become edematous [14].

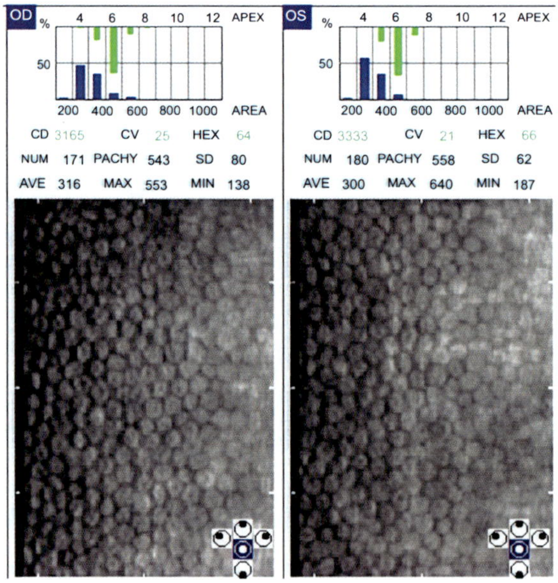

Fig. (15). Specular microscopy images and statistics of normal endothelium for both right and left eyes.

Abnormalities discovered by specular microscopy include a reduction of the percentage of hexagonally shaped cells (pleomorphism), an increase in variation of cell size from cell to cell (polymegathism), and a reduction of the normal age-related values for cell counts. Additionally, specular microscopy will provide an optical pachymetry measurement taken at a specific location and allow for direct image observation for the detection of abnormalities such as guttata and endothelial cell inclusion bodies [15]. The causes of what are best described as "endotheliopathies" are numerous and include Fuch's corneal dystrophy, age-related corneal endotheliopathy, surgically induced endotheliopathy, uveitis-induced endotheliopathy, glaucoma-induced endotheliopathy (from long-term damage from elevated intraocular pressure), and, most pertinent to this text, contact lens-induced endotheliopathy. All types of endotheliopathies can lead to corneal edema (Fig. **16**). The primary reason for contact lens-induced endotheliopathy is corneal hypoxia. Contact lens wear can produce both acute and chronic changes in corneal endothelial morphology. Increases in polymegathism are commonly found as the initial abnormality in contact lens-induced endotheliopathy. If not addressed, continued chronic corneal hypoxia can lead to more dramatic abnormalities revealed with specular microscopy, such as reduced cell count, and can also result in both corneal vascularization and edema. Addressing the offending contact lens-induced hypoxia will often result in improvements in endothelial findings with specular microscopy. However, it may take extended periods of time for such recovery to occur. In many cases, endothelial morphological changes may be permanent [16].

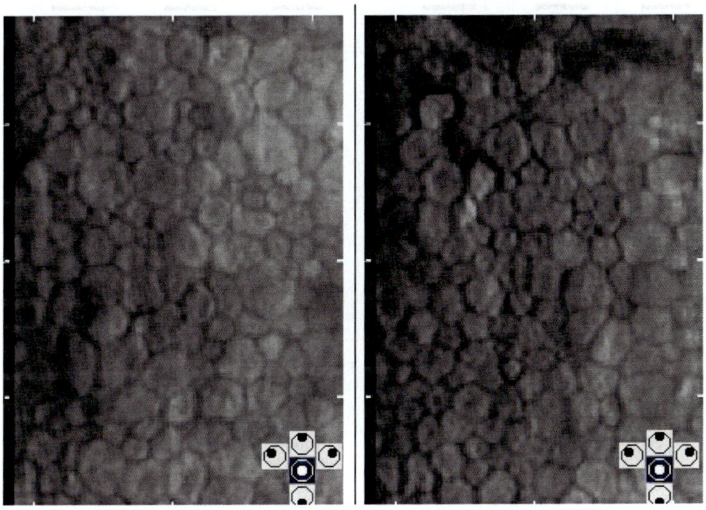

Fig. (16). Specular microscopy of a case of contact lens-induced endotheliopathy due to over a decade of continuous overnight wear of low-oxygen-permeable contact lenses.

Baseline specular microscopic imaging and analysis is a useful technique for all contact lens wearers. Periodic repeat imaging is dependent on the risk factors for the development of corneal hypoxia. These risks include continuous or overnight wear of contact lenses, thick lens designs, and/or lenses fabricated from lower-oxygen-transmissible materials and corneas at risk for hypoxic sequelae and other causes of endotheliopathies.

Confocal Microscopy

Confocal microscopy is an imaging technology that developed as a highly useful technique for the detailed study of corneal cellular structure. Minsky developed the original confocal microscope in 1955 to image brain tissue [17]. Confocal microscopy was further developed during the 1980s and 1990s [18]. The basic principle of a confocal microscope comprises a single point source of illumination on a single point of tissue that is simultaneously imaged by a camera in the same plane, hence the term "confocal." This produces an image with a very high resolution but with virtually no depth of field. To address this problem, the instrument simultaneously illuminates a small region of tissue with thousands of spots of light that are reconstructed to create a usable field of view with exquisitely high resolution and magnification [19].

Confocal microscopy is a powerful diagnostic technique that allows non-invasive microscopic examination of the cornea. However, until recently, use in clinical practice has been limited to research centers. New developments in technology have made confocal microscopy available to clinical practitioners. The applications of confocal microscopy in ophthalmic practice are numerous and expanding as the value of these high-resolution images is realized. For example, confocal microscopy can be used in the identification of the causative organism in patients with infective keratitis such as *Acanthamoeba* keratitis [20] and other causes of contact lens-related keratitis [21]. There is also a role for confocal microscopy in the deeper understanding of keratoconus, glaucoma, and dry eye/ocular surface disease. Confocal microscopy has been shown to be highly applicable to the detection of corneal anomalies induced by contact lens wear (Fig. **17**). For example, continuous wear of contact lenses can cause a loss of keratocytes [22]. The physical presence of a contact lens may induce the release of inflammatory mediators that may cause keratocyte dysgenesis or apoptosis [23]. Additionally, a study of long-term contact lens wearers discovered that a type of chronic corneal stromal change was observed in all subjects with long-term contact lens wear. What was described as highly reflective pan-stromal microdot deposits in the corneal stroma were found in all long-term contact lens wearers (both soft and rigid gas permeable subjects) and not in the control patients. Because patients with soft contact lens wear had more pronounced corneal degeneration than those with gas permeable contact lens wear, the authors assumed that the deposits were induced by chronic hypoxia. The condition of stromal microdot degeneration as observed with confocal microscopy may indicate the early stage of a significant corneal disease, which eventually may affect large numbers of patients after decades of contact lens wear [24]. In a pilot study, *in vivo* confocal microscopy was useful for detecting an elevated immune response associated with soft contact lenses and for identifying lens-related and solution-related immune responses [25]. The researchers found that differences in central corneal dendritic immune cell densities associated with various combinations of soft contact lens materials and lens care solutions could be detected by *in vivo* confocal microscopy.

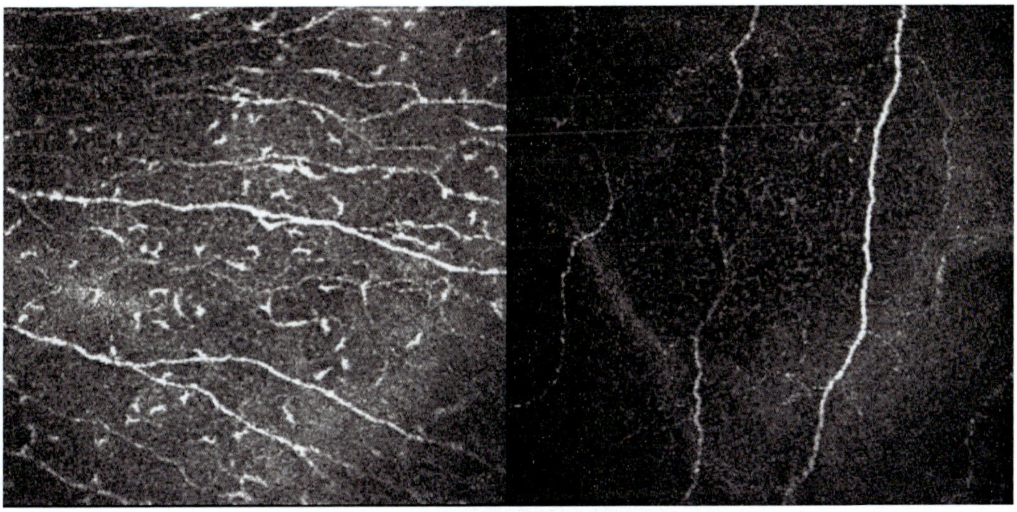

Fig. (17). Confocal corneal microscopy images showing dendritic cell upregulation of the immune response in a patient wearing silicone hydrogel contact lenses (A) versus a non-contact lens wearing patient (B). Images courtesy of Christine Sindt.

As confocal microscopy continues to develop, researchers are discovering more about a variety of diseases and conditions with the use of this technology.

Placido-Based Corneal Topography

Imaging systems for measuring corneal shape, power, and elevation are generically described as topographers. The most common subset of these instruments is Placido, or reflective imaging technology. These topographers are sold in large numbers due to their relatively low cost and software oriented for contact lens application. Typically, topographers measure the cornea alone, which would appear inadequate to aid in scleral lens fitting. Surprisingly, they provide numerous benefits in a large-diameter scleral lens practice.

One of the most important questions a corneal topographer can answer is: which patients need a scleral lens, and which do not? When is the asymmetry of the cornea so severe that custom soft, corneal gas permeable, or hybrid lenses are doomed to failure? The elevation map of topographers can guide practitioners to determine when the height changes across the corneal surface are beyond a specific threshold, requiring a scleral lens to vault the asymmetry. Using the elevation map display, ensure that the best fit spherical radius is <±10 µm from the corneal surface at the apex. Next, find the axis of greatest elevation change from the highest point (red) to the lowest point (blue). The micron change in height from the highest to the lowest points along this axis indicates the elevation differential (Fig. **18**). Zheng *et al.* determined that corneal gas permeable lenses could be successful 88% of the time when the elevation differential was <350 µm [26]. However, when the differential was >350 µm, a corneal gas permeable lens did not successfully fit the asymmetry, and a scleral lens was required. This fast and efficient analysis can help to guide the decision-making process when choosing a lens modality for challenging corneal shapes.

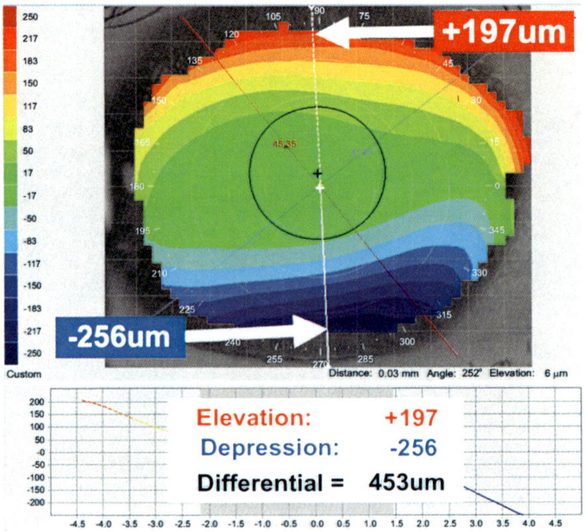

Fig. (18). On the elevation display with the Medmont E300 corneal topographer, find the highest and lowest elevation, then calculate the differential between them to determine whether a corneal GP or scleral lens is best suited for the eye.

When a practitioner chooses a scleral lens as the appropriate modality for the patient, it is beneficial when only one diagnostic lens is needed to achieve success, reducing chair time significantly. Selecting the correct initial diagnostic lens is challenging, especially for an irregular cornea. Considering that keratometry readings are captured over a very small surface area, they are of limited value in scleral lens fitting. However, measuring the height of the cornea can be very helpful in determining the initial sagittal depth of the scleral lens required. Numerous topographers provide the measurement of corneal sagittal depth over a specified chord diameter (Fig. **19**). Caroline *et al.* showed that the height of the normal cornea was approximately 1750 µm over a 10mm chord [27, 28]. By comparison, keratoconic patients averaged a height of 1960 µm, or approximately 200 µm higher, over the same chord diameter [28, 29]. Practitioners should increase the height of the selected diagnostic lens when the depth of the cornea is higher than average. Conversely, when the measured height is below the mean, practitioners should choose a lower-depth diagnostic lens to obtain an appropriate apical clearance.

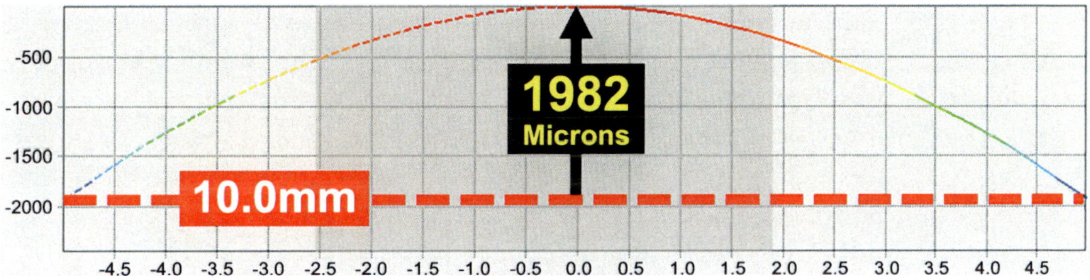

Fig. (19). The sagittal depth of the cornea can be calculated from a chord diameter of 10mm with the Medmont E300 corneal topographer, then the height of the eye in microns is measured. This height calculation can be used to determine the relative depth of the cornea and can aid in scleral lens selection.

Scleral Sag Factor Table

Diameter (mm)	Microns (µm)
14.0	1700
14.5	1800
15.0	2000
15.5	2200
16.0	2400
16.5	2600
17.0	2800
17.5	3000
18.0	3200

Fig. (20). The scleral sag factor table can be used in combination with the measured corneal sag at 10mm. Determine the diameter that the scleral lens height is calculated over, then add the appropriate sag factor depth along with the measured corneal sag and desired posterior fluid layer clearance. The combination of depths added together will aid in the selection of the initial scleral diagnostic lens.

This method can be improved upon by using the "scleral sag factor." If the topographer can measure the sagittal depth of the cornea across a chord diameter of 10mm, the scleral sag factor provides the depth from the 10mm chord to the point at which the scleral lens height is measured and labeled [28, 30]. The table (Fig. **20**) can be used to determine the scleral sag factor for various scleral lens diameters. For example, if the corneal sagittal depth is 1800 µm and the chosen lens depth is calculated to a 15 mm chord, then a scleral sag factor of 2000 µm should be added. Next, the manufacturer's recommended apical clearance is included in the sum to provide the lens depth required. For example, 1800 + 2000 + fluid thickness in microns = required lens sag. Rather than using keratometry readings, which calculate the measurement at 3 mm, this formula considers the entire anterior chamber depth and is a more scientific approach to selecting the initial diagnostic scleral lens.

The scleral sag factor provides an estimation of the anterior chamber depth from 10 mm across the cornea to the calculated diameter from which the selected scleral lens sag may be measured. This calculation assumes that the peripheral cornea and scleral angle as described by Achong-Coan is an average 38 degrees [29]. As expected, the range of scleral angles falls within a natural bell shape curve, so not all patients will accurately fit into this estimation. To measure and not assume the angle, topography companies can determine the peripheral corneal angle and use it to predict the anterior chamber depth and ideal scleral lens height. After measuring the corneal height across 10 mm, the peripheral corneal angle is assessed and an algorithm is applied (Fig. **21**). The depth of the anterior chamber can be estimated based on the measured height of the cornea and the angle of the periphery [3]. In a study by Harkness *et al.*, this estimated height agrees with other imaging technologies that measure beyond the limbus [31]. Therefore, this may be a more accurate formula for measuring the initial scleral lens depth.

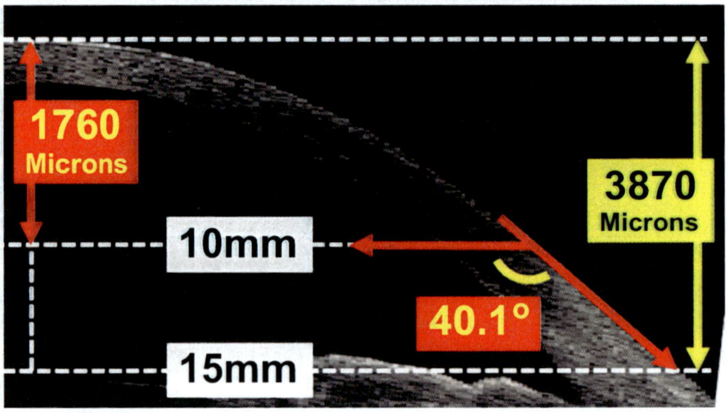

Fig. (21). Measuring corneal sag with the Zeiss Visante OCT across a 10 mm chord, then calculating the scleral angle from 10 mm and beyond allows for the estimation of anterior chamber depth and accurate scleral diagnostic prediction.

Another function of a corneal topographer is the ability to map over a scleral lens with the lens on the eye [32]. When patients manifest residual astigmatism with their scleral lens, the practitioner cannot be certain whether it is internal cylinder or due to lens flexure or warpage. Performing topography or keratometry over the lens can determine whether the anterior surface is spherical, indicating that the residual astigmatism must be internal, which would require front surface optical toricity (Fig. **22**). However, if the anterior surface of a symmetric, spherical scleral lens appears toric, then it must be flexing to create an astigmatic topography or simulated keratometry readings. In some cases, manufacturers recommend increasing the center thickness to reduce lens flexure.

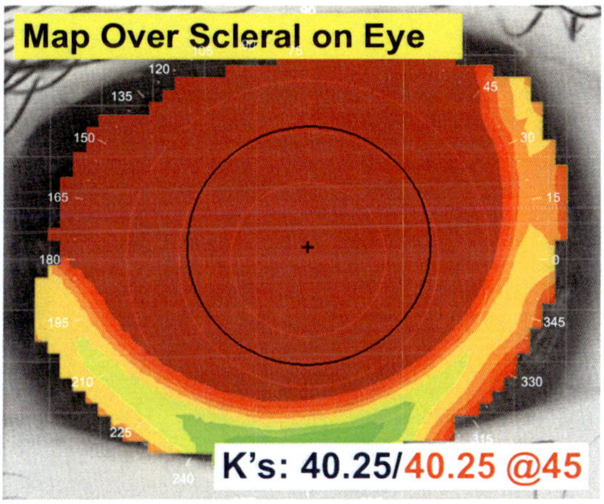

Fig. (22). Performing topography with the Medmont E300 corneal topographer over the scleral lens on eye can be beneficial in determining whether any warpage or flexure may exist. Should residual astigmatism be present in the over-refraction, this method can be used to diagnose whether cylinder is internal or on the anterior surface of the lens.

It seems counter-intuitive that a corneal topographer could benefit the practitioner when fitting a lens that is larger than the cornea. However, corneal topography can be employed at every stage of the scleral lens fitting process. The elevation of the cornea can be assessed to determine whether a patient is ideally suited for a scleral lens. Then the height of the cornea can be predictive of the initial lens to be selected. Coupled with algorithms to estimate the entire anterior chamber depth, the topographer can improve the efficiency of lens selection even beyond its measured capture area. Additionally, topography can be employed with the lens on the eye to understand problems with visual acuity. These units have a wide scope in general practice, but also specifically related to scleral lenses.

SUMMARY

Innovations and advances in modern imaging technology have enhanced traditional methods of scleral lens fitting. While not every piece of equipment is required for fitting scleral lenses, any additional information provided by unique instrumentation aids the practitioner in achieving scleral lens fitting success.

DISCLOSURES

Jeffrey Sonsino
Consultant or research support by: Alcon, Art Optical, Contamac, Johnson & Johnson Vision Care, Optovue, Shire, SynergEyes, Visionary Optics
Shareholder: LVR Technology

S. Barry Eiden
Consulting or research support by: Alcon, Allergan, Bausch + Lomb, Cooper Vision, Oculus, Oasis, Optovue, Shire, Special Eyes, SynergEyes, Vistakon
Financial Interest: EyeVis Eye & Vision Research Institute, International Keratoconus Academy of Eye Care Professionals

Randy Kojima
Consulting or research support by: Precision Technology Services, Cardinal Contact Lens, Medmont International Pty, Alcon, Bausch + Lomb, Contamac and Paragon

CONFLICT OF INTEREST

The authors declare no conflict of interest, financial or otherwise.

ACKNOWLEDGEMENTS

Declared none.

REFERENCES

[1] Gemoules G. A novel method of fitting scleral lenses using high resolution optical coherence tomography. Eye Contact Lens 2008; 34(2): 80-3. [http://dx.doi.org/10.1097/ICL.0b013e318166394d] [PMID: 18327042]

[2] Luo ZK, Jacobs DS. Current and potential applications of anterior segment optical coherence tomography in contact lens fitting. Semin Ophthalmol 2012; 27(5-6): 133-7. [http://dx.doi.org/10.3109/08820538.2012.708814] [PMID: 23163267]

[3] Sonsino J, Mathe DS. Central vault in dry eye patients successfully wearing scleral lens. Optom Vis Sci 2013; 90(9): e248-51. [http://dx.doi.org/10.1097/OPX.0000000000000013]

[4] Michaud L, van der Worp E, Brazeau D, Warde R, Giasson CJ. Predicting estimates of oxygen transmissibility for scleral lenses. Cont Lens Anterior Eye 2012; 35(6): 266-71. [http://dx.doi.org/10.1016/j.clae.2012.07.004] [PMID: 22878418]

[5] Khaja WA, Grover S, Kelmenson AT, Ferguson LR, Sambhav K, Chalam KV. Comparison of central corneal thickness: ultrasound pachymetry *versus* slit-lamp optical coherence tomography, specular microscopy, and Orbscan. Clin Ophthalmol 2015; 9: 1065-70. [PMID: 26109840]

[6] Kuerten D, Plange N, Koch EC, Koutsonas A, Walter P, Fuest M. Central corneal thickness determination in corneal edema using ultrasound pachymetry, a Scheimpflug camera, and anterior segment OCT. Graefes Arch Clin Exp Ophthalmol 2015; 253(7): 1105-9.

[http://dx.doi.org/10.1007/s00417-015-2998-y] [PMID: 25896108]

[7] Soeken TA, Apsey DA, Townley JR, Haas RW, Caldwell MC. Comparison of pachymetry measurements between the Alcon Wavelight EX500 and Sonogage Corneo-Gage plus platforms. J Refract Surg 2015; 31(5): 328-32. [http://dx.doi.org/10.3928/1081597X-20150423-06] [PMID: 25974972]

[8] Scheimpflug T. Der photoperspektrograph und seine anwendung. Photogr Korr 1906; 43: 516-31.

[9] Tomidokoro A, Oshika T, Amano S, Higaki S, Maeda N, Miyata K. Changes in anterior and posterior corneal curvatures in keratoconus. Ophthalmology 2000; 107(7): 1328-32. [http://dx.doi.org/10.1016/S0161-6420(00)00159-7] [PMID: 10889107]

[10] Dharwadkar S, Nayak BK. Corneal topography and tomography. Jour of Clin Ophthalmol and Research 2015; 3(1): 45-62. [http://dx.doi.org/10.4103/2320-3897.149379]

[11] Villavicencio OF. Independent Population Validation of the Belin/Ambrósio Enhanced Ectasia Display: Implications for Keratoconus Studies and Screening. International Journal of Keratoconus and Ectatic Corneal Diseases 2014; 3(1): 1-8.

[12] Belin MW, Asota IM, Ambrosio R Jr, Khachikian SS. What's in a name: keratoconus, pellucid marginal degeneration, and related thinning disorders. Am J Ophthalmol 2011; 152(2): 157-162.e1. [http://dx.doi.org/10.1016/j.ajo.2011.03.028] [PMID: 21708379]

[13] Hill WE. IOL power calculations after keratorefractive surgery. Supplement to Cataract and Refractive Surgery Today 2008; 13-5.

[14] McCarey BE, Edelhauser HF, Lynn MJ. Review of corneal endothelial specular microscopy for FDA clinical trials of refractive procedures, surgical devices, and new intraocular drugs and solutions. Cornea 2008; 27(1): 1-16. [http://dx.doi.org/10.1097/ICO.0b013e31815892da] [PMID: 18245960]

[15] The Konan Cell Book Vol 2 Torrance: Konan Medical USA.

[16] Thomas C. Use Specular Microscopy to Diagnose Corneal Disease. Review of Optometry 2009; 146(6).

[17] Minsky M. Memoir on inventing the confocal scanning microscope. Scanning 1988; 10: 128-38. [http://dx.doi.org/10.1002/sca.4950100403]

[18] Masters BR, Thaer AA. *In vivo* real-time confocal microscopy of wing cells in the human cornea: A new benchmark for *in vivo* corneal microscopy. Bioimages 1995; 3: 7-11.

[19] Efron N, Perez-Gomez I, Mutalib HA, Hollingsworth J. Confocal microscopy of the normal human cornea. Cont Lens Anterior Eye 2001; 24(1): 16-24. [http://dx.doi.org/10.1016/S1367-0484(01)80005-9] [PMID: 16303449]

[20] Kaufman SC, Musch DC, Belin MW, *et al.* Confocal microscopy: a report by the American Academy of Ophthalmology. Ophthalmology 2004; 111(2): 396-406. [http://dx.doi.org/10.1016/j.ophtha.2003.12.002] [PMID: 15019397]

[21] Kaufman SC, Laird JA, Cooper R, Beuerman RW. Diagnosis of bacterial contact lens related keratitis with the white-light confocal microscope. CLAO J 1996; 22(4): 274-7. [PMID: 8906387]

[22] Efron N, Perez-Gomez I, Morgan PB. Confocal microscopic observations of stromal keratocytes during extended contact lens wear. Clin Exp Optom 2002; 85(3): 156-60. [http://dx.doi.org/10.1111/j.1444-0938.2002.tb03028.x] [PMID: 12033976]

[23] Kallinikos P, Efron N. On the etiology of keratocyte loss during contact lens wear. Invest Ophthalmol Vis Sci 2004; 45(9): 3011-20. [http://dx.doi.org/10.1167/iovs.04-0129] [PMID: 15326115]

[24] Böhnke M, Masters BR. Long-term contact lens wear induces a corneal degeneration with microdot deposits in the corneal stroma. Ophthalmology 1997; 104(11): 1887-96. [http://dx.doi.org/10.1016/S0161-6420(97)30011-6] [PMID: 9373122]

[25] Sindt CW, Grout TK, Critser DB, Kern JR, Meadows DL. Dendritic immune cell densities in the central cornea associated with soft contact lens types and lens care solution types: a pilot study. Clin Ophthalmol 2012; 6: 511-9. [http://dx.doi.org/10.2147/OPTH.S28083] [PMID: 22536045]

[26] Zheng F, Caroline P, Kojima R, Lampa M, Kinoshita B, André M. Corneal Elevation Differences and the Initial Selection of Corneal and Scleral Contact Lens (Poster). Las Vegas: GSLS 2015.

[27] Copitestz L, Kinoshita B, Caroline P, Lampa M, Kojima R, André M. Are You Scared of Heights? (Poster Global Specialty Lens Symposium. Las Vegas. 2012.

[28] Kojima R, Caroline P, Graff T, *et al.* Eye shape and scleral lenses contact lens spectrum 2013; 38-43.

[29] Achong-Coan R, Caroline P, Kinoshita B, *et al.* How Do Normal and Keratoconic Eyes Differ in Shape? (Poster Global Specialty Lens Symposium. Las Vegas. 2015.

[30] Caroline P, Kojima R, So K, Kinoshita B, Lampa M, André M. Sagittal Height Uncovered (Poster Global Specialty Lens Symposium. Las Vegas. 2012.

[31] Harkness B, *et al.* Comparison of Sagittal Height Measurement Methods (Poster). American Academy of Optometry 2015.

[32] Kojima R, Caroline P, Kinoshita B, Lampa M, André M, Rosen C. Applications of Corneal Topography Beyond Corneal Shape. Contact Lens Spectr 2013; (28 November): 36-51.

CHAPTER 8

Initial Lens Selection

Jason Jedlicka*

School of Optometry, Indiana University, Bloomington, IN, USA

Abstract: This chapter will cover the process of choosing an initial lens for evaluation when fitting a scleral lens. Topics that will be discussed include what pre-selection factors are helpful with lens selection, what essential design and diameter to select, which lens within a given fitting set to select, as well as alternative methods of lens selection utilizing technology such as OCT and topography.

Keywords: Benefits, Corneal Graft, Diagnostic lens, Diameter, Fit, Initial lens, Lens bearing, Limitations, Oblate, OCT, Post-surgical, Prolate, Refractive Surgery, Sagittal Depth, Sagittal Height, Scleral shape, Software-Guided, Topography, Vault.

INTRODUCTION

The process of fitting scleral lenses can be laborious if done without consideration for the patient's unique ocular characteristics, the various lens designs, and how to select the initial lens for application. Bypassing this process will result in a lens that is less likely to be successful and will require more modification to reach an optimal endpoint. Prior to commencing, thoughtful consideration and insight can ensure that the scleral lens fitting process will be enjoyable for both practitioner and patient. This can yield impressive results. Understanding what initial data is required can help select the ideal design and diagnostic lens. Additionally, utilization of technology to determine the initial lens is explored.

PRE-LENS SELECTION CONCEPTS: WHAT CONSTITUTES AN IDEAL FIT?

When fitting a scleral lens, there are some basic goals to achieve; these enable the selection of the proper lens for that individual from the outset. It is important to understand both the eye being fitted as well as what constitutes an ideal fit. There

* **Corresponding author Jason Jedlicka:** School of Optometry, Indiana University, Bloomington, IN, USA; Tel: (812) 855 - 4651; Fax: (812) 856 - 0934; E-mail: jajedlic@indiana.edu

Melissa Barnett & Lynette K. Johns (Eds.)

are three essential aspects of a good scleral lens fit: proper corneal vault, limbal clearance, and scleral alignment.

Proper Corneal Clearance: Recognize the Corneal Shape

Proper corneal clearance is required for a successful scleral lens fit, as insufficient clearance can result in corneal epithelial compromise and excessive clearance may result in corneal hypoxia and difficulty with application. It is speculated that scleral lenses and the tear reservoir that they hold reduce oxygen transmission to the cornea [1]. Scleral lens materials have a Dk value of approximately 88-140. Scleral lens thicknesses typically range from 250 microns to greater than 500 microns. In addition, the fluid reservoir, which has a Dk itself of approximately 80 [2], limits oxygen transport to the cornea and is also thickness dependent. One may argue that there is solubilized oxygen already in the fluid reservoir contributing to corneal oxygen delivery. An optimal lens fit that provides an acceptable level of oxygen to the cornea should maintain a fluid reservoir that is not excessive and also maintain adequate corneal clearance.

How much clearance is ideal? As mentioned, no clearance at all results in lens bearing, which is damaging to the corneal epithelium and should be avoided. Some speculate that thinner fluid reservoirs will also lead to thin film adhesion, not to be confused with lens to cornea adhesion, between the eye and the lens due to the adhesive forces between the fluid reservoir and the lens, and this is also not a desirable outcome. In theory, thin film adhesion may create suction and cause scleral lens removal difficulty. Future studies may confirm if this phenomenon is present. A tear reservoir of 100-200 microns appears to be the proper balance between too little and too much clearance, which negatively impacts oxygen transmission. However, scleral lenses "settle" or sink into the conjunctiva and sclera, and that over several hours, lenses will lose anywhere from 75 to 175 microns of clearance [3 - 5]. An appropriate amount of clearance at initial lens fitting might fall in the range of 250-400 microns. Further studies need to investigate ideal clearance as it is still debated and speculated at the time of this publication.

In addition to the amount of clearance, there is the consideration for the distribution of clearance beneath the entire scleral lens surface. Clearance will decrease toward the limbus, and will vary with an irregular cornea. Ideally, a fluid reservoir will be as symmetric as possible to minimize the risk of contact over the most elevated point of the cornea, as well as avoiding areas of excessive clearance, which may impact oxygen transmission in those regions. Therefore, a fairly symmetric fluid reservoir should be considered an optimal outcome. This can be achieved by recognizing the shape of the cornea prior to fitting and matching the profile. Steep central corneas (Fig. **1**) will require different lens geometries than corneas that are flat centrally and steep peripherally (Fig. **2**).

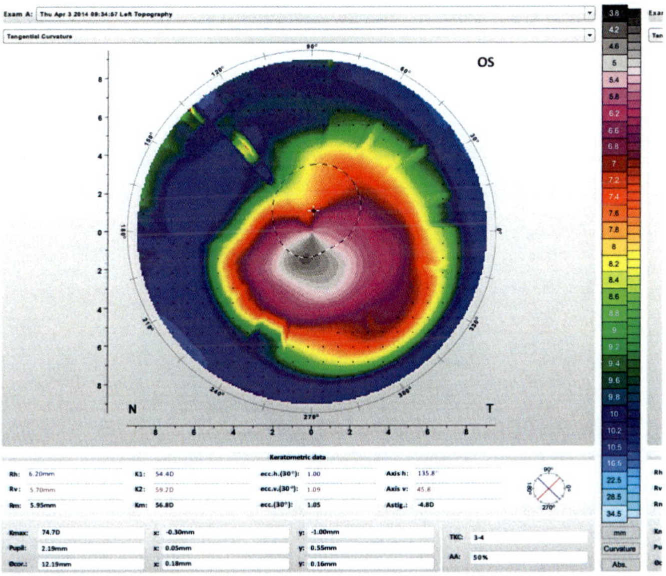

Fig. (1). Steep central topography will require a lens design that is steepest centrally and flattens rapidly.

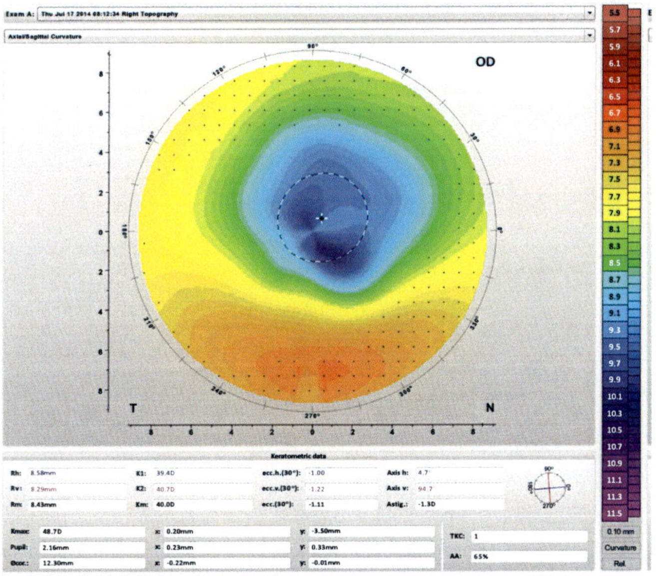

Fig. (2). Flat central corneal topography typical for a post-surgical eye. This eye will require a lens that is reverse geometry in design for optimal fit.

Achieving Limbal Clearance: Recognize the Corneal Diameter

The limbus, the border of the cornea and sclera, is a vital region as it gives rise to new corneal epithelial cells [6]. Scleral lenses that are improperly fit can bear their weight on this region and negatively impact function. A well-fit scleral lens will demonstrate clearance or non-bearing over the limbus of the eye. One of the main methods for accomplishing this is to choose a proper lens diameter. Scleral lenses are designed to provide clearance before landing on the scleral conjunctiva. Therefore, larger corneas will likely require a somewhat larger overall diameter, while smaller corneas may fare better in a smaller overall diameter. If a lens diameter is too small relative to the diameter of the cornea and limbus, then it is likely that the lens will rest on the limbus. In order to obtain proper limbal clearance, the choice of a proper diameter may reduce the fitting process complexity and the number of reorders required to reach an optimal fit.

Prior to initial lens selection, time should be taken to evaluate the corneal diameter. The importance of corneal diameter is often underestimated in the fitting process. It is perhaps the crucial component in determining which lens diagnostic set, diameter, and sagittal depth to start with. The impact of corneal diameter on corneal sagittal depth was described in an article by Andre, Davis, and Caroline in 2001 [7]. The authors reported that when calculating the sagittal depth values instead of corneal curves, the difference in sagittal depth between the flattest, smallest cornea segment and the steepest, largest cornea segment is 2.81 mm. Numerical analysis shows that the variations in diameter account for 62 percent of this difference, while the variations in radius are responsible for a little more than a third of the difference in soft lenses. It is mathematically apparent that diameter is significantly more influential than curvature in determining sagittal depth.

Measuring corneal diameter can be done with instrumentation such as corneal topography (Fig. **3**), tomography, handheld rulers (Fig. **4**), reticules on slit lamps, slit lamp cameras with measuring capabilities, comparison to lenses of known diameter, or simply through estimation with a trained eye. Once the corneal diameter is estimated or measured, the proper lens diameter range can be determined which will narrow down the choices for the initial lens selection.

Scleral Alignment: The Next Frontier

The final component to a successful scleral lens fit is achieving alignment to the sclera. This is necessary to avoid an excessively tight or loose fit circumferentially or focally. A tight scleral lens fit will lead to discomfort, hyperemia, rebound hyperemia after lens removal, conjunctival staining, and sometimes conjunctival laceration and conjunctival hypertrophy. A loose lens fit will lead to lens awareness, lens movement, and accumulation of debris or even air bubbles under the lens and may exacerbate giant papillary conjunctivitis. Analyzing scleral shape has historically been impossible, as instrumentation was not available to measure the shape of the sclera. Therefore, scleral alignment had to be evaluated based upon a diagnostic lens on the eye. However, with the introduction of new instrumentation developed to measure scleral shape, scleral lens fitting can now be evaluated in the pre-fitting process.

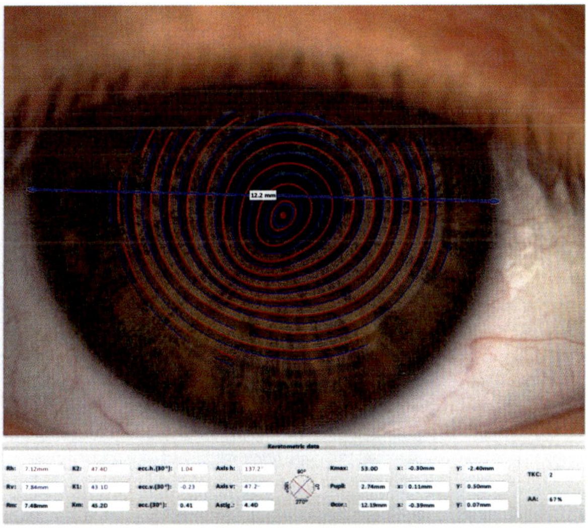

Fig. (3). Corneal topography display demonstrating a corneal diameter of 12.19 mm, confirmed by manual measurement of 12.2 mm.

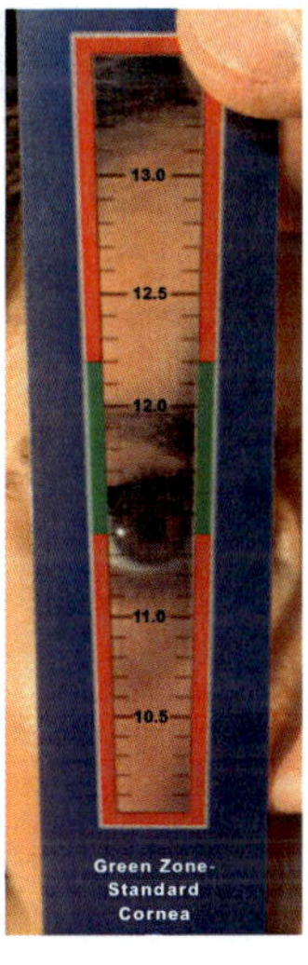

Fig. (4). HVID ruler for measuring horizontal corneal diameter.

Scleral profilers utilize height data from multiple projectors or by stitching multiple images to create a broad view of up to 22 mm of the ocular surface. With this broad view of the sclera, it is easier to visualize the need for toric or quadrant specific scleral landing zones (Fig. **5**). If the sclera is highly toric, a diagnostic lens that employs toric landing zones would be appropriate to use for an initial lens evaluation. Currently, these instruments are not common in practice. As increasing penetration into the ophthalmic market occurs, this information will aid in the pre-fitting process.

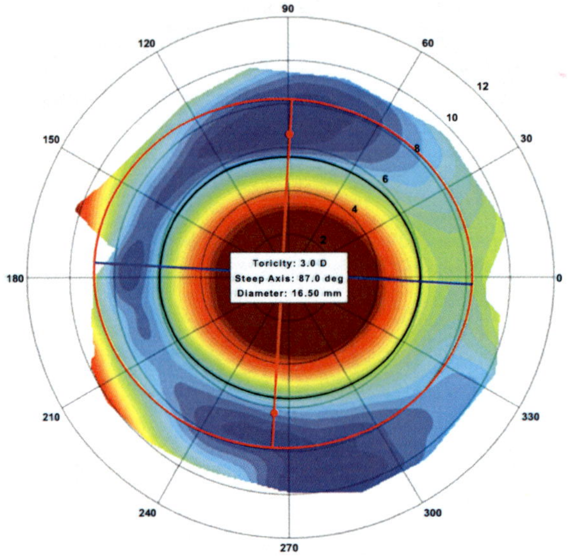

Fig. (5). Scleral profilometry demonstrating 3 diopters of scleral toricity. A scleral lens with toric landing curves may be indicated from the outset with this information. (Greg DeNaeyer, OD)

Choosing a Diagnostic Set

There are many excellent scleral lens designs available for the practitioner to choose. In general, they vary based upon diameter, geometry of the central and limbal regions, and the landing zone. To be successful, a scleral lens needs a minimum width of scleral conjunctival landing to avoid problematic compression of the vessels. It is suggested this width should be no narrower than 1 mm on each side of the eye. Additionally, it is recommended that the lens should land beyond the limbus by at least a few tenths of a millimeter. To then calculate a minimum diameter for a scleral lens, the corneal diameter can be added to the limbal clearance width and the landing zone. Assuming a small corneal diameter of 10.5 mm, allowing for limbal clearance and a minimum landing zone by the above recommendations, the smallest a scleral lens with corneal and limbal clearance may be is roughly 13.5 mm. Microcorneas are an exception to this diameter. On the other end of the spectrum, scleral lenses may also be fit as large as 23 mm. In North America, the majority of scleral lenses are fit in the range of 14.5 - 18.5 mm. In Europe, even larger diameters are used in the range of 20-23 mm [8, 9]. The choice of diameter is based typically on corneal diameter, but can also depend on aperture size, fornix integrity, conjunctival irregularities, corneal regularity, and patient dexterity. Knowing these parameters and adding approximately 4-5 mm to the known corneal diameter may determine an optimal initial scleral lens diameter. This diameter helps determine which fitting set is most appropriate to choose for the initial diagnostic lens.

Diagnostic sets also have different geometries. Within this set the lenses will follow a progression from shallowest to deepest. These geometries may start with the flattest curve as the base curve and progressively steepen (standard geometry). These designs are utilized for a variety of corneas, including keratoconus or normal corneas. Other designs may be intended for plateau corneal profiles that have a flatter central curve that steepens in the mid-periphery before flattening again across the sclera. These lenses are described as having a reverse geometry design, and are utilized in the post refractive surgery or post corneal transplant eye. Understanding history prior to fitting, topography and profilometry, a lens design can be selected that will provide the most even clearance across the ocular surface (Fig. **6**). This avoids contact in areas of inadequate clearance, and may prevent corneal hypoxia in areas of excessive clearance (Fig. **7**).

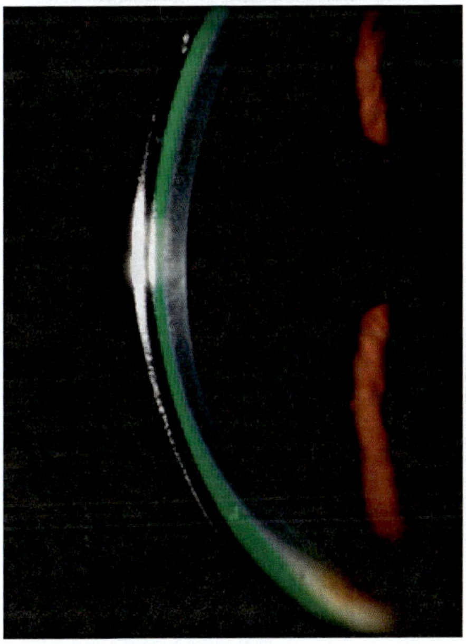

Fig. (6). Scleral lens with even clearance across the ocular surface.

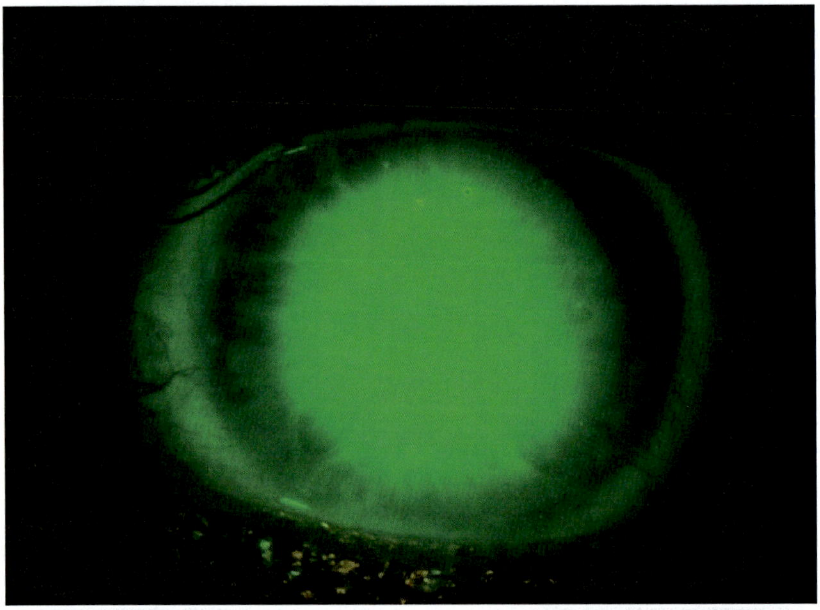

Fig. (7). Scleral lens with excessive central clearance and inadequate peripheral clearance, due to improper lens geometry selection.

Some diagnostic sets may also include different peripheries (flat, standard, steep) to aid in alignment of the initial diagnostic fit. As discussed in previous chapters, the sclera can often be asymmetric and a lens with scleral misalignment may create discomfort, awareness, debris, or other issues. To better manage these individuals, manufacturers can fabricate lenses with toricity in the landing zone [10, 11]. Some manufacturers build in toricity into their base lens design. If diagnostic testing is available to demonstrate scleral toricity to a significant degree, then a diagnostic set with toric peripheries would also be appropriate. Once the choice of proper diameter and geometry is made, and a toric scleral pattern is discovered in the scleral zone, then a diagnostic fitting set is selected. At this point, the first diagnostic lens can be chosen, and the fitting is underway.

Preparing for Initial Lens Selection: Considerations

Scleral lens diagnostic sets typically have eight-24 lenses within the set. Once a diagnostic fitting set has been selected based upon the desired diameter and geometry, how is the first lens selected? Can selection of the first lens with a bit of early effort increase the odds of initial success? If so, what are the benefits to the practitioner and the patient? Prior to selecting the first lens, choices within the set may be narrowed down by taking extra steps.

Measuring Sagittal Depth of the Eye

To quickly select the proper initial lens is to determine the sagittal depth of the eye at the same chord length as the diameter of the diagnostic lens. For example, using a 16 mm diameter diagnostic lens, calculate the corneal-scleral region of the eye out to 16 mm. This will determine which sagittal depth diagnostic lens to select first. Not all practitioners have access to instrumentation that easily calculates sagittal depth. It is possible to estimate this value with instruments that many practitioners already have.

Sagittal Height at 10mm

One useful measurement to aid in optimizing the initial lens selection process is the corneal sagittal height at a 10 mm chord. This value is found on many corneal topographers (Fig. **8**). With this information, a starting point for the sagittal height of the diagnostic lens can be determined.

A technique for utilizing this information was described in an article by Kojima *et al.* [12]. They found that the average sagittal height of the chord from 10-15 mm for all eye types was approximately 2000 microns, with a range from 1630 to 2360 microns. By using the 10 mm chord depth and adding 2000 microns for the sag of the 10-15 mm chord plus the desired amount of clearance, an approximate sagittal depth of the lens can be determined.

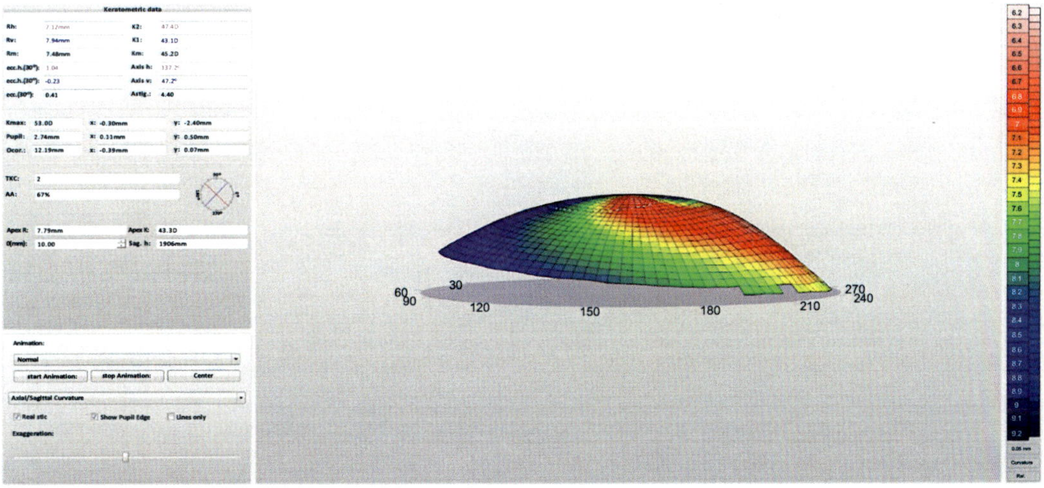

Fig. (8). Three-dimensional display of corneal topography demonstrates corneal sagittal height measurement at 10.0 mm of 1906 microns.

As an example, in Fig. (**8**), where a 10 mm chord demonstrates a sagittal height of 1906 microns, the desired clearance is 350 microns centrally, then the initial diagnostic lens of a 15 mm diameter would be:

1906 microns (measured) + 2000 microns (estimate) + 350 microns for vault = 4256 microns starting point for a 15 mm lens.

If the lens is larger than 15 mm, incrementally increase the sagittal height by roughly 300 microns per millimeter of lens diameter. For an example, a 17 mm lens will require 600 (300 x 2) additional microns:

4256 microns + 600 microns (for a 2 mm larger lens) = 4856 microns sagittal height for a 17 mm diameter lens. The final lens that this patient currently wears has a sagittal height of 4900.

Using this method to help determine the best lens based upon sagittal height can be done quickly with a topographer, and allow the practitioner to get very close with the initial lens selection.

Sagittal Height by OCT or Tomographer

Another method for obtaining a starting point for an initial diagnostic lens is use of imaging equipment such as an Optical coherence tomographer (OCT), or a Pentacam® tomographer. These instruments can provide a cross sectional image of the anterior segment and measure a variety of heights and widths (Fig. **9** and **10**). Use of this technology can streamline fitting to provide a starting point for initial lens selection (again, adding approximately 300 microns for each millimeter larger than the measured chord).

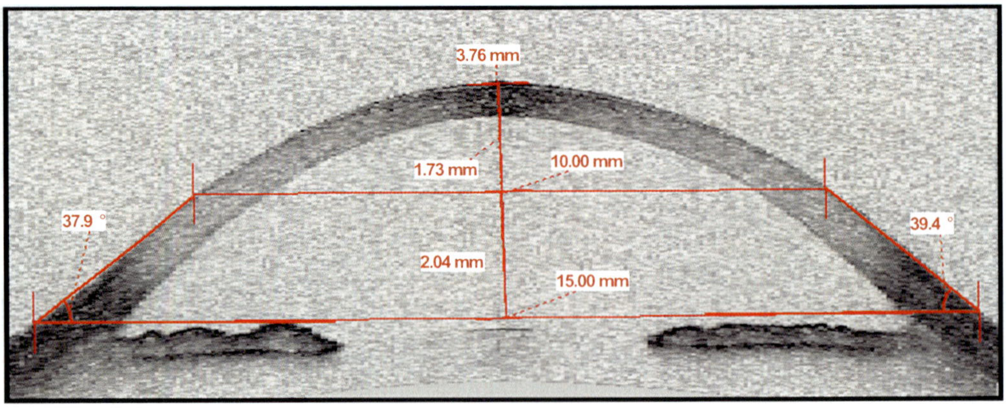

Fig. (9). OCT image demonstrating a sagittal height of 3760 microns at a 15mm chord. Image courtesy of Randy Kojima.

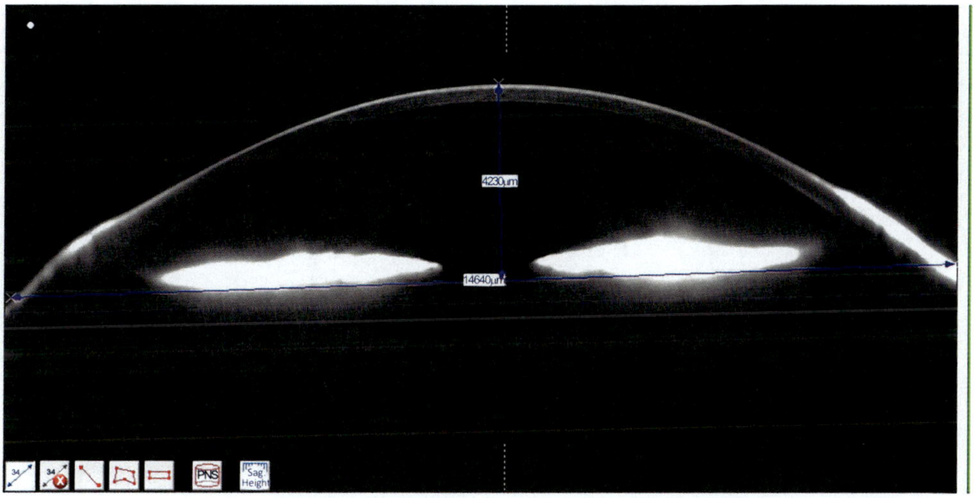

Fig. (10). Pentacam image demonstrating a sagittal height of 4230 microns at a chord of 14.64 millimeters.

In the example in Fig. (**10**) of a sagittal height of 4230 microns at 14.64 millimeters, the patient was fit with a 17 mm lens design. To calculate, we would add approximately 750 microns for the increased size and then add 350 microns for our desired clearance to our measured sagittal height of 4230:

4230 microns + 750 microns for the diameter increased to 17.0 (300 x 2.5 = 750) + 350 microns for clearance = 5330 microns.
The final lens that this individual currently wears is 5400 microns.

Again, using this type of estimation can yield results that can get the practitioner very close to the final sagittal depth needed for an optimal fit.

Putting in the Effort: Benefits to the Practitioner and Patient

Contact lens fitting is often considered an art and a science. However, the more science applied to the process, the less art is required to achieve an optimal fit. Utilizing a scientific approach and a pre-fitting protocol allows the practitioner to delegate much of the process to technical staff. By using these techniques, the initial lens selection and application can be standardized. This allows a technician to perform diagnostic testing, select the appropriate fitting set, determine the calculated sagittal depth, and select the initial lens. The technician can then apply the lens before the practitioner needs to become involved. This saves valuable time, and demonstrates to the patient an efficient, well thought out process which builds patient confidence.

There is also the aspect of applying multiple lenses on the eye of a patient new to scleral lenses. Scleral lenses may be intimidating, and the patient may be reluctant to try on a large lens. When an initial lens is nearly optimal, it minimizes the number of lenses and applications that are placed on the eye to determine an ideal fit. This reduces patient anxiety. This aspect of investing time when considering the initial lens should not be dismissed. It has a major impact on everyone involved in the fitting process. In addition, an unacceptable initial diagnostic lens may fit so poorly that it causes patient discomfort, and makes future lens application and evaluation more difficult. Finally, a suboptimal fitting lens becomes almost useless as a diagnostic lens. Acknowledging that there is a psychological aspect for both patient and practitioner when fitting scleral lenses, investing time in the initial diagnostic lens selections is time well spent.

Opening up the Fitting Set: Which Lens to Select?

Once the diameter, geometry and calculations have been determined, select the best choice based on those criteria. When selecting a lens, there are several methods. First, follow the diagnostic fitting guide recommendation for initial lens selection. Second, utilize the measured sagittal depth of the cornea. Third, simply choose a lens based on practitioner experience of the diagnostic set. It is worth noting that not all lenses are labeled with their sagittal height. If using measured sagittal depths to determine the initial lens, contact the laboratory for the sagittal height data.

Use of Fitting Guides

Fitting guides are supplied with all diagnostic lens sets in an attempt to provide a simple process to obtain a reasonably accurate outcome. Fitting guides are the result of practitioner experience with laboratory collaboration. If unable to obtain the previously explained data, the advantage to using the fitting guide will likely provide an initial lens that is acceptable for evaluation.

Diagnostic fitting guides may utilize either corneal curvature readings or categorize eyes based upon the ocular condition. When using keratometry readings, steeper corneas will require deeper lenses. Progressing from flattest to steepest base curves, the lenses have increasingly deeper sagittal heights. Fitting guides may assume certain things about the cornea, such as the general shape of the eye (prolate shape), or average corneal diameter when the diagnostic set is not labeled for a specific corneal geometry or condition.

Using the general condition or geometry is another approach. This method will assume that certain types of eyes will have an approximate shape and depth. Post-surgical eyes will often be flatter centrally and steeper in the mid-periphery, and shallower in depth. Keratoconic eyes will generally be steepest paracentrally and have more depth than an average cornea. Without considering the impact of corneal diameter on sagittal depth, excessive or shallow corneal clearance may occur. Experience with a diagnostic set and fitting guide facilitates an initial recommendation, but other factors impacting corneal sagittal depth may influence the lens fit and a second diagnostic lens may be required.

Software Guided Fitting for Initial Lens Selection

A final approach to initial lens selection is to use software aided scleral lens design. There are two options within this modality: first, the use of software utilizing corneal topography with diagnostic sets; second, utilizing corneal and scleral topography software for lens design.

Corneal Topography Guided Software

Roughly 10 mm in diameter of the corneal shape can be determined by corneal topography. As discussed previously, the shape of this zone can be influential in determining an initial diagnostic lens. Determination of corneal apex, sagittal height at the 10 mm chord, and corneal diameter readings can be used to determine a reasonably accurate initial scleral lens. Utilizing lens design software can incorporate this data to initiate the fitting process and can be a time saver. Eyespace™ is one example of a topographer that has scleral lens design software which incorporates corneal topographical information, refractive error, and corneal diameter to design an initial diagnostic lens. Once the scleral lens is ordered and dispensed, the software also guides the fitter through modifications depending on the issues with the initial lens.

Eyespace™ works with Medmont and Oculus® Topographers. Once topography is taken, the software can be launched. After selecting the appropriate map, the practitioner then chooses the type of lens to be fit among the menu options (Fig. **11**).

Once the lens design has been selected, refractive error is entered along with corneal diameter. From there, the software presents an initial lens along with a schematic of the lens (Fig. **12**). The lens can be electronically ordered directly from this screen.

Another software that utilizes corneal topography to design initial scleral lenses is Wave Contact Lens System® software. Wave software has been robust for many years, and recently incorporated scleral lens design using topography. The lens edge and angle modification can be manipulated with the software. To use Wave, topography is captured and the spectacle prescription is entered. Then, the software will automatically design the first lens. When a scleral design option is selected, the software will recalculate the diameter of choice (Fig. **13**). The lens is then displayed in profile as well a simulated fluorescein pattern. Modifications can be made at this stage if needed. From this point, a lens can be ordered electronically.

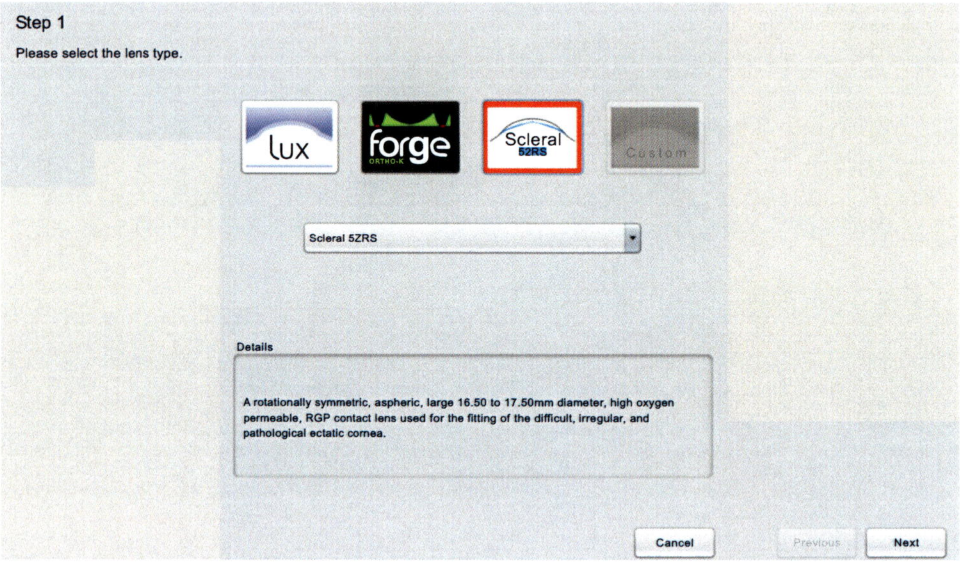

Fig. (11). Eyespace™ software lens selection menu.

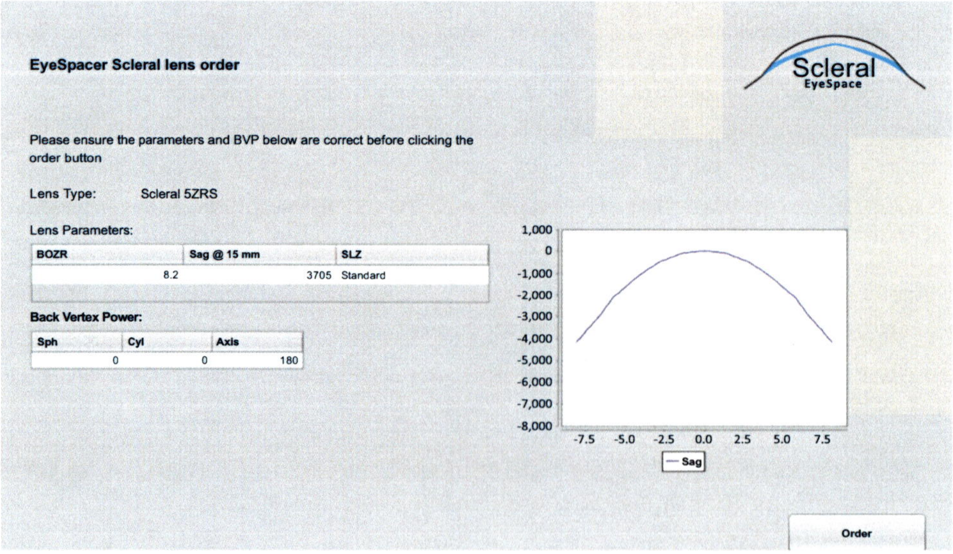

Fig. (12). Eyespace™ software with initial scleral lens design based upon topography and spectacle prescription.

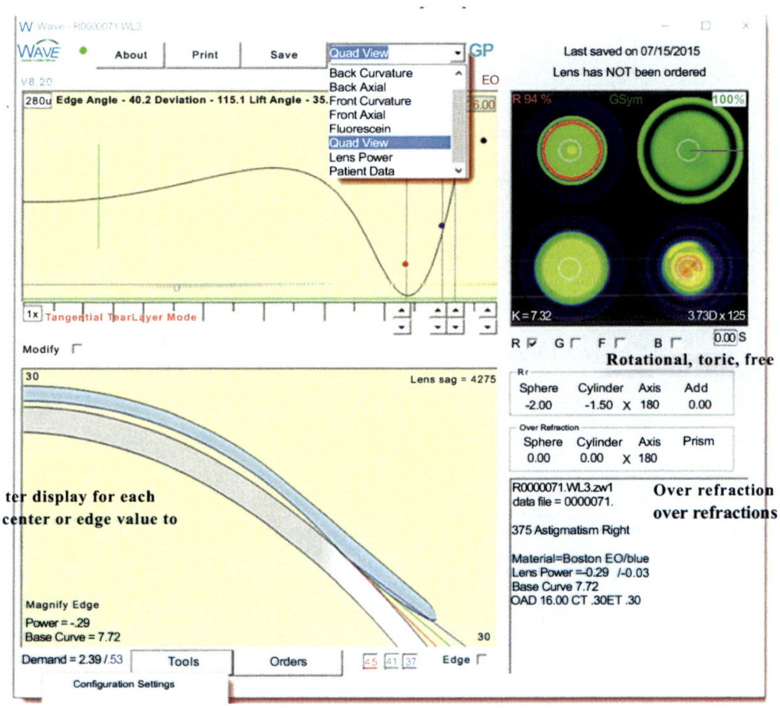

Fig. (13). Initial scleral lens design using Wave Contact Lens System® software.

As with Eyespace™, modification to this initial lens can be made using the software to guide the practitioner.

Scleral Topography Guided Software

The final method for initial lens selection with scleral lenses is using scleral topographers, or profilers. These instruments image the cornea and scleral topography. They reveal the depth and shape of the cornea, as well as the shape of the sclera, and whether toricity is needed in the landing zone. There are currently two instruments that are capable of obtaining scleral topography and use the map to create scleral lenses, the sMap3D by Precision Ocular Metrology (New Mexico, US) and the Eye Surface Profiler by Eaglet Eye (Netherlands).

The sMap3D takes 3 images of the ocular surface using fluorescein to obtain optimal data collection, and then stitches the images together to create a single image of the ocular surface. From this point, after spectacle refraction entry, a lens can be designed using the software. The lens design software will identify the amount of scleral toricity, integrating this information into the landing curves if needed. The software will also design the best fit lens based upon the Europa

Scleral® lens (Visionary Optics) to determine initial lens parameters (Fig. **14**). After scleral lens evaluation on the patient, modifications can be made by using the software.

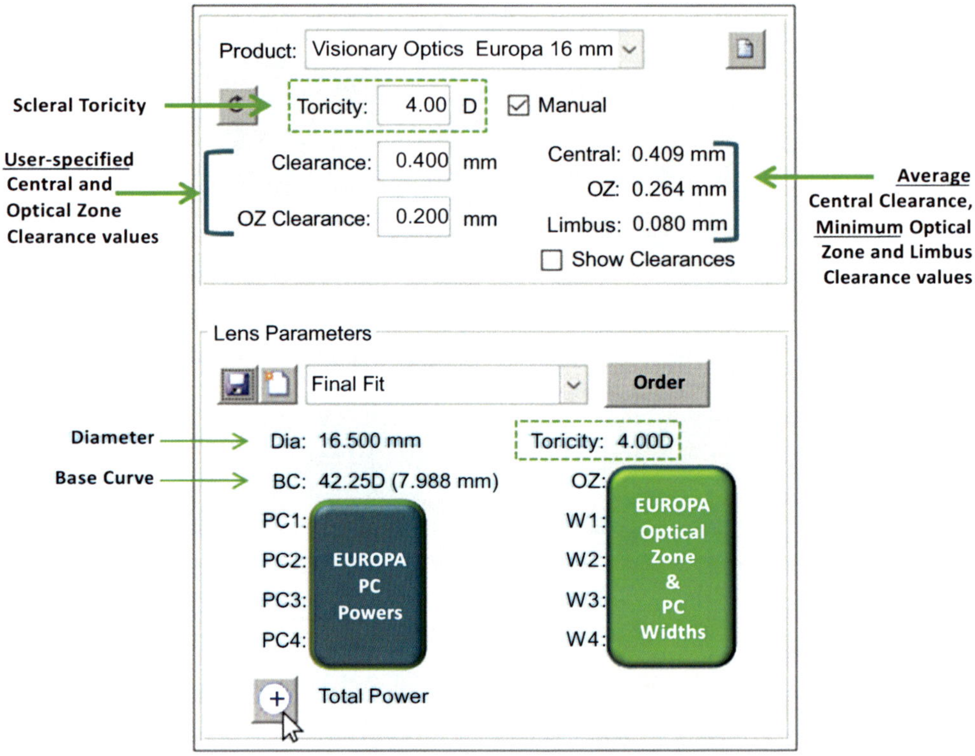

Fig. (14). Scleral lens design software on the sMap3D scleral profiler.

The Eye Surface Profiler (ESP) captures a single image of the cornea and sclera in primary gaze. Corneal and scleral curvature and height data is then used to select a lens from the available designs in the software. With a single click, the instrument generates the initial lens diameter based on the size of the cornea, as well as the suggested initial lens SAG value and the amount of toricity recommended in the scleral landing zone for optimal fit (Fig. **15**). The toricity in the landing zone is derived not just from scleral shape alone, but also from the total SAG of each of the major meridians of the eye, allowing for precise landing in each meridian. The suggested lens can then be placed on eye and an over refraction completed to finalize the initial lens order.

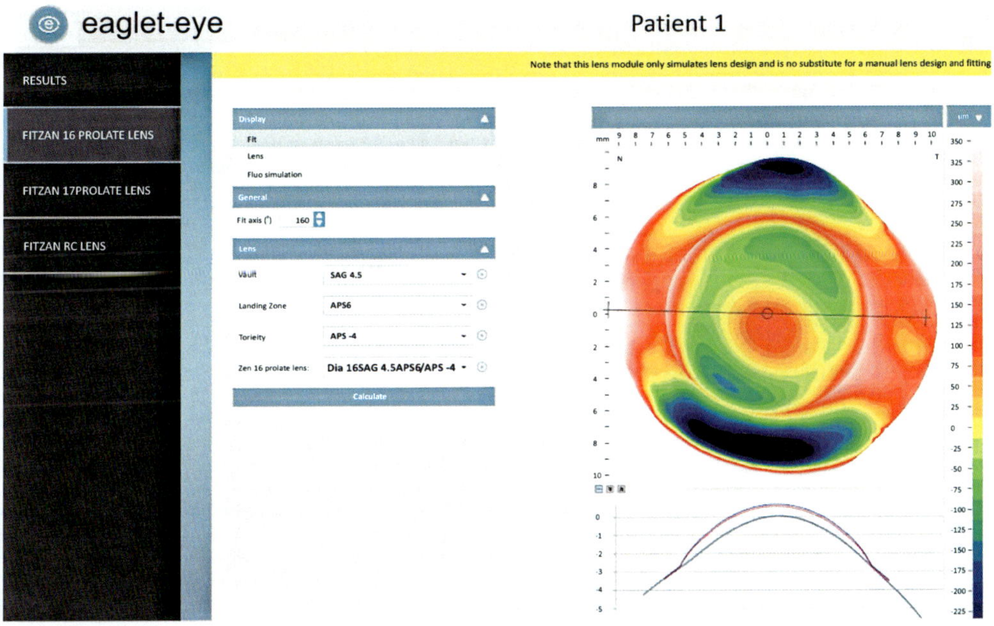

Fig. (15). The Eye Surface Profiler Initial Lens Selection screen provides the desired lens SAG, diameter, and the peripheral curves for the two major meridians.

SUMMARY

Starting the fitting process with a scleral lens can be a bit daunting to the novice practitioner. One may ask, "How do I select the lens design? Which diameter is best? Which lens do I first select?" The inexperienced scleral lens practitioner may encounter all of these questions. Determining an initial lens to apply can be simplified with either the use of lens design software, or with a methodical approach to initial lens selection. This approach includes gathering data such as corneal diameter, corneal topography, scleral topography, as well as available sagittal height measurements. Even if the initial diagnostic lens is suboptimal, evaluation of that lens will help determine which lens to use next. By designing a protocol with strategic follow through, much of the guesswork can be taken out of initial lens selection. This will save the practitioner, staff and patient time and will create a favorable impression towards scleral lenses and the scleral lens process in general.

CONFLICT OF INTEREST

The authors declare no conflict of interest, financial or otherwise.

ACKNOWLEDGEMENTS

Declared none.

REFERENCES

[1] Michaud L, van der Worp E, Brazeau D, Warde R, Giasson CJ. Predicting estimates of oxygen transmissibility for scleral lenses. Cont Lens Anterior Eye 2012; 35(6): 266-71. [http://dx.doi.org/10.1016/j.clae.2012.07.004] [PMID: 22878418]

[2] Benjamin WJ. Oxygen transport through contact lenses.Contact Lens Practice. Chapman Hall Medical Publishers 1994; pp. 47-69.

[3] Mountford J. Scleral contact lens settling rates. 10th Congress of the Orthokeratology Society of Oceania (OSO). Queensland, Australia. 2012.

[4] Michaud L. Variation of clearance with mini-scleral lenses. Global Specialty Lens Symposium. Las Vegas, NV. 2014.

[5] Kauffman Matthew J, Gilmartin Christopher A, Bennett Edward S, Bassi Carl J. A comparison of the short-term settling of three scleral lens designs. Optometry and Vision Science 2014; 91(12): 1462-6.

[6] Secker GA, Daniels JT. Limbal epithelial stem cells of the corneaThe Stem Cell Research Community 2009.

[7] Andre M, Davis J, Caroline P. A new approach to fitting soft contact lenses. Eyewitness 2001; 4: 1-4.

[8] Visser ES, Visser R, van Lier HJ, Otten HM. Modern scleral lenses part I: clinical features. Eye Contact Lens 2007; 33(1): 13-20. [http://dx.doi.org/10.1097/01.icl.0000233217.68379.d5] [PMID: 17224674]

[9] Tan DT, Pullum KW, Buckley RJ. Medical applications of scleral contact lenses: 2. Gas-permeable scleral contact lenses. Cornea 1995; 14(2): 130-7. [http://dx.doi.org/10.1097/00003226-199503000-00001] [PMID: 7743793]

[10] Visser ES, Visser R, Van Lier HJ. Advantages of toric scleral lenses. Optom Vis Sci 2006; 83(4): 233-6. [http://dx.doi.org/10.1097/01.opx.0000214297.38421.15] [PMID: 16614579]

[11] Visser ES, Van der Linden BJ, Otten HM, Van der Lelij A, Visser R. Medical applications and outcomes of bitangential scleral lenses. Optom Vis Sci 2013; 90(10): 1078-85. [http://dx.doi.org/10.1097/OPX.0000000000000018] [PMID: 23974663]

[12] Kojima R, Caroline P, Graff T, *et al.* Eye shape and scleral lenses. Contact Lens Spectrum 2013; 28(4): 38-43.

CHAPTER 9

Scleral Lens Evaluation

Lynette K. Johns[1,*], **Jennifer Anne McMahon**[2] and **Melissa Barnett**[3]

[1] *The New England College of Optometry, Boston, Massachusetts, USA*

[2] *Great Western Hospitals NHS FT, Swindon, UK*

[3] *University of California, Davis, Sacramento, CA, USA*

Abstract: Systematic evaluation of scleral lens fitting is essential to identify and address areas of concern at the outset with a view to minimizing the risk of potential physiological complications. Thorough and consistent evaluation ensures proper functionality, comfort and safety for the patient. This chapter details scleral lens evaluation techniques ranging from immediately after application to subsequent fitting evaluations. Scleral lens evaluation can be intimidating relative to other contact lens modalities since the lenses are much larger and have more variables that can be changed. Systematic and methodical evaluation ensures that practitioners do not overlook key findings of ill-fitting scleral lenses. After scleral lenses are removed, the ocular surface tells its story as well. At every evaluation, practitioners should always remember to evaluate the eye without the lens to ensure that the patient is not compromised and can continue to enjoy all the properties that a scleral lens offers.

Keywords: Blanching, Bubbles, Clearance, Compression, Conjunctiva, Conjunctival hypertrophy, Evaluation, Fluorescein, Hyperemia, Impinging, Inside-out evaluation, Light, Limbus, OCT, Scleral compression, Settling, Slit lamp, Staining, Surface wettability, Toricity, Vessels.

Systematic evaluation of scleral lens fitting is essential to identify and address areas of concern at the outset with a view to minimizing the risk of potential physiological complications. Thorough and consistent evaluation ensures proper functionality, comfort and safety for the patient. This chapter details scleral lens evaluation techniques ranging from immediately after application to subsequent fitting evaluations.

GROSS EVALUATION OUTSIDE OF THE SLIT LAMP

Simply examining the lens outside of the slit lamp shortly after application

* **Corresponding author Lynette K. Johns:** The New England College of Optometry, Boston, Massachusetts, USA; Tel: 617-262-2020; Fax: 617-236-6323; E-mails: johnsl@neco.edu; lynettekjohns@gmail.com

provides initial information that directs the practitioner to further investigate the slit lamp.

Once the scleral lens is *in situ*, the practitioner can establish if any bubbles are trapped in the tear reservoir, detect wettability issues, observe the initial fluorescein pattern, observe lens movement and identify early conjunctival compression patterns using a pen light or a transilluminator outside of the slit lamp (Fig. **1**). Cobalt blue LED lights also help identify bubbles when using fluorescein and provides an initial fluorescein pattern. A simple handheld LED blue light (often found as a keychain) can be used (Fig. **2**), as well as the blue filter on an ophthalmoscope. The practitioner should be ready to immediately remove the lens if it is decentered.

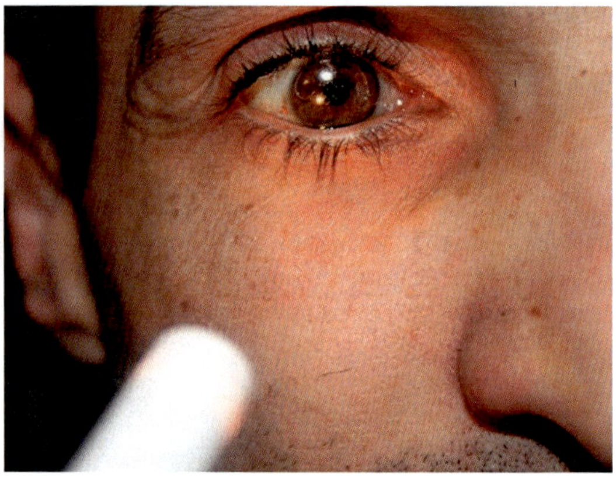

Fig. (1). Initial evaluation of a scleral lens using a penlight. An application bubble and surface wetting defects are present.

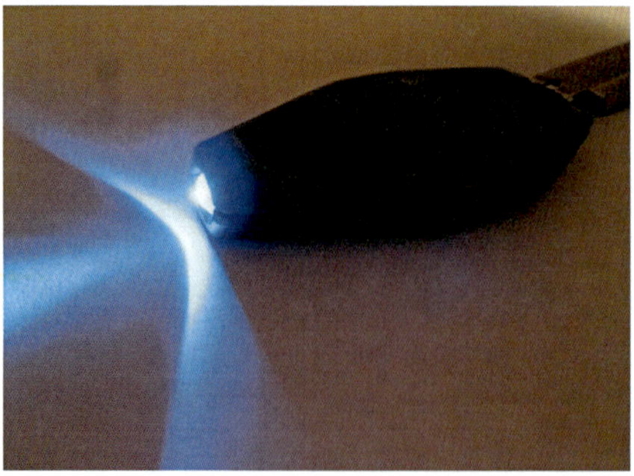

Fig. (2). An example of a cobalt blue LED keychain light that can be used for gross examination of a scleral lens.

Bubble Check

To assess for bubbles the eyelids are retracted as wide as is feasible and a light is directed tangential to the surface of the lens. Bubbles are easily recognizable in the presence of fluorescein with both white and cobalt blue light (Fig. **3**). Sometimes, without fluorescein, bubbles can very easily be missed. For example, a large bubble may fill the whole reservoir of vaulted space (Fig. **4**). The boundary of the bubble may align with the very edge of the fluid reservoir. Wearers commonly complain almost immediately of blurry vision and/or discomfort. Over time, the back surface of the lens may fog, or steam up with condensation, confirming the presence of a bubble (Fig. **5**) and at this point, lens removal and reapplication is necessary.

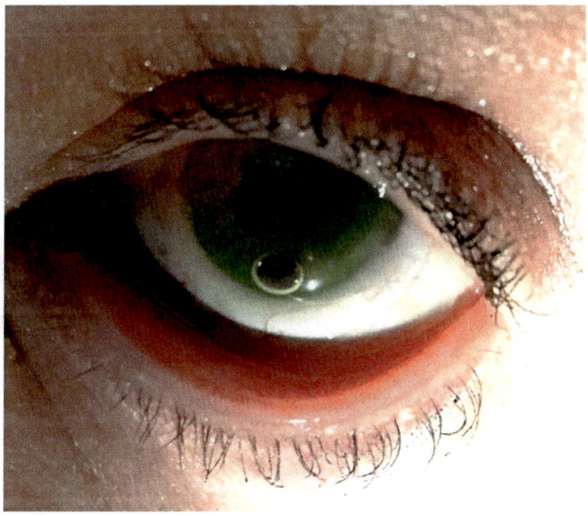

Fig. (3). A bubble can easily be identified using a penlight or transilluminator outside of the slit lamp.

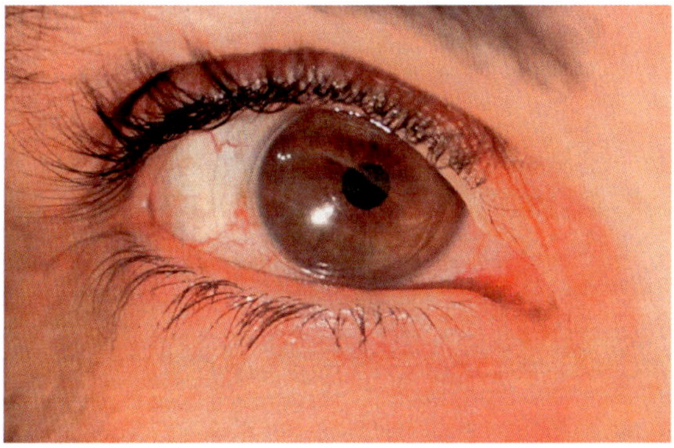

Fig. (4). Example of a large application bubble that fills the entire chamber of the scleral lens reservoir. To visualize the bubble, the practitioner needs to scan the penlight/transilluminator across the entire surface of the lens to highlight the edges of the bubble. Often, a large bubble can be overlooked.

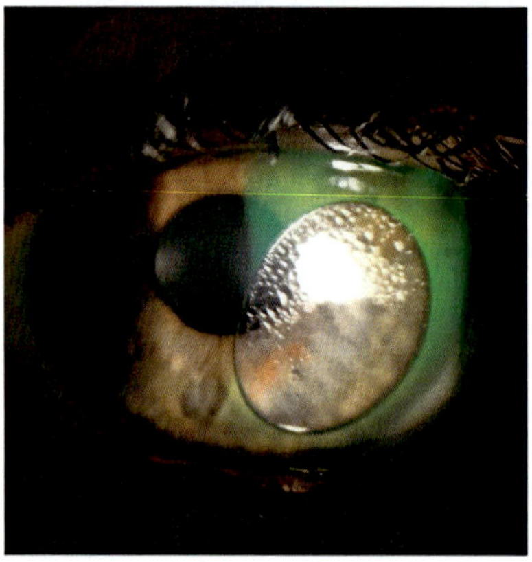

Fig. (5). Condensation forming on the back surface of a scleral lens from an application bubble.

Surface Wettability

If there is no bubble, then the lens surface quality can be evaluated. The reflection of the light on the surface should exhibit a nice sharp reflex (Fig. **6**). Quickly scanning the surface of the lens with the light will show an inconsistency of the reflex if there is a wetting defect. The lens can still be evaluated with the wetting defect; however, it will impair the best corrected visual acuity. The lens can either be removed or cleaned prior to reapplication or the front surface can be conditioned whilst on the eye. To condition the lens surface *in situ*, moisten a cotton swab or DMV remover with either gas permeable conditioning solution or preservative free saline. While off-label, sometimes using a multipurpose soft contact lens solution can also be effective. Gently rub the conditioner over the surface of the lens with the swab or the edge of the DMV remover, especially over the wetting defect. When using the DMV remover, only use the edge of the remover as the "squeegee," and care should be taken to not apply the remover directly to the surface of the lens; otherwise, the remover may inadvertently adhere the plunger to the surface of the lens and affect removal (Fig. **7**). If the surface quality remains poor, the lens should be removed, cleaned and reapplied.

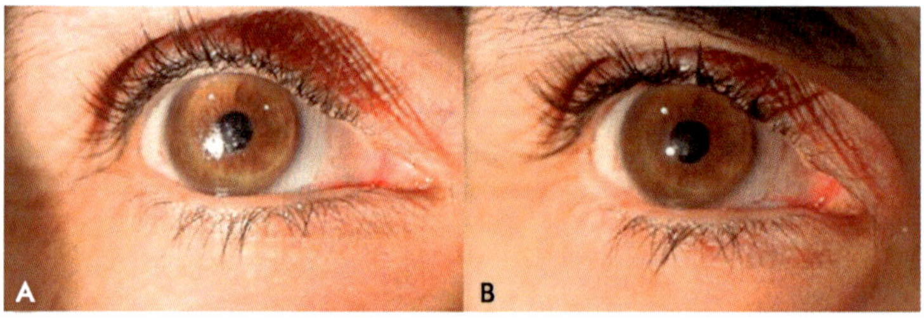

Fig. (6). Evaluation of the surface of a scleral lens. A wetting defect disperses the light reflex from the penlight on the surface of the lens (A). A smooth and wetting surface will reflect a distinct reflex from the penlight (B).

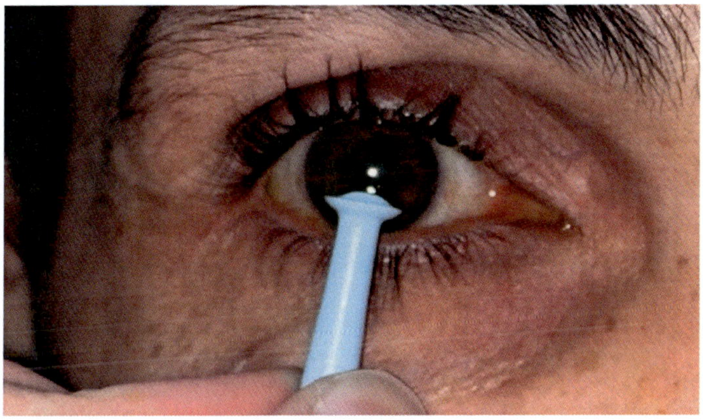

Fig. (7). Example of using a DMV removal plunger as a squeegee. A drop of solution either a re-wetting solution, artificial tear or conditioning multipurpose solution is placed on the face of the plunger and the edge of the plunger rubs the surface of the lens.

Movement

Typically, scleral lenses demonstrate minimal movement on eye. The following are possible causes of unexpected lens movement:

- Poor wetting of the lens surface may cause the inner surface of the upper eyelid to temporarily stick to the dry portions causing the lens to lift during a blink excursion. The wetting defect is usually quite large in such cases and can be confirmed with the procedure described earlier. Lens removal and thorough cleaning is necessary to improve surface wettability. A well-conditioned lens surface should feel smooth to the touch when it is gently rubbed and this can be demonstrated to the wearer.
- If there is significant contact of the lens on the cornea, the lens edge is lifted off the bearing surface and the lens is destabilized much like a Frisbee resting on a basketball (Fig. **8**). If fluorescein is used in the reservoir of the lens, it will confirm this possibility.
- Conversely, if the lens landing zone is too steep for the scleral topography and the lens is balanced on the very rim or edge of the lens, it may exhibit movement. Further investigation of the scleral lens with the slit lamp will determine if the periphery is too steep or the landing zone is too narrow.
- A toric or asymmetric scleral topography may cause movement as the lens is unstable. The movement can be explained by the lens teetering on the flat meridian with the blink, like a seesaw.

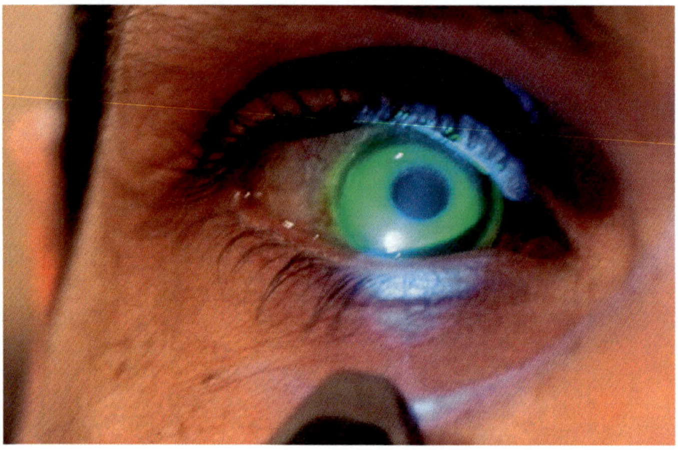

Fig. (8). Example of a diagnostic lens with insufficient central clearance observed outside the slit lamp with a blue LED light.

Scleral Landing Zone Patterns

Compression patterns, evidenced by conjunctival blanching, are easily detected outside of the slit lamp. Due to the mechanical manipulation of the eye when the lens is applied, the eye may be more injected than usual. As a result, compression of the conjunctiva will be readily observed. If compression is observed 360 degrees around the far periphery of the scleral lens landing zone, the periphery is likely too tight/steep and lens removal should be considered if it is excessive to prevent suctioning of the lens. An extremely tight and suctioned lens is not only uncomfortable and difficult to remove but may also cause the cornea to become edematous. If the patient has a history of a penetrating keratoplasty, LASIK surgery or radial keratotomy, the scleral lens should be carefully removed to prevent dehiscence of the graft, loosening of the flap or wound gap of the incisions, respectively. It is likely that compression of the lens landing zone 360 degrees will create increasing suction of the lens and difficulty removing the lens over increased wearing time. A diagnostic lens with a looser or flatter periphery, if available, should be applied.

When blanching is meridional the sclera may be toric. The ability to have a gross overview outside of the slit lamp allows the total meridian of compression to be observed and can be quite beneficial (Fig. **9**). Additionally, movement of the lens may also be concurrently observed. These findings require further investigation with the slit lamp.

Information and fitting cues gleaned from multiple methods of observation aid the fitting and optimization of scleral lenses. While a scleral lens cannot be fit properly and effectively with gross evaluation outside of a slit-lamp, many features of the fit are revealed that direct further investigation by other techniques such as slit lamp and OCT evaluation.

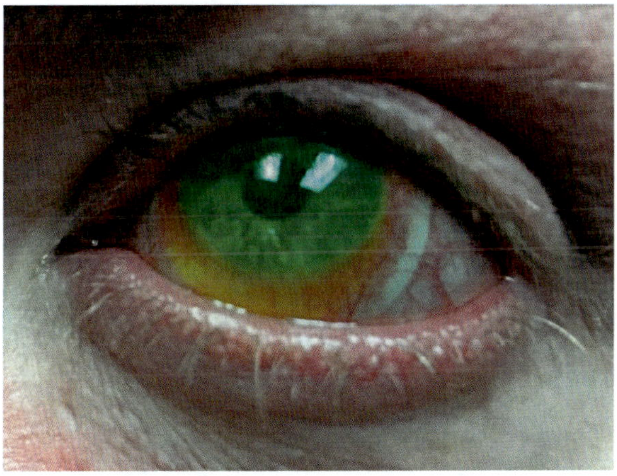

Fig. (9). Meridional compression can be observed with a penlight or transilluminator outside of the slit lamp.

SLIT LAMP EVALUATION OF THE SCLERAL LENS

Systematic evaluation of scleral lenses aids the practitioner to develop a consistent routine. Following the same methods during each examination prevents inadvertent mistakes by omission. Scleral lens assessment styles include the "inside-out" and "outside-in" methods. "Inside-out" evaluation refers to examining the central clearance first and continuing to evaluate the lens more peripherally. A challenge with using the "outside-in" method is that the landing zone may be considered very loose with excessive edge lift when the lens is actually touching the cornea. In this example, if the practitioner ordered a lens based on this assessment and increased the sagittal depth, the periphery may be tightened as well. However, the edge lift may be secondary to the lens landing on the cornea (Frisbee on a basketball analogy) and a diagnostic lens with increased central clearance may provide adequate landing zone alignment. The following describes the "inside-out" scleral evaluation method.

Apical Clearance with Fluorescein and Diffuse Cobalt Illumination

A scleral lens by definition clears the cornea in its entirety; therefore, it is important to establish the location of the most elevated portion of the cornea is cleared by the scleral lens and to ensure that the lens is not in contact with this region. The addition of fluorescein to the lens reservoir prior to applying the scleral lens to the eye allows the fluorescein pattern to be observed with ease. The fluorescein pattern can be viewed using low magnification and a broad/diffuse beam of cobalt blue illumination. A Wratten #12 filter further enhances the subtleties of the fluorescein pattern (Fig. **10**). The glow of the fluorescein will be brighter in areas of greater corneal clearance and darker in areas where the clearance is shallower. When scanning the cornea with the diffuse beam, the angle of the beam should be continually adjusted. The sharp demarcation of the beam on the lens surface may give the appearance of contact, particularly in the limbal zone, when, in fact, there is none. (Fig. **11**, A arrow and 11 B). Adjusting the angle of the beam will prevent mistaking this finding for insufficient clearance (Fig. **11B**). If necessary the patient can be asked to look slightly to the side to verify the presence of clearance. If definite apical contact is identified the lens can be removed and replaced with a lens of increased sagittal height.

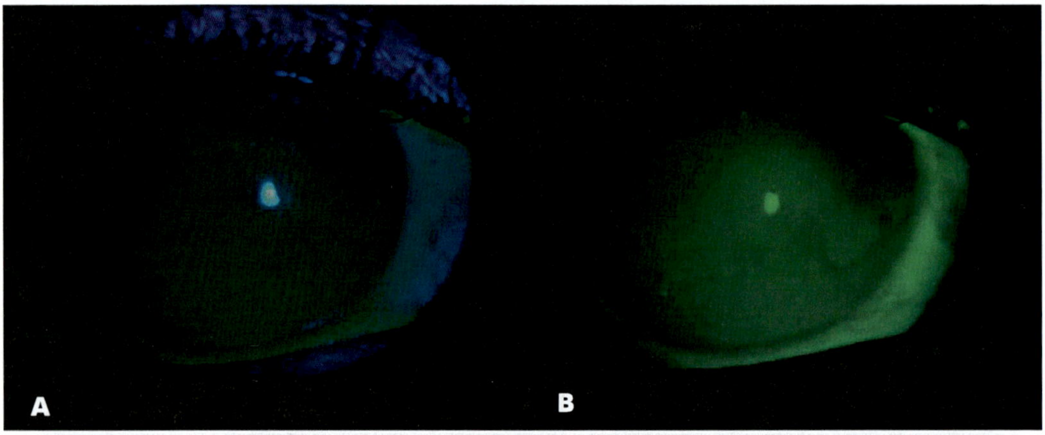

Fig. (10). Example of a scleral lens on a right eye with narrow superior-nasal clearance (A). The same view with the use of a Wratten #12 filter (B).

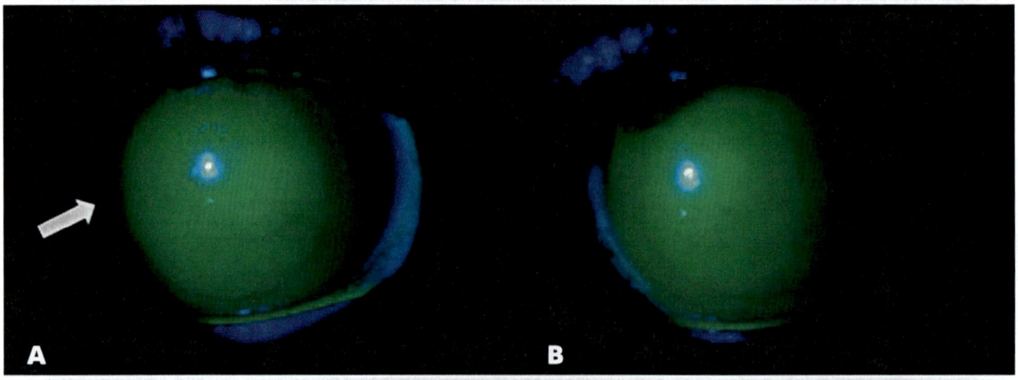

Fig. (11). (A) The demarcation of the cobalt blue diffuse beam on the surface of the lens (white arrow). The dark band around the edge of the beam can be mistaken for insufficient limbal clearance. The angle of illumination is adjusted temporally (B) and the fluorescein pattern extends to the edge of the cornea.

Apical and Limbal Clearance with Fluorescein and Optic Section

Areas identified as having shallow clearance or possible corneal contact using a diffuse/ broad cobalt blue filter can then be evaluated in more detail. A narrow beam of white light (optic section) with high magnification can be used to demonstrate the presence or absence of clearance and to make an estimation of the amount. A layer of fluorescein observed between the back surface of the lens and the anterior surface of the cornea indicates corneal clearance. The cornea is carefully scanned by viewing the optic section superiorly to inferiorly and nasally to temporally (Fig. **12**). The most elevated portion of the cornea typically will have the narrowest fluorescein band overlying it (Fig. **13**). It should be remembered that the corneal apex may not be located at the center of cornea particularly in conditions such as keratoconus.

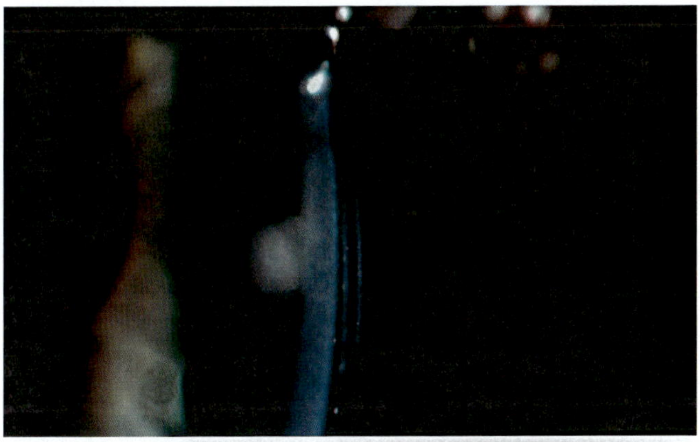

Fig. (12). Observing the optic section superiorly to inferiorly, while scanning the entire cornea may highlight areas where clearance is shallow or absent.

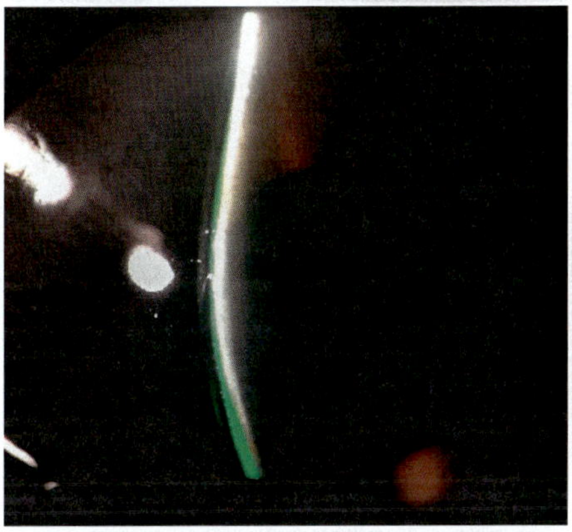

Fig. (13). The scleral lens is vaulting over Salzmann's nodules. It is important to vault over the most elevated portion of the cornea which may not always be central.

The limbal zone should also be assessed using the same optic section. Ideally, fluorescein should extend beyond the corneal borders, over the limbus and taper gradually towards the adjacent sclera.

Measurement of Apical Clearance

The amount of corneal clearance can be precisely measured using ocular coherence tomography (OCT). Alternatively, an approximate measurement can be made using biomicropscopy. Measuring the amount of corneal clearance at each visit provides valuable information about the interaction of the lens and the eye. Typically, cobalt blue light is used for assessing fluorescein patterns, however when assessing clearance with an optic section, white light highlights the fluorescein band well. White light produces reflexes on the front and back surfaces of the lens that highlight lens thickness to which the thickness of the fluorescein band can be compared. As most laboratories specify the thickness of diagnostic lenses or will provide this information on request, the thickness of the tear layer can be estimated from the comparison. It should be remembered that the thickness of the final ordered lens may not be the same as the diagnostic lens. The thickness of the cornea may also be used as a basis for comparison to estimate clearance; however, it may be less reliable particularly in cases of corneal ectasia. In many cases, scleral lenses are used for irregular corneas, and the corneas have variable thicknesses. The center thickness of the lens is fixed and provides a consistent comparator.

When estimating the clearance using a slit lamp, the beam should be at an angle of 45 degrees from the observation system. If the beam is positioned closer to 180 degrees (at a wider angle), the clearance may be overestimated; conversely, the clearance can be underestimated if the beam is at a lesser angle closer to 90 degrees. To begin, increase the magnification and the illumination of the beam. Narrow the optic section until all the surfaces of the lens and cornea are visible. Anteriorly, the first illuminated surface will be the tear film overlying the anterior/front surface of the lens. Posterior to that will be a black band which is the center thickness of the lens bordered by a reflection from the posterior surface of the lens (not always easily visible). The bright green band of fluorescein is the clearance over the corneal surface bordered posteriorly by the corneal surface (Fig. **14**).

To estimate the corneal clearance, compare the fluorescein band to the center thickness of the lens (black transparent band). Since the value of the center thickness is known or readily available, the clearance can be estimated as a ratio to that value. For example, if there is a 1:1 ratio of the clearance to the center thickness, then the clearance is roughly the same amount in microns of depth.

In Fig. (**15**), the lens thickness is 0.2 mm or 200 μm thick. The clearance band is between one and a half to two times as thick as the lens thickness. Therefore, the clearance of this lens is 350 to 400 μm. It is important to remember that the thickness should be measured over the most elevated portion of the cornea. Topography maps, specifically elevation maps, may cue practitioners on the location of the highest elevation. As stated previously, it is particularly important to measure the clearance over this region of the cornea.

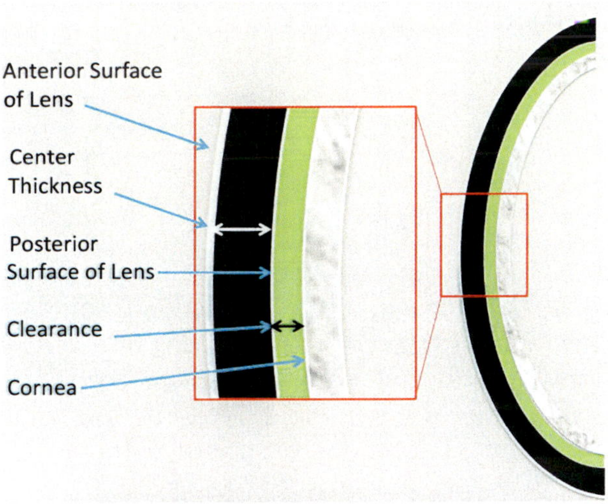

Fig. (14). Diagram of an optic section of clearance using fluorescein.

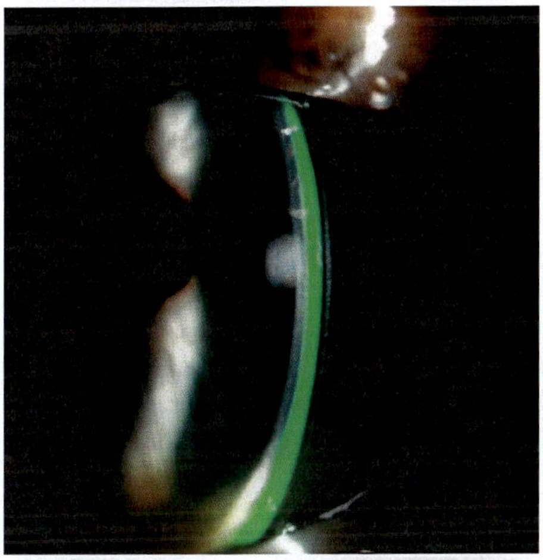

Fig. (15). Image of optic section of clearance using fluorescein.

Scleral lenses may decenter infero-temporally (down and out) for a variety of reasons especially with larger diameter lenses [1], therefore, it is not uncommon to find that the clearance is narrower supero-nasally than elsewhere on the lens. Often this decentration is a result of scleral anatomy described in detail in Chapter 3. Over time, it is possible that the lens settles back during wear to contact the cornea and then mechanical trauma/corneal staining may ensue. Therefore, areas of initial narrow or nonexistent clearance should be monitored carefully for corneal staining after the lens is removed. Fortunately, scleral lenses are also dynamic and exhibit some movement. As a result, the cornea that demonstrates contact in primary gaze may be fully vaulted/cleared by the lens in downgaze because the lens is shifted upward. If that is the case, there is less risk of mechanical complications such as lens adherence or epithelial damage.

Fluorescein is a tremendous asset to assist practitioners when evaluating corneal and limbal clearance. However, patients do not apply fluorescein into the eye prior to their visits. Practitioners must also develop the skill of visualizing and assessing corneal clearance without the use of fluorescein. Certainly, a patient may be dispensed a fluorescein strip and instructed to apply the lens with fluorescein the day of their visit, but that depends on the laws where the practitioners are located. However, patients do not always appreciate the appearance of fluorescein during the day under their lenses cosmetically. Alternatively, OCT can be used if available. Nevertheless, not every practitioner owns an OCT. Therefore, evaluating the clearance without the use of fluorescein is an essential skill. Visually, the only difference without fluorescein is that clearance will be transparent. The practitioner must clearly identify the front and back surface of the lens and the anterior surface of the cornea (Fig. **16**).

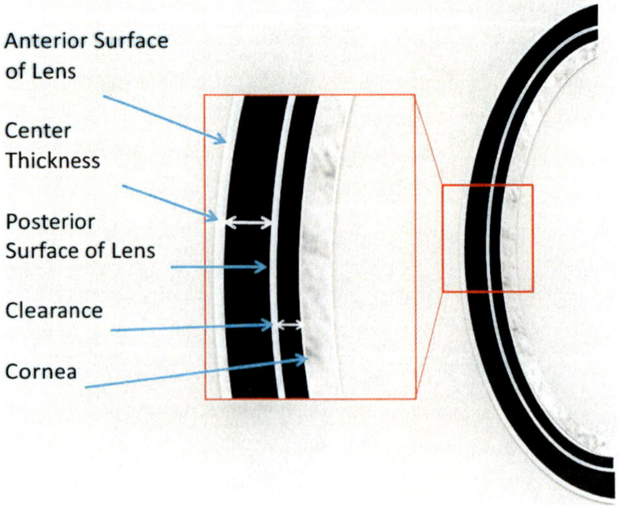

Fig. (16). Diagram of optic section of clearance without fluorescein.

The challenge of this skill is to correctly identify both surfaces. The posterior surface of the lens can be quite difficult to illuminate and observe, and it becomes increasingly difficult with smaller amounts of clearance. Positioning the slit lamp beam between 90 and 75 degrees, the back surface sometimes elicits a significantly bright reflection and once identified, the anterior surface can be confirmed. Sometimes, the reflex on the anterior surface can be distracting (Fig. **17**). It is important to maintain both reflexes while carefully adjusting the angle of the beam to be 45 degrees to measure the clearance (Fig. **18**).

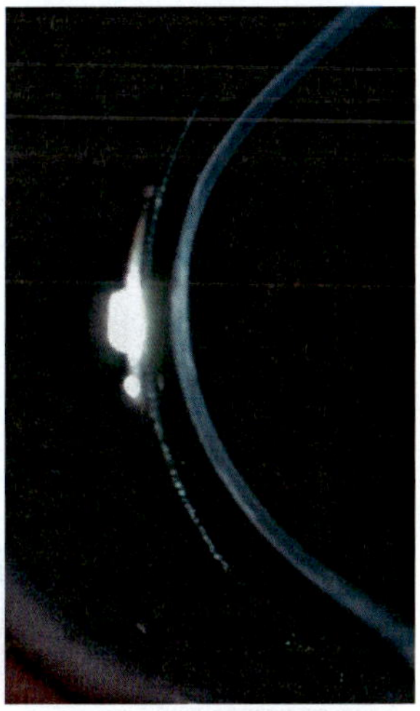

Fig. (17). Measuring the clearance without fluorescein. Note the bright reflex of the slit lamp beam on the anterior surface.

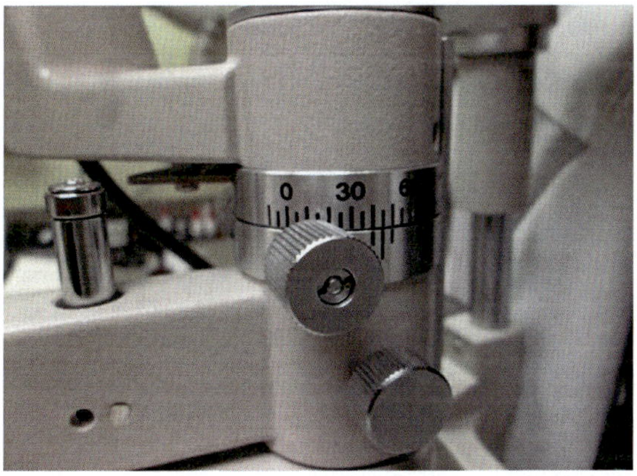

Fig. (18). Aligning the slit lamp beam at 45 degrees ensures optimal measurement of the clearance.

In both scenarios, with and without fluorescein, the clearance should be evaluated superiorly to inferiorly while also scanning laterally. When scanning over the limbus, it may be difficult to identify both lens surfaces. The slit lamp housing and binoculars can be angled to the side of the patient to maintain the appropriate angle of illumination (Fig. **19**).

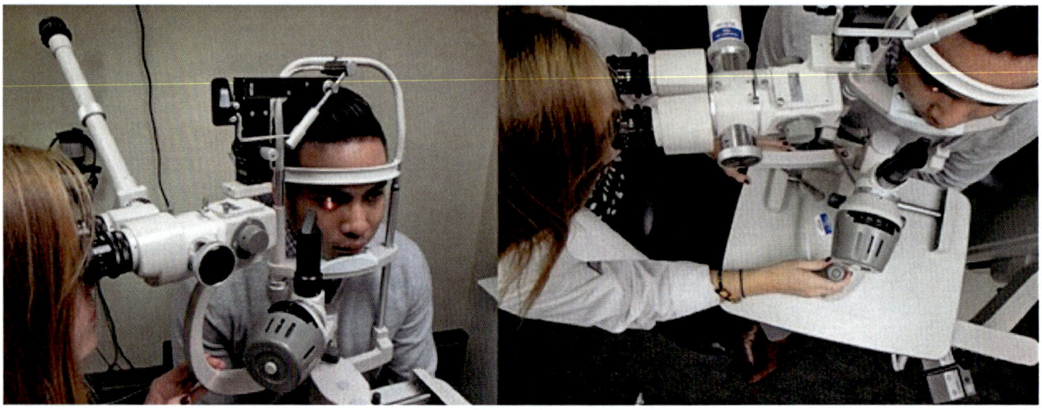

Fig. (19). Manipulating the slit lamp alignment may aid in observing limbal clearance.

How Much Clearance is Ideal?

To date there has been no clear consensus on the ideal clearance and each lens design tends to have its own optimum recommendation. It has been suggested that 200μm central clearance and 50μm limbal clearance with a lens thickness of 250 μm may optimize oxygen transmission to the cornea [2].

Scleral lenses settle back on the eye during wear presumably due to the pliable nature of the conjunctiva so the clearance will reduce gradually over the day from its maximum amount at application. Caroline reported settling of 96 μm (ranging from 70 to 180 μm) over the course of eight hours in 15 subjects wearing a 16.5 mm lens [3]. Kauffman *et al.* evaluated the settling of three different designs; 14.3, 15.8 and 18.2 mm lenses settled by 113.7, 133.7, and 88.1μm, respectively. Both showed that settling is nonlinear and that the majority happens soon after lens application [4]. In a study by Esen *et al.*, two lens diameters (16.5 and 17.5 mm) were tested with initial clearances between 100-200, 200-300, and >300 μm [5]. They reported that 80% of the settling occurred within the first 4 hours. The 16.5 mm diameter lenses demonstrated more settling than the 17.5 mm lenses and lower initial clearances settled less than the higher clearances. However, there was significant inter and intrasubject variability. Whilst an average increase in central corneal thickness of 1.3% occurred, it was not statistically different in any clearance category and remained within physiological limits. A 2016 study of 16 patients evaluated how the change in fluid reservoir depth affects the total refractive power of the scleral lens/reservoir system, it was determined that settling appeared to have a relatively small impact (0.25D) on lens power needed to provide optimal visual acuity in this group of patients [6]. These studies are consistent with clinical observations especially in terms of the significant inter and intra subject variability.

Based on the previously described studies, it appears that larger diameter scleral lenses settle less than smaller diameter scleral lenses. Therefore, it is advisable to fit the lens with slightly greater clearance than is the final goal to allow for settling. Wherever possible, the first follow up appointment should be after a minimum of four hours of scleral lens wear to evaluate this patient-specific settling effect. If there is insufficient clearance at the four-hour fit evaluation, then an increased sagittal height and /or limbal clearance should be made to account for further settling with longer wear times.

Additionally, if the patient has a progressive ectatic disorder, the lens can be dispensed with extra clearance to allow for corneal progression.

Scleral Landing Zone Evaluation

Once the corneal and limbal clearance are established, the practitioner can evaluate the scleral landing zone. Ideally, the landing (also known as the scleral or haptic) zone of the lens should align with the conjunctiva overlying the sclera (Fig. **20**). It is known that the sclera is irregular and asymmetric in shape and that there is a wide inter-subject variation in scleral topography therefore true alignment is unlikely with preformed/diagnostic lenses. However, there is certainly a range of clinically acceptable scleral zone fittings that minimize the risk of physiological complications. Suboptimal scleral zone fittings usually present with either conjunctival compression and/or impingement (or both) into the conjunctiva. Conversely, if the landing zone is too loose, there may be edge lift/standoff. These features may be circumferential, meridional or localized.

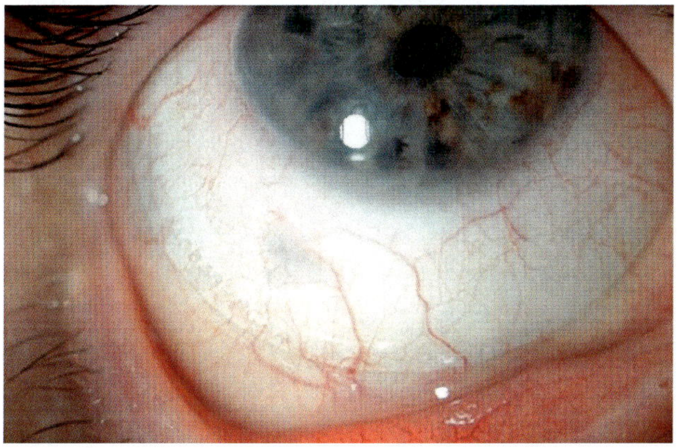

Fig. (20). Large and small conjunctival vessels should flow underneath an aligned scleral lens unimpeded.

There is confusion, and even debate, in the scleral lens field about compression and impingement. For clarification, in this text, compression and impingement are defined with respect to the conjunctival surface.

Compression

Blanching of the conjunctival vessels that occurs because of excessive bearing/pressure of the scleral lens peripheral curves. Compression may occur anywhere under the landing zone of the lens, not just at the edge. The location of the compression indicates where the landing zone is bearing too harshly and thus directs the type and zone of modification required. Compression may cause hyperemia adjacent to the area of blanching with the lens *in situ*, and on lens removal, rebound hyperemia may occur where the vessels had previously been compressed. Compression does not typically result in conjunctival staining.

Compression can be identified outside of the slit lamp as described earlier. If there is meridional compression and blanching, then a toric periphery may be indicated. The lens always must bear its weight somewhere, so it is not uncommon to have some form of blanching since the conjunctival tissue is easily compressible and soft. Ideally, the bearing should be evenly balanced throughout the landing zone of the lens to minimize long term complications and prevent symptoms of discomfort.

Compression may be exaggerated on application, especially if the eye has a degree of baseline hyperemia, for example in eyes with known ocular surface disease. The differential between the hyperemia and the blanching often reduces as the eye adapts to the presence of the lens. Over time, a hyperemic and inflamed eye may adapt to a scleral lens. Effectively, the hyperemia and inflammation resolves and the landing zone now becomes too loose. Similar to fitting a shoe to a swollen foot, once the swelling goes down, the shoe becomes too loose. Therefore, careful and close monitoring in the early phases of the fitting process is necessary. This will ensure that the fit remains appropriate for the patient in the long term. If the lens becomes too loose, then exogenous tear debris is more likely to seep under the lens into the post lens tear reservoir. In extreme cases, there can be a significant gap between the landing zone and the ocular surface that can allow air to seep under the lens and create a bubble.

When evaluating scleral lens landing zones, it is important to examine the patient after extended wearing times (three hours or more), as areas of compression may appear or become obvious once the lens has settled onto the conjunctiva. If compression is evident 360 degrees, the lens may suction to the eye (Fig. **21**). Where the conjunctiva is blanched underneath the lens, the same vessels will demonstrate rebound hyperemia after lens removal (Fig. **22**). The patient usually describes a sensation of tightness and/or tiredness if the compression is significant. Also, the patient will report that there is immediate relief once the lens is removed although the eye may remain tender to the touch. Rebound hyperemia is a sign that suggests loosening of the lens. The conjunctiva can be probed using the eyelids. Manipulating the eyelid to press on the tissue peripheral to the hyperemia causes the patient to report pressure rather than pain, tenderness or discomfort. If it is similarly manipulated to press on the region of hyperemia, the patient often describes a sore sensation. A moistened cotton tipped applicator can also be used for this purpose. If symptoms occur from palpation, then a change of the landing zone is required to alleviate the compression.

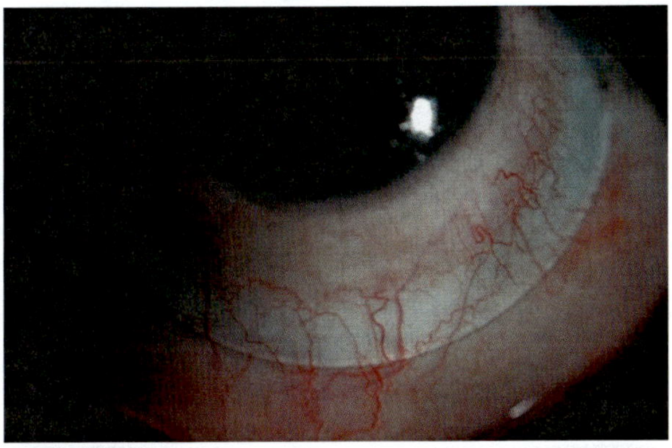

Fig. (21). An example of scleral compression all around the edge of the lens. This can create suction. Image courtesy of Lynette Johns, Optometry Times (July 2016).

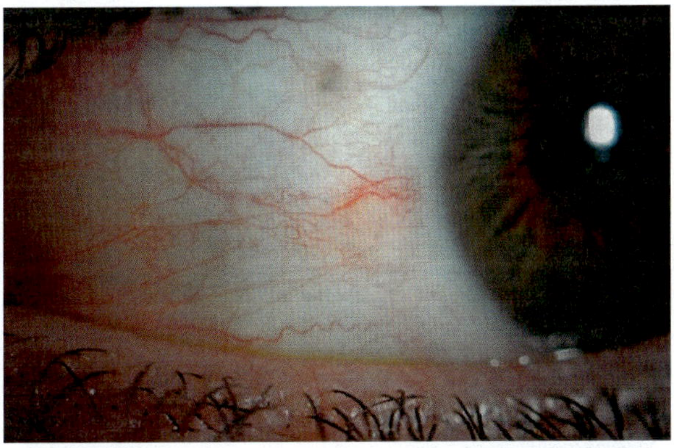

Fig. (22). Sectoral Rebound hyperemia over a pinguecula. Image courtesy of Lynette Johns, Optometry Times (July 2016).

Compression needs to be addressed early in the fitting process as the longer the patient is wearing a compressed landing zone the more symptomatic he will likely become. It is not uncommon for a patient to drop out of scleral lens wear due to intolerance as a result of compression three to six months after the initial fitting.

Any redness, especially after lens removal, requires further investigation once handling errors have been ruled out. If the practitioner experiences significant resistance when removing the lens, it is likely that compression is the culprit. If the lens comes out easily for the practitioner and the eye remains white and quiet, more training for the patient is indicated.

Compression is not always obvious as some patients have naturally white and "quiet" eyes, and if the landing zone is small, it can be easy to miss compression. To determine the degree of compression, gentle pressure can be exerted on to the globe using the eyelid or a moistened cotton tipped applicator just adjacent to the lens edge. Where blanching is present, the greater the amount of pressure required to perfuse the vessels under the lens means that a larger degree of compression is present. If fine caliber vessels re-perfuse immediately, the degree of compression is minimal, and only small changes to the lens design are indicated.

Compression is reduced or eliminated by redesigning the landing zone of the lens. Compression in the mid periphery of the landing zone may require the far peripheral curves to be steepened and/or the curves closest to the transition to be flattened to make for a gentler slope (Fig. **23**). Compression at the far periphery, or the very edge of the lens, requires the peripheral curves to be flattened. Determining the amount to adjust a compressed periphery is an art, which practitioners become more skilled with experience. In the initial stages, or when using a new design for the first time, it is advisable to take advantage of the laboratory consultation team who know the intricacies of their lens design intimately including the proprietary curves.

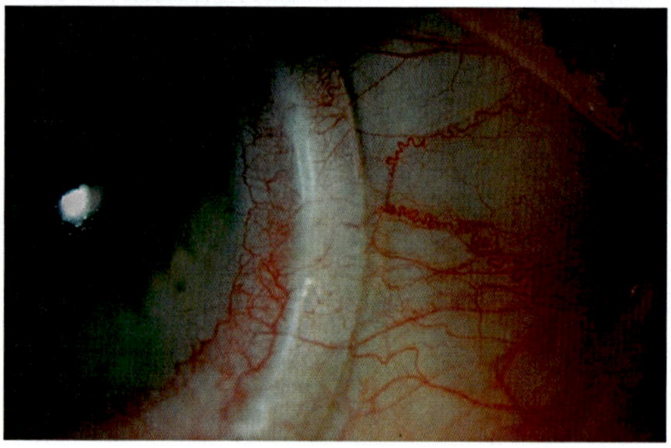

Fig. (23). Compression of conjunctival tissue with significant localized blanching of the vessels and adjacent circumlimbal hyperemia. This compression resulted from a harsh junction of midperipheral and peripheral landing zone curves.

Impingement

The edge of the lens focally pinches into the conjunctival tissue. Impingement can occur as a result of a very steep landing zone with minimal contact with the conjunctiva except for the very edge of the lens. Essentially, the edge of the lens acts as a cookie-cutter into the conjunctival tissue and in extreme cases, the conjunctiva can lacerate at which point lens wear must be discontinued until it has healed.

Impingement can be difficult to observe especially when it occurs in the absence of compression (Fig. **24**) as vascular blood flow may not be impacted. A subtle observation is that the adjacent tissue outside the edge of the lens may bow forward.

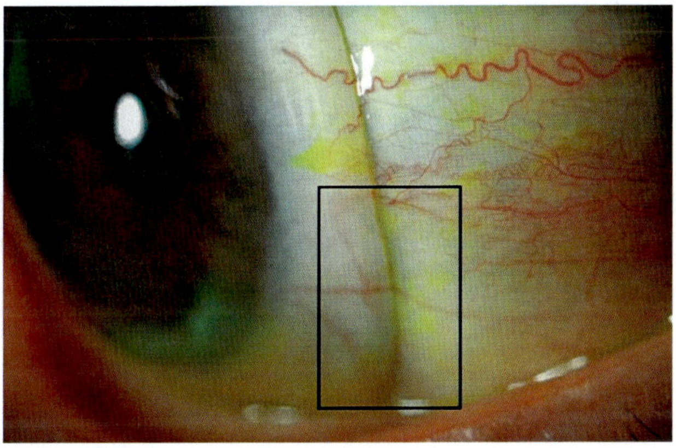

Fig. (24). Example of impingement without compression. Note the ocular surface tissue appears to be pinched along the edge of the lens causing the tissue outside of the edge to bow outward. The vessel featured in the box retains its blood flow beside and underneath the edge of the lens; however, the vessel is not coursing straight through.

It is not uncommon that subtle impingement is missed during initial evaluation, although the appearance may become more obvious with increased wearing time. If the impingement is significant, the patient usually experiences symptoms of discomfort with the lens *in situ* and tenderness is often accompanied by tearing on lens removal. These symptoms increase throughout the wearing time and can cause long term intolerance of the lens. Impingement results in arcuate conjunctival staining after lens removal (Fig. **25**). Long term impingement may result in conjunctival hypertrophy (Fig. **26**).

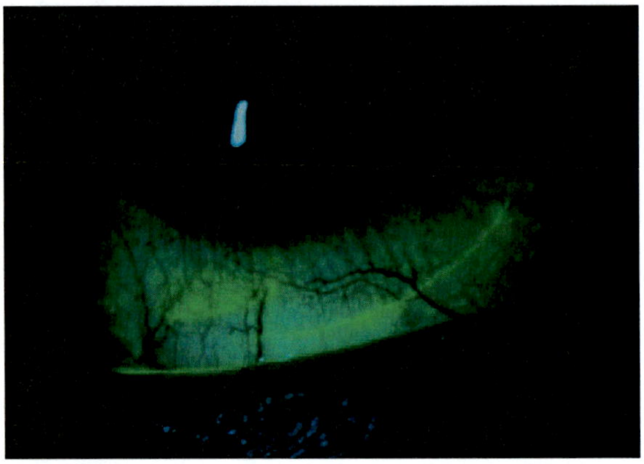

Fig. (25). Example of conjunctival staining resulting from short term (<3 hours) impingement of the landing zone of the lens.

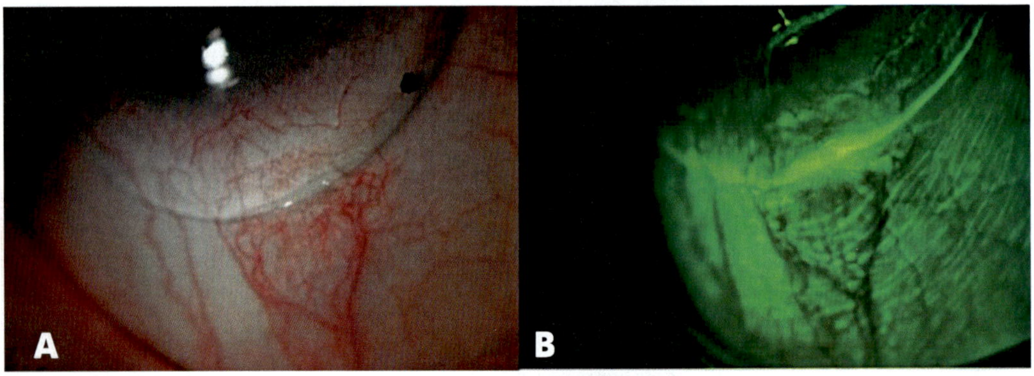

Fig. (26). Scleral impingement of a tight scleral lens infero-nasally (A) A small band of compression is also present at the edge. (B) Associated conjunctival hypertrophy created by the impingement from the same lens in A. In this image, the scleral lens had been removed and the ridge was created by the tight landing zone edge. Image courtesy of Lynette Johns, *I-Site e-newsletter* (March 2016).

While the long-term effects of impingement can be quite dramatic, hypervigilance and careful observation/documentation during the initial stages of the fitting can highlight some of the potential signs of impingement. Therefore, it is strongly advised to always remove the scleral lens and evaluate the conjunctiva (and cornea) with fluorescein. Fortunately, troubleshooting impingement is straightforward. Impingement is relieved by lifting the lens edge away from the scleral surface which may be specified by either flattening of the peripheral curves or an increase in the edge lift. If both compression and impingement are observed together, the modification to the lens is similar, but may be of a larger magnitude.

The practitioner must be aware that flattening the peripheral curves by larger amounts can result in the conversion of a far peripheral compression/impingement zone to a mid-peripheral compression zone unless compensatory adjustments can also be made from the transition zone outwards.

Edge Lift/Standoff

The edge of the lens is lifted off the ocular surface creating tear pooling, or in extreme cases, an air meniscus. Edge lift is seen as a shadow, fluorescein pooling, tear frothing, or an air meniscus at the edge of the lens (Fig. **27**).

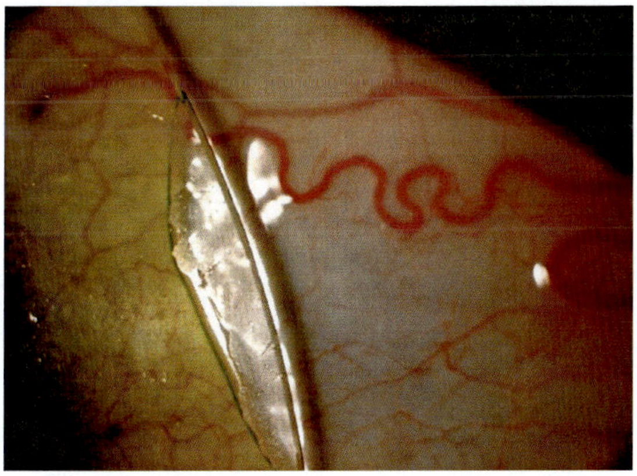

Fig. (27). Example of extreme edge-lift with fluorescein pooling and an air meniscus.

Edge lift is arguably the most common cause of lens awareness for the patient upon lens application. Patients may report a "tight" sensation, irritation or sharpness. Patients can be quite specific about the location of the awareness or discomfort, especially with significant edge lift, and this can direct the practitioner's investigation. The sensation may be exacerbated by squeezing the eyelids tightly shut. This can assist the practitioner in the initial location of a compromised landing zone. If there is edge lift, the pressure generated from their eyelids will increase the lens awareness because the edge lift is affecting their palpebral conjunctiva. Impingement may also be identified because the edge is being pushed into the bulbar conjunctiva. Basically, if the patient can further identify a region of increased awareness, the practitioner can more easily identify landing zone misalignment either being too loose (edge lift) or too tight (impingement and some cases compression). Typically, compression does not create a sensation immediately after application unless it is quite severe. However, with increased wearing time, compression can be symptomatic and may illicit a response when squeezing the eye.

Short term consequences of edge lift are primarily symptoms of lens awareness. Bulbar conjunctival findings are unlikely since the far peripheral landing zone is not aligned to the surface. However, edge lift can occur in conjunction with mid-peripheral compression in which case conjunctival blanching may be seen in the mid-periphery of the landing zone. Superior edge lift may induce or exacerbate giant papillary conjunctivitis (Fig. **28**). Inferior edge lift may cause the lens to snag on the lower lid during blink and can destabilize the lens as well as creating a more acute sensation for the wearer. Edge lift/standoff is remedied by redesigning the landing zone specified by either steeping the peripheral curves or reducing the lift in microns.

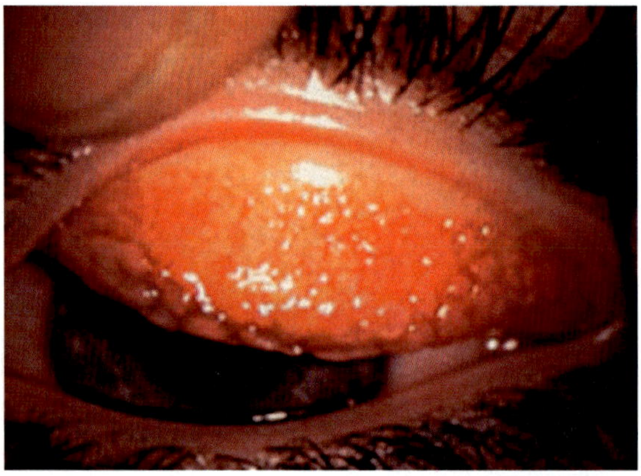

Fig. (28). Example of giant papillary conjunctivitis in a scleral lens wearer.

With excessive edge lift, there will be increased tear exchange; this may create a path for a bubble and tear film debris entry. The amount of edge lift can potentially be measured with an OCT. Without an OCT, edge lift highlights well with fluorescein. If a tighter scleral lens is designed, there will be less fluorescein pooling at the edge. On the other hand, when a lens is too tight, it is difficult to determine how much to loosen the landing zone. Using the eyelid to press the conjunctiva adjacent to the edge of the lens where compression is present can help determine how tightly the lens is compressing. The more pressure it takes to re-perfuse the blanched vessels under the scleral lens, the more step changes the landing zone requires to loosen the fit in that region or overall.

How much looser or tighter should the landing zone be changed? It often depends on the steps of change that can be made by the manufacturer. Steps of change may be listed in microns, angles, radii, or diopters. One step may be 25 microns by one manufacturer and 100 microns from another manufacturer. It is always advisable to discuss slit lamp observations with laboratory consultants. When determining the magnitude of landing zone changes, it is important to view the scleral landing zone in all extreme gazes (superiorly, inferiorly, nasally and temporally) since compression and impingement are often exaggerated. Then observe the landing zone in primary gaze. If the findings are still significant or present in primary gaze, loosen the landing zone in larger steps. However, if the findings are eliminated in primary gaze, either no change is required, or a minimal step change can be designed.

Utilizing Toric or Quadrant-Specific Designs

Scleral asymmetry increases from the limbus to the equator of the globe. Recently OCT analysis has been used to show that the transition between the cornea and sclera is a tangential [7]. It is also known that the nasal meridian is flatter than the rest of the scleral meridians. Scleral shape is discussed in detail in Chapter 3.

Most diagnostic lenses are rotationally symmetric, but in view of the known nature of scleral topography, rotationally asymmetric designs are frequently required in scleral lens practice to approximate alignment of the landing zone with the sclera. Careful and detailed documentation and schematic drawing of findings in each quadrant can aid in identifying patterns (Fig. **29**).

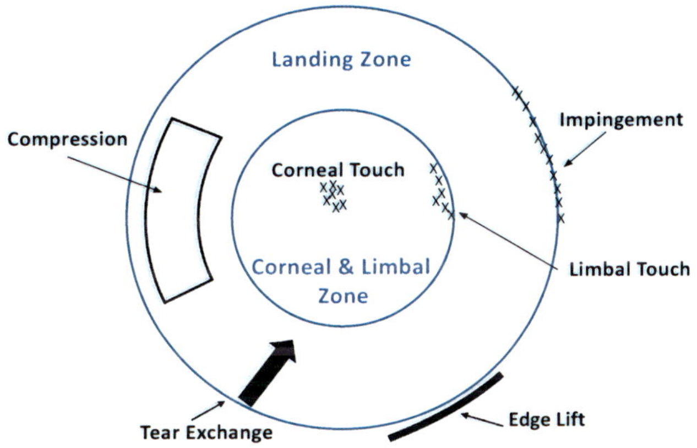

Fig. (29). A schematic example of scleral lens documentation. The scleral lens fit is divided into two zones: the corneal and limbal zone and the scleral landing zone. Corneal or limbal contact is labeled with Xs. A band of compression is drawn where there is blanching. Edge lift is highlighted where fluorescein would pool. An arrow demonstrates the directionality of tear exchange. Impingement is designated with Xs at the edge of the lens.

Many modern scleral lens designs are available with back surface toric and quadrant specific peripheral designs.

Modern anterior segment topographers and OCT devices can provide information about scleral toricity but in their absence, rotationally symmetric diagnostic lenses themselves act as topographical aids. If the sclera is asymmetric, the diagnostic lens may demonstrate alignment, edge lift, compression or impingement (or both) in different meridians.

The fitting characteristics of a rotationally symmetric landing zone applied with-the-rule to scleral topography (the flatter/elevated meridian is horizontal) vary depending on the relationship between the actual scleral curvature and the landing zone configuration. There are three possible appearances if the lens periphery is **too tight**:

1. Alignment in the vertical meridian with compression and/or impingement in the horizontal.
2. Circumferential compression/blanching but the degree of blanching greater in the horizontal meridian than the vertical (Fig. **30** and **32** left eye).
3. Peripheral curves appear compressed and/or impinged in the horizontal meridian but with edge lift/standoff in the vertical (Fig. **31** right eye).

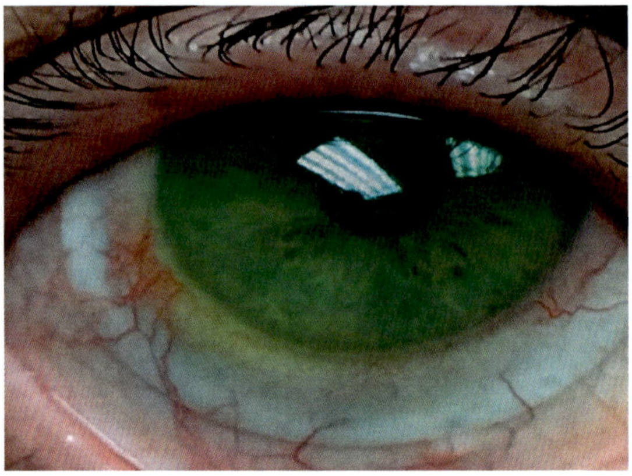

Fig. (30). Tight rotationally symmetric lens on a with-the-rule sclera. At first glance, the lens appears tight 360 degrees around. However, there is significantly more compression horizontally than vertically. Image courtesy of Lynette Johns.

It is always important to determine the flattest or most elevated meridian of the eye. If the lens appears too tight along the eye's flat meridian, then the lens should be redesigned to alleviate the compression and impingement observed.

Conversely, consider a loose-fitting lens with a rotationally symmetric landing zone applied to a with-the-rule sclera. Then the landing zone may demonstrate edge lift/standoff 360 degrees, but there would be substantially more edge lift/standoff along the vertical meridian. Additionally, fluorescein exchange will be more prominent along the vertical meridian.

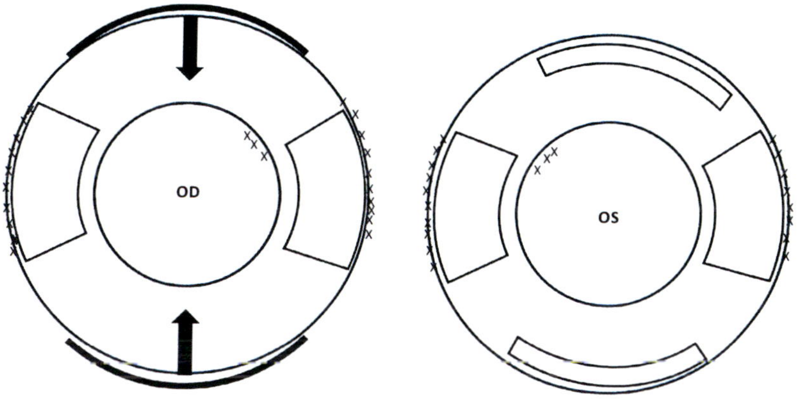

Fig. (31). Documentation of tight rotationally symmetric diagnostic lenses on with-the-rule scleras. The right lens is compressing and impinging along the horizontal (flat) meridian, but is demonstrating edge lift with tear exchange along the vertical meridian. There is superior-nasal limbal contact. The left lens is tight all around, but tighter along the horizontal (flat) meridian as evidenced by broader compression and impingement. There is no tear exchange and compression along the vertical meridian. The left lens is also touching the superior-nasal limbus which may also suggest decentration. The landing zone in the lens in Fig. **30** would be documented like the left lens in this diagram.

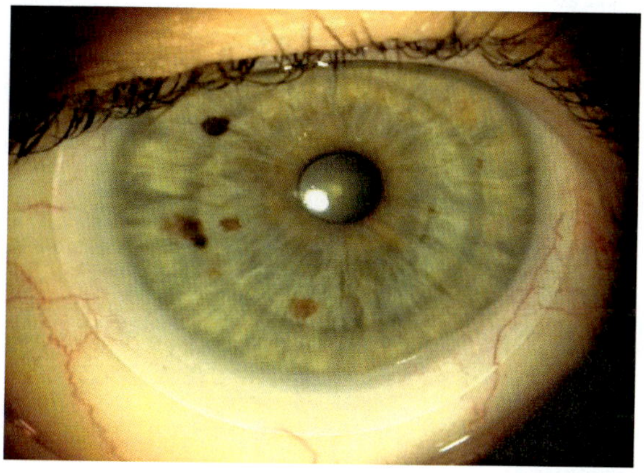

Fig. (32). Example of a right scleral lens that is mildly decentered infero-temporally. Note the width of the landing zone superior-nasally compared to the width of the landing zone infero-temporally. Image courtesy of Maria Walker.

It has been shown that incorporating toricity into the landing zone gives improved lens comfort. If a (back surface) toric scleral lens is rotated more than 45 degrees either clockwise or counter-clockwise, it will return to its original position on average within four seconds [8]. Improved patient satisfaction and increased wearing times were also statistically significant. A bitangential toric scleral lens design, that is tangents at perpendicular meridians, improved comfort while demonstrating stability [9].

In some cases, the fitting pattern is asymmetric within a single meridian, for example, there may be more edge lift inferiorly than superiorly, with alignment in the horizontal meridian. A toric scleral landing zone can be utilized as it will perform much better than a rotationally symmetric design giving better comfort and reduced tear exchange and subsequent debris intrusion. However, asymmetry along the vertical meridian will remain with either the inferior quadrant demonstrating edge lift while the superior quadrant is aligned, or the superior quadrant demonstrating compression and/or impingement while the inferior quadrant is aligned. Quadrant specific designs allow a modification to the landing zone to be made in any quadrant independently of the others to improve overall alignment, comfort, and tear exchange. Unfortunately, not every lens design is capable of quadrant specific modifications; therefore, if it is apparent at an early stage that this may be necessary, then a compatible design can be chosen.

Some scleral lens designs have toric and/or quadrant specific landing zones built into diagnostic lenses. Like a bitoric corneal gas permeable lens, they will rotate and orientate themselves on the corresponding meridians. Rotationally asymmetric diagnostic lenses always have one meridian labeled and when evaluating, it is important to document the rotation of the marking for lenses that require front surface optical toricity. The axis of optical toricity is modified to compensate for the rotational orientation of a lens in a similar manner to soft toric contact lenses. The quantity of degrees of rotation is added if the lens is rotated to the left / clockwise and subtracted if the lens rotated to the right / counter-clockwise (Left Add Right Subtract - LARS, Clockwise Add Anticlockwise Subtract - CAAS). Back surface toricity and quadrant specific lenses are stable and return to their original orientation rapidly if rotated [8], therefore, no further stabilization feature (prism ballasting, double slab off prism, dual thin zone, truncation) is required.

To optimize application of the lens in the proper orientation, lenses may be dotted or engraved. The convention is either one dot for the right lens and two dots for the left lens or a dot of one color for the right lens and a different color for the left lens. The engravings are usually on the vertical meridian, although some laboratories routinely mark the steep or flat meridian, therefore the practitioner needs to understand the design they are using. If the lens is intended to be marked in the vertical meridian but the scleral toricity is oblique, then the engravings will appear rotated *in situ*. The patient must be educated about this rotation, otherwise the patient may continue to remove and reapply the lens trying to have the dot placed at 6 o'clock. Similar to a soft toric contact lens, the back surface always rotates to the same orientation, therefore any front surface toricity must be adjusted to compensate for this.

Movement

There is little intentional movement associated with scleral lenses. Any movement observed usually signifies that the landing zone may be misaligned, the lens has too narrow a landing zone, the lens is resting on the cornea or poor wettability is causing the lid to adhere to the surface of the lens on blink. The lens fit should be checked immediately for corneal contact and then for suboptimal landing zone alignment.

Asymmetric compression zones can force the lens to rock with the blink and can be remedied by incorporating back surface toricity or quadrant specific designs described earlier. Optimizing the diameter to minimize the effect of irregular scleral zones can also help to stabilize the lens.

Another scenario that may induce lens rocking and movement is the presence of bilateral pinguecula. The lens lifts over the pinguecula in the horizontal meridian resulting in unwanted edge lift in the vertical meridian. Remedies include toric peripheral curves, edge notching, localized vaulting or using an alternative diameter to land either closer to the cornea than the pinguecula or to land beyond the pinguecula.

Lens Decentration

Lenses may decenter on the eye typically inferiorly or infero-temporally (Fig. **32**). Decentration is likely multifactorial in most cases but contributing factors include lens thickness, lens weight and eyelid tension; all of which cause the lens to drop inferiorly. Asymmetry and irregularity of the scleral landing zone causes the lens to locate infero-temporally, especially with larger diameter lenses as the nasal sclera is flatter and more elevated and has a smaller potential bearing zone.

Refining the peripheral curves including toric and quadrant specific modifications can provide improved alignment with the ocular surface and center the lenses better. Smaller diameter lenses tend to center better than larger diameters as they land on a more regular part of the sclera. Lenses fit with a very narrow landing zone are also prone to decentration. This can be seen using fluorescein which will extend well past the limbal clearance zone, over the conjunctiva and towards the far periphery of the lens (Fig. **33**). The start of the landing zone will be observed where the fluorescein ends. In cases of extreme scleral asymmetry, there may be no landing zone contact with the ocular surface (Fig. **34**). In such cases, the peripheral curves and angles must be manipulated to lower or flatten the lens in these regions to more closely align to the ocular surface and extend the landing zone inward toward the limbus.

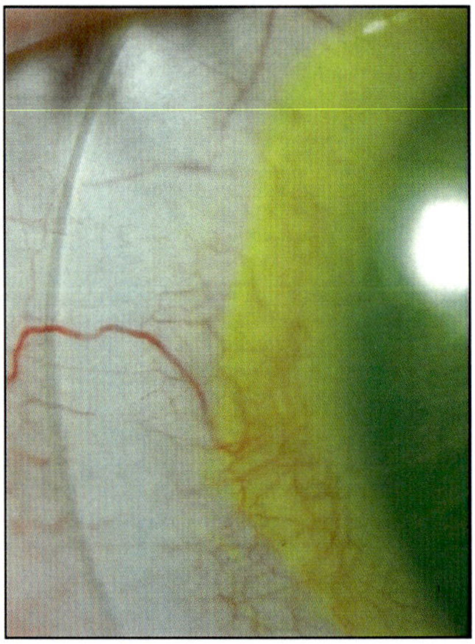

Fig. (33). Example of a scleral lens that demonstrates clearance over the adjacent sclera. If the landing zone was significantly smaller with the same amount of scleral clearance, the lens would be prone to instability, movement and decentration. Image courtesy of Michael Lipson.

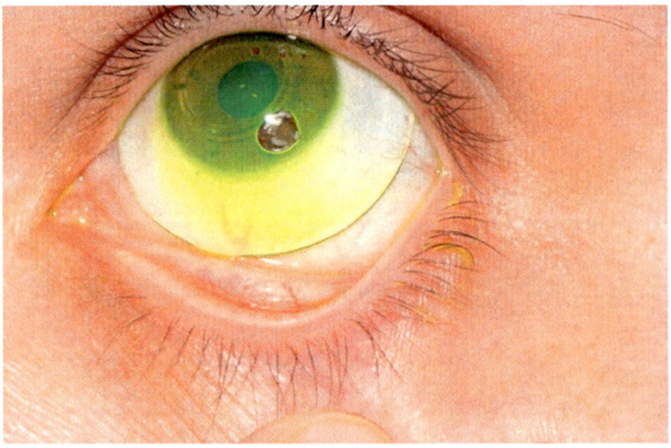

Fig. (34). An extreme example of a scleral lens that demonstrates significant clearance over the adjacent sclera inferiorly. Figure courtesy of Jennifer McMahon.

Altering the overall thickness profile of the lens can reduce the bulk of the lens reducing the decentration effect caused by the lens weight or the downward pressure of the upper eyelid. Excessive clearance particularly at the limbus can also create a bulge of the optic zone that can force the upper lid to push the lens downward. Ensuring an optimum clearance pattern and modifying the curves to give smooth transitions can reduce decentration issues and improve comfort.

Decentration is particularly problematic when fitting scleral lenses with multifocal optics. Scleral lenses can provide an optimal platform for such designs because of their limited movement, however, good centration is essential for correct alignment of the optics. In the correction of higher order aberrations, the optics are decentered to align and compensate for the decentration; otherwise, there would be no point to the correction. Decentration of optics is possible, but not readily available.

Conjunctival Prolapse

Since some scleral lenses decenter inferiorly and also have asymmetric limbal clearance, there is a tendency for the conjunctiva to be drawn and pulled underneath the scleral lens (Fig. **35**). Eyes with excessive conjunctival tissue, conjunctivochalasis, and loose conjunctiva are particularly prone to this phenomenon. Also, lenses that exhibit excessive inferior or peripheral clearance can also create the space for the conjunctiva to be pulled into.

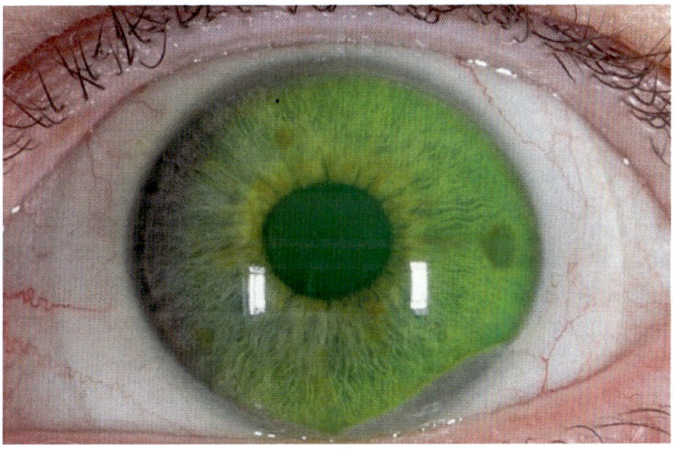

Fig. (35). Example of inferior conjunctival prolapse. Image courtesy of Tom Arnold.

Many designs incorporate shape profiles into their optic or clearance zone. These shapes can be prolate, oblate, reverse geometry and asymmetric. Incorporating shapes that more closely align to the corneal and limbal surface can reduce the excessive clearance and gap into which the conjunctiva can be drawn. Improving overall alignment and extending the alignment of the landing zone can also reduce this phenomenon. In larger diameter lenses (greater than 20 mm in diameter), the phenomenon appears to reverse and it is more common to see conjunctival prolapse if a fitting has insufficient circumferential limbal clearance.

FOLLOW-UP SCLERAL LENS AND EYE EVALUATION

Once the final lens has been dispensed, it is crucial to reassess the lens fit regularly to ensure that it remains optimal. During follow up visits, a careful history is taken, a detailed evaluation of the lens is performed, photos and OCT, if necessary, are obtained, and finally an ocular surface evaluation following lens removal is undertaken.

Follow-up Case History

The report of comfort, wearing time, handling issues, and care systems are all crucial pieces of information for the scleral lens practitioner. Some patients are reluctant to report any discomfort with scleral lenses since they are concerned that practitioners will determine that they are no longer candidates for scleral lenses. This can be very disconcerting since, oftentimes, a scleral lens is a treatment of last resort. Patient reassurance is very important when developing an honest dialogue during the case history.

At the time of publication, there is no documented and validated measure of scleral lens success. Wearing time and comfort are two critical determinants of patient success. Since the goals of scleral lens wear include visual rehabilitation, attenuation of ocular surface disease symptoms, and ocular surface support, both the patient and practitioner should be cognizant of the original treatment goals at each follow-up visit to ensure the lenses are meeting both of their expectations.

There are a variety of reasons for reduced wearing time of scleral lenses. In the beginning, shortly after dispensing scleral lenses, handling is one of the primary reasons patients reduce wear or discontinue entirely [9]. Patients may be ashamed that they are having difficulty applying and removing the lenses. Fortunately, reinstruction and supervised trainings are simple remedies.

Patients may also state that they experience intermittent discomfort with scleral lenses. They have “good days” and really “bad days.” Patients may say that they were comfortable when they left the office wearing their scleral lenses, but when wearing them at home they hurt. Application bubbles are often the cause of this intermittent symptom. A patient leaves the office comfortable because the practitioner ruled out that no bubbles were present before the patient left. However, when the patient is home and unable to identify application bubbles, their cornea desiccates from the bubble (Fig. **36**). Bubble identification should be a part of scleral lens training. Patients can purchase a high magnification mirror and a penlight or flashlight to aid recognizing a bubble. The best solution to alleviate the discomfort from a bubble is to reapply the lens without one. However, patients are often very reluctant to reattempt lens application.

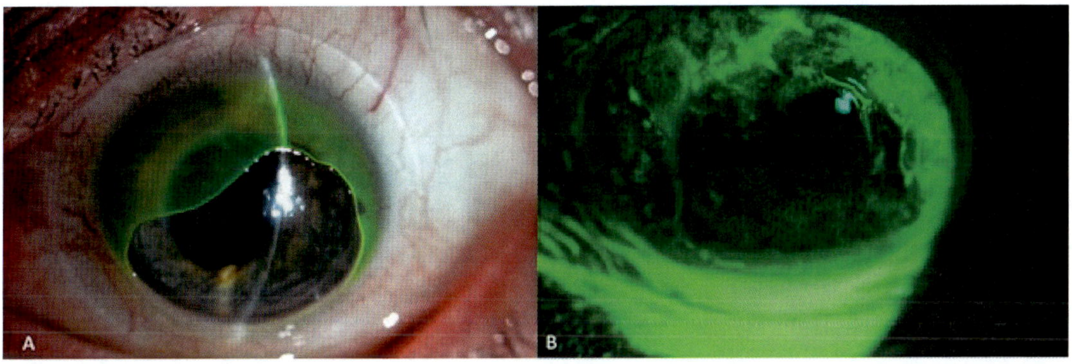

Fig. (36). Example of a large application bubble (A) and the associated desiccation staining after removal (B). Image courtesy of Andy Taddeo.

Symptoms of improperly fitting scleral lenses vary depending on the type, magnitude and location of the problem. Much attention is focused on clearing the cornea, although, in reality, patients do not experience significant discomfort from corneal contact while the scleral lens is worn. Patients may complain of a vague nonspecific discomfort at the end of the day or as the day goes on. This can be particularly significant if the lens settles back further than expected. One of the hallmark symptoms of corneal touch and contact is a foreign body sensation that may be associated with tearing after the lens is removed. The practitioner should carefully examine the cornea for punctate epithelial erosions shortly after the lens is removed.

Compression of the landing zone can lead to discomfort with increased hours of wear. It is always important to ask the patient what type of symptoms they experience and when they occur. Symptoms may be described as tight, sore, tired, tender or achy to name a few. Patients will often describe relief after lens removal. There may be sectoral or complete rebound hyperemia.

"Redness" can be a very common complaint with many etiologies. A hyperemic response signifies a problem and it is up to the practitioner to determine the cause. Solution toxicity induces hyperemia and is usually accompanied by punctate epithelial erosions. Therefore, it is important to determine which solutions the patient is using with their scleral lenses. In some cases, the patient may be using an appropriate filling solution, but a thick and viscous gas permeable conditioner may remain on the inside of the lens creating a mild toxicity reaction. Patients may complain about redness after removal as described previously. It is important to rule out improper removal techniques. If a patient applies the removal plunger to the center of the lens and pulls directly out, a significant amount of suction is created that can induce hyperemia after removal. It is important to ask if the lenses can be removed easily, is there suction, or even a noise when removing.

The practitioner should remove the scleral lens after an extended wearing time to determine the amount of resistance or suction (after the lens had been thoroughly evaluated). If the lens is removed easily for the practitioner and no hyperemic response occurs, the patient simply needs removal reinstruction. If the redness complaint occurs while wearing the lens and worsens with increased wearing time, then the fit should be carefully assessed.

The symptoms and complaints described in the history can cue the practitioner where to evaluate the lens carefully. Typically, each symptom corresponds to a unique location of the lens fitting relationship. Not only can the location be isolated, but the timing of the symptom can indicate if the fitting relationship is too tight or too loose.

The patient may also have visual complaints. "Midday fogging" is a very common and typically the patient presents describing "hazy" or "misty" after 3-4 hours of lens wear. Possible causes include poor wetting, front surface deposits, debris in the tear reservoir, and corneal edema. It is important to ask the patient if they see rainbows around lights, indicative of microcystic epithelial edema (Fig. **37**) or Sattler's veil.

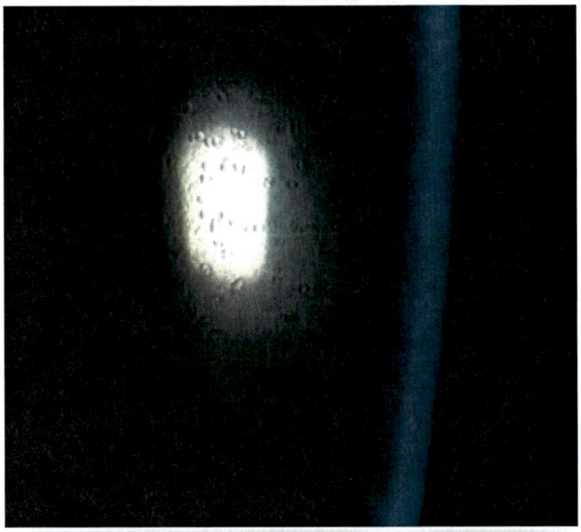

Fig. (37). Example of microcystic corneal edema in a failing graft that is retroilluminated from the reflection off an intraocular implant.

Patients often describe a sensation of heat under these circumstances and in extreme cases severe, migraine-like headaches have been reported. Practitioners should be hypervigilant about corneal edema especially with corneal transplant patients. During the fitting process, a penlight can be dispensed to patients for hourly "rainbow checks." Patients should be instructed to pay attention to how many hours of wearing time before the onset of fogging and/or rainbows. If such symptoms occur the patient should be encouraged to remove the lens, clean and reapply immediately. If the vision is clear on reapplication the cause is more likely related to the lens/fit than to the corneal response.

Lastly, an inquiry about solutions should be documented. Cleaning, disinfection, filling solutions, rewetting drops, topical and systemic medication changes may cue the practitioner to explanations when atypical ocular findings are discovered.

Visual Acuity

The visual acuity and over-refraction should be measured at each visit. Sometimes it is helpful to shine a penlight or transilluminator to check the front surface reflex quality and evaluate for bubbles prior to obtaining visual acuities. If the front surface has debris or wetting defects, topical rewetting drops or a gentle surface cleaning/squeegee can be done to the lens (Fig. **7**). Any atypical results of visual acuity may need to be revisited after evaluation of the scleral lens. Sometimes, best-corrected visual acuity measurements with the scleral lens may need to be taken after the lens is removed, cleaned, and reapplied. However, removing the lens to refresh the solution should be discouraged because it will negate the settling effect of the lens.

Follow-up Slit Lamp Evaluation of Lens

When evaluating the scleral lens on a follow-up evaluation, a similar systematic approach to evaluation and documentation as the initial fitting assessment is crucial. The inside-out approach is straightforward and develops a routine when evaluating a scleral lens either during the fitting or the follow-up evaluations.

Front Surface

The front surface of the scleral lens can develop deposits which may be either lipids, proteins or both. In patients that have lagophthalmos or incomplete blinks, the surface of the lens dries out in the exposed area. Fortunately, the ocular surface is protected and lubricated with the saline in the lens reservoir, but the exposure is transferred to the front surface of the lens. When there is exposure, the deposits bind to the surface of the lens and are not easily rinsed off. Grading the amount, location, and type of deposits is important to monitor different treatment and cleaning regimens between visits.

The quality of the surface also should be evaluated. The surface can become scratched, chipped or crazed. Often right lenses are labeled with one dot and the left lenses have either no dots, two dots or one dot of a different color. If a patient has a history of recent and sudden vision (or comfort) changes, it is important to verify that the patient has the lenses in the proper eyes. Document the order number of the lens if labeled on the lens.

If a lens has front surface toricity for the correction of astigmatism, it will be stabilized with either prism ballasting, dual thin zones, double slab-off prism, back surface toricity or quadrant specific or asymmetric peripheries to orient the optical axis. Always check with the lens manufacturer where the dot should be placed (either on the top or on the bottom). If the patient applies the lens dot in the wrong orientation, the optics may be misaligned and result in poor vision. Other markings in addition to the dot may also be present. Similar to soft toric lens markings, each manufacturer labels their orientation markings differently. For example, they may align to the flat axis of back surface toricity or to the axis that more closely aligns to the horizontal. It is important at every visit to determine the orientation of the markings. This can simply be done by rotating the slit lamp beam and "connecting" the markings. This angle of the beam is the axis of scleral lens stabilization that should be consistent between visits. If the beam and markings are rotated, just like a soft toric lens, the amount of rotation is measured and can be optically compensated if necessary.

Measurement of Clearance

The amount of corneal and limbal clearance should be assessed and considered against the wear time that day. Lens evaluations should be scheduled at different wearing time intervals to ensure proper all-day clearance. Clearance is measured with the same techniques as described previously; however, patients will not arrive with fluorescein under their lenses. *A scleral lens should NOT be removed and refilled with fluorescein to measure the clearance.* If a scleral lens is removed and reapplied, the lens will not return to its settled position. Therefore, learning to evaluate clearance without fluorescein is an important skill (Fig. **16** and **17**). If a practitioner relies on fluorescein for determining the clearance, OCT measurements are very useful.

Evaluating the limbus without fluorescein can be quite challenging. Manipulating the slit lamp housing to position the light at various angles can aid illumination of the peripheral corneal and limbal clearance. Sometimes, a hazy ring in the peripheral cornea suggests limbal contact. After lens removal, there is corneal staining, tiny microcysts or bullae. There may also be a sharp ridge of demarcation that suggests that the contact is along a peripheral curve or optic zone junction. Practitioners should be reassured that if a finding suggesting a poor fitting relationship is missed, the ocular surface will demonstrate a finding associated with the lens fit. If corneal contact is present, oftentimes, corneal staining is left behind.

Evaluation of the Post-Lens Tear Reservoir

Midday fogging is a common complaint and troublesome challenge to overcome when fitting scleral lenses. If front surface debris is ruled out as a source of fogging, the next most common location is in the scleral lens reservoir. Here particulate matter of different sizes and consistencies may be present. Practitioners can grade the amount of debris and describe the debris for future reference. Various remedies are described in the problem-solving and challenges chapters (Chapters 12 and 14).

Landing Zone Evaluation

Compression and impingement both become more prominent with increased wearing time and lens settling at the follow-up evaluation. Hyperemia increases adjacent to the area of compression, and the contrast between the hyperemia and conjunctival blanching can be striking. Symptoms of tightness and awareness with increased wearing time suggest compression, impingement or both. Patients often can localize their symptoms that cues the practitioner which section of the landing zone requires further investigation. Symptomatic patients with white and quiet conjunctivae can be challenging when determining the cause of the symptoms. Careful views with high magnification of the path of small caliber vessels may reveal the sectors of compression. In some cases, the impact of suboptimal landing zone alignment is more pronounced after lens removal due to rebound hyperemia which highlights the location of the blanched compressed conjunctiva. Depending on the severity of the compression, palpation may illicit a significant response of tenderness or pain.

Impingement may or may not have associated hyperemia. Long-term impingement demonstrates hypertrophic raised ridges. Lacerated conjunctiva can overlay the edge of the lens. Impingement over time will make the conjunctiva and sclera appear sharply dented with the ocular surface adjacent to the lens edge appearing to bulge forward. Sometimes it can be subtle just outside the very edge of the lens. When the lens is removed, arcuate staining will highlight where the impingement was located. This tissue can be quite tender if palpated.

Fluorescein Assessment

Fluorescein can be applied to the front surface of the lens. After a few blinks, practitioners can look for fluorescein uptake or exchange underneath the lens. Asymmetric or circumferential suboptimal alignment patterns can be more easily identified using this technique. In particular, rapid fluorescein exchange may signify the location of the landing zone that requires improved alignment in cases where "midday fogging" is a problem.

Edge lift will be highlighted with fluorescein. Without fluorescein, a shadow around the periphery of the lens indicates edge lift. However, the orientation of the illumination is very important to see the shadow (Fig. **38**). If there is edge lift, patients will be aware of the lens as soon as it is applied if they are symptomatic. Symptoms may improve with wearing time because the lens settles. Often, they describe the lens as feeling "tight." Patients can be quite specific when localizing these symptoms. Just like compression and impingement, edge lift can also be meridional. A scleral lens with toric peripheries where the meridian of edge lift is designed steeper/tighter will reduce symptoms of edge lift and may also reduce excessive tear exchange.

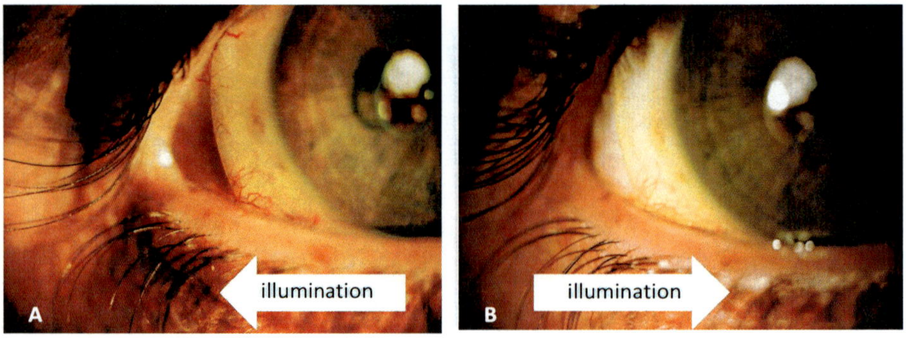

Fig. (38). The same right lens is featured in A and B with significant edge lift. The difference is the angle of illumination. When the slit lamp arm is nasal and the beam is illuminating temporally, the shadow of the edge lift appears. However, if the slit lamp arm is temporal and illuminating nasally, there is no shadow and it is difficult to appreciate the edge lift.

In general, edge lift is more of a nuisance for the patient. Over time, patients eventually adapt to edge lift if the lens is not redesigned. It rarely creates long term complications. However, as stated earlier, superior edge lift may exacerbate giant papillary conjunctivitis (GPC). When evaluating the lids for GPC, it is more comfortable for the patient to evert the eyelids for tarsal plate evaluation when the lens is removed.

Assessment of Lens Removal

Since scleral lenses are semi-sealed to the ocular surface, practitioners should ensure that the lens does not suction to the eye. The presence of tear exchange is a good indicator that the lens has not adhered on the eye. In most cases, a well fit scleral lens does not demonstrate clinically significant tear exchange without mechanical manipulation. Therefore, the only way to prove it is not suctioned is to test removal resistance and it is important for the practitioner to remove the lens as part of the evaluation. If a patient is complaining of difficulty with lens removal or hyperemia after the lens is removed, both may be caused by a tight lens or improper removal technique. If the lens comes out easily for the practitioner but not for the patient, then the patient may require re-instruction. Similarly, if the eye does not have reactive hyperemia after lens removal when the practitioner removes the lens, the patient may need re-instruction. However, if the practitioner experiences resistance from the lens during removal, the lens landing zone may require loosening/flattening.

Assessment of the Cornea

Once the lens is removed, the cornea should be carefully evaluated. Corneal staining and punctate epithelial erosions are atypical findings after wearing a scleral lens. Scleral lenses reduce or eliminate corneal epithelial erosions in severe dry eye patients (Fig. **39**) [10]. Therefore, the presence of punctate erosions may suggest contact of the cornea with the back surface of the scleral lens. Unfortunately, reapplying the lens after the lens had settled may not demonstrate corneal touch since the settling effect is lost; however, shallow clearance may be observed confirming the potential for corneal contact.

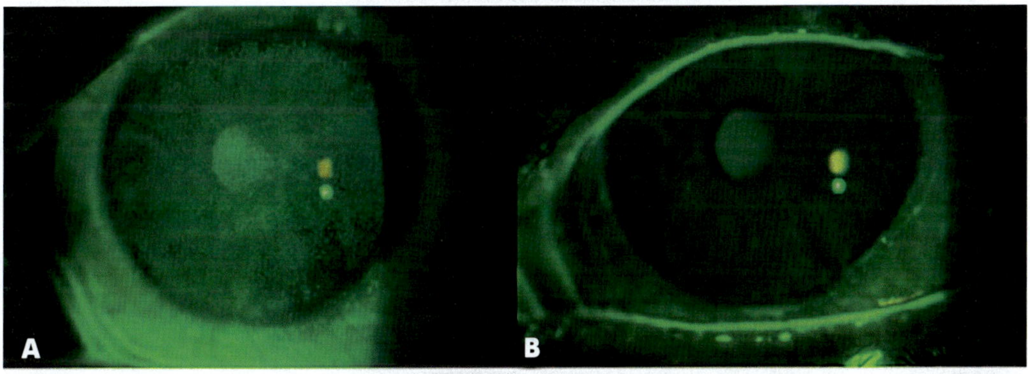

Fig. (39). This patient has keratoconjunctivitis sicca combined with lagophthalmos. A shows the baseline punctate epithelial erosions, whereas B is the same cornea after almost five hours of scleral lens wear. Image courtesy of Lynette Johns, Contact Lens Spectrum (July 2011).

It is helpful to photodocument neovascularization either at the baseline visit or one of the follow-up evaluations. If photo capability is unavailable, careful documentation of radial location, depth and extent of the neovascularization is important for careful monitoring. If there is an increase in neovascularization with scleral lens wear, practitioners should carefully evaluate the clearance in those areas. Oftentimes, neovascularization relates to hypoxia, but mechanical events can also stimulate neovascularization. For that reason, overlying corneal staining should be ruled out.

Edema can also occur or worsen with scleral lens wear. Tiny microcysts and bullae can appear at the limbus. Re-evaluation of the lens after settling may reveal limbal compression and congestion. Modifications to the limbal clearance area in the intermediate zone and anterior scleral landing zone curves may eliminate or reduce this occurrence.

Bullae may form over the surface of a dense stromal scar. If a bulla is observed before the lens is removed, the lens should be carefully and cautiously removed so as not to rupture the bulla. A ruptured bulla will result in a persistent epithelial defect and can be a nidus for infection.

Penetrating keratoplasty is an indication for scleral lens fitting. After lens removal, ensure that there are no areas of corneal staining/punctate erosions, increases in neovascularization, epithelial microcystic edema, loose sutures, or stromal edema.

Any atypical finding of the cornea or limbus that was not present prior to initiating scleral lens wear should be carefully investigated. Some findings are transient, some require lens modifications, and others may require complete discontinuation of lens wear. Careful documentation is crucial in baseline and follow-up evaluations.

Assessment of Conjunctiva and Sclera

The conjunctiva reveals a great deal about the fitting relationship of the scleral lens landing zone. Therefore, it is important to carefully evaluate all quadrants of the conjunctiva after lens removal.

Hyperemia

Compression underneath the scleral lens landing zone results in blanching and impingement of the flow of the vessels. Occasionally, the conjunctiva is hyperemic surrounding the area of compression. When the lens is removed, however, the blanched area becomes hyperemic (Fig. **21**). In cases where the patient reports hyperemia after removal, it is important to rule out any removal difficulties. If the practitioner removes the lens easily, and rebound hyperemia occurs then compression was the likely culprit.

The conjunctiva of some patients can be mechanically hypersensitive and inevitably inject with even mild manipulation. It can be challenging to determine if the rebound hyperemia was due to significant compression that requires loosening of the scleral lens landing zone. Probing the area of rebound hyperemia by using the eyelid may illicit a symptom of tenderness or soreness. If a patient is symptomatic during this manipulation, they probably also experience discomfort while wearing the lens. Symptoms of discomfort with scleral lenses from compression worsen over time. Thus, it is prudent to adjust the lens early in the fitting process. Ideally, the eye should remain white and quiet during wear and after the lens is removed.

Conjunctival Staining

A tight lens edge impinges into the conjunctival tissue. This results in conjunctival arcuate staining (Fig. **40**). Impingement is easily remedied by loosening/flattening the scleral lens landing zone either in a meridian, quadrant or all around. Impingement increases with wearing time. Therefore, it is important to evaluate the lens and eye after a wearing the lens for many hours.

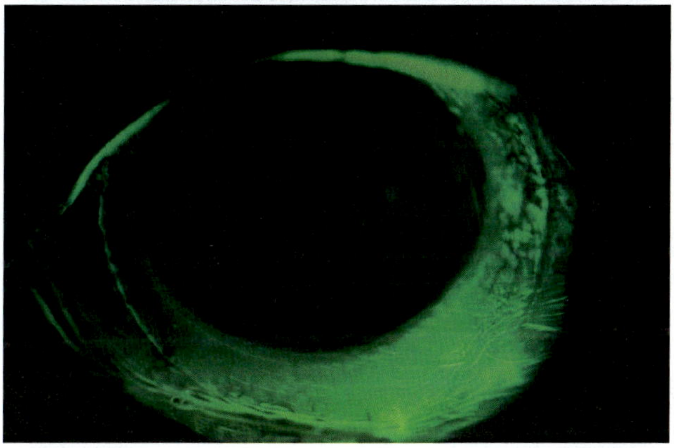

Fig. (40). Example of impingement arcuate staining pronounced at 3 and 9 o'clock. In this case, designing the lens with a flatter horizontal meridian, making the lens toric, will alleviate the staining. Image courtesy of Andy Taddeo.

Impression Ring

Not as extreme as conjunctival staining, scleral lens landing zone compression can also create an imprint or a trenchlike impression into the conjunctival tissue (Fig. **41**). Depending on the depth of the impression ring, fluorescein may pool. If the eye is white and quiet, and there are no symptoms of tenderness after palpation, practitioners should monitor the patient. If the lens is redesigned with a larger landing zone, the intensity of the impression ring can be reduced or eliminated. In some cases, this finding is unavoidable since the conjunctival tissue can be soft and spongy.

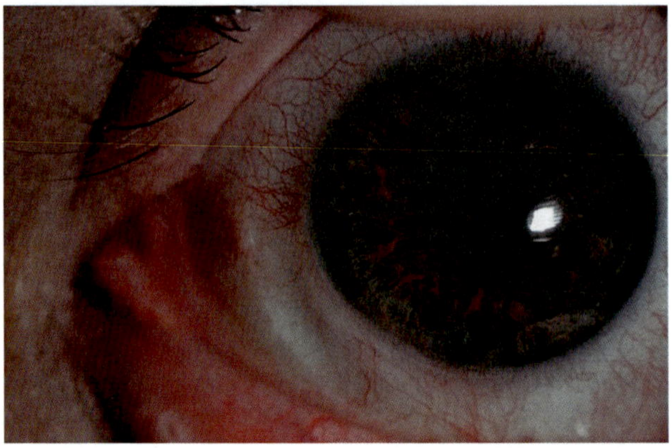

Fig. (41). Example of conjunctival impression infero-nasally. Also present is superior-nasal rebound hyperemia inside the conjunctival impression. Note that the impression is not present inferiorly. Image courtesy of Andy Taddeo.

Once the initial fit is established, it is valuable to evaluate the lens fitting relationship in the late afternoon or early evening. If after 6-8 hours of wearing, there is no corneal staining, edema, rebound hyperemia, conjunctival staining or compression rings, the fit of the scleral lens is most likely not compromising the ocular surface. There still remains a lot to learn about the impact of scleral lenses on the ocular surface, as well as long term effects of scleral lens wear. For now, careful evaluation, documentation and close monitoring should be exercised for maintaining clear vision and comfortable wear as long as the patient requires a scleral lens.

Determination of Quality of Lens Optics

If the visual acuity of the patient does not match the previous records, the patient may be wearing the wrong lens in their eye, there may be a refractive change for the patient, or the lens has warped. Over-refracting may not always help explain the discrepancy. Scleral lenses can warp over time. Performing an over-topography or an over-keratometry can reveal curvature changes with the lens on the eye. If available, a radiuscope measures curvature changes as well off the eye. Warpage is slightly more difficult to determine with lensometry, but it still can be useful. When in doubt, practitioners can return to the diagnostic lens set and recheck the over-refraction as long as the diagnostic lens is not warped.

SUMMARY

Scleral lens evaluation can be intimidating relative to other contact lens modalities since the lenses are much larger and have more variables that can be changed. Systematic and methodical evaluation ensures that practitioners do not overlook key findings of ill-fitting scleral lenses. After scleral lenses are removed, the ocular surface tells its story as well. At every evaluation, practitioners should always remember to evaluate the eye without the lens to ensure that the patient is not compromised and can continue to enjoy all the properties a scleral lens offers.

CONFLICT OF INTEREST

The authors declare no conflict of interest, financial or otherwise.

ACKNOWLEDGEMENTS

Dr. Johns wishes to thank Drs. Perry Rosenthal and Amy Watts who invested time, patience and imparted their great wisdom and experience when introducing her to the art of evaluating and designing scleral lenses.

Ms. McMahon would like to acknowledge the invaluable teaching and support of Ken Pullum to whom she is indebted for her love of medical contact lenses.

REFERENCES

[1] Van der Worp E. A Guide to Scleral Lens Fitting (English) Version 20 Book 2015.http://commons.pacificu.edu/mono/4/

[2] Caroline P, André M. Contact lens case reports scleral lens settling. Contact Lens Spectrum 2012; 27: 56.

[3] Kauffman Matthew J, Gilmartin Christopher A, Bennett Edward S, Bassi Carl J. A comparison of the short-term settling of three scleral lens designs. Optometry and Vision Science 2014; 91(12): 1462-6.

[4] Esen F, Toker E. Influence of apical clearance on mini-scleral lens settling, clinical performance, and corneal thickness changes. Eye Contact Lens 2016.

[5] Britton S, Bray C, Yeung D, Haines L, Sorbara L. Changes in over-refraction after scleral lens settling. Global Specialty Lens Symposium. Las Vegas NV. 2016.

[6] Van der Worp E, Graf T, Caroline PJ. Exploring beyond the corneal borders. Contact Lens Spectr 2010; 6: 26-32.

[7] Visser ES, Visser R, Van Lier HJ. Advantages of toric scleral lenses. Optom Vis Sci 2006; 83: 233Y6.

[8] Visser ES, Van der Linden BJ, Otten HM, Van der Lelij A, Visser R. Medical applications and outcomes of bitangential scleral lenses. Optom Vis Sci 2013; 90(10): 1078-85. [http://dx.doi.org/10.1097/OPX.0000000000000018] [PMID: 23974663]

[9] Schornack MM, Pyle J, Patel SV. Scleral lenses in the management of ocular surface disease. Ophthalmology 2014; 121(7): 1398-405. [http://dx.doi.org/10.1016/j.ophtha.2014.01.028] [PMID: 24630687]

[10] Johns L. Fitting scleral lenses for ocular surface disease. Contact Lens Spectr 2011.

CHAPTER 10

Documentation

Bruce Baldwin*

Department of Ophthalmology, University of North Carolina, Chapel Hill, NC, USA

Abstract: Detailed and careful documentation is crucial for all aspects of the scleral lens patient's medical care. A thorough medical and ocular history details the patient's past medical treatments, outcomes, and previous contact lens modalities. This information serves as a platform to diagnose, monitor and initiate new management strategies including scleral lenses. Proper documentation may also aid the patient with government services and insurance reimbursement. Since scleral lens fitting is intricate and complex, detailed observations assist the practitioner with changing parameters, lens designs, and supplemental ocular management. Due to the progressive nature of ocular conditions that require scleral lenses, photodocumentation of baseline findings, topographies, OCT images, and careful notetaking aid practitioners in optimizing management strategies. When communicating with the patient's medical team, a careful summary of ocular findings may also aid their medical decision making. Lastly, appropriate documentation may be necessary in medical-legal circumstances.

Keywords: Documentation, consultation, patient, ocular history, medical history, penetrating keratoplasty, anterior segment disease, treatment, visual acuity, refraction, slit lamp, eyelids, cornea, conjunctiva, Stevens-Johnson syndrome (SJS), graft *vs* host disease (GvHD), landing, toricity, debris, dispense, imaging.

INTRODUCTION

Documentation of patient encounters is important for many reasons. For the practitioner, comprehensive documentation regarding the medical history, habitual contact lens history and parameters is critical for following progress and may indicate a refit for the patient. Complete consultation notes are helpful when communicating with the referring provider when coordinating care for subsequent visits. Comprehensive notes are required prior to the visit in order to obtain authorization from insurance providers and other financial agencies that support patient care. This chapter will review examination data that should be recorded for patient encounters. Much of the information discussed would apply to any

* **Corresponding author Bruce Baldwin:** Department of Ophthalmology, University of North Carolina, Chapel Hill, NC, USA; Tel: 919-428-0698; Fax: 919-595-9553; E-mails: bbaldwin@med.unc.edu; bruce.uncod@gmail.com

Melissa Barnett & Lynette K. Johns (Eds.)

"routine" patient encounter. However, many scleral lens patients have unique histories, treatment plans and require specialized care.

Initial Encounter - New Patient

Patients seen for the first time from any source (self-referral, consultation, *etc.*) inevitably require more time and documentation. Many practitioners will do a preliminary or diagnostic examination on the initial visit. Depending on the first visit, further testing may be required prior to initiating a scleral lens fitting. The patient may return on a subsequent visit in order to finish the comprehensive initial evaluation and begin or complete a lens fitting. There are many exceptions including patients traveling from a long distance, patients with limited access to transportation, their support network or other resources such as translation. The examination may be two to four times longer than a standard new patient visit. When possible, communication with a new patient prior to the examination is especially important so they can expect and prepare for longer than standard examination times.

Ancillary testing such as photography, corneal topography and optical coherence tomography and other testing may take significant time to acquire in addition to time spent with the technician, staff and practitioner. Patients who are new to specialty lens fitting are often unaware of the considerable amount of time for initial and some subsequent visits. Form letters sent to patients, or a webpage dedicated to instructions to new patients can be very important to notify patients of realistic expectations.

Consultation

A true consultation according to insurance requirements involves a request from one provider for an examination by another provider. The examination includes adequate testing and evaluation to render an opinion to the referring provider regarding diagnosis and treatment plans. A consultation may also involve initiation of treatment. However, "consultation" by definition would involve at some point returning the patient to the referring provider for continued care. Comprehensive notes for the referring provider or insurance carrier would include many of the details discussed below. In the United States, Medicare no longer recognizes a specific billable consultation code; however, other insurance carriers still accept consultation codes. Requirements for documentation of a billable consultation are more extensive than other office visits.

Generally speaking, practitioners often use the terms consultation and referral interchangeably. If a patient is expected to return to the referring provider, then comprehensive and understandable visit notes are essential for continuation of patient care. In addition to legible notes, consideration should be given to the quality of digital imaging. Black and white or faxed copies of corneal topography or anterior segment photography have limited value. Consideration should be given to transferring digital full color imaging when available.

Self-Referral

Some patients may seek care with a scleral lens provider after a recommendation from a friend, an internet search, or specific websites where providers have registered as having experience with scleral lens fitting. Internet search terms such as "scleral lens fitter," or specific disease entities like "keratoconus doctor" will locate practitioners on websites such as The Scleral Lens Education Society (www.sclerallens.org), The Gas Permeable Lens Institute (www.gpli.info), The National Keratoconus Foundation (www.nkcf.org), scleral lens manufacturers or private provider websites. These "self-referred" patients will have a range of lens wearing experiences from recently diagnosed but never fit to a multi-year history of fitting and refitting by one or more practitioners. These self-referred patients will usually require a comprehensive examination including imaging and other testing. Previous eye examination records may not be available. When previous records are available, updated testing such as corneal topography or ocular coherence tomography is at the discretion of the provider.

Fitting After Examination by Another Provider

In a multi-provider or multi-specialty clinic, documentation of a referred patient for scleral lens fit need not be extensive. For example, in a large private practice or university practice, a patient may have been followed for some time by one or more providers. Extensive history, notes, and imaging are likely to be already documented. In this case, minimal information can be obtained to begin a new scleral lens fitting. However, existing data may need to be compiled from the record to communicate with an insurance provider.

Medical and Ocular History

A patient presenting for a scleral lens fitting will usually have a significant ocular history ranging from a "normal" cornea with symptomatic dye eye symptoms, to a disfigured cornea due to degeneration, disease, trauma, or surgery. The medical history can be equally or more important than the ocular history. For example, in patients with Sjögren's disease or rheumatoid arthritis, ocular signs and symptoms may flare as a result of the systemic condition. Therefore, systemic treatment or modifications in the current treatment may be required to alleviate ocular manifestations. Additionally, risk factors for contact lens wear may include soft, corneal gas permeable and hybrid contact lens incompatibility and handling issues with different systemic conditions. Furthermore, scleral lens wear is becoming popular for "normal" corneas with regular astigmatism to better correct refractive error, improve stability of vision, and lens stability for athletes. Multifocal scleral lenses are also available for presbyopia [1]. When fitting scleral lenses for "normal" corneas, practitioners should not overlook systemic medical conditions such as diabetes or hypertension that could lead to potential long term ocular health and systemic complications.

As previously stated, many scleral lens patients will have an ocular condition that originated secondary to a systemic medical condition. Severe exposure keratopathy secondary to Stevens-Johnson syndrome (SJS), chronic graft *vs.* host disease (GvHD), or stroke are a common indication for scleral lens wear [2]. A thorough knowledge of the underlying medical condition is important for long term care of these patients. Knowledge and understanding of treatment is also important for communication with the patient's medical team including the internal medicine physician, rheumatologist, oncologist, or neurologist. Aspects of the medical and ocular history that are important for documentation are described in more detail.

History of Present Illness (HPI) and Medical History

There are many contributing factors that lead to symptoms that may be outside the realm of scleral lens fitting. These include the main complaint of poor visual acuity, significant discomfort, or both. Patients with a new diagnosis may have been unable to obtain a driver's license due to poor visual acuity, or recently ineligible due to a reduction in acuity. Patients may experience disabling discomfort due to severe dry eye, lens intolerance from a small diameter rigid gas permeable (RGP) lens or contact lens intolerance. It is particularly important on an initial encounter to discover the primary complaint along with unexpressed difficulties affecting the patients' quality of life. Patients with no previous lens wear are often confused about why they have poor vision and require considerable education before proceeding with treatment. Other patients who have seen multiple providers with limited treatment success may have a long list of problems, perceived or real, that they want addressed. These patients may be skeptical at this visit. Patient education is important so that a prioritized treatment plan can be established to address each of their problems. Documentation of patient education in the medical record should include the patients' concerns and possible treatment options that were discussed. The practitioner should always be aware that patients have a legal right to information in the medical record and are much more likely in recent years to request those records. Careful wording in the chart of discussions about patients' HPI is prudent in order to not upset a patient who later reads comments that may be taken out of context or misinterpreted.

Patients' concerns and treatment goals are critically important to carefully document in a way that are quickly reviewed at subsequent visits. This is especially important if a patient calls on the phone or emails days or weeks later inquiring about their care. Well written notes documenting the provider/patient plans will help alleviate further miscommunication.

Ocular Trauma

Trauma involving the anterior segment is a common indication for scleral lens wear. Important components of the history include blunt *vs.* penetrating aspects of the injury. With blunt trauma, the patient is at risk for retinal damage and if not documented, a dilated fundus examination should be completed with imaging as indicated [3]. Examination of the anterior chamber angle may reveal angle recession, which increases the lifelong risk of glaucoma [4]. Patients with corneal or corneal-scleral lacerations often use scleral lenses for visual rehabilitation. Early documentation and long term surveillance of the nature of the injury is important. Wound integrity and intraocular pressure are important to document when fitting an eye with recent corneal or corneal-scleral sutures. Loose corneal sutures can place a patient at risk for infection [5]. Broken sutures can cause redness and irritation that may be masked by the scleral lens; however, examination of the eye after scleral lens removal will determine if medical intervention is necessary.

Ocular Surgery

Penetrating keratoplasty (PK) is a major indication for scleral lens wear. Depending on the surgical technique and elapsed time from surgical date, patients may have a variable number of corneal sutures. Documentation of the type of suture (running and/or interrupted) is important. Similar to sutures in ocular trauma, a loose suture carries the same risks. Corneal neovascularization along a suture track can potentially lead to complications like graft rejection and careful notes or photographs are valuable.

Patients who have had glaucoma, retinal, or oculoplastic surgery may have concomitant conditions treated by scleral lens wear. The indications for the surgery may be unrelated to the reason for scleral lens wear. However, the scleral lens practitioner must be aware of complications that may arise from surgery or the underlying condition that resulted in surgery. A good relationship with referring surgeons will ensure optimal coordination of care between providers. For example, patients with severe exposure keratopathy are often managed by an oculoplastic surgeon with a lid weight and tarsorrhaphies (temporary or permanent) [6, 7]. If a patient presents with a temporary tarsorrhaphy, it may need to be removed prior to fitting a scleral lens. Careful observation and documentation of eyelid health can lead to prompt referral for surgical intervention.

Neurological and Motility Disorders

Any condition that results in paralysis or partial paralysis of the normal blink reflex can cause significant exposure keratopathy. Disorders of the VIIth cranial nerve [8], including Bell's palsy, trauma, or surgical trauma from brain tumor surgery can lead to incomplete blink and corneal exposure keratopathy. Documentation of blink excursion and corneal findings is important to determine the severity of the condition and monitoring for improvement. Slit lamp photography is recommended when significant keratopathy is present. Baseline photography is helpful prior to commencing a scleral lens fitting. Corneal epitheliopathy and fluorescein staining should improve with scleral lens wear [9]. If the epitheliopathy is worse than baseline photography on subsequent examination, a lens design change or additional therapeutic intervention may be indicated. Careful examination notes and photographic documentation are crucial for objective measures of therapeutic efficacy.

With long term loss of vision in one eye, strabismus may be present [10]. Documentation of the features of strabismus should include but is not limited to the magnitude and direction, consistency, and most importantly if fusion or diplopia is present. Documentation of constant *vs.* intermittent strabismus will correspond with the level of vision, as a patient with constant strabismus will have worse vision. Comitancy *versus* non-comitancy can be documented; with existing strabismus, comitancy spreads over time. In recent onset strabismus, comitancy is helpful to narrow down the muscle/cranial nerve involved. Fusion or diplopia is particularly important if the patient has symptomatic diplopia. It is important to educate and discuss treatment options with patients as even an ideal scleral lens will not always resolve fusional diplopia.

All of these variables can help determine if an eye should be fit with a scleral lens and for counseling a patient. A patient may not understand why scleral lens fitting is indicated for their strabismic eye. Several of the author's patients with large, long-standing exotropia developed cosmetic and/or sensory fusion a short time after starting scleral lens wear. Patient education can guide visual and cosmetic expectations during the scleral lens fitting process. A period of diplopia may be present, which may lead to "straightening" of the eyes after adaptation to the scleral lens.

Anterior Segment Disease

There are numerous indications for treatment of anterior segment disease with scleral lenses. Documentation is similar in most conditions. Documentation of history should include family history, age of onset, lifestyle impact, level of disability and previous treatments. The family history can be particularly important for conditions with a genetic component, such as keratoconus or Fuchs' endothelial corneal dystrophy. Patients with a new diagnosis and no known family history may want to consider having family members examined to detect early manifestations. Imaging can be obtained as indicated by the condition. Scarring with corneal thinning secondary to herpetic or bacterial keratitis is an example where anterior segment OCT is important. Documentation of thinning and surveillance of the thin area is advisable. Scleral lenses can provide remarkable improvement in acuity of a scarred cornea.

Past Ocular Treatments

Other than scleral lenses, many patients may have tried other treatment modalities. An attempt should be made to investigate and document all prior treatment modalities, both successful and unsuccessful. Various types of over-the-counter and prescription medications are used for dry eye to increase lubrication with contact lens wear. There are dozens of types of lubricant artificial tears, gels and ointments. Patients may prefer a particular brand or ingredient. Any allergies or sensitivities to a known ingredient should be documented. Most scleral lens providers prefer preservative free artificial tears for use with scleral lenses. When recommending particular products, either prescriptions, handouts and/or photographs aid patients in finding the recommended type of lubrication eyedrops.

Prescription drops may include cyclosporine 0.05%, lifitegrast 5% and a variety of topical steroids to control inflammation and treat dry eye. Due to the possibility of steroid induced elevated intraocular pressure, any patient taking a topical steroid eyedrop should have baseline intraocular pressure recorded and monitored during the time a steroid is used [11]. Even so called "mild" steroids like fluorometholone (FML) can cause elevated IOP when used long term [12]. When maintaining these topical medications in combination with scleral lenses, patients should be advised to remove lenses for optimal penetrance. Topical medications used twice a day can be instilled prior to lens insertion and after lens removal.

Autologous serum eyedrops are used for rehabilitation in severe ocular surface disease such as severe dry eye, epithelial defects, and exposure keratopathy [13]. A scleral lens patient may have used or are currently using autologous serum eye drops. Documentation of the duration of serum drop use and the patient's perceived benefit should be recorded. When deciding to maintain a patient on autologous serum drops with scleral lenses, documentation demonstrating the past benefit of autologous serum is useful. Additionally, it is helpful to document the location of the clinic or compounding pharmacy where the blood draw and preparation occur.

Fish oil supplements are effective for managing dry eye in patients wearing conventional contact lenses [14]. There are numerous brands of non-prescription fish oil capsules, chewable and liquid. Documentation of the brand, quantity and compliance of fish oil consumed is important to monitor efficacy. Precautions for fish oil supplementation include but are not limited to allergy to fish, diabetes, liver disease or current use of a blood thinner [15]. If a patient reports little effect from a store brand of fish oil, pharmaceutical quality omega-3 fatty acids purified from fish oil can be prescribed. To date there are no studies evaluating fish oil supplementation specifically for scleral lens wearers. Benefits have been clearly established for other contact lens wearers [14].

There are multiple indications for amniotic membrane grafts [16]. Like autologous serum eyedrops, eye disease for which amniotic membrane grafts are used overlap with conditions where scleral lenses are used. An amniotic membrane can be sutured in place or positioned directly on the cornea for pain control or to enhance wound healing. The type of graft, date of application and outcome should be documented.

Punctal occlusion is a common treatment for dry eye disease. There are various types of punctal plugs including collagen, silicone and intracanalicular. Consider punctal cautery when punctal plugs have shown to be beneficial. Documentation of the status of all four punctae is important. For example, if the lower punctae are plugged or cauterized but the upper punctae are open, the patient may benefit from additional occlusion of the upper punctae. Of particular importance is any history of a retained silicone plug that is below the surface of the lid, or previous placement of intracanalicular plugs. Silicone plugs that are trapped in the canaliculus and intracanalicular plugs have been associated with infections of the lacrimal drainage system [17]. A patient who presents with signs of eyelid or lacrimal sac infection who also has a documented history of retained plugs below the surface, may need a surgical referral for removal of the plug and treatment of lid cellulitis.

A history of eyelid procedures is common in patients who present for a scleral lens evaluation. Eyelid surgeries that are not uncommon in scleral lens patients include tarsorrhaphies and placement of gold or platinum weights. The goal of a tarsorrhaphy procedure is to reduce exposure by surgically bolstering, connecting, or suturing the superior and inferior eyelids together. The most common tarsorrhaphy is partially sewing the outer third lateral eyelids together. A tarsorrhaphy is used to manage a variety of conditions such as non-healing epithelial defects and other exposure keratopathies [18]. The size of the horizontal palpebral aperture is measured and recorded. Small apertures may limit the size of a scleral lens selected for fitting. A tarsorrhaphy that results in a palpebral aperture less than 15mm makes scleral lens fitting difficult, if not impossible. If scleral lens wear is deemed critical for the patient, a request could be made to the surgeon to reduce the size of the tarsorrhaphy by an amount that would allow adequate insertion and removal of the desired lens. After the tarsorrhaphy is taken down, the fitting process is delayed until the eyelids have healed. In the absence of the tarsorrhaphy, these patients are vulnerable and require aggressive lubrication, especially at bedtime.

Patients with exposure from eyelid motility disorders leading to incomplete blinks, lagophthalmous, and corneal exposure may have a gold or platinum weight implanted in the upper lid [6, 7]. This allows for more complete blinks and reduced corneal desiccation. Gold weights can be quite bulky and may interfere with scleral lens wear. Low profile platinum weights may be more physically compatible with blinking over a scleral lens. In a patient with a cranial nerve palsy, careful measurement and documentation of the interpalpebral exposure height is important to document the current state of their condition. Gold and platinum weights can be surgically removed if the eyelid palsy improves [6].

Contact Lens History

Many patients presenting for a scleral lens fitting evaluation will have a past or current history of contact lens wear. This includes soft, corneal gas permeable, piggyback, hybrid, and scleral lenses. Some patients may still be wearing PMMA lenses. When possible, current lens parameters should be entered into the examination record. For gas permeable designs, overall diameter, base curve, and power can be verified in office and recorded. It is not unusual for patients self-referred or referred by other providers to have several unsuccessful contact lens fittings including scleral lenses. If the parameters of the unsuccessful lenses can be determined, this might avoid unnecessary chair time when refitting a lens. Since scleral lenses have multiple important parameters, obtaining previous invoices or examination records with lens parameters is useful. Unlike standard contact lenses, a patient is unlikely to have a copy of the complete scleral lens prescription.

The use of scleral lenses for "normal" eyes without a history of disease, trauma, or surgery is becoming increasingly common as more manufacturers are producing smaller lens designs. Potential scleral lens patients with high spherical or astigmatic refractive error may have been unsuccessful with traditional lenses due to discomfort, visual acuity, or visual stability. Documentation of failure with previous contact lenses may support refitting to a scleral design.

Visual Function

Improvement of visual acuity is one of the most significant advantages of scleral lenses and may be an upmost concern for most patients. Documentation of visual improvement can also be important for legal and insurance purposes.

Determination of best corrected visual acuity (BCVA) with manifest refraction with and without rigid lenses can establish visual function for driving standards, disability for low vision and potential visual improvement.

Visual Acuity

Uncorrected visual acuity (UCVA) should always be obtained on a new patient. In addition to sound medical practice, UCVA may be needed for driver license standards or to establish improvement in acuity with a scleral lens. Due to irregular astigmatism and ocular surface disease, BCVA may be poor and unable to be improved with manifest refraction.

Any improvement in acuity with pinhole can be recorded but should not be used as a measure of best corrected acuity. If there is improvement in pinhole acuity, it should not be used as a measure of BCVA. Despite the best refractive measures, spectacle or contact lens acuity may not match the pinhole acuity. If the UCVA is worse than the largest symbol on a standard projection chart, a patient can be moved toward the chart or the chart moved toward the patient, then the Snellen acuity can be calculated with simple ratios. Alternatively, acuity levels such as count fingers at xx feet or hand motions at xx feet can be recorded. The World Health Organization (WHO) classifies levels of visual impairment in stages noted by Snellen acuity [19]. For example, "severe visual impairment" is worse than 20/200 and equal to or better than 20/400. Most eyecharts will have letters or numbers as large as Snellen 20/400. However, the next WHO level of visual impairment includes a 20/1200 Snellen equivalent, unlikely to be found on a standard chart. If a patient has this level of impairment, a closer viewing distance and calculation of the Snellen equivalent would be necessary. Per WHO classification, "counts fingers (CF) at 1 metre" is equivalent to 20/1200. The World Health Organization is currently working on a revision of vision standards for impairment that includes levels of impairment for refractive error.

Best-corrected visual acuity as measured with glasses or contact lens prescription is usually used to determine the legal status of visual impairment. Practitioners should be aware that visual acuity measured with an eyechart in optimum conditions can establish a level of documented visual impairment based on established references. However, visual function in daily life can be determined by other factors. For example, a patient with 20/50 vision and a severely restricted visual field, or significant history of optic neuritis and poor contrast vision can have more disability than a patient with 20/150 vision due to refractive error.

Manifest Refraction

The manifest refraction without a contact lens on is extremely important for a number of reasons. As described above, the best corrected visual acuity (BCVA) can determine if a patient meets the standard for visual impairment at the "legal blindness" level. The method of best correction should be documented if BCVA is with spectacle or contact lens correction. In the United States, a BCVA in the better eye of worse than 20/200 meets government standards for legal blindness and affords the patient access to help with rehabilitation and training, vision aids, and tax exemption [20]. A patient could have vision worse than 20/200 with glasses, however pass a driver licensing visual acuity test with scleral lenses. The revised IRS codes state that an individual might not qualify for the legal blind exemption if contact lenses are comfortably worn: "If your vision can be corrected beyond these limits only by contact lenses that you can wear only briefly because of pain, infection, or ulcers, you can take the higher standard deduction for blindness if you otherwise qualify." This highlights the importance of documenting the manifest refraction and associated BCVA, as well as habitual wearing time and any contact lens related complications.

The manifest refraction can also determine the type of contact lens to select, and whether to recommend glasses instead of contact lenses. Glasses are a sufficient recommendation if visual acuity meets driving standards and if the patient is comfortable wearing glasses. However, glasses may not optimally correct their acuity or reduce glare and haloes, therefore practitioners should discuss and adequately document contact lens options. In a situation where a patient has an aging corneal graft with very low endothelial cell count or recurrent herpetic disciform keratitis and can see well with glasses, the practitioner may recommend glasses instead of scleral lenses due to the risk of complications.

On the other hand, if the manifest refraction shows a large anisometropia or very high refractive error likely to cause discomfort or diplopia with glasses, then a scleral lens would be an option, despite a potential risk of complications. The results of the manifest refraction and a trial frame demonstration can be used for the patient to decide whether or not to be fit with scleral lenses.

The manifest refraction while wearing a diagnostic scleral lens (over-refraction) can determine the final lens power or the need for cylindrical correction in a scleral lens. Flexure may cause residual astigmatism with a diagnostic lens if the lens is thin or if there is significant corneal-scleral or scleral toricity. Measuring the anterior lens curvature with keratometry can reveal flexure in the lens which may be reduced with a lens design change such as increased center thickness or toric peripheries [21]. If there is residual astigmatism and no lens flexure, then a toric lens design could be considered.

Another use of a diagnostic scleral lens over-refraction is to determine a scleral lens power that is combined with a particular glasses prescription worn over the scleral lens. As an example, a patient with poor vision in the right eye is fit with a scleral lens resulting in much improved acuity. If the patient was wearing glasses with -4.00 diopters in both eyes where the right lens was formally a balance lens, the practitioner can over-plus the scleral lens so the requirements for the -4.00 spectacle lens is maintained. This can save the patient money by not purchasing additional pairs of glasses and also keep the glasses prescription nearly equal in each eye avoiding anisometropia and aniseikonia. In a busy practice, careful documentation of the diagnostic lens over-correction can be used later to order the power to match the glasses prescription. Alternatively, the diagnostic over-refraction can be done with the patient wearing their habitual spectacle correction.

Eye Examination Data

Some of the information in this section has already been covered in previous chapters. All patients should have had a recent comprehensive examination including intraocular pressure and dilated fundus examination. While important, these examination components will not be discussed in this chapter. For the typical scleral lens patient, anterior segment findings are the most important examination results to document. These parameters that can be measured and documented may provide decision-making information for the practitioner.

Slit Lamp Findings

Modern slit lamps have a number of components that can be utilized to aid in the examination of the anterior eye, thus assisting the fitting and evaluation of scleral lenses. A thin optic section may be used to estimate corneal thickness. Corneal abnormalities may be observed with a parallelepiped beam. High magnification and indirect lighting are used to identify corneal endothelial changes such as guttata, which might indicate a low endothelial cell count. Diffuse illumination is used to observe the eyelids, conjunctiva, and punctae.

Eyelids and Eyelashes

Healthy eyelids can contribute to successful scleral lens wear. Scleral lens surface debris on the anterior surface of the lens and particulate matter and debris accumulation underneath the lens are some of the more common complications of scleral lens wear. The presence of blepharitis, meibomian gland dysfunction, or Demodex will often lead to lens deposits and debris. When possible, aggressive treatment of these conditions is advisable prior to a lens fit or refit.

A tarsorrhaphy will reduce the size of the palpebral aperture and possibly preclude fitting of a larger diameter scleral lens. Both the horizontal and vertical diameter of an open eye can be measured in infants, children or adults, especially when a tarsorrhaphy is present or when a patient has small apertures.

These parameters can be measured directly by holding a millimeter ruler next to the eye. Alternatively, uncooperative, or wheelchair/bed bound patients can be photographed while holding a millimeter ruler adjacent to the eye. The photographed imaged of the ruler can be used as a scale, and the ocular features can then be measured precisely (Fig. **1**).

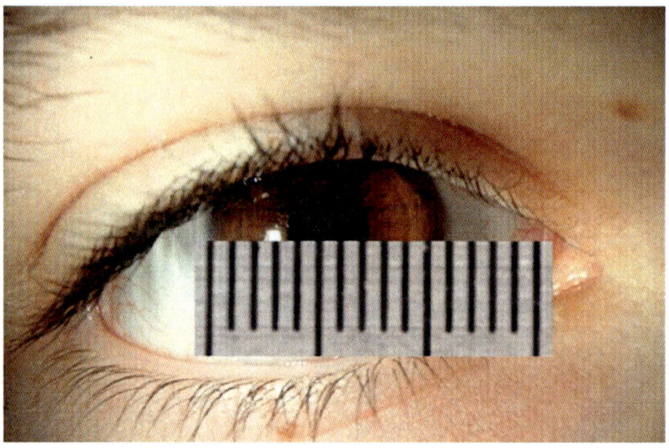

Fig. (1). Example of using a photograph of a millimeter ruler to scale the size of eye structures. In this example, the child's eye and ruler were photographed separately at the same magnification and combined.

Conditions of the eyelashes are important to document. A patient with a history of GvHD, SJS, chemical burn or radiation therapy may have scant or no eyelashes (Fig. **2**). These lashes tend to grow aberrantly and become trichiatic, which may lead to recurrent eye pain and corneal or conjunctival abrasions. The scleral lens protects the cornea when the lens is on and eye pain is significantly reduced. Once the scleral lens is removed, pain resumes due to abnormal lashes rubbing on the cornea. Distichiasis also produces the same discomfort. These abnormal eyelashes can be epilated or cauterized, however upon regrowth, they tend to be sharp and cause more discomfort than a fully grown eyelash. The decision to epilate can be left to the patient to decide. If a scleral lens patient calls the clinic reporting that the eye is irritated after scleral lens removal, the record notes may indicate trichiasis or distichiasis as a possible reason for the irritation. Slit lamp inspection and documentation of all four puncta including the presence of punctal plugs or cautery should be noted.

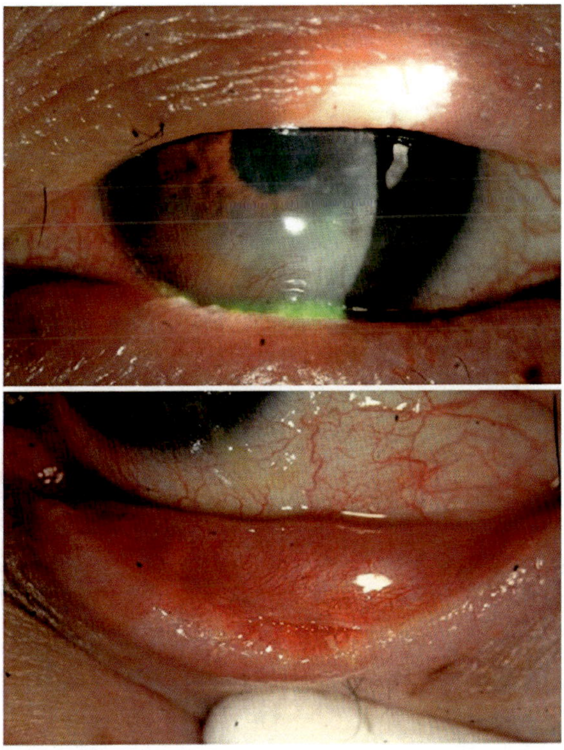

Fig. (2). Patient with Stevens-Johnson syndrome/toxic epidermal necrolysis (SJS-TEN) patient with loss of eye lashes, scarring of the palpebral conjunctiva and corneal neovascularization with scarring.

Cornea

Complications from corneal disease, trauma, or surgery are the most common indications for scleral lens wear [22]. This could possibly change over time as the numbers of normal eyes fit with scleral lenses for refractive error continue to increase. For all patients, careful documentation of the cornea is imperative. The location, extent and activity of neovascularization should be well-documented in the initial examination. Even the smallest opacity or endothelial abnormality needs to be documented in order to demonstrate a pre-existing condition. Slit lamp findings that could be documented are too numerous to list. Regardless of the corneal condition, appearance of the cornea after instillation of sodium fluorescein dye should be described. It is also important to instill sodium fluorescein after lens removal. If an atypical fluorescein pattern or staining is observed after scleral lens wear, it is important to determine if the findings are better or worse than before lens wear. Similarly, other corneal conditions such as scarring or edema should be documented pre and post scleral lens wear.

Ideally, the corneal appearance should be documented with slit lamp photography. Recommended settings include a low magnification with diffuse illumination that captures the cornea, conjunctiva and eyelids. Additionally, images with higher magnification of the corneal structures can be photographed. Slit lamp cameras can be expensive, but there are a number of affordable slit lamp eyepiece attachments used with smart phone cameras [23].

Conjunctiva

While called scleral lenses, they obviously land on the conjunctiva overlaying the sclera, thus the conjunctiva is an important structure to document. A boggy conjunctiva, or conjunctivochalasis, may lead to conjunctival prolapse, where the conjunctiva is drawn and entrapped underneath the lens (Fig. **3**). The presence of significant conjunctivochalasis, a pinguecula, pterygium or a shortened fornix from symblepharon (Fig. **4**) should be documented in the record or photographed. These findings might influence the choice of lens design, such as a smaller lens diameter or customized peripheries.

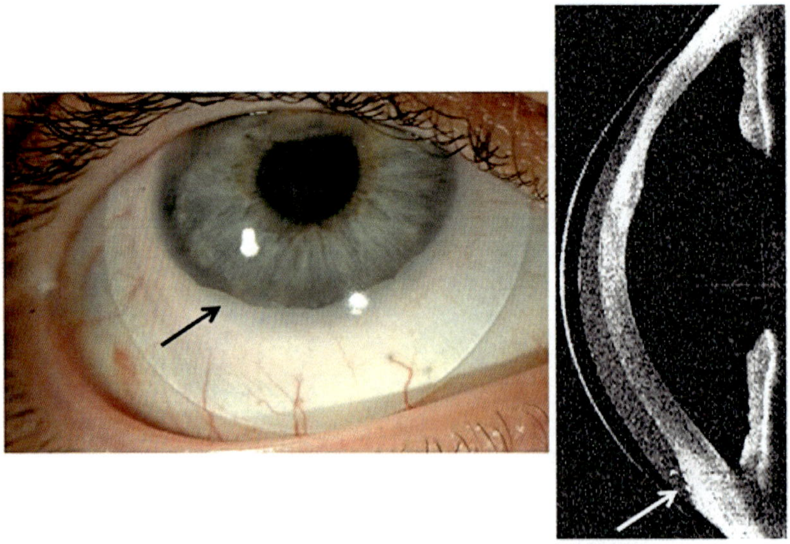

Fig. (3). Excessive conjunctiva drawn and trapped underneath a scleral lens is also known as conjunctival prolapse. This is common finding is usually benign but may lead to adherence or corneal neovascularization.

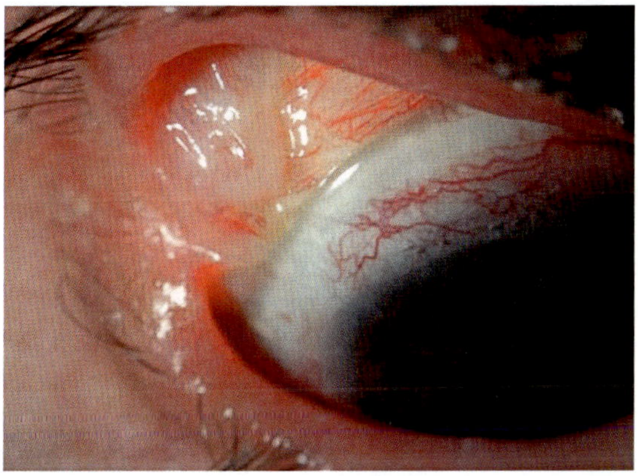

Fig. (4). Symblepharon adjacent to a scleral lens edge can be an obstacle to scleral lens fitting. Image courtesy of Lynette Johns.

The superior palpebral conjunctiva, more than the lower, is associated with giant papillary conjunctivitis (GPC). It is recommended to evert the superior lids on the initial visit to note the presence or absence of papillae. A patient with evidence of papillary conjunctivitis should ideally be treated before initiating lens wear. Periodic inspection of the superior palpebral conjunctiva may be necessary if GPC is suspected. When assessing dry eye, desiccation of the conjunctiva with dye staining is often overlooked. Lissamine green will often stain the conjunctiva heavily in conditions like Sjögren's disease and superior limbic keratitis when only minimal fluorescein staining is present. A large diameter scleral lens may be beneficial when desiccation of the conjunctiva is present.

Assessment and Documentation of Common Conditions in the Scleral Lens Practice

The medical history and objective findings are important for forming a treatment plan, determining the frequency of follow-up visits, and the level of involvement with other members of the health care team. The ocular history is directly related to the scleral lens fit. Lens parameters such as size, shape, material, and other design criteria can be selected, in part by the ocular history. Below some common anterior segment conditions and past treatments that are important to document as the fitting process proceeds are described.

There are numerous systemic conditions with co-morbidities involving the eyes. A smaller subset of these conditions affects the anterior segment in ways that can be managed with scleral lenses. The referring doctor may explain the patients' diagnosis and current treatments to date. In new patients that were not referred, after establishing a diagnosis and patient discussion, a treatment plan needs to be established and followed.

Other Systemic Conditions

Besides diabetes and hypertension that are important in eye care, conditions that are important to a scleral lens practice include autoimmune disease, dry eye, medication reactions, transplant complications, radiation therapy, genetic disorders and other medical conditions. Usually, the medical history will be known to the patient and previous documentation is available. A brief review of some of the more common conditions managed with scleral lenses is discussed.

Autoimmune Conditions

Autoimmune conditions including rheumatoid arthritis, Sjögren's disease, systemic lupus erythematosus, and thyroid eye disease (TED) commonly induce signs and symptoms of dry eye (keratoconjunctivitis sicca) or exposure keratopathy [24]. A practitioner should consider a referral or workup for an autoimmune disorder for a patient presenting with significant dry eye without a previous diagnosis of an autoimmune disease. A review of systems (ROS) during the patient history should include specific questions inquiring about personal or family history of an autoimmune disorder. Specifically ask for symptoms of dry mouth and arthritis if autoimmune disorders are suspected. The objective portion of the examination should encompass corneal and conjunctival staining, tear quality and tear meniscus, tear break up time (TBUT) and Schirmer's testing. Evaluation of the hands and joints, motility, dexterity and grip strength can influence application and removal training strategies. It is important to question the patients' social status and whether they live alone or have a companion. Companions can aid in application and removal of scleral lenses. Coordination of care with the patient's rheumatologist is critical for long term management of these patients.

Stevens-Johnson Syndrome (SJS)

Stevens-Johnson syndrome (SJS) or the more severe form toxic epidermal necrolysis (TEN), is a severe hypersensitivity reaction, usually to a systemic medication, with cutaneous and ocular manifestations [25], including severe dry eye and exposure keratitis due to loss of eyelashes, lack of lacrimal gland and mucus membrane function, and in some cases, cicatrized eyelids. Keratinization of the conjunctiva or eyelid margins leads to recurrent or persistent corneal epithelial defects. These patients will always have a history of a hospital admission, usually to a burn ward due to skin lesions. Review of the admission notes is important to document the causative agent, often an oral antibiotic or anti-epileptic medication. With slit lamp examination, document the presence of trichiasis, distichiasis, and keratinization of the eyelid margins. Measure the extent of corneal neovascularization and pannus. Document the location and extent of the symblepharon. These patients can be quite photophobic, and a full slit lamp examination may not be possible until a scleral lens is placed on the eye. If symblepharon leads to the corneal surface, a scleral lens is contraindicated (Fig. **4**). Practitioners should practice extreme caution when prescribing any topical medications to these patients. Patients with a history of SJS may suffer a recurrence from a different causative agent.

Graft vs Host Disease (GvHD)

Graft-*versus*-host disease (GvHD) is a complication that can occur after a stem cell or bone marrow transplant. With GvHD, the newly transplanted donor cells attack the transplant recipient's healthy tissue [26]. Ocular symptoms, when present, cover a wide range of severity and can be found in acute and chronic GvHD. Ocular signs range from mild dry eye to severe exposure keratopathy, scarring and symblepharon formation [27]. Scleral lenses can provide symptomatic relief from eye pain and promote epithelial healing [28]. These patients often have a depleted immune system from the bone marrow transplant or post-transplant anti-rejection medications. Thus, the patient may be more susceptible to an eye infection. Careful documentation of current medications and allergies, appearance of the eye and adnexa, and telephone/pager numbers of the patient's hematologist or oncologist are critical for long term management of these patients. Any ocular flare up of GvHD can indicate a systemic etiology. Discussion with the patient's medical team should precede any topical ocular treatments since changes in systemic medications may be required. A periodic summary letter may be sent to the medical team. Special testing includes Schirmer's testing, corneal and conjunctival staining and tear break up time.

Radiation Therapy

Radiation therapy of the orbit, head, or neck often causes destruction of the lacrimal system, eyelashes, and conjunctival accessory glands [29]. Radiation therapy can lead to scarring, exposure keratopathy, and eye pain quite similar to SJS and GvHD (Figs. **5** and **6**). These signs and symptoms can be managed with large diameter scleral lenses. Documentation of the total amount of radiation exposure is important because the severity of dry eye signs and symptoms can be directly related to total exposure [29]. Tumors of the orbit, head, or neck can recur and require periodic imaging by the treating physician. The eyecare practitioner should encourage the patient to return to their oncologist for routine visits, even when in remission. Any atypical finding should be documented and coordination of care can be initiated. This could literally be a lifesaving referral in the case of a recurrent malignant tumor. It is critical to document staining, loss of lashes and corneal scarring. If the eye is pre-phthisical, measuring palpebral aperture and exopthalmometry are beneficial for monitoring and scleral lens selection.

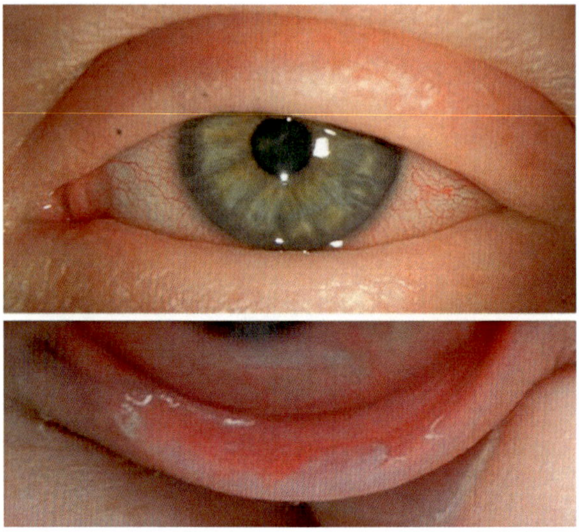

Fig. (5). Loss of eyelashes (madarosis) and eyelid keratinization and scarring in a patient with a malignant orbital tumor with a history of radiation.

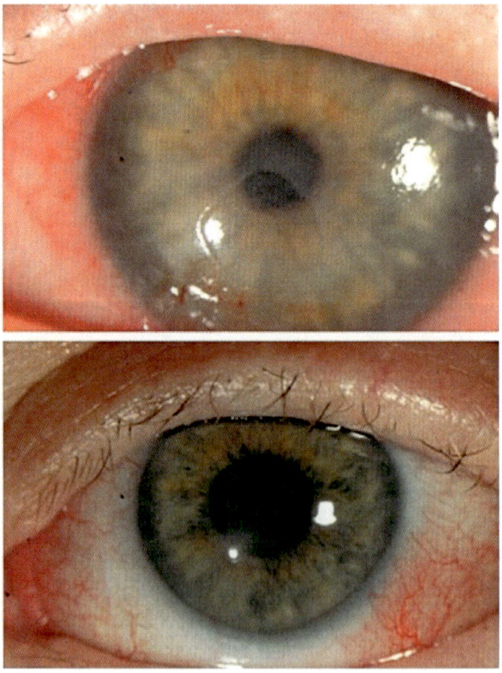

Fig. (6). Same patient as in Fig. (**5**). The patient developed a neurotrophic corneal ulcer that responded to treatment. Note some regrowth of the upper lashes over time.

Other Systemic Conditions

There are numerous other systemic conditions where a patient may be wearing a scleral lens directly related to the condition, for example, dry eye. Alternatively, a patient may have an eye condition requiring a scleral lens that is unrelated to the systemic condition. Understanding and documentation of other systemic conditions is important. A good example would be ensuring appropriate dilated fundus examinations of a diabetic patient with testing of blood glucose and HbA1c. Genetic syndromes often cause anterior segment conditions treatable with scleral lenses. Examples include keratoconus in Down syndrome [30] and corneal scarring in aniridia [31].

Documentation of Scleral Lens Fit

During a diagnostic lens fitting session, it is very important to keep track of the different diagnostic lenses used including the physical fit observations, over refraction, and visual acuity for each eye. Undoubtedly, all busy lens practitioners have on occasion lost track of what diagnostic lenses were used and had to have the patient return for a revisit to complete the fit process. Practitioners should develop a consistent system for annotating enough information in the chart so that final lens parameters can be calculated and lenses ordered, often long after the patient has left the clinic. For example, a diagnostic lens that did not fit well could be noted with minimal information like "diagnostic lens X, needs much more vault," or "diagnostic lens X, severe limbal impingement 360."

A lens with a suboptimal fit should be noted and immediately removed from the eye and documented. It is helpful to separate suboptimal lenses from the immediate work area. A diagnostic lens with an acceptable fit will have additional information recorded including the fit and over refraction.

Once a lens for one or both eyes is determined to have an acceptable fit, lens parameters should be recorded with additional notes such as any planned adjustments to the fit. During the examination, it is advisable to record the over-refraction in the chart and calculate the final power later, thus avoiding a hasty math error.

Sometimes it is helpful to verify the parameters before calculating the final lens order. Additionally, this prevents diagnostic lenses from being mixed up. Some scleral lens manufacturers put lens identification markings on the trial lens making verification quick and easy.

There are numerous details that comprise a well-fitting scleral lens. Three broadly defined fitting parameters to evaluate and document during a fitting are the clearance/vault, the landing, and tear exchange. These three parameters are equally important for a good fit. Below we will review details of each of these parameters.

Lens Clearance (Vault)

Scleral lenses are designed to completely vault over the central cornea and limbus. Synonyms for vault include clearance and fluid chamber. The vault of a lens is determined by the overall sagittal depth of the lens. The sagittal depth is driven by a combination of effects from the central base curve, the overall diameter, and other curves peripheral to the base curve. Central and limbal vault should be carefully evaluated and documented. The depth of central vault can be estimated by several techniques. If the center thickness of the diagnostic lens is known, a direct comparison of the lens central clearance can be estimated quite easily with an optic section of the slit lamp microscope. Sodium fluorescein dye instilled into the bowl of the lens prior to insertion, or after insertion, can aid in visualizing the clearance. Sometimes the post-lens tear reservoir with fluorescein is easier to visualize with a bright white slit beam than the cobalt blue light of the slit lamp.

If the center thickness of the diagnostic lens is not known, the vault can be compared to the estimated corneal thickness. Prior knowledge of the corneal thickness is important. Corneal grafts can be over 600 microns and keratoconic corneas less than 400 microns. An estimate of the vault in microns can be recorded, and if corneal thickness not immediately known, a note such as "one half central corneal thickness" can be noted and corneal pachymetry reviewed later.

Practitioners with anterior segment ocular coherence tomography (OCT) instrumentation can image the lens on eye to get a high magnification image of the lens to cornea relationship. Most OCT models have software that can measure and graphically display the magnitude of the central and limbal vault in microns.

When documenting the central clearance, note the settling time of the diagnostic lens. Research has shown that standard scleral lenses can settle more than 100 microns during the first three hours of wear [32]. This phenomenon of lens settling can lead to underestimation of the clearance of a completely settled lens. Lens to cornea contact could have grave consequences. For example, after dispensing, the scleral lens settles and creates central bearing on a keratoconic eye. Fig. (7) shows a patient with central bearing of a scleral lens with acute hydrops. Fortunately, the poor fitting lens was photo documented and the findings were discussed with the patient prior to developing hydrops. She was refit but decided against medical advice to continue to wear her ill-fitting lens. When a patient refuses to follow medical orders or advice, it is important to have thorough documentation from a legal standpoint.

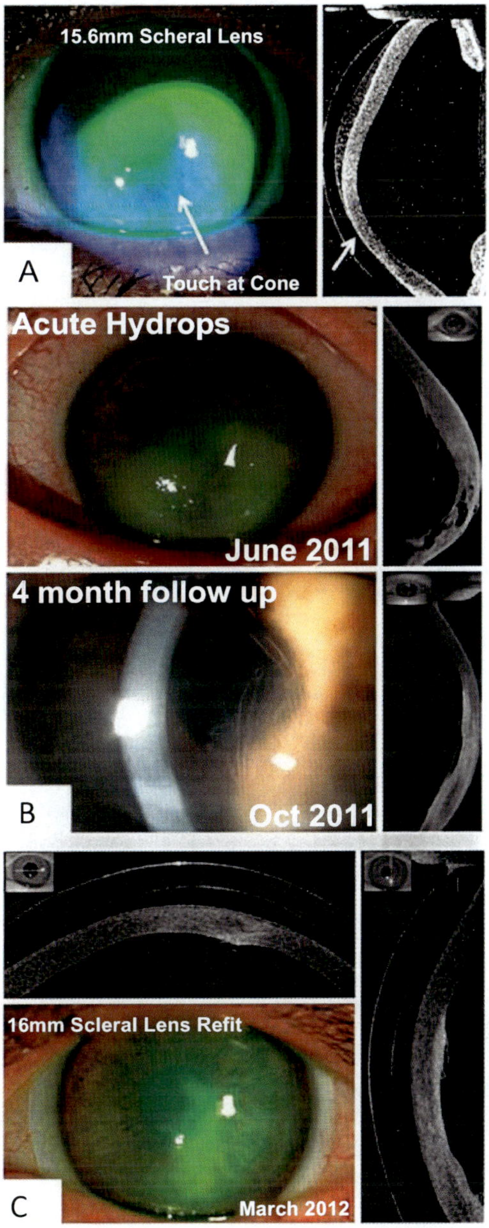

Fig. (7). Patient with advanced keratoconus wearing a scleral lens with corneal touch. A. Photograph and OCT of corneal touch, B. Photograph and OCT of acute corneal hydrops, C. Well fit scleral lens after recovery of hydrops.

Estimating the clearance of a lens can be difficult for a novice fitter. However, with experience and documentation of the techniques above, practitioners become proficient in evaluating the vault and sagittal depth of a lens with the slit lamp. Fig. (**8**) demonstrates how the slit lamp observation correlates with an anterior segment OCT image.

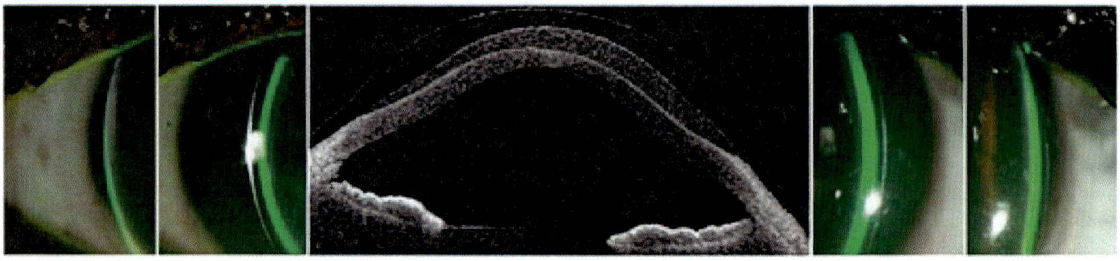

Fig. (8). Composite images of a patient with keratoconus of asymmetrical sagittal depth over the horizontal meridian. Note that the thickness of the fluorescein layer correlates with the vault seen in the OCT. Central corneal thickness was measured at 310 and 330 µm by two different instruments. Based on the known corneal thickness, the estimated vault at the corneal apex is about 300 µm. Image courtesy of Bruce Baldwin and Sarah Moyer. Review of Cornea and Contact Lenses. April 2012.

The Landing/Landing Zone

The peripheral portion of a scleral lens and how the lens rests on the sclera (or technically the conjunctiva) is usually referred to as the landing or landing zone. This physical area of the lens contains one or more curves or tangents with associated widths and is often referred to as the haptic, the peripheral curve system or scleral lens periphery. The landing is extremely important for lens centration and tear flow under the lens. Careful assessment of the landing and documentation of the alignment of the landing on the sclera will determine the suitability of the fit and drive any recommended modifications during the fitting or refitting process.

Ideally, the landing should rest aligned with the sclera without edge lift or compression (impingement). Good alignment is often referred to as a "soft" landing. A well aligned, soft landing is seen in Fig. (**9**). Note that there is no blanching of the conjunctiva (compression of superficial blood vessels), or edge lift. A diagnostic lens that demonstrated ideal clearance with compression 360 degrees is shown in Fig. (**10**) along with the OCT image of the edge. A lens with this much edge compression will certainly lead to stagnation of tears, poor tear flow under the lens, and mechanical irritation and redness.

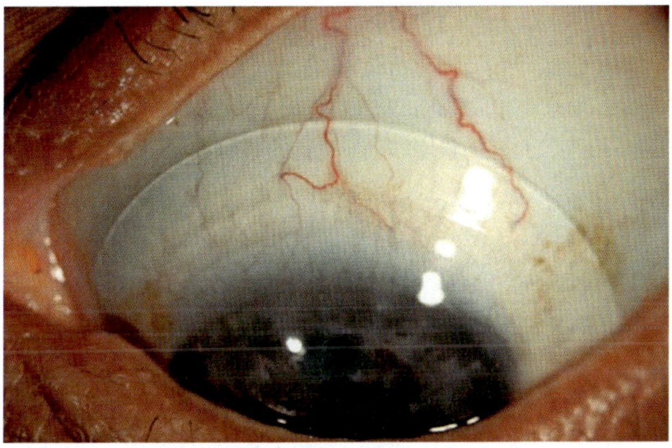

Fig. (9). Large diameter scleral lens vaulting over a corneal graft showing an aligned or "soft" landing without conjunctival blanching or compression of blood vessels.

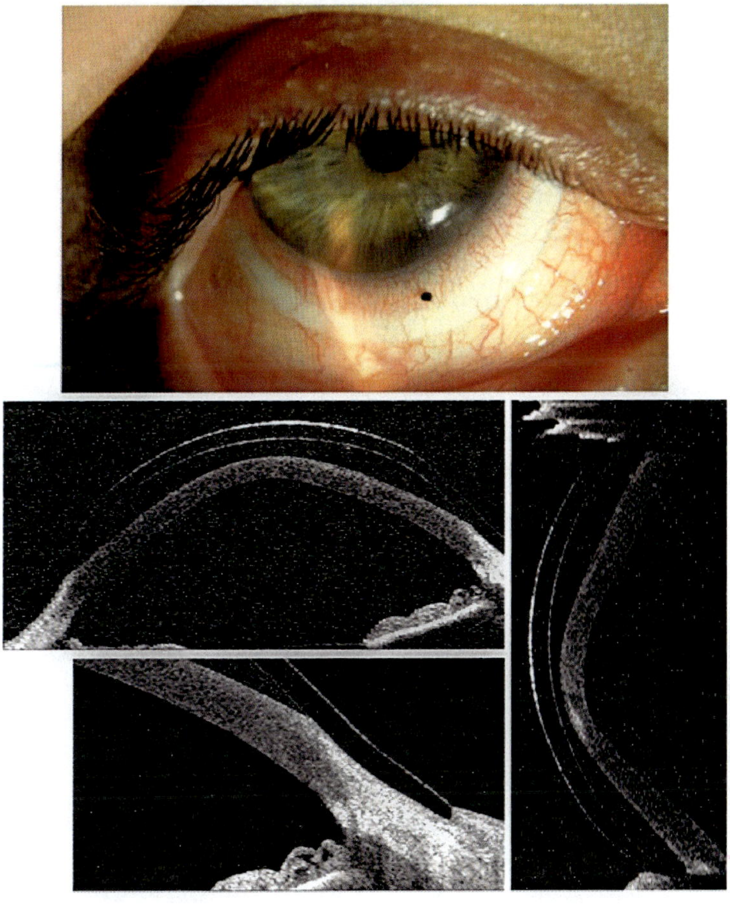

Fig. (10). Scleral lens with a "tight" landing resulting in blanching of the conjunctival blood vessels. Note adequate central and limbal vault.

One cause for lens decentration downward is poor alignment of the landing with the sclera. Without a good 360 degree “semi-seal” of the lens, the lens will have some movement with blinking and will decenter down. The topic of decentration is addressed elsewhere, but careful observation and documentation of the landing can help with lens design decisions. It can be difficult, even for experienced practitioners, to determine where the landing is misaligned. Fig. (**11**) shows a corneal graft patient with extreme toricity of the sclera and resultant extreme edge lift of a scleral lens. Most scleral landing misalignments are much more subtle and require special slit lamp techniques or fluorescein dye tests to observe.

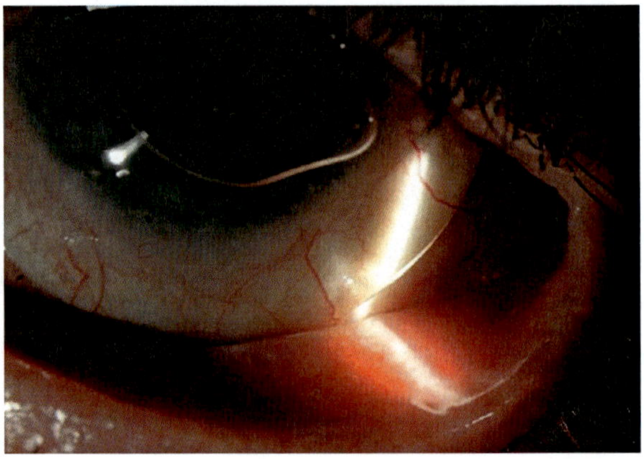

Fig. (11). Extreme edge lift over a corneal graft with high scleral toricity after surgery. The visual acuity was 20/30, however with eye movements a large bubble would form due to the lack of peripheral seal from edge lift.

As an example, practitioners can place the slit beam perpendicular to the edge of the lens and look for subtle lift of the edge often at 12:00 and 6:00 o’clock. If there is edge lift at 12:00 and 6:00 o’clock, there is often light compression 90 degrees away at 3:00 and 9:00 o’clock. This is an example of with-the-rule scleral toricity. Just like corneal toricity, not all scleral toricity is with the rule.

Notes in the chart about the magnitude of landing misalignment can be useful for designing the lens or when speaking with a consultant. For example, descriptions like “subtle edge lift at 12:00 and 6:00” or “heavy compression and blanching at 3:00 and 9:00” can be useful for making decisions on how to modify the lens edge, or whether to refit to another lens diameter or lens type.

In addition to simple observation of the lens edge, the practitioner can assess the differential flow of fluorescein under the lens at different locations. After placing the lens on eye without fluorescein, followed by applying the fluorescein to the inferior cul-de-sac, on the lens surface, or above the lens, it may flow into the fluid chamber faster in one or more locations. This may indicate excess edge lift or peripheral clearance at that location. If there is very rapid inflow of dye under the lens, this suggests that the lens is too loose and there is not a seal in that location. Large amounts of particulate matter may also flow along this pathway causing midday fogging. Often there is excess movement of tears or chamber debris in the fluid chamber with each blink indicating an inadequate peripheral seal.

There are other causes for a scleral lens to decenter. A bulky, high plus lens with a deep sagittal depth on an eye with a tight upper lid might tend to decenter down from mechanical forces of the upper lid. Documentation of a "tight" or "floppy" upper lid will help to determine the cause of a downward decentered lens. Large diameter lenses can decenter horizontally due to the differential anterior insertion of the lateral rectus muscles [33]. A scleral lens that decenters vertically or horizontally does not necessarily indicate a poor fit or need for refit. If other aspects of the lens including vault, tear flow, comfort, acuity, wearing time, and corneal physiology after lens wear are reasonable, then a decentered lens is acceptable.

Careful documentation in the notes of any of the above phenomena will aid in an eventual design of a well-fitting lens. Slit lamp photography and anterior segment OCT are also valuable in designing a lens or evaluating a lens to be refit. Scleral lens manufacturer consultants appreciate comprehensive notes from slit lamp observations, and many will accept images emailed as an aid to lens design.

Tear Exchange

A scleral lens with adequate vault and a good landing will usually have acceptable tear exchange. However, a lens may appear to fit very well but not have adequate tear exchange. During a diagnostic fitting, a technique often used is to place sodium fluorescein dye with saline in the bowl of the lens for insertion. This allows immediate assessment of the corneal and limbal vault. With dye already under the lens, tear *outflow* can be assessed, but this can take hours for a "tight" landing [34]. To assess tear *inflow*, one recommended technique is to place the lens on the eye in the usual manner, then put a copious amount of fluorescein in the inferior cul-de-sac. With normal blinking and eye movements, some fluorescein may be visible under the lens after a few blinks and much of the post lens tear reservoir filled after several minutes. Fig. (**12**) shows an example of a lens that appeared to have a good fit but had poor tear flow under the lens. After manually finger pumping dye under the lens the chamber was not completely filled after fourteen minutes. This indicates poor inflow of tears. This lens had been dispensed to the patient because at the dispensing visit it appeared to fit well except that slow tear exchange was noted. On follow-up, the patient complained of discomfort and redness after a few hours of wear. Since the slow tear flow had been well documented at the dispensing visit, there was an easy decision to redesign the landing to allow for better tear exchange.

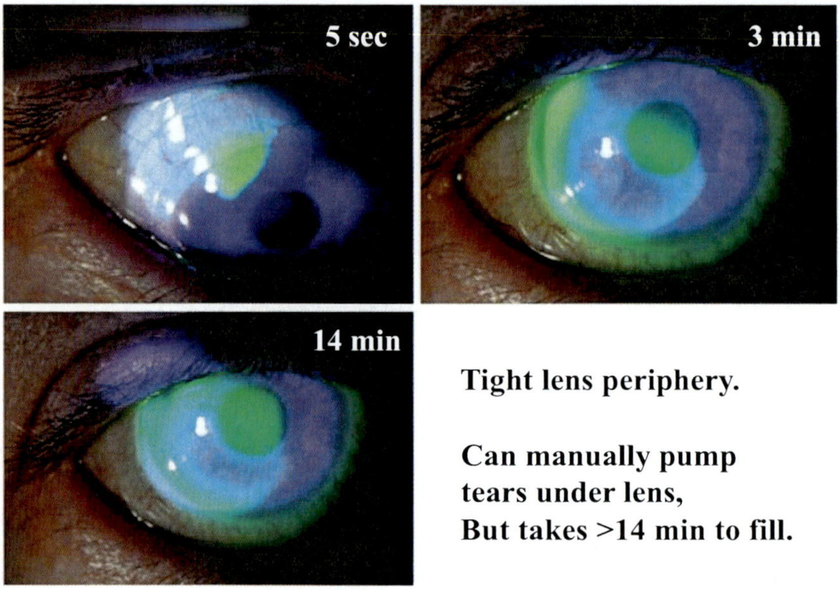

Fig. (12). Example of a lens with poor tear exchange due to the design of the landing zone.

As described in Chapter 3, some patients' globes have a toric shape profile and require a toric peripheral design for an adequate semi seal of the landing while preserving good tear exchange. As noted above, if excess fluorescein can be seen entering the lens in some locations, such as the 12:00 position, and no inflow in other locations, the landing could be custom designed for optimum tear exchange. Careful observation and documentation will aid the practitioner or consultant in a custom design.

A patient with poor wearing time, despite a seemingly well designed and well fit lens, may benefit from dry eye therapy. As noted earlier, documentation of the appearance of the lacrimal punctae and dry eye findings may indicate that punctal occlusion or other aggressive dry eye therapy is indicated. Dry eye therapies can be initiated before redesigning the scleral lens or at any time after dispensing if improved tear exchange is desired.

Additional Fit Parameters and Observations

If the lens vault, the landing, and tear exchange are well fit, there is a likely chance the fit will be successful. There are a number of additional observations to document for a complete assessment of the fit that will be briefly discussed below.

Centration and Movement

Centration and movement were mentioned above but deserve additional discussion. Decentration alone is not necessarily a problem. A patient with a lens that is decentered in any direction but has good comfort, visual acuity, and meets the other requirements of acceptable vault, landing and tear exchange does not have to be redesigned. However, a diagnostic lens that decenters more than 1 mm will often have undesired movement, lens awareness, and excessive tear exchange due to a poor semi-seal. It would be rare if a lens with any movement did not have some problem with comfort or physiology. Due to excess fluid on insertion of a diagnostic lens, some minimal movement may be observed initially. A chart note such as "Lens moved with blink after insertion but settled after five minutes" would alert the practitioner to observe for lens movement at the follow up visit. It can sometimes be difficult to determine the cause of decentration, and also to determine which lens parameters to change to improve centration.

A scleral lens with a high plus power or a deep sagittal depth (Fig. **13**) placed on a patient with a tight upper lid is more likely to decenter downward. Many have observed the phenomenon where the palpebral aperture on a unilateral lens wearer is much larger due to the bulky lens interacting with the lids. Fig. (**14**) shows this eye opening effect in a keratoconus patient. Scleral lenses have been used to treat ptosis because of the ability to increase the palpebral aperture [35]. If the lid-lens interaction causes a problem with the fit, some attempt at redesign may be needed. Documenting the relative palpebral fissure heights and the upper lid tonicity will aid in diagnosing a cause for lens decentration.

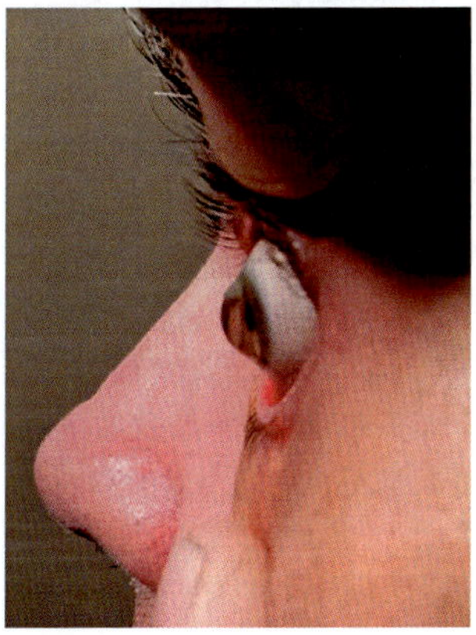

Fig. (13). Profile of a patient with a corneal graft with a deep sagittal depth. In order to vault this cornea, a scleral lens with a deep sagittal depth will be required to vault over this cornea. This lens will likely be bulky.

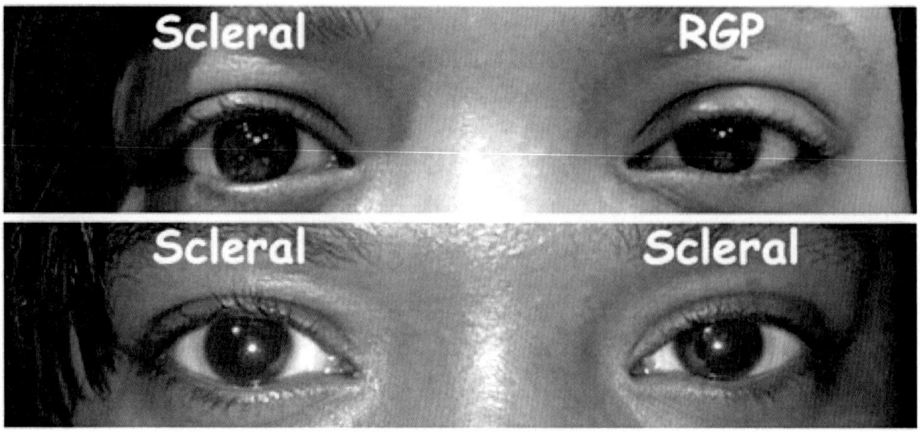

Fig. (14). Example of how a scleral lens can reduce ptosis or increase the palpebral aperture due to the physical bulk of the lens.

A lot of scleral toricity might cause a lens to decenter down, and/or move on blinking. If a patient has a toric sclera and the diagnostic lens has a standard periphery the practitioner may be able to see some differential edge lift or compression. Again, a decentered lens may not be a problem but careful observation and documentation of other fit parameters is important to record an otherwise good fit.

Surface and Chamber Debris

Some lenses appear to have a "textbook fit" at the dispensing visit, but the patient complains about foggy vision after a few minutes or hours of wear. This fogging can be due to deposits and poor wetting of the lens surface, or to trapping and collecting tear film debris or metabolic waste under the lens. Sometimes a brief diagnostic fitting will show deposits or debris after just a few minutes of wear. These are two of the most common, but difficult, problems to solve. A systematic investigation of the symptoms and documentation of the findings can help find a solution.

If deposits are collecting on the lens surface, there has to be some kind of interaction of the tear film components with the surface of the lens. If deposits or poor wetting is observed, there is a long list of questions to ask the patient. Practitioners should ask if there is a history of dry eye, meibomian gland dysfunction (MGD), or giant papillary conjunctivitis (GPC). Are there signs of these conditions? What is the lens material, lens cleaner, hand soap, eye makeup, age/condition of rubber plunger, age and condition of the lens including any scratches? Are any eyedrops of any kind including medications used and when?

When does the lens fog? Is fogging constant or intermittent? Is fogging associated with activities like reading, computer, outdoor activities, or exposure to airborne particles or vapors? Any of these factors can be associated with surface deposits or poor wetting and obviously reducing the problem is dependent on the cause.

There can also be many causes of debris trapped under the lens, some that overlap with causes of surface deposits. Patients with dry eye and MGD typically have more tear film debris. Therefore, there is a greater chance of some debris getting under the lens. Very fine particulate matter may be from corneal, conjunctival, or eyelid metabolic debris including microscopic lipid spheres [36]. These tiny particles can become trapped under even a well fit lens. Treating dry eye, MGD, or GPC can help reduce this cause for chamber fogging. Sometimes a few weeks of adaptation will reduce the debris. However, if there are large globs of mucus that move a lot with each blink or eye movement, then there is most likely an area of the landing where there is too much space or edge lift.

As noted above, there are many potential causes of problems with surface debris, poor wetting, and fogging from trapped debris. The many potential solutions are beyond the scope of this chapter. To determine any solution, the first step is investigation and careful observation and documentation of the signs and symptoms.

Documentation of Ordered Lens Parameters

After a new fitting session or sessions, there should be enough data in the record to order all the final lens parameters, or, there should be enough observations to discuss with a laboratory lens consultant to design and order a lens. Sometimes a diagnostic lens from a fitting set will fit well enough that there is a reasonable certainty that the first lens ordered will be successful. In that case, a full set of parameters can be ordered. This set of parameters will differ somewhat depending on the proprietary parameters of the scleral lens manufacturers available worldwide. A minimum set of parameters includes lens material, overall diameter, base curve and power. Be aware that back and front vertex powers can differ by greater than one diopter for high plus lenses. Other parameters commonly available to specify include sagittal depth, center thickness, optic zone diameter, limbal and peripheral edge design. These parameters should be recorded in the chart and compared after arrival with a verified lens and/or the lens invoice. Adequately recorded lens parameters can be easily copied over at the dispensing visit.

If an adequate fit cannot be obtained from a diagnostic set, then observations from the fitting session can be recorded on the order form and relayed to the laboratory lens consultant. An example would be: "The diagnostic lens with X mm, X base curve and X sag requires an over-refraction of –4.75 (non-vertexed) and would need about 100 microns of additional sagittal depth. The lens decentered down about 1.5 mm and might center better with a toric periphery." Contemporaneous notes like these can be very valuable if a lens is ordered after the patient has left the clinic. A scleral lens that is ordered with parameters outside the standard diagnostic lens set can be considered a "custom diagnostic, lens" and the patient briefed that further modifications in the lens are possible. After receiving the lens, all the parameters can be recorded in the chart making them readily available for comparison of fit observations at the dispensing visit.

A few custom lens manufacturers do not rely heavily on diagnostic lenses. Impression molded, OCT computer aided, and CAD computer designed scleral lenses have unique proprietary methods for designing a lens. However, because the base curve of a rigid lens is partly responsible for the effective power, some lens with a known base curve and power needs to be placed on the eye with an over-refraction in order to determine the relative base curve to power relationship of the final lens.

Subsequent Encounter – Dispensing or Follow-up

Dispensing a New Lens

Prior to dispensing a new lens, it is advisable to verify all of the possible lens parameters. Diameter and power can be easily verified. The base curve can be easily verified if a radiuscope is available. For efficiency, the lens care products can be selected and packaged when dispensing a lens. An interval history should be recorded with any changes in general health, eye health, or eye problems. Uncorrected visual acuities, or if possible, best corrected spectacle visual acuities should be recorded prior to dispensing a lens. It is a good medical-legal practice to observe the anterior segment, including the cornea with fluorescein dye, to be sure there are no significant problems that might be exacerbated during an application/removal training session. When severe anterior segment disease is present, slit lamp photographs will document the appearance of the eye before training.

Some practitioners will dispense the lens, record the visual acuity, observe the fit, obtain an over-refraction, then have the patient train with application and removal. If the patient is trained first, their eyes may become red and irritated during training making documentation of the fit unreliable. Observing and recording the fit will include all the observations discussed above at "Documentation of a scleral lens fit." One major parameter to accurately record is the central and limbal vault. Recall that a lens can settle up to 100 microns or more during the first three hours of wear [32]. If a lens does not have an additional 100 microns greater than the desirable sagittal depth at the initial dispensing, a practitioner may want to consider having the patient return after three hours of wear that same day to reassess the clearance.

After successful training, the patient is typically dispensed a small supply of lens solutions including cleaning and storage, and insertion saline and plungers along with their scleral lens(es). A handout is often given with the listed solutions and alternative solutions as well as sources to purchase those solutions. Solutions are recorded in the record in a location easily available to office staff so that phone calls about solutions and prescription renewals can be quickly answered. If solutions such as non-preserved inhalation saline are recommended, and use of that brand is "off label" (not FDA approved for U.S. providers) then a note about the risks and benefits of using an off label product should be documented.

A recommended first follow-up appointment will vary by practitioner and the nature of the patient's eye condition. For example, a long time RGP lens wearer dispensed with a very well fitting scleral lens could probably be safely followed in a month or more. On the other hand, a patient with no lens experience and severe exposure keratopathy from Bell's palsy might need a follow-up after one day of wear. Careful documentation and instructions to the patient are important regardless of the follow-up schedule. It is always a good idea to have a recall system in place to track patients who do not show for a follow up appointment. Fig. (**15**) shows severe corneal neovascularization and scarring from a patient who returned three years after scheduling a three month follow-up. He had slept in the lens almost continuously for three years. This illustrates the importance of proper follow-up and documented attempts to contact a patient who fails to keep an appointment.

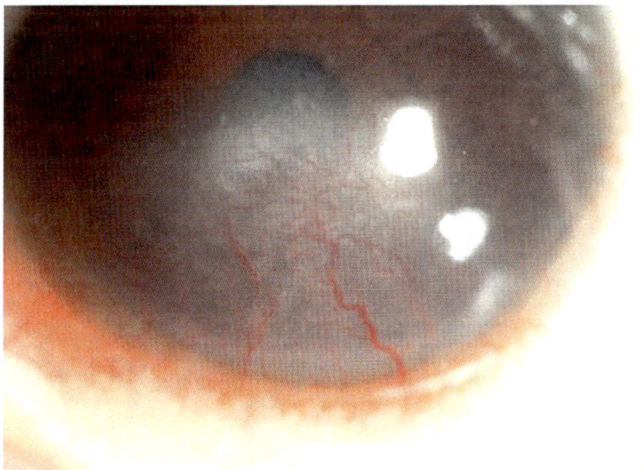

Fig. (15). Patient with keratoconus who wore scleral lenses almost continuously for three years and developed corneal neovascularization and scarring.

Documentation with Imaging

There are many sophisticated instruments available for evaluation, documentation and management of scleral lens patients. Some instruments like corneal topographers and slit lamp cameras have become quite common. Other instruments such as anterior segment optical coherence tomographers (OCT) are readily available but less common in private practice clinics due to cost. Novice scleral lens practitioners ask, "Do I need a topographer or an OCT to fit scleral lenses?" The answer is a qualified "no." Corneal topography is useful for defining the severity of keratoconus or irregular astigmatism and following changes with treatment and progression. However, as noted by Schornack and Patel [37], the ability of topography simulated keratometry readings to predict the base curve of the final scleral lens fit was not strong. This is certainly because large diameter scleral lenses are fit based on overall sagittal depth not central base curve. Likewise, OCT can be very helpful for novice scleral lens practitioners to learn how to interpret what is visualized the slit lamp. However, after a number of successful scleral to fittings, expert use of the slit lamp will minimize the dependence on OCT. Anterior segment cameras are extremely important for documenting the eye before and after a scleral lens fitting. In this section, case reports will briefly discuss the use of Scheimpflug imagery, ocular photography, and OCT. More detailed discussions are found in other chapters.

Scheimpflug Imagery

A Scheimpflug camera captures images of multiple slit beams on the cornea and the computer reconstructs anterior and posterior corneal topography as well as 2D corneal pachymetry [38]. Some instruments also utilize a Placido disc image for improved anterior topography. Fig. (**16**) shows one of many possible screen outputs for a Scheimpflug instrument. This keratoconus patient, with no corneal scarring, was only corrected to 20/50 in this eye with several type lenses including scleral lenses. In the upper left, the anterior axial simulated keratometry readings showed moderate keratoconus. The pachymetry (upper right) was reasonable at about 460 microns. The lower right posterior corneal topography, available in Scheimpflug images, showed compact and significant posterior corneal changes. This may be why the scleral lens acuity was only 20/50, and why the retinoscopy reflex was very irregular even with a well fit scleral lens. Scheimpflug instruments are valuable to documenting eyes of scleral lens patients because they can produce several useful measurements with one quick capture session.

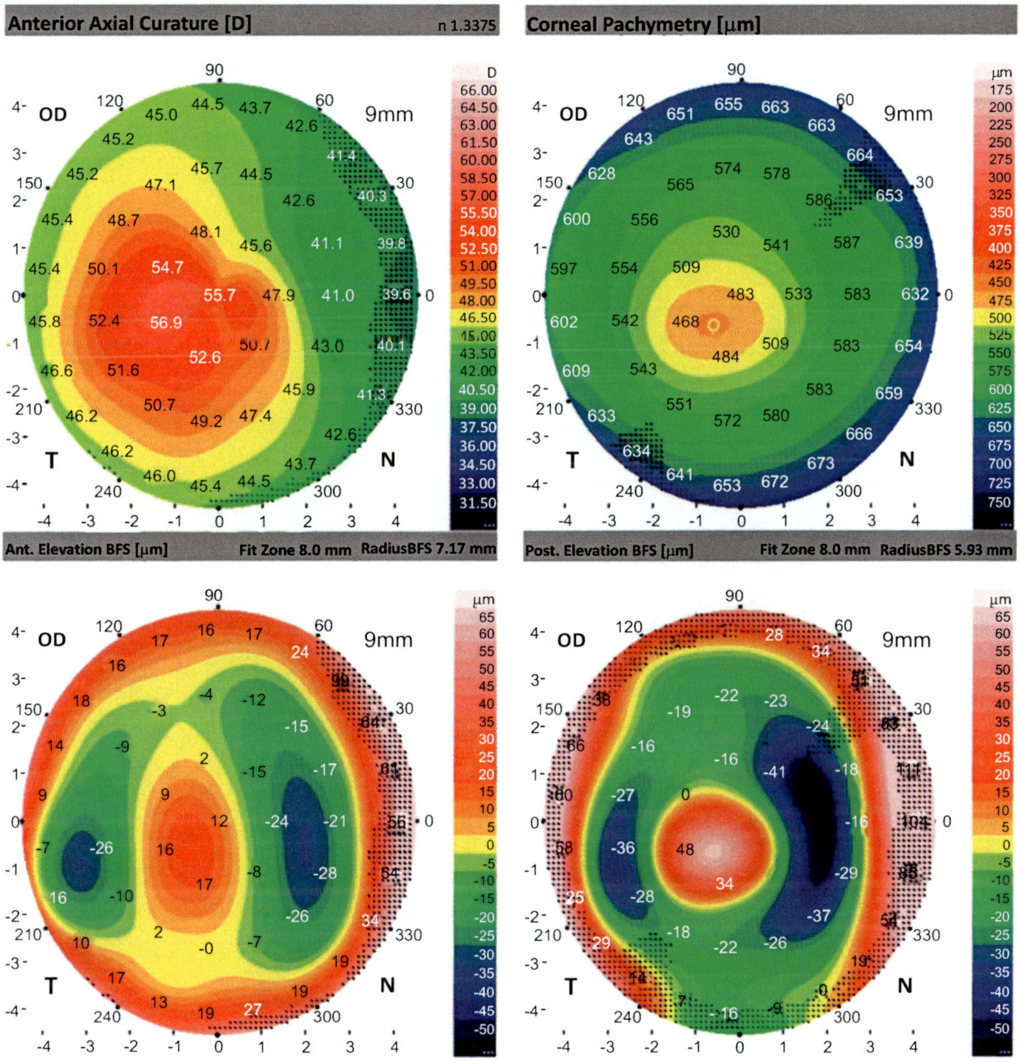

Fig. (16). Representative output from a Scheimpflug instrument. Other available output images include 2D Cornea/Iris/Lens Image, Wavefront Report, and Placido Disk Image.

Slit Lamp Camera

There is probably no more important optical instrument than a slit lamp camera. As noted previously, anterior segment attachments are available for smart phones, but a dedicated slit lamp camera can image in greater magnification and depth. Corneal transplants are one of the more common uses of scleral lenses. Practitioners must be aware that a patient with a corneal transplant can develop graft rejection at any time after surgery. Photographic documentation of signs of rejection is extremely valuable, especially in multi-provider practices where a patient may see a different practitioner on follow-up. Fig. (**17a**) shows a patient who developed endothelial graft rejection on post-op day 172. Photodocumentation demonstrated resolution of the rejection six weeks later, which is important clinically and potentially legally. As seen in Fig. (**17b-c**), this patient developed three more episodes of rejection during the first 413 days of his post-operative course. This illustrates the need for hypervigilance in observation and documentation of signs (or lack of signs) of rejection on every visit of a patient who has had a corneal transplant. The sclera lens was dispensed at post-operative day 55 because he needed to renew his commercial truck driver license.

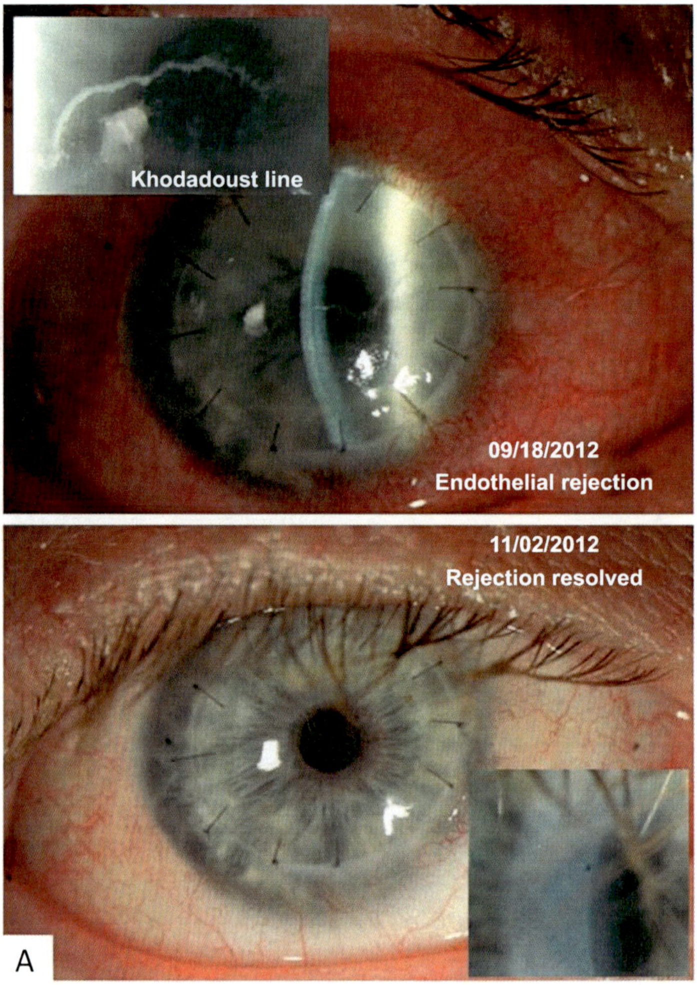

Fig. (17a). (Top) Endothelial rejection in a post-penetrating keratoplasty patient and scleral lens wearer. (Bottom) Resolution of rejection episode after aggressive topical steroid treatment.

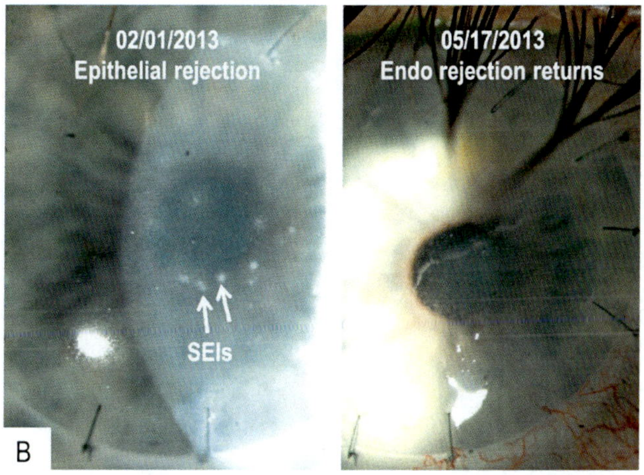

Graft Rejection History

PK 3/30/2012	PO Days
Endo 1	172
Epi 1	249
Epi 2	308
Endo 2	413

C

Fig. (17b). One of two epithelial rejection episodes and recurrent endothelial rejection episode. 17c. History of four graft rejection episodes while wearing a scleral lens during the first post-operative year.

Anterior Segment Optical Coherence Tomography (OCT)

OCT is very useful for learning how to fit scleral lenses. Correlating slit lamp observations with OCT (Fig. **8**) can quickly help a practitioner to become a scleral lens expert. While OCT is not necessary for scleral lens fitting, it becomes a management tool.

Fig. (**18**) is the same patient in Fig. (**17**). This graphically shows the healing and rounding of a new penetrating keratoplasty over the first year. Note the top image with a "plateau" or sunken graft. The scleral lens was fit with excessive vault, so the expected rounding of the graft would not cause corneal touch. In fact, the same scleral lens was used most of the first year.

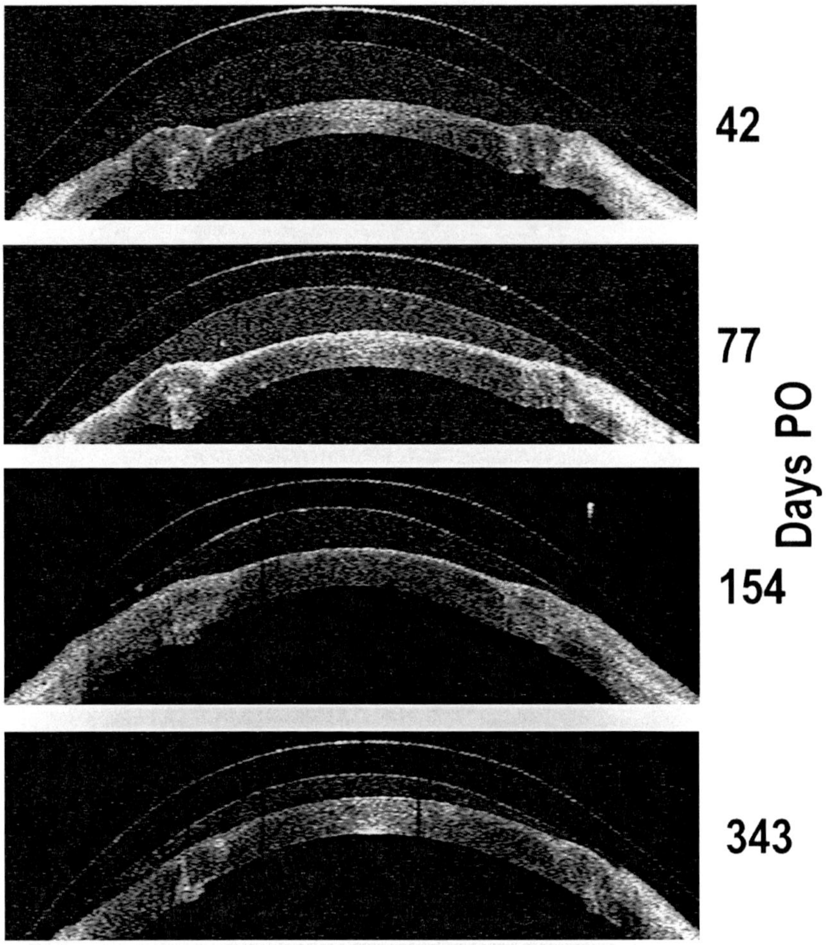

Fig. (18). Composite image of corneal graft changes during the first 343 days after surgery. Note that the first scleral lens was fit with "generous" clearance so that the lens would not need to be refit as the corneal shape normalized during recovery. This is the same patient as Fig. (**17**).

Vaulting a scleral lens over the cornea and limbus is one of the most important concepts when fitting a scleral lens. A scleral lens that rubs the limbus can disrupt the normal epithelial physiology and cause a range of complications (Fig. **19**). The top image was emailed to the laboratory consultant asking for advice on how to increase the limbal clearance relative to the diagnostic lens. The lens was made larger with a reverse geometry curve. As seen in the lower images, there is adequate limbal clearance with this lens. OCT can be used to diagnose and manage poorly fitting scleral lens characteristics, as well as to document the fit for communication and consultation with a laboratory.

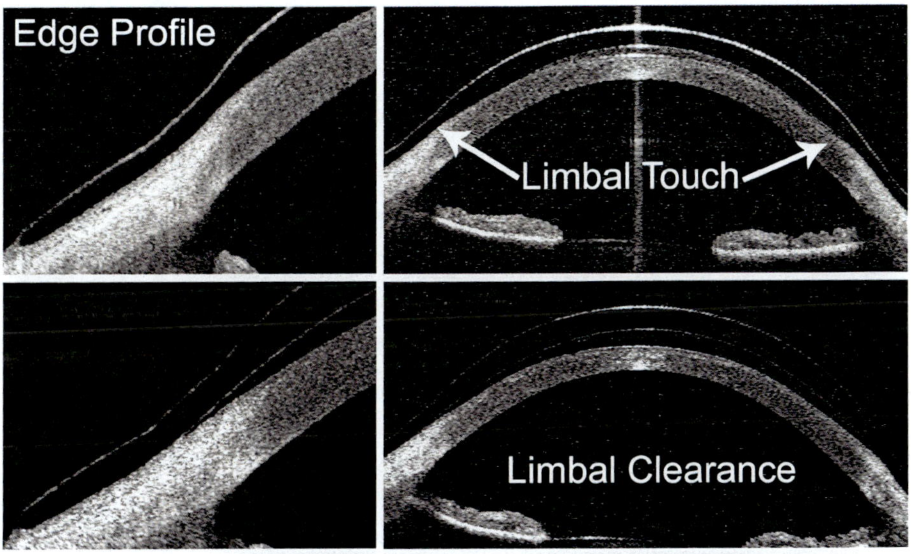

Fig. (19). Top: Trial lens with inadequate limbal clearance. Bottom: Redesigned lens with a larger diameter and reverse curve design with adequate limbal clearance.

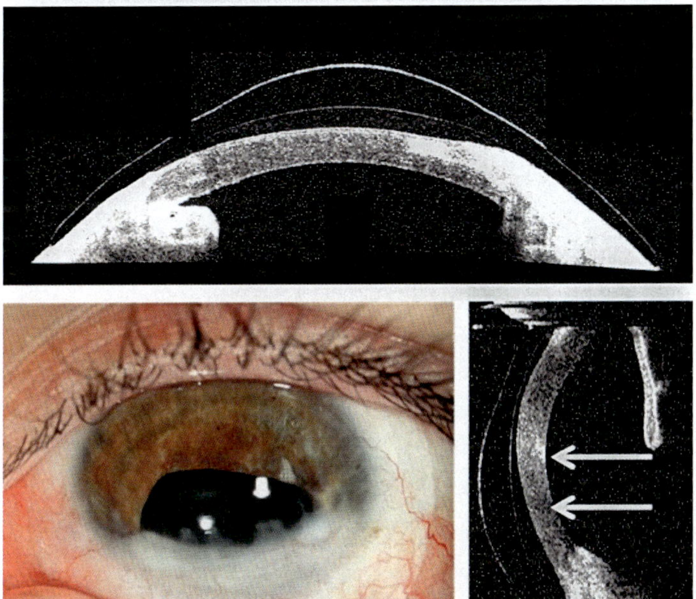

Fig. (20). Top: Custom manufactured scleral device from an impression molding procedure. Note precise alignment of the "soft" landing on this disfigured eye. Bottom right: Arrows show pupil center indicating slight downward decentering of the lens.

Another example of communication with a scleral lens laboratory is shown in Fig. (**20**). The upper image is a composite of a scleral device manufactured from an eye mold. This is an aphakic patient who suffered an open globe from a knife injury. In the lower two images, it is evident that even though the lens is centered on the eye, the optical center of the lathe cut lens is decentered inferiorly. This resulted from the eye mold following the contours of the extremely disfigured cornea. Guided by the photograph and OCT, the laboratory manufactured the lens and moved the optical center over the visual axis.

There are a number of optical instruments and cameras that are useful for diagnosing, treating, and managing scleral lens patients. The examples above show uses for photography, Scheimpflug imaging, and anterior segment OCT. Ultimately, the practitioner is most valuable asset for documenting the scleral lens patient.

SUMMARY

Detailed and careful documentation is crucial for all aspects of the scleral lens patient's medical care. A thorough medical and ocular history details the patient's past medical treatments, outcomes, and previous contact lens modalities. This information serves as a platform to diagnose, monitor and initiate new management strategies including scleral lenses. Proper documentation may also aid the patient with government services and insurance reimbursement. Since scleral lens fitting is intricate and complex, detailed observations assist the practitioner with changing parameters, lens designs, and supplemental ocular management. Due to the progressive nature of ocular conditions that require scleral lenses, photodocumentation of baseline findings, topographies, OCT images, and careful notetaking aid practitioners in optimizing the management strategies. When communicating with the patient's medical team, a careful summary of ocular findings may also aid in their medical decision making. Lastly, appropriate documentation may be necessary in medical-legal circumstances.

CONFLICT OF INTEREST

The author declares no conflict of interest, financial or otherwise.

ACKNOWLEDGEMENTS

Thanks to our highly skilled and professional ocular photographers Sarah M Armstrong, CRA, OCT-C, FOPS, Rona Lyn Esquejo-Leon, CRA, Debra Cantrell, COA and Houston Sharpe, COA, OCT-C.

REFERENCES

[1] Barnett M. Multifocal scleral lenses. Contact Lens Spectrum 2015; 30: 26-31.

[2] Shikari H, Antin JH, Dana R. Ocular graft-*versus*-host disease: a review. Surv Ophthalmol 2013; 58(3): 233-51.
[http://dx.doi.org/10.1016/j.survophthal.2012.08.004] [PMID: 23541042]

[3] Eagling EM. Ocular damage after blunt trauma to the eye. Its relationship to the nature of the injury. Br J Ophthalmol 1974; 58(2): 126-40.
[http://dx.doi.org/10.1136/bjo.58.2.126] [PMID: 4820984]

[4] Ng DS, Ching RH, Chan CW. Angle-recession glaucoma: long-term clinical outcomes over a 10-year period in traumatic microhyphema. Int Ophthalmol 2015; 35(1): 107-13.
[http://dx.doi.org/10.1007/s10792-014-0027-5] [PMID: 25520267]

[5] Hood CT, Lee BJ, Jeng BH. Incidence, occurrence rate, and characteristics of suture-related corneal infections after penetrating keratoplasty. Cornea 2011; 30(6): 624-8.
[http://dx.doi.org/10.1097/ICO.0b013e3182041755] [PMID: 21282987]

[6] Tan ST, Staiano JJ, Itinteang T, McIntyre BC, MacKinnon CA, Glasson DW. Gold weight implantation and lateral tarsorrhaphy for upper eyelid paralysis. J Craniomaxillofac Surg 2013; 41(3): e49-53.
[http://dx.doi.org/10.1016/j.jcms.2012.07.015] [PMID: 22901733]

[7] Silver AL, Lindsay RW, Cheney ML, Hadlock TA. Thin-profile platinum eyelid weighting: a superior option in the paralyzed eye. Plast Reconstr Surg 2009; 123(6): 1697-703.
[http://dx.doi.org/10.1097/PRS.0b013e3181a65a56] [PMID: 19483568]

[8] Sohrab M, Abugo U, Grant M, Merbs S. Management of the eye in facial paralysis. Facial Plast Surg 2015; 31(2): 140-4.
[http://dx.doi.org/10.1055/s-0035-1549292] [PMID: 25958900]

[9] Schornack MM, Pyle J, Patel SV. Scleral lenses in the management of ocular surface disease. Ophthalmology 2014; 121(7): 1398-405.
[http://dx.doi.org/10.1016/j.ophtha.2014.01.028] [PMID: 24630687]

[10] Sidikaro Y, von Noorden GK. Observations in sensory heterotropia. J Pediatr Ophthalmol Strabismus 1982; 19(1): 12-9.
[PMID: 7069561]

[11] Kersey JP, Broadway DC. Corticosteroid-induced glaucoma: a review of the literature. Eye (Lond) 2006; 20(4): 407-16.
[http://dx.doi.org/10.1038/sj.eye.6701895] [PMID: 15877093]

[12] Nagy ZZ, Szabó A, Krueger RR, Süveges I. Treatment of intraocular pressure elevation after photorefractive keratectomy. J Cataract Refract Surg 2001; 27(7): 1018-24.
[http://dx.doi.org/10.1016/S0886-3350(01)00889-6] [PMID: 11489570]

[13] Soni NG, Jeng BH. Blood-derived topical therapy for ocular surface diseases. Br J Ophthalmol 2016; 100(1): 22-7.
[http://dx.doi.org/10.1136/bjophthalmol-2015-306842] [PMID: 26178904]

[14] Bhargava R, Kumar P. Oral omega-3 fatty acid treatment for dry eye in contact lens wearers. Cornea 2015; 34(4): 413-20.
[http://dx.doi.org/10.1097/ICO.0000000000000386] [PMID: 25719253]

[15] Bays HE. Safety considerations with omega-3 fatty acid therapy. Am J Cardiol 2007; 99(6A): 35C-43C.
[http://dx.doi.org/10.1016/j.amjcard.2006.11.020] [PMID: 17368277]

[16] Liu J, Sheha H, Fu Y, Liang L, Tseng SC. Update on amniotic membrane transplantation. Expert Rev Ophthalmol 2010; 5(5): 645-61.

[http://dx.doi.org/10.1586/eop.10.63] [PMID: 21436959]

[17] Hill RH III, Norton SW, Bersani TA. Prevalence of canaliculitis requiring removal of SmartPlugs. Ophthal Plast Reconstr Surg 2009; 25(6): 437-9. [http://dx.doi.org/10.1097/IOP.0b013e3181b80d63] [PMID: 19935244]

[18] Pakarinen M, Tervo T, Tarkkanen A. Tarsorraphy in the treatment of persistent corneal lesions. Acta Ophthalmol Suppl 1987; 182: 69-73. [PMID: 2837065]

[19] International Statistical Classification of Diseases and Related Health Problems 10th revision (ICD-10--WHO version for; 2016. Diseases of the eye and adnexa. Visual disturbances and blindness (H53-H54) 2016.http://apps.who.int/classifications/icd10/browse/2016/en#/H53-H54

[20] Internal Revenue Service, definition of blindness. https://www.irs.gov/publications/p501/ar02.html#en_US_2015_publink1000221051

[21] Visser ES, Visser R, Van Lier HJ. Advantages of toric scleral lenses. Optom Vis Sci 2006; 83(4): 233-6. [http://dx.doi.org/10.1097/01.opx.0000214297.38421.15] [PMID: 16614579]

[22] Schornack MM. Scleral lenses: a literature review. Eye Contact Lens 2015; 41(1): 3-11. [http://dx.doi.org/10.1097/ICL.0000000000000083] [PMID: 25536528]

[23] Lee WW. Slit lamp adapters turn smartphones into clinical cameras http://www.ophthalmologyweb.com/Featured-Articles/136817-Slit-Lamp-Adapters-turn-Smartphons-into-Clinical-Cameras/2016.

[24] Gomes BA, Santhiago MR, Jorge PA, Kara-José N, Moraes HV Jr, Kara-Junior N. Corneal involvement in systemic inflammatory diseases. Eye Contact Lens 2015; 41(3): 141-4. [http://dx.doi.org/10.1097/ICL.0000000000000141] [PMID: 25794330]

[25] Fritsch PO, Sidoroff A. Drug-induced Stevens-Johnson syndrome/toxic epidermal necrolysis. Am J Clin Dermatol 2000; 1(6): 349-60. [http://dx.doi.org/10.2165/00128071-200001060-00003] [PMID: 11702611]

[26] Shikari H, Antin JH, Dana R. Ocular graft-*versus*-host disease: a review. Surv Ophthalmol 2013; 58(3): 233-51. [http://dx.doi.org/10.1016/j.survophthal.2012.08.004] [PMID: 23541042]

[27] Mian SI, De la Parra-Colín P, De Melo-Franco R, Johnson C, Barrientos-Gutierrez T. Dry eye disease incidence associated with chronic graft-host disease: Nonconcurrent cohort Study (An American Ophthalmological Society Thesis). Trans Am Ophthalmol Soc 2015.

[28] Jacobs DS, Rosenthal P. Boston scleral lens prosthetic device for treatment of severe dry eye in chronic graft-*versus*-host disease. Cornea 2007; 26(10): 1195-9. [http://dx.doi.org/10.1097/ICO.0b013e318155743d] [PMID: 18043175]

[29] Finger PT. Radiation therapy for orbital tumors: concepts, current use, and ophthalmic radiation side effects. Surv Ophthalmol 2009; 54(5): 545-68. [http://dx.doi.org/10.1016/j.survophthal.2009.06.004] [PMID: 19682622]

[30] Woodward MA, Blachley TS, Stein JD. The association between sociodemographic factors, common systemic diseases, and keratoconus: An analysis of a nationwide heath care claims database. Ophthalmology 2016; 123(3): 457-65.e2. [http://dx.doi.org/10.1016/j.ophtha.2015.10.035] [PMID: 26707415]

[31] Kojima T, Hasegawa A, Nakamura T, Isogai N, Kataoka T, Ichikawa K. Five-year PROSE treatment for aniridic keratopathy. Optom Vis Sci 2016; 93(10): 1328-32. [http://dx.doi.org/10.1097/OPX.0000000000000942] [PMID: 27668496]

[32] Kauffman MJ, Gilmartin CA, Bennett ES, Bassi CJ. A comparison of the short-term settling of three scleral lens designs. Optom Vis Sci 2014; 91(12): 1462-6.

[http://dx.doi.org/10.1097/OPX.0000000000000409] [PMID: 25279781]

[33] van der Worp E, Bornman D, Ferreira DL, Faria-Ribeiro M, Garcia-Porta N, González-Meijome JM. Modern scleral contact lenses: A review. Cont Lens Anterior Eye 2014; 37(4): 240-50. [http://dx.doi.org/10.1016/j.clae.2014.02.002] [PMID: 24631015]

[34] Morrison S, Walker M, Caroline P, *et al.* Tear exchange beneath scleral lenses. Global Specialty Lens Symposium.

[35] Shah-Desai SD, Aslam SA, Pullum K, Beaconsfield M, Rose GE. Scleral contact lens usage in patients with complex blepharoptosis. Ophthal Plast Reconstr Surg 2011; 27(2): 95-8. [http://dx.doi.org/10.1097/IOP.0b013e3181d07408] [PMID: 21057345]

[36] Walker M, Morrison S, Caroline P, *et al.* Laboratory analysis of scleral lens tear reservoir clouding. Global Specialty Lens Symposium. Las Vegas. 2014.

[37] Schornack MM, Patel SV. Relationship between corneal topographic indices and scleral lens base curve. Eye Contact Lens 2010; 36(6): 330-3. [http://dx.doi.org/10.1097/ICL.0b013e3181eb8418] [PMID: 20631627]

[38] Piñero DP. Technologies for anatomical and geometric characterization of the corneal structure and anterior segment: a review. Semin Ophthalmol 2015; 30(3): 161-70. [http://dx.doi.org/10.3109/08820538.2013.835844] [PMID: 24175646]

CHAPTER 11

Examination Flow for Scleral Lens Fitting

Brooke Messer[1,*] and **Stephanie Woo**[2]

[1] *Cornea and Contact Lens Institute of Minnesota, Edina, MN 55436, USA*

[2] *Havasu Eye Center, Lake Havasu City, AZ 86403, USA*

Abstract: Most practitioners will agree in that fitting scleral lenses is a very rewarding and fulfilling experience. As the awareness of scleral lenses becomes widespread, the number of patients seeking scleral lenses continues to grow. Due to the rise in demand, proper preparation by the practitioner and the clinic can optimize the patient experience. Patients who wear scleral lenses often have complex and unique ocular conditions. It is important to educate patients on their condition and the scleral lens fitting process to avoid frustration when multiple follow up visits are necessary. Examination flow of scleral lenses is an evolving process, and current standards will continue to change as technology, lens designs and research develop.

Keywords: Adaptor, authorization, care, case history, contact lens, deep, dispense, examination, evaluation, medically necessary, OCT, patient, phone, practitioner, refraction, shape, slit lamp, testing, topography, visual acuity.

THE INITIAL EXAMINATION

Most practitioners will agree in that fitting scleral lenses is a very rewarding and fulfilling experience. As the awareness of scleral lenses becomes widespread, the number of patients seeking scleral lenses continues to grow. Due to the rise in demand, proper preparation by the practitioner and the clinic can optimize the patient experience. There will be many questions about the fitting process when patients first present to the office. To maximize office efficiency, it can be helpful to obtain previous ocular records and verify insurance benefits prior to patient arrival.

Insurance Authorization

Obtaining pre-authorization from insurance companies for medically necessary contact lenses can be a frustrating and tedious process for all parties involved. The information required and time it takes to receive an authorization can be a long,

* **Corresponding author Brooke Messer:** Cornea and Contact Lens Institute of Minnesota, Edina, MN 55436, USA; Tel: 952-300-2151; Fax: 952-657-5745; E-mail: drbmesser@gmail.com

Melissa Barnett & Lynette K. Johns (Eds.)

drawn out task. Vision insurance plans are typically much easier to work with and find actual information about the patient's benefits and fitting and material allowances. When the patient calls to set up an appointment, it is important to gather all the necessary information required to determine their coverage for medically necessary contact lenses. Helpful information includes whether the patient is eligible, the initial eligibility date and obtaining a prior authorization for medically necessary contact lenses. Keeping in mind, some insurances require a prior authorization, while others do not require this step. A prior authorization often requires information from the examination to verify that patient qualifies for medically necessary contact lens coverage. The insurance may request information like best corrected visual acuity with glasses compared to specialty contact lenses, the diagnosis requiring contact lenses and the corresponding diagnosis, procedure and material codes. Some insurance companies may also request the usual and customary fees, as well as visit documentation. A contract between the patient and the practitioner is recommended to assist in outlining fees, fitting timeframe and potential patient responsibilities. Reviewing insurance eligibility prior to the patient visit is ideal, when possible, so both the patient and provider are informed of potential costs involved.

Case History

Some of the most important moments with the patient are in those first conversations when obtaining the patient history. The appropriate questions and explanations can establish trust and confidence in skill and decision making process of the practitioner.

At the initial encounter, determining the patient's reason for visit will establish the strategy for future care and possible co-management. Has this patient been referred from another provider? Is this patient self-referred or someone from the current practice looking for an improvement in comfort or vision from the current modality? It is important to establish a relationship with the patient's other providers, if any, to optimally manage the patient. For example, other conditions like corneal transplants or glaucoma require ophthalmic specialty care, whereas Sjögren's disease may require rheumatology consultation. The optimal scleral lens design and prescribed wearing time should reflect the patient's need for topical medications and overall corneal health.

A diagnostic medical and ocular history should also be obtained. The history, if known, should include the onset of the condition and if there are other associated ocular findings. Requesting records from previous providers can be helpful in trying to determine onset of ocular findings like corneal opacities, cataracts or retinal problems. If previous records are unavailable, a detailed documentation of the initial visit findings is helpful to monitor long term ocular health.

When first diagnosing the patient with a condition, be sure to explain the disease in detail, along with the prognosis and management options. For instance, in keratoconus, the practitioner should review treatments such as corneal cross-linking, intrastromal ring segments, corneal transplantation, spectacle correction, and all appropriate contact lens options.

Many patients seek scleral lens practitioners for improved comfort compared to their previous lens modality. A contact lens history should be reviewed, including previous lens designs worn and the success, or lack thereof, with each type. If the patient is currently wearing contact lenses, discussing their current experience can provide insight for future fitting goals. Some patients desire a new lens design with better comfort and optical options, such as toric or multifocal. Other patients seek a small improvement in their current modality, like improved lens stability or vision. Discussing the fitting goals of the patient enhances lens design selection.

Occupational needs and hobbies may require an extra stable lens, or one with very precise optical properties. Questions should also include: current vision quality, ease of insertion and removal of their contact lenses, care system, dependency on artificial tears, average lens wearing time compared to hours of comfortable wearing time and areas of their wearing experience that could be improved. Problems with their current lenses should be reviewed such as lens dislodgment, dryness and fluctuating vision.

Visual Acuity

When assessing visual acuity, if the patient has an irregular cornea, it can be reassuring if you acknowledge that they may see double or triple images out of one eye. Encourage them to give their best effort. It is also helpful to take notes of their description of the visual quality. Direct the patient to observe if they see the visual acuity chart as doubled, haloed or distorted. These are also qualities that can be compared once fit in a scleral lens. Pinhole visual acuity can help determine if a prescription change may be necessary or if vision can be improved with scleral lenses. If the vision cannot be improved with over-refraction or a contact lens change, then the discrepancy in pinhole visual acuity is likely due to higher order aberrations.

Refraction

A good attempt at baseline refraction can be valuable in managing patients that wear scleral lenses. If the patient has an irregular cornea, it can be a piece of the data that can contribute to the overall management picture. For insurance purposes, to validate the need for medically necessary contact lenses, a refraction is sometimes needed. For patients with regular corneas, routine refractions are helpful in monitoring overall corneal health and detecting any corneal warpage. Patients with irregular corneas are easily frustrated during a refraction due to their poor quality of vision. Be sure to remind the patient that the main purpose is to demonstrate the insurance company how important scleral lenses are in improving their vision.

All contact lens wearers should have a backup pair of glasses, even patients with irregular corneas, despite having less than satisfactory vision through spectacle lenses. Measured visual acuity does not reflect the quality of vision in an irregular cornea patient. Although patients may meet the legal standard for driving, they should be dissuaded from driving with spectacles if their visual acuity is best corrected with contact lenses.

Slit Lamp Evaluation and Photodocumentation

A detailed slit lamp evaluation of the anterior segment is essential in the initial experience with the patient. At this time, all details of the anterior segment should be evaluated and recorded. Photodocumentation with an anterior segment camera of any abnormal findings aids in monitoring for changes over time. Photodocumentation of pre-existing conditions prevents attributing any significant findings to a poor fitting scleral lens. During the slit lamp evaluation, document findings that could limit scleral lens success. Some examples of significant findings would include:

Eyelids and Lashes

Evaluate the eyelids and eyelid margins for various conditions including infectious, inflammatory, physiologic issues (lagophthalmos or eyelid tonicity), blepharitis, meibomian gland dysfunction (Fig. **1**), lid-wiper epitheliopathy and eyelid lesions. Meibomian gland dysfunction is the most frequent cause of dry eye [1], and could contribute to compromised lens wettability.

Conjunctiva

Evaluate and measure the presence of conjunctival anomalies such as cysts, pingueculae, pterygium, papillae, giant papillary conjunctivitis (Fig. **2**), conjunctival concretions, allergic conjunctivitis and surface altering glaucoma procedures (*i.e.*, filtering tubes and trabeculectomies).

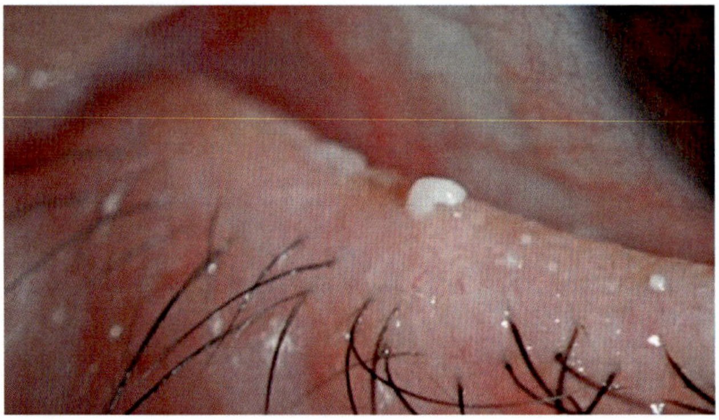

Fig. (1). Eyelid with severe meibomian gland dysfunction after manual expression. Image courtesy of Lynette Johns.

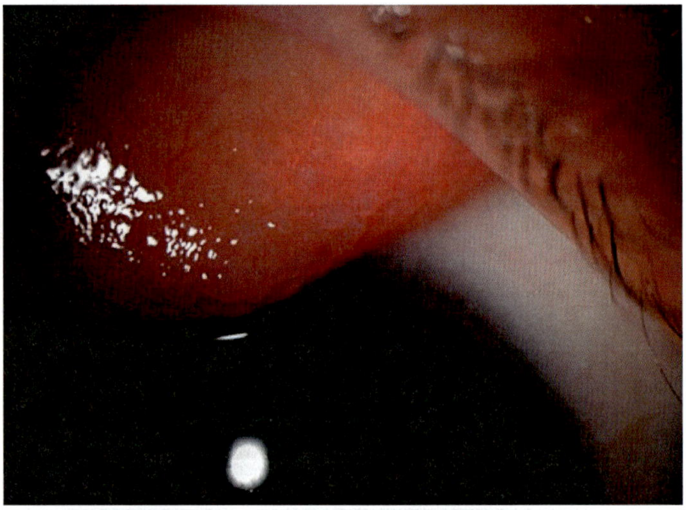

Fig. (2). Giant papillary conjunctivitis on superior palpebral conjunctiva.

Anterior Chamber and Iris

Assess the depth of the anterior chamber and any iris anomalies such as irregular pupils, synechiae and iris pigmentation or nevi.

Lens

Rule out any media opacities of the natural crystalline lens or intraocular lens implant that may limit best corrected visual acuity (BCVA).

Cornea

Document findings including any epithelial irregularities or corneal staining, stromal opacities, and the presence of endotheliopathies Fig. (**3**). It is very important to note any presence of limbal irregularities like pannus or corneal neovascularization. Scleral lenses can have a large impact on the limbal health.

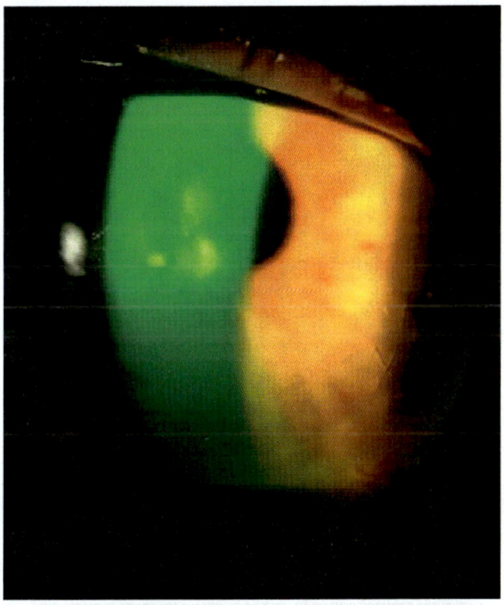

Fig. (3). Slit lamp photodocumentation of corneal scarring in keratoconus.

Retina

A dilated examination to evaluate the retina is pertinent for all patients. If the patient was referred from another provider, it may not be necessary to perform the dilated examination at the time of scleral lens fitting. Pay close attention to the macula for fine irregularities. Identifying any areas of the eye that could lead to the potential for decreased vision is essential for outlining patient expectations. For instance, if a patient has keratoconus (without cornea opacities) with 20/70 vision, many practitioners would assume that a gas permeable contact lens should improve vision. However, if the patient has a retinal defect such as a macular hole, vision may not be improved with the lens. Due to corneal irregularity, completing a dilated fundus examination can be difficult. Applying a gas permeable contact lens can improve resolution of retinal findings.

Contact Lens Evaluation

When the patient arrives wearing contact lenses, evaluate vision and assess the fit of the contact lens. This can yield helpful troubleshooting information, and explain reasons for the specialty lens fitting referral.

Evaluate soft lenses without fluorescein for coverage, centration and alignment. Over-refraction is helpful to determine best corrected visual acuity with the habitual lens. Be mindful that depending on the length of use and handling, the habitual lens parameters may be altered. This information can aid in the decision to maintain or change lens designs and materials.

Examination of hybrid contact lenses includes the lens centration, skirt alignment and the alignment of the inner and outer landing zones. If improperly fit, these zones can contribute to lens seal off and spectacle blur. Include evaluation of the surface for scratches or deposits. Imaging the lens with optical coherence tomography (OCT) can document the amount of corneal clearance and the relationship to the corneal surface at the junction of the gas permeable lens and soft skirt.

When evaluating gas permeable lenses, the first evaluation should be without sodium fluorescein. The lens surface, wettability, edge quality and deposits or biofilms are better viewed without fluorescein. Next, fluorescein is helpful to evaluate lens alignment, centration and movement. An OCT image in scleral lens fittings can be particularly helpful to evaluate corneal and limbal clearance, as well as edge alignment. An over-refraction can assist in determining best corrected visual acuity, as well as an over-topography or keratometry to rule out lens flexure or warpage. With all lens designs, pinhole acuity can determine if a refractive change is indicated, or if ocular conditions are limiting the patient's best corrected visual acuity. If the vision cannot be improved with over-refraction or a contact lens change, then the discrepancy in pinhole visual acuity is likely due with higher order aberrations.

Special Testing

While it could be argued that special instrumentation is not always needed to fit specialty contact lenses, including scleral lenses, certain instrumentation is essential to monitor the entire ocular surface.

An anterior segment camera is very helpful in contact lens fittings and documenting the current status of corneal findings. Photodocumentation of findings including fluorescein patterns of gas permeable lens fittings, tortuous conjunctival vessels, pingueculae, corneal opacification and the baseline appearance of the limbus assists in monitoring over time. In addition, it is beneficial to document acute findings like corneal staining, abrasions, foreign bodies and inflammatory events.

Currently, there are a variety of methods and equipment available for taking anterior segment photographs. The technology ranges from basic, such as an adapter that attaches a camera or cell phone to the ocular on the slit lamp, to advanced methods of elite digital imaging software connecting and uploading to electronic health records (Fig. **4** and **5**).

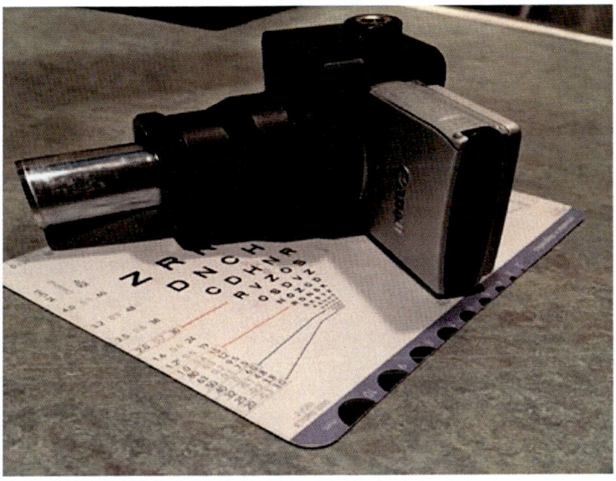

Fig. (4). Example of a slit lamp adaptor for a personal camera.

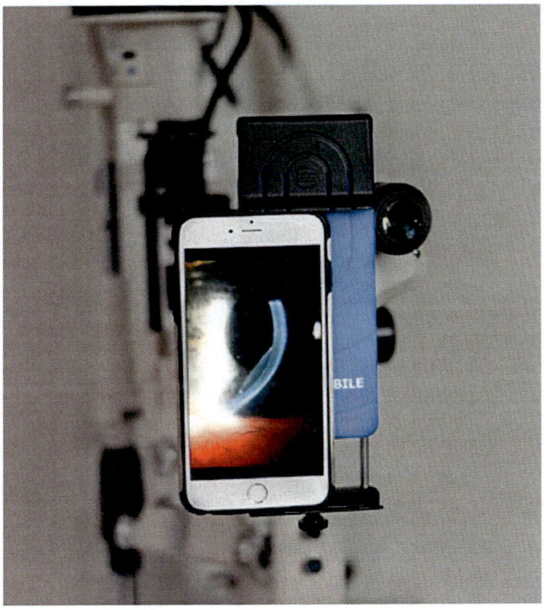

Fig. (5). Example of a slit lamp adaptor for a mobile phone.

Obtaining high quality photographs takes practice. First and foremost, allowing adequate time for optimal patient fixation and refining the amount of lighting and magnification is important. Utilizing a diffusing filter softens the slit lamp beam and improves visualization of the conjunctival vessels when evaluating scleral lens landing zones. A direct light beam may bleach out the conjunctival vessels. Since diffusers produce an even light over a larger area of the ocular surface, these aid in a low magnification, global scleral lens view. Subtle corneal findings, or other findings with depth, like a nodule or cyst, are best captured with a slit beam. Another tip is to begin focusing with a low magnification, then increase magnification as needed, keeping in mind that more light is needed with increased magnification. Perhaps the most important thing to obtain good photographs is to allocate enough time and not rush the procedure. If it is difficult to keep the eye open, consider using a drop of topical anesthetic to keep the patient comfortable.

Corneal topography can be very helpful in scleral lens fitting and management. Keratometry and topographical elevation readings are useful to understand the corneal layout as a whole in order to guide our evaluation for optimal scleral lens clearance and design. Be mindful that the steepest portion of the cornea does not always correspond with the highest elevation of the cornea. A study from Mayo clinic concluded that a scleral lens base curve has no correlation to the corneal keratometry readings [2]. For example, when comparing a patient with Salzmann's nodular degeneration and a patient with keratoconus, they both may have steep keratometry findings, but in very different locations on the corneal surface. During the fitting process, a topographer can also assist in troubleshooting unsatisfactory vision. If the over-refraction is revealing astigmatism, topography over a scleral lens can rule out lens flexure [3]. Topography can also assist in scleral multifocal lens fitting if front surface add powers are utilized. With multifocal lenses, the practitioner can determine if the lens optical center lines up with the visual axis; this may help troubleshoot and determine if scleral lens centration needs to be adjusted.

The use of OCT for the anterior segment has more recently become a key tool in successful scleral lens fitting and troubleshooting. An OCT can be utilized to determine the amount of corneal clearance and scleral lens center thickness with accurate precision (Fig. **6**). Without anterior segment OCT, practitioners estimated the amount of scleral lens clearance by comparing the thickness of the tear layer to the center thickness of the scleral lens. OCT technology has allowed practitioners to confidently fit scleral lenses with shallower clearances. This can potentially optimize oxygen transmissibility and decrease debris build-up in the post-lens tear layer. Anterior segment OCT images are particularly helpful in confirming proper limbal clearance. Corneal pachymetry and ocular surface tomography are valuable tools when monitoring various corneal conditions, like nodules, opacities and the positioning of intrastromal ring segments. The progression of corneal ectasia. The progression of corneal ectasia includes corneal thinning that can be monitored with ease using corneal pachymetry and tomography since the amount of thinning may vary in different locations of the cornea. Global pachymetry *via* tomography provides the practitioner valuable information regarding the variable corneal thickness of the entire surface. A baseline central corneal thickness measurement before initiating a scleral lens fit can be repeated and compared after lens removal to determine if corneal edema is suspected, especially post penetrating keratoplasty [4, 5].

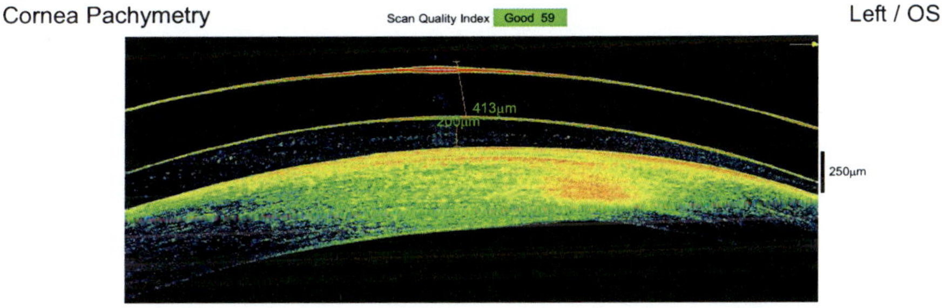

Fig. (6). Image of OCT (Optovue, Inc) demonstrating central corneal clearance.

Lastly, specular microscopy provides helpful information about the corneal endothelium. Polymegathism and pleomorphism can be detected and quantified before the initial scleral lens fitting. Epithelial basement membrane dystrophy, guttata, Fuch's corneal dystrophy and other corneal dystrophies can be detected and monitored during the scleral lens care. Endothelial cell count can be especially useful in managing patients with corneal transplants. Patients with reduced endothelial cell counts may be at higher risk to develop corneal edema and may not be ideal candidates for scleral lenses.

INITIAL SCLERAL LENS FITTING

Both practitioners and patients are seeking scleral lenses because of their superior comfort and stable vision. Ocular indications have expanded for scleral lenses, and have grown to assist a large variety of patient populations. The growing number of patients has created a demand for several scleral lens designs, including a range of lens diameters, sagittal depths, edge designs, and lens shapes.

Lens Diameter

During the initial evaluation, specialized testing, refraction and slit lamp findings will aid in selecting a lens design. Viewing the profile of the cornea outside of the slit lamp may also assist the practitioner with selecting an initial diagnostic lens. Selecting the scleral lens diameter is the first step in the initial scleral lens fitting process. Considerations when selecting lens diameter are corneal diameter, disease severity, the condition being treated and availability of diagnostic lenses.

Larger corneas, with horizontal visible iris diameters of 12.0 millimeters (mm) or greater,will need larger lens diameters to sufficiently clear the limbus. Patients with corneas that are very ectatic and have large sagittal depths will also need large diameter scleral lenses to adequately bear the weight of the lens and post-lens tear layer. A wider scleral lens landing zone on the scleral conjunctiva will create a more even surface area, rather than sinking into the soft conjunctiva with a smaller landing zone.

Lastly, patients with ocular surface disease may appreciate a larger lens acting as a shield to protect a larger area of the eye's surface from the outside environment. In a study done at Pacific University, scleral shape was measured in a variety of subjects; it was determined that scleral curvature becomes increasingly asymmetric shape further from the limbus [6]. Larger scleral lens designs may require toric peripheral curves due to the change in scleral shape [7].

Smaller diameter scleral lenses will be the lens of choice for most patients with small palebral fissures, mildly irregular and normal corneas. Smaller diameter scleral lenses, around 15 mm, have a similar diameter to soft contact lenses, so they may be less intimidating for patients who already wear soft lenses. Insertion and removal may be easier with smaller diameters. Finally, smaller diameter lenses may center better over the cornea, which may improve optical performance in front toric and multifocal scleral lens wearers.

Lens Shape

Scleral lenses are now available in prolate lens shapes, for normal and ectatic corneas, as well as oblate or reverse geometry lens designs, for post-surgical corneas. By selecting a lens shape that best matches the corneal profile, the post-lens tear layer thickness may be optimized, therefore limiting unwanted side effects like tear layer debris and conjunctival prolapse.

Some corneas can be a combination of oblate and prolate shapes, creating a more challenging starting point for lens selection. For example, a patient with keratoconus that has intracorneal ring segments, or a patient with recurrent keratoconus after a corneal transplant may demonstrate aspects of both prolate and plateau corneal shapes. A topographical elevation map can assist lens shape profile selection. Nevertheless, the decision can easily be made by placing a lens design of either shape on the eye to evaluate the optimal post-lens tear layer thickness.

Scleral lens peripheral zone designs, also known as the landing zone or lens haptics, are also improving in design. Most scleral lens manufacturers can modify the peripheral zones to be steeper or flatter than standard designs. Many can incorporate back surface toric and quadrant specific peripheries, which can dramatically improve the fit and comfort of the lens.

Diagnostic Lens Selection

Selecting the initial lens from a diagnostic set can be a hurdle for new practitioners. Proper lens selection can dramatically improve the experience for a new patient and streamline the fitting process. The lens manufacturer will include a fitting guide to assist in selecting the initial lens from the diagnostic set. Other exam findings can also be helpful in lens selection. When viewing the corneal profile, observe the steepest portion of the cornea. If the ectasia is viewable with the naked eye, the cornea is likely "sagittally deep," and a "steeper" or "deeper" lens from the fitting set would be a good first choice. Larger corneas typically have deeper sagittal depths than smaller diameter corneas. A patient with a normal cornea, or small area of irregularity that is not viewable with the naked eye likely requires a less deep lens. The diagnostic lenses for these patients will likely be flatter or shallower.

Once the initial lens is selected, it needs to be prepared before application. If the diagnostic lenses are stored dry, be sure and clean and condition the lens very generously before application, or else unstable wettability may occur. Place the lens onto the application device of your choice, then fill the lens with preservative-free saline and sodium fluorescein.

To apply the lens, have the patient tuck their chin to their chest and point their nose to the floor keeping their face parallel to the ground. Have the patient assist by pulling down their lower lid, while the practitioner controls the upper lid. Swiftly place the scleral lens directly centered over the cornea. If the scleral lens catches an eyelid or the patient moves their eye, this could result in an air bubble behind the lens. Check for air bubbles immediately after application and remove if a bubble is observed.

As experience is gained from fitting more scleral lenses, the initial lens selection becomes dramatically easier and less overwhelming. Another helpful tip in working with a diagnostic fitting set is to be aware of the differences between each lens in the set. The difference in sagittal depth, peripheral zone and diameter will guide the practitioner to efficiently navigate through the diagnostic set. After evaluating the lens on the eye, the practitioner will more easily select the next diagnostic lens.

For new scleral lens fitters, it is recommended to start with one or two lens designs. It is also recommended to communicate with the consultation team to learn about the unique aspects and terminology of each lens. After fitting a few patients successfully, then consider branching out to other lens designs and learn what makes each lens unique. Before gathering too many scleral lens sets, consider fitting a few patients successfully, and then reach out to the laboratory.

Lens Evaluation

For optimal efficiency, evaluate the initial scleral lens fit immediately after application. This will give the practitioner an overall view before allowing the lens to settle. Assessing the lens on low magnification with a cobalt blue filter will give the practitioner a general view of the lens clearance (Fig. **7**). If any areas of black are seen, this would indicate corneal touch and the selected lens is too shallow. Remove the lens and select another diagnostic lens with a deeper sagittal depth.

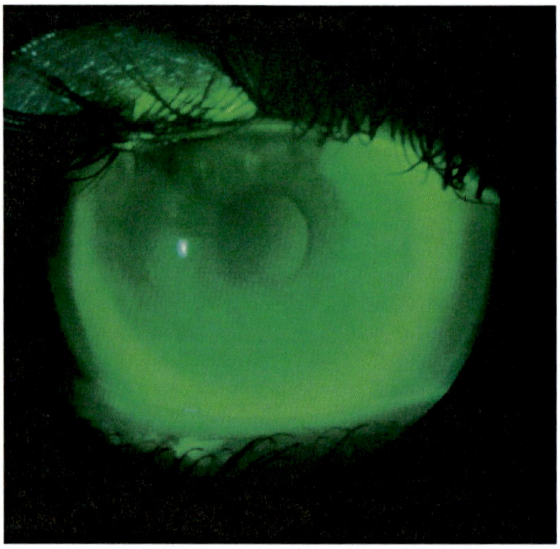

Fig. (7). Image of overall fluorescein pattern demonstrating areas of shallow corneal clearance.

After achieving complete corneal clearance, create a thin optic section with white light and adjust the beam to 45 degrees (Fig. **8**). Scan the entire cornea to evaluate the fluorescein tear layer beneath the scleral lens. Be sure and examine the central, mid-peripheral, and limbal areas for complete clearance, keeping in mind that the most deepest area of the cornea is not always central, nor does it always correspond to the area with steepest keratometry readings. Using the center thickness of the scleral lens as a guide, estimate the thickness of the tear layer between the back surface of the lens and the cornea. For instance, if the diagnostic lens has a known center thickness of 300 μm, and the fluorescein layer looks to be about the same thickness, it can be estimated that the thickness of the tear layer is approximately 300 μm. This should be evaluated at the most elevated point on the corneal surface. Also evaluate the limbal clearance with an optic section to ensure adequate coverage and clearance. Limbal clearance is importance to protect corneal stem cell production.

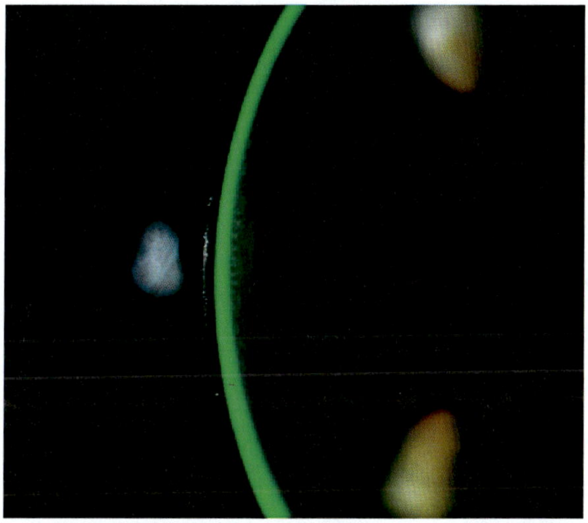

Fig. (8). Image of optic section of fluorescein under a scleral lens demonstrating central corneal clearance.

With low magnification and low illumination, evaluate the landing curves of the scleral lens. The blood vessels of the conjunctiva should travel under the edge of the lens without impediment. Evaluate lens peripheral alignment of the superior, inferior, nasal, and temporal conjunctiva. Documenting the areas of impingement, compression or edge lift, as well as the severity, is helpful in designing the lens periphery. Peripheral designs can be steepened for a tighter alignment or flattened for a looser fit. More complex designs can include toric peripheral curves, which are steeper in one meridian and flatter in the other, to better align to asymmetric scleral shapes.

When possible, allow the diagnostic lens to settle on the eye in office for 20-40 minutes. This settling can reveal some potential areas for adjustment, such as increased sagittal depth or looser lens peripheries. Evaluating the lenses too quickly can lead to an inaccurate assessment of lens fit.

Historically, scleral lens powers were typically spherical. Now that lens designs can incorporate front surface toric corrections, a sphero-cylindrical over-refraction can maximize acuity for those patients with residual astigmatism. If astigmatism is found in the over-refraction, further assessing the lens with over-keratometry or over-topography can help identify lens flexure (Fig. **9**). This determines if a front toric optics are truly necessary to correct internal astigmatism, or if the lens fit needs to be modified to negate lens flexure.

After the diagnostic fitting is complete, remove the lenses and soak in hydrogen peroxide for 10 minutes to disinfect, per the guidelines from the Center for Disease Control [8].

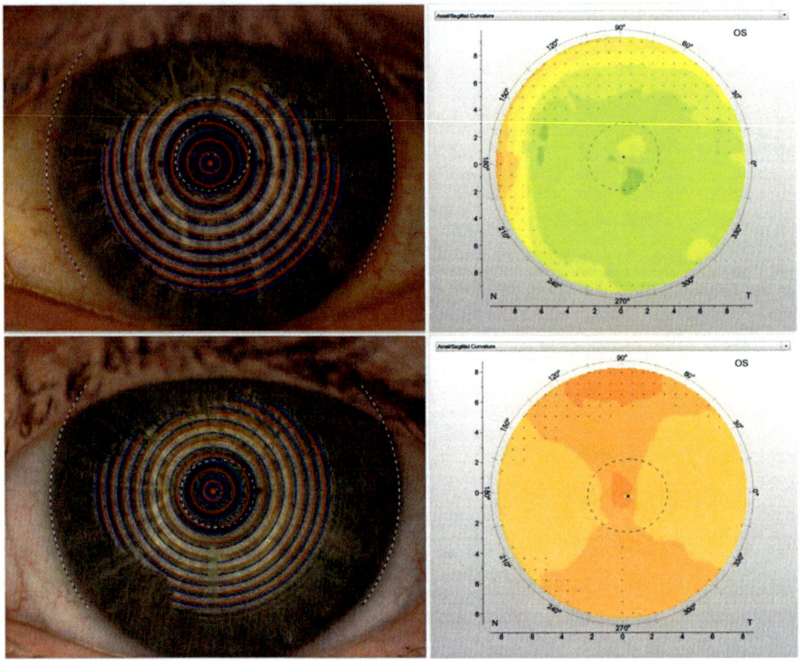

Fig. (9). (Top) Example of a scleral lens with front surface spherical optics without flexure. Note the spherical pattern of the topography. (Bottom) Over-topography of scleral lens exhibiting flexure. Note the front surface against the rule astigmatism of a scleral lens that is known to have front surface spherical optics.

Ordering scleral lenses is straightforward. Practitioners can call the laboratory to place the order over the phone, or can speak with a consultant who can help design a lens based on the information collected during the fitting. Some laboratories promote electronic orders either through email or an online ordering portal.

FOLLOW UP EXAMINATIONS

Initial Dispensing Visit

When the scleral lens arrives from the laboratory, place the lens in a lens case with gas permeable conditioning solution to improve initial application wettability if the lens has been shipped in a dry state. When the patient arrives, briefly confirm that there are no changes in the patient history, obtain visual acuities and confirm with the slit lamp that there are no contraindications.

Apply the scleral lens with sodium fluorescein and evaluate similar to the diagnostic lens process. The evaluation should include initial visual acuity, over-refraction and slit lamp evaluation. If vision is acceptable and the lens fit is appropriate to dispense, the patient is trained in the application and removal process, lens care and handling, and a follow-up visit is scheduled. The patient is also instructed about a wearing schedule which allows for a gradual increase in wearing time. Patients are educated if they experience redness, pain, foreign body sensation, discharge, change in vision, or light sensitivity to remove the lens immediately. If symptoms do not resolve on their own, patients are given emergency contact information and are advised to contact the practitioner immediately. If the lens is deemed unacceptable at this visit and requires changes to the lens design or power, allow the lens to settle in the office before rechecking lens fit and over-refraction. Reorder the lens with the new changes accordingly.

Continuation of Care Schedule

Appropriate follow up care is extremely important to monitor ocular health and prevent complications. While each visit is similar in examination flow, patients may present with different comments or complaints as they continue to adapt to their new scleral lenses. For new scleral lens wearers, a repeat evaluation should be completed 1-2 weeks after the initial dispensing visit. Depending on the lens fit and the patient's report of comfort and vision, a new lens may need to be ordered after that visit. If the lens still performs well and demonstrates a good fit, some practitioners also recommend another visit 1-2 months later, to ensure optimal vision and ocular health. In addition, practitioners should be aware of the timeframe of a scleral lens warranty from the laboratory. Each laboratory has different policies that may dictate the timeframe between follow up visits. Certain patients may require a four to six month follow up appointment, to ensure the disease processes has remained stable and the scleral lens fit remains optimal. Established scleral lens wearers with stable corneas may have a more relaxed schedule, with evaluations scheduled annually.

The amount of follow up care varies by practitioner and condition being treated. New scleral lens practitioners will likely follow their patients more closely, until they develop an understanding for lens adaptation, and when certain problems develop. For example, a patient wearing scleral lenses with high astigmatism will likely need less follow up care than a patient with a corneal transplant. As the practitioner gains more experience with scleral lenses and different corneal conditions, they will adopt a follow up care plan that is acceptable for both their office and their patients.

At each visit, a case history should be performed. To prevent confusion with lens wearing schedule, care or expectations, ask the patient how they are adjusting to their new lenses and if they have any problems while wearing their scleral lenses.

Also discuss vision, wearing time, level of comfort and if they are sleeping in their lenses. What care system and filling solution are they using? Do they sleep in the lenses? Asking open ended questions is a helpful tip for an accurate patient history. For example, ask the patient what brand of solution they are using, rather than asking, "Are you using Brand X?"

Visual acuities should also be monitored at each visit, both monocularly and binocularly. When needed, perform an over-refraction to ensure the lens is providing the best corrected visual acuity. Keep in mind, vision may change very quickly in some disease processes; for example, a young patient with keratoconus who has not been crosslinked and is progressing. This patient may require more lens modifications in order to increase the clearance over the progressing ectasia and compensate for any visual changes.

During the slit lamp evaluation, assess the condition of the scleral lenses for scratches, deposits, and tear chamber debris. Also examine the surface of each lens for unstable wettability. Evaluate the peripheries of the lens with white light to observe scleral alignment. Then finalize the lens clearance assessment with a white light optic section, measuring the central and limbal clearance. Lastly, apply fluorescein to the conjunctiva or lens surface to see how quickly it is pumped into the tear chamber, if at all. Assessing tear exchange can help troubleshoot debris in the post-lens tear layer. During the fitting period, a slit lamp evaluation of the ocular surface without the lens can help highlight areas of the lens design that need to be adjusted. Use sodium fluorescein to stain the cornea for any epithelial defects or microcystic corneal edema. Areas of epithelial staining may be a clue that the lens is touching the cornea or limbus and lens alterations are necessary to ensure a healthy lens fit. Also, examine the cornea for any evidence of hypoxia, endothelial changes, and changes in corneal thickness. Evaluate the conjunctiva for evidence of lens compression, impingement, irritation to conjunctival lesions (*i.e.* pinguecula) or excessive conjunctival staining. During visits after the initial fitting period, observe the cornea for any new neovascularization, opacities, or changes to the corneal thickness and endothelium.

If deemed necessary, evaluate central and limbal clearance and peripheral alignment with OCT imaging (Fig. **10**). Scleral lenses may settle over time, which will change the central and limbal clearance. The peripheral alignment may also change due to lens settling. When a patient returns to the office for an evaluation during the fitting period, recommend four hours or more of wearing time prior to the visit; this can assist changing the lens design accurately and efficiently.

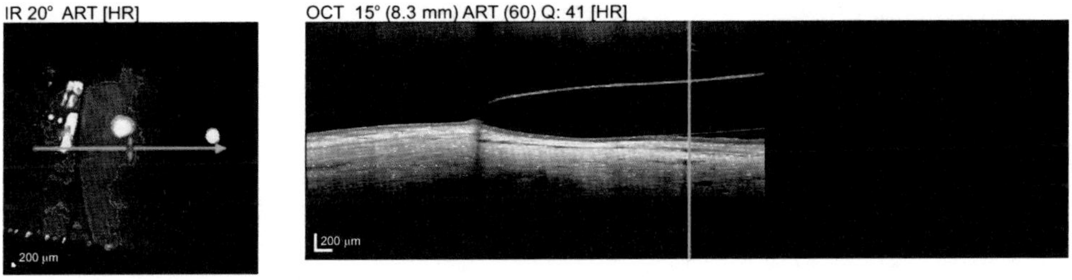

Fig. (10). OCT image of scleral lens landing zone and edge.

Prior to completing the follow up visit, inform the patient that minor changes may be required to obtain the optimal lens fit. Explain the importance of proper lens care and follow up visits necessary to ensure that the ocular health is maintained. If a patient is transitioning from corneal lenses or soft lenses with an improper fit, it may take a few weeks to obtain an accurate prescription due to changes in corneal shape. It may be advisable to postpone releasing the glasses prescription until the patient's refraction has stabilized on two or more occasions. Performing comparison topography maps at each visit will also aid in determining when the cornea has stabilized.

Patients who wear scleral lenses often have complex and unique ocular conditions. It is important to educate patients on their condition and the scleral lens fitting process in order to avoid frustration when multiple follow up visits are necessary.

Examination flow of scleral lenses is an evolving process, and current standards will continue to change as technology, lens designs and research develops.

CONFLICT OF INTEREST

The author declares no conflict of interest, financial or otherwise.

ACKNOWLEDGEMENTS

None Declared.

REFERENCES

[1] Nichols KK, Foulks GN, Bron AJ, *et al.* The international workshop on meibomian gland dysfunction: executive summary. Invest Ophthalmol Vis Sci 2011; 52(4): 1922-9. [http://dx.doi.org/10.1167/iovs.10-6997a] [PMID: 21450913]

[2] Schornack MM, Patel SV. Relationship between corneal topographic indices and scleral lens base curve. Eye Contact Lens 2010; 36(6): 330-3. [http://dx.doi.org/10.1097/ICL.0b013e3181eb8418] [PMID: 20631627]

[3] DeNaeyer G. Modern Scleral Contact Lens Fitting. Contact Lens Spectr 2010.

[4] Barnett M, Lien V, Li JY, Durbin-Johnson B, Mannis MJ. Use of Scleral Lenses and Miniscleral Lenses After Penetrating Keratoplasty. Eye Contact Lens 2015.
[PMID: 26214530]

[5] Lee JC, Chiu GB, Bach D, Bababeygy SR, Irvine J, Heur M. Functional and visual improvement with prosthetic replacement of the ocular surface ecosystem scleral lenses for irregular corneas. Cornea 2013; 32(12): 1540-3.
[http://dx.doi.org/10.1097/ICO.0b013e3182a73802] [PMID: 24145631]

[6] van der Worp E, Graf T, Caroline P. Exploring beyond corneal borders. Contact Lens Spectr 2010.

[7] Visser ES, Visser R, VanLier H. Advantages of Toric Scleral Lenses. Optometry & Vision Science 2006; 83(4): 233-6.
[http://dx.doi.org/10.1097/01.opx.0000214297.38421.15]

[8] Smith CA, Pepose JS. Disinfection of tonometers and contact lenses in the office setting: are current techniques adequate? Am J Ophthalmol 1999; 127(1): 77-84.
[PMID: 9933004]

CHAPTER 12

Scleral Lens Complications and Problem Solving

Karen G. Carrasquillo[1,*], **Michael J. Lipson**[2], **Damon J. Ezekiel**[3], **Lynette K. Johns**[4] and **Melissa Barnett**[5]

[1] *BostonSight, Needham Heights, MA, USA*

[2] *Department of Ophthalmology and Visual Science, University of Michigan, Northville Health Center, Northville, MI, USA*

[3] *Ezekiel Eyes, Nedlands WA, Australia*

[4] *New England College of Optometry, Boston, MA, USA*

[5] *University of California, Davis, Sacramento, CA, USA*

Abstract: Scleral lenses have become a mainstream option for the treatment of distorted corneas and ocular surface disease. Well-fit scleral lenses vault the cornea and are supported entirely by the sclera. They create a tear layer reservoir which helps neutralize an irregular, damaged or diseased cornea while creating constant lubrication and necessary oxygen supply. They provide optics comparable to corneal gas permeable lenses, with equivalent comfort to soft contact lenses. Like any type of medical treatment, there must be first and foremost an understanding of the disease process and pathology being treated when fitting scleral lenses. Without true understanding of the disease process and its limitations, practitioners may inadvertently induce complications. A comprehensive understanding of the intended scleral lens design and fitting parameters is paramount. Equally important is establishing a close relationship with the lens manufacturing laboratory and their consultants. This is particularly critical when troubleshooting challenging cases. Establishing appropriate scleral lens follow up and close communication with the referring corneal or medical specialist is very important. Proper understanding of the disease process and its limitations are important to avoid scleral lens induced complications. Appropriate follow up and adequate collaboration with specialists is also essential to ensure successful treatment with scleral lenses. From the care and handling aspect as well as disease management strategies, patient communication and involvement can improve compliance and favorable outcomes.

Keywords: Abrasion, Application, Comfort, Corneal abrasion, Corneal Neovascularization, Edema, Fogging, Graft Rejection, Hyperemia, Impression ring, Injection, Keratitis, Neovascularization, Non-wetting, Pain, Problem Solving, Prolapse, Redness, Removal, Visual Acuity.

* **Corresponding author Karen G. Carrasquillo:** BostonSight, Needham Heights, MA 02494, USA; Tel: 781-72--7337; Fax: 781-726-7310; E-mail: kcarrasquillo@bostonsight.org

Melissa Barnett & Lynette K. Johns (Eds.)

INTRODUCTION

Scleral lenses have become a mainstream option for the treatment of distorted corneas and ocular surface disease. Well-fit scleral lenses vault the cornea and are supported entirely by the sclera. They create a tear layer reservoir which helps neutralize an irregular, damaged or diseased cornea while creating constant lubrication and necessary oxygen supply. They provide optics comparable to corneal gas permeable lenses, with equivalent comfort to soft contact lenses.

Like any type of medical treatment, there must be first and foremost an understanding of the disease process and pathology being treated when fitting scleral lenses. Without true understanding of the disease process and its limitations, practitioners may inadvertently induce complications. Examples include fitting corneas with an incorrect type of polymer material, with inadequate limbal clearance, not offering proper follow up and medical management after fitting, or simply fitting a patient that is an inappropriate candidate.

Next, a comprehensive understanding of the intended scleral lens design and fitting parameters is paramount. Equally important is establishing a close relationship with the lens manufacturing laboratory and their consultants. This is particularly critical when troubleshooting challenging cases. Establishing appropriate scleral lens follow up and close communication with the referring corneal or medical specialist is very important. Complications rarely arise immediately after fitting scleral lenses, but weeks or months later. Consequently, if a patient is lost to follow up, complications may become more severe.

Patient education is essential for a successful outcome with scleral lenses. A scleral lens, whether fluid-ventilated or air-ventilated (fenestrated), will settle over time. Once the wearing time has been increased to eight to 12 hours on a daily basis, potential complications can develop. Proper corneal clearance is required for a successful scleral lens fit, as insufficient clearance can result in corneal epithelial compromise and excessive clearance may result in corneal hypoxia and difficulty with application. A well-fit scleral lens will demonstrate clearance or non-bearing over the limbus. Overall, tightly fitting lenses can lead to lens suction, and impinging lenses can cause acute or chronic hypertrophic ridges on the conjunctival tissue. In addition, thoughtful material selection would address the need for added oxygen permeability and improve front surface wettability.

Poor patient compliance may also lead to complications such as extended wear and/or over wear. In some cases, extended wear of scleral lenses is medically necessary; however, these require close monitoring and follow up. Patient education is crucial to ensure proper compliance.

It is helpful to have a standardized routine of evaluating lens fit, corneal health and troubleshooting when problem solving scleral lens complications. Techniques should be developed to rule out the most common complications first and progress through a diagnostic routine that covers all potential issues.

At each step of the fitting process from baseline evaluation, initial lens dispense, and subsequent examination, a strategic and routine approach is necessary. As previously stated, understanding the patient's diagnosis and scleral lens goals can prepare the practitioner to monitor potential complications.

Prior to initiating the scleral lens fitting, baseline examination should include a thorough assessment of the eyelids, cornea, conjunctiva and tear film. Begin by evaluating the eyelids and meibomian glands. Document signs of blepharitis, meibomitis, telangiectasia, irregular eyelid margins and Demodex. Perform meibomian gland expression or meibomography if available. Corneal evaluation including topography, staining, scarring, nodules and edema should be evaluated. The length and depth of corneal neovascularization should be well documented at baseline examination. If epithelial defects are present, note location and measure the size. Assessment of the conjunctiva including staining, hyperemia, pingueculae, pterygia, glaucoma drainage devices or blebs, conjunctivochalasis, symblepharon and giant papillary conjunctivitis should be documented. Measurement of tear film quantity and quality can be performed by assessing tear meniscus height, Schirmer's test, tear break-up time (TBUT), osmolarity, topography and tomography. Once applying a diagnostic lens, document any areas where the lens may interact with abnormal findings as mentioned above.

When first dispensing scleral lenses, verify that assessment of patient comfort, application and removal, fit and vision is sufficient in order to dispense lenses to the patient. At each follow up visit, maintain a consistent routine. During the patient history, inquire about comfort, wearing time, quality of vision and success with handling and lens care. Ensure they are using preservative free filling solution. Objective measurements including visual acuity, scleral lens fit, lens removal to ensure suction is not present; slit lamp examination after lens removal to rule out corneal and conjunctival staining should systematically be performed. Atypical findings that differ from baseline should be well documented and monitored.

An overview of some of the most common complications, their causes, manifestations, and overall management strategies will be covered in this chapter. Long-term success for practitioners and their patients is dependent on having the tools, knowledge of lens parameters and observational skills to solve those problems. This chapter will also detail how to make changes to troubleshoot complications.

Corneal Edema

The cornea provides two thirds of the total refractive power of the eye; thus, its transparency is necessary in order to provide adequate vision. When there is a lack of corneal transparency, visual rehabilitation will be limited using the rigid optics of a corneal or scleral gas permeable lens.

One of the causes for loss of transparency is the development of corneal edema. This could develop from physical factors at any of the corneal cell layers. For example, compromised epithelial gap junctions may lead to a barrier breach, inducing intracellular edema. This is a result of homogeneous loss of the refractive index of cells throughout the epithelial layer [1]. Consequently, a compromise to the endothelial layer leads to loss of transparency. The mechanism by which the endothelium contributes to corneal transparency is bimodal. One mode acts as a barrier to aqueous components. The second mode is that the endothelium uses sodium-potassium adenosine triphosphatase pumps, which actively removes fluid that leaks into the stroma from the aqueous compartment [1].

In order to minimize or avoid complications of microcystic corneal edema (MCE) associated with the use of scleral lenses, it is crucial to first rule out any underlying pathology or causes that predispose the cornea to develop edema at baseline. A true understanding of scleral lens indications and complications would prevent a patient with contraindications from unnecessarily being fit with a scleral lens. For example, a patient with Fuchs' endothelial dystrophy with compromised endothelial function may become more edematous with scleral lens wear.

One of the most common causes of MCE could be elevated intraocular pressure (IOP). Persistent elevated IOP drives fluid across the endothelium, creating both epithelial and stromal edema [2]. Primary or secondary endothelial disease can also cause MCE, for example, Fuchs' dystrophy and pseudophakic bullous keratopathy (PBK). Obtaining an endothelial cell count can help monitor endothelial disease. Patients with these conditions are typically not good candidates for scleral lenses, unless they had a penetrating keratoplasty or Descemet's stripping endothelial keratoplasty (DSEK). Secondary endothelial disease could also be a consequence of trauma to the eye. Old corneal grafts or grafts that have a low endothelial cell count at baseline may be predisposed to develop MCE with a fluid-ventilated scleral lens (Fig. **1**) and may at times require an air-ventilated lens in order for the treatment to be successful.

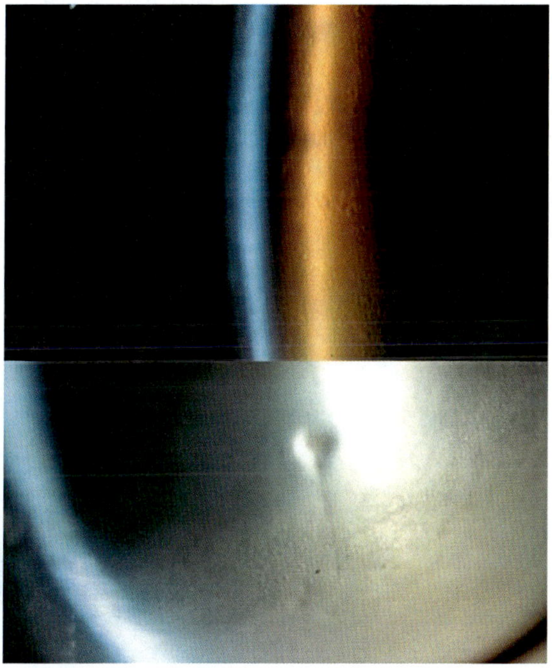

Fig. (1). Microcystic corneal edema in two cases post penetrating keratoplasty after 8 hours of scleral lens wear. Images courtesy of Karen Carrasquillo.

It is important to rule out mechanical complications from scleral lens fitting that could lead to the development of MCE. With corneal swelling, transparency is lost and edema could induce irregular astigmatism and affect vision. Once underlying contraindicated pathologies are ruled out, appropriate candidacy is determined.

Even though studies are needed in order to determine all the factors leading to mechanically induced MCE from scleral lens wear, one of the causes could be reduced or inadequate clearance at the limbus (Fig. **2**).

While much has been hypothesized about the adequate amount of theoretical apical clearance with scleral lenses, clinical observations of patients wearing scleral lenses for more than twenty years has shown that the amount of central apical clearance might not necessarily be the key factor in the development of MCE. In the authors' experience with apical clearance up to 400 microns, the development of MCE was not observed with this clearance. These same patients demonstrated limbal clearance, and lack of conjunctival compression without a compromised endothelium. This may suggest that if the height of the lens is distributed over an adequate surface area and there is no suction and compression at the limbus, then the risk of developing MCE is low. If inadequate limbal clearance is accompanied with excessive apical clearance and the overall surface area of the landing zone where the weight of the lens is distributed is small, for example in a small diameter lens, then complications are often witnessed. Thus, if a grafted or non-grafted cornea with an endothelial cell count of ≥ 1000 cells/mm^2, develops MCE, a practitioner should consider increasing limbal clearance and overall lens diameter in order to distribute the weight over a larger surface area and avoid compression over the limbus.

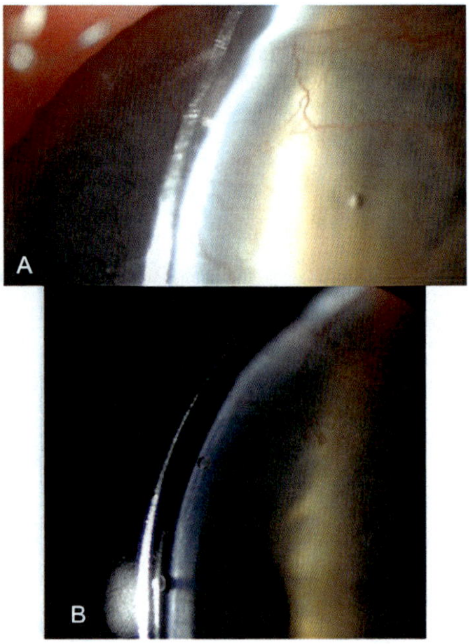

Fig. (2). Microcystic edema (A) in a Stevens-Johnson patient wearing a 19mm lens as a consequence of low limbal clearance (B). MCE was resolved by increasing clearance at the limbus. The apical clearance remained unchanged. Images courtesy of Karen Carrasquillo.

Another potential cause could be peripheral curves that are too steep/tight, causing the lens to seal-off. Flattening the peripheral curves will overcome this issue. Sometimes, if the optic zone is too small, it may crowd the limbal area causing compression which may induce corneal edema; a larger optic zone could improve the lens fit.

Even when the scleral landing zone is successfully aligned, there is adequate limbal clearance and the material is optimized, center thickness of the lens should not be overlooked. If the center thickness of the lens is too thick, (≥0.4mm), despite working with a hyper-permeable material, oxygen permeability could be compromised and lead to the development of corneal edema. This is particularly of concern when dealing with aphakic eyes or high plus prescriptions. In some cases, it may be necessary to split the plus power between the scleral lens and spectacles in order to reduce the center thickness of the scleral lens.

Despite using all of the considerations mentioned above, if the corneal endothelium lacks an effective pump mechanism, then corneal edema will likely develop with scleral lens wear. In the short term, patients should remove their scleral lens at the first sign of haloes with rainbows. Hypertonic sodium chloride drops or topical steroids may be recommended immediately post lens wear. Wearing schedule should be reduced and modified. Mid-day breaks may need to be scheduled. After ruling out mechanical triggers, an air-ventilated (fenestrated) lens may be helpful (Fig. **3**), although success cannot be guaranteed.

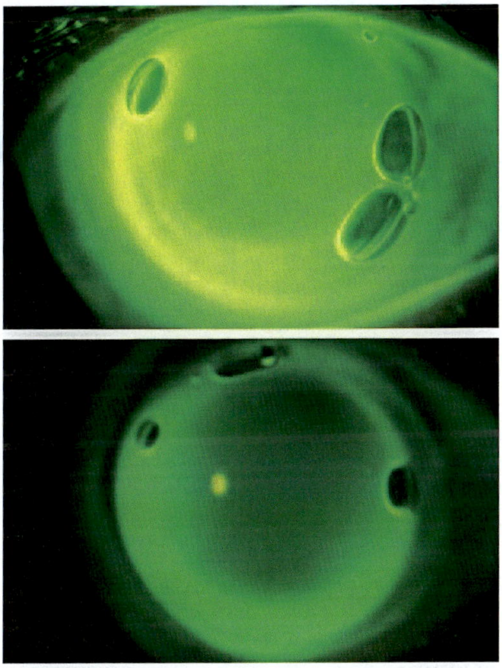

Fig. (3). Fenestrated scleral lens fit in two different cases post penetrating keratoplasty with ≤700 cells/mm^2 in the corneal endothelium that developed MCE with fluid-ventilated scleral lenses. Attempts were made to troubleshoot the fit by ruling out mechanical triggers and failed. Both cases were successful with fenestrated lenses. Images courtesy of Karen Carrasquillo.

When choosing an air-ventilated (fenestrated) design or approach to fitting, there are still considerations that should be followed in order to avoid complications. In order to shift the air bubble from the visual axis, apical clearance is greatly minimized. Lens settling and duration of scleral lens wear may contribute to corneal contact that causes superficial keratitis (Fig. **4**).

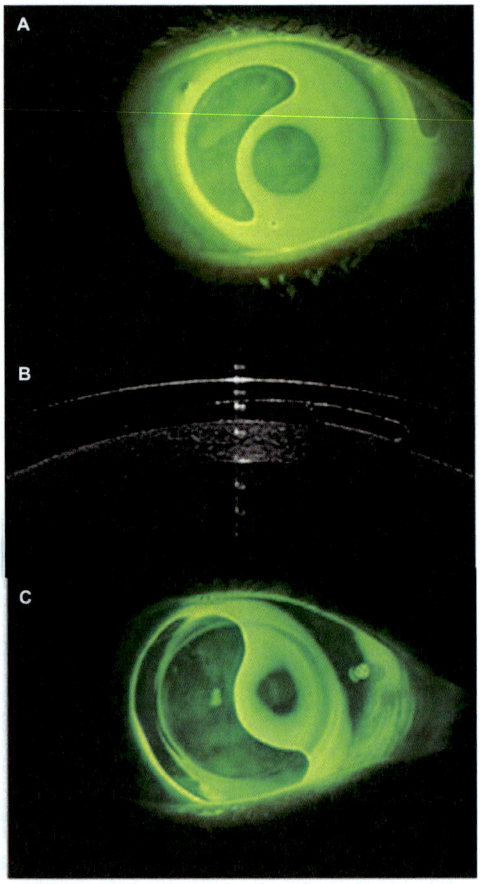

Fig. (4). A) Significant corneal touch and (B,C) bubbles encroaching visual axis having a detrimental effect in vision in air-ventilated (fenestrated) designs. Images courtesy of Damon Ezekiel.

Adequate follow up and close monitoring is necessary for fenestrated scleral lenses. Significantly large bubbles encroaching on the visual axis could have detrimental effects in vision, either causing significant glare at night or simply reducing best corrected vision.

Often scleral lenses are used to treat ocular surface disease (OSD). These corneas have compromised surfaces that in many cases have loose gap junctions; the development of intracellular edema at the epithelial layer is possible which may be exacerbated by scleral lens wear. For example in the case of concomitant glaucoma, changing topical medications to preservative-free versions may be required. This is one prime example where working closely with specialists is imperative.

The table below summarizes key aspects to consider in order to minimize or avoid complications of corneal edema with scleral lenses.

Potential ocular causes for corneal edema
• Elevated intraocular pressure (IOP)
• Primary or secondary endothelial disease
  - Poor candidates for scleral lenses unless s/p keratoplasty
• Poor endothelial cell count
• Topical medications which may contain toxic preservatives
  - Special consideration in OSD
 	
Potential scleral lens-related causes for corneal edema
• Inadequate limbal clearance
  - May require larger diameter
  - Independent limbal area manipulation of lens design
  - Increase optic zone diameter
• Polymer material with poor oxygen permeability
  - In some cases hyper-permeable materials are warranted
• Lens center thickness
  - Avoid high center thickness
  - Special consideration in aphakia
  - High plus prescriptions

Problem Solving Corneal Edema

• If corneal edema is from mechanical contact at the limbus (as evidenced by corneal staining), increase the limbal clearance. • If excessive apical clearance is observed, reduce apical clearance or consider increasing the overall diameter of the lens to distribute the weight of the lens over a broader surface area making sure that the limbus is not compressed. • If corneal edema is caused by steep peripheral curves and lens seal off, flatten the peripheral curves and ensure fluorescein exchange and reduce the amount of peripheral toricity if present. • Increasing the optic zone diameter aids in reducing limbal congestion and compression. • Optimize oxygen to the cornea by reducing the center thickness and selecting a hyper Dk material. Consider reducing a high plus prescription in the scleral lens to be distributed between glasses and the lens. • If all options fail, reduce wearing time and specify a detailed wearing schedule for the patient. • Manage persistent corneal edema with hypertonic sodium chloride drops and consider topical steroids in extreme cases. • Fenestrating the scleral lens may also help extend wearing time prior to the onset of edema. Control the location of the bubble and reduce the impact of it centering over the visual axis by reducing central clearance and flattening the base curve. Monitor the bubble. If the bubble is mobile, there is less of a risk for the cornea to desiccate. Monitor fenestrated patients closely for lens settling, bubble desiccation and corneal edema. • Consider changing topical ocular medications to preservative free formulations.

Bullae

Bullae are caused by the failure of the corneal endothelial layer to perform its normal pump function. The pump function failure is due to poor cell function or the number of endothelial cells decreasing below a critical level to maintain corneal clarity. This would be a sequela as stated above from primary or secondary endothelial disease. These conditions should be identified before initiating treatment with a scleral lens, as scleral lens success will be limited.

Sub-epithelial fluid-filled bullae could form at the ocular surface as a result of stromal swelling after trauma, persistent epithelial defects (PED) or in some cases, as a result of intracellular edema from loose gap junctions in the context of ocular surface disease. It is not rare to see the formation of bullae during the re-epithelialization of a persistent epithelial defect (Fig. **5**) [3, 4]. Bullae may sometimes rupture causing a transient setback. Ultimately, even recalcitrant persistent epithelial defects tend to heal by the appropriate microenvironment that scleral lenses offer [3, 4]. If bullae develop under these circumstances, then daily monitoring and patient education is warranted. As the epithelium heals and regenerates, the entire ocular surface improves.

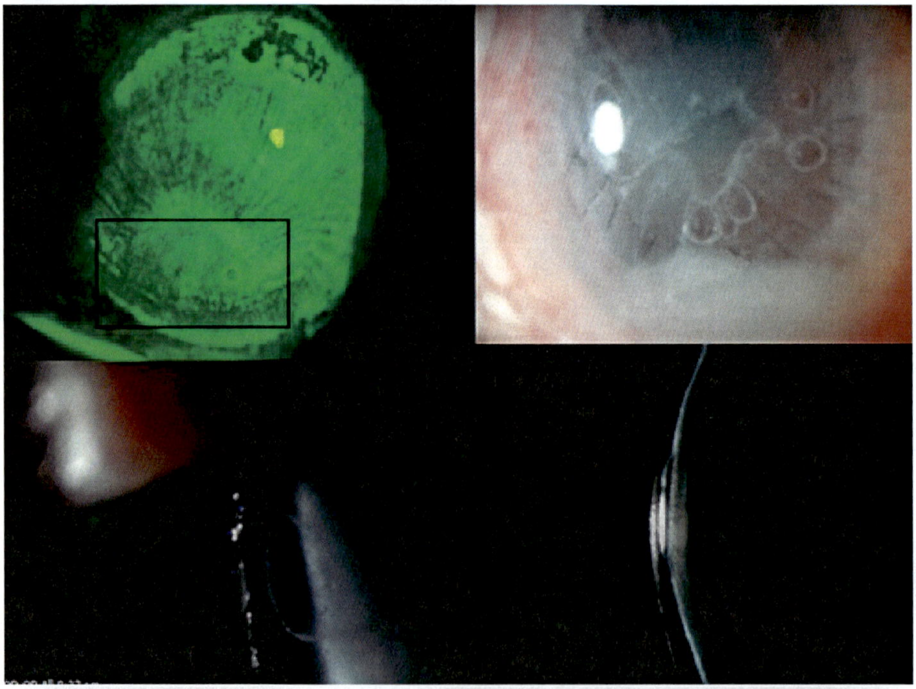

Fig. (5). Subepithelial bullae after persistent epithelial defects in different cases. Images courtesy of Karen Carrasquillo.

If subepithelial bullae develop in the absence of trauma or PED, then the choice of polymer material should be explored and suction from tight fitting lenses should be ruled out.

Problem Solving Bullae

- If bullae are pre-existing, scleral lens fitting is contraindicated.
- Consider changing the polymer material.
- If the lens is suctioned, loosen the peripheral curves and reduce the amount of peripheral toricity to ensure fluorescein exchange and no resistance upon removal.

Epithelial Bogging

With a sealed scleral lens, it has been demonstrated that there is little or no tear exchange throughout the day [5]. Therefore, preservative-free saline or preservative-free artificial tears placed into the bowl of the lens upon application will remain in contact with the ocular surface throughout the wearing time.

When the sealed scleral lens is removed and biomicroscopy is performed, the ocular surface is irregular with a corrugated surface and appears "water-logged," otherwise known as epithelial bogging (Fig. **6**). The exact etiology and mechanism for this phenomenon is unknown. The condition appears to be transient and with time, the epithelium adjusts to the environment and resumes a more normal and regular appearance.

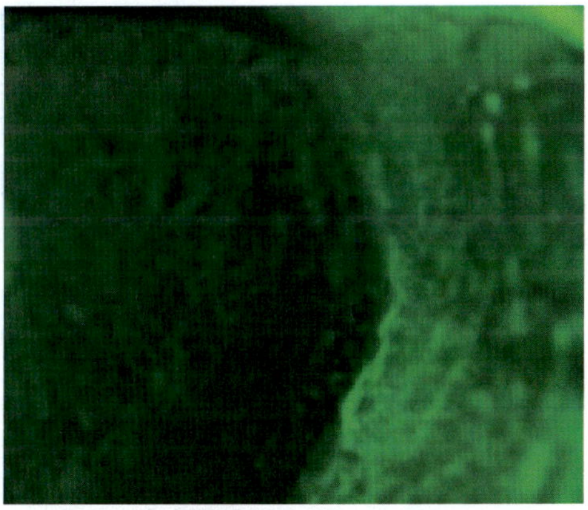

Fig. (6). Presentation of corneal surface after 6 hours of wearing time. Note the uneven pattern of fluorescein appearing wavy or corrugated, suggesting epithelial bogging. Image courtesy of Lynette Johns.

Currently, epithelial bogging is perceived as a benign scleral lens complication. Additional research is recommended to provide insight into this phenomenon.

Problem solving Epithelial Bogging

- Always advise patients to use preservative free solutions when filling their lenses.
- If the epithelial bogging corneal finding does not resolve, discontinue scleral lens use for one day and re-evaluate.

Corneal Neovascularization

Corneal neovascularization is the ingrowth of blood vessels from the limbal vascular plexus into the cornea, caused by deprivation of oxygen or limbal stem cell deficiency (LSCD). Causes of LSCD include sequela from trauma, chemical injury, tumours, infections, immunological disorders, Stevens-Johnson syndrome (SJS) and ocular cicatricial pemphigoid. There is a delicate balance of pro-angiogenic and anti-angiogenic factors in a healthy cornea along the palisades of Vogt where corneal stem cells reside. This delicate balance maintains an avascular state in a healthy cornea. When this balance is compromised, there could be a decrease in anti-angiogenic factors leading to corneal neovascularization [6]. LSCD and corneal neovascularization can also be caused by soft or rigid gas permeable contact lens wear [7, 8]. Typically, the causes are contact lens over-wear and extended wear. With contact lens wear, superficial neovascularization is more common than deep stromal neovascularization.

Superficial neovascularization with scleral lenses can be caused by high plus powered lenses (aphakia) with excessive center thickness compromising oxygen permeability, extended wear, poor compliance, low oxygen permeable polymer materials, and/or poor follow-up care. Hence, all of the above should be carefully evaluated and managed.

In reports of contact-lens induced LSCD and corneal neovascularization, medical therapy (topical corticosteroids, topical cyclosporine, topical vitamin A, oral doxycycline, punctal occlusion, or a combination of these) reversed the effects [9]. Clinical observations of patients with LSCD in conditions like SJS demonstrated a reduction of hyperperfusion of corneal neovascularization, otherwise termed as ghosting when there was limbal clearance (Fig. 7).

Deep stromal neovascularization is a serious condition, possibly leading to loss of optical transparency. In these cases, working closely with a corneal specialist will ensure proper medical management.

In general, tight fitting lenses should be refit to achieve scleral alignment in order to avoid suction and further complications. A looser fitting lens will release pressure around the limbus. Aside from ensuring adequate clearance at the limbus, increasing the Dk of a gas permeable material may ultimately be needed to increase the amount of oxygen to the cornea.

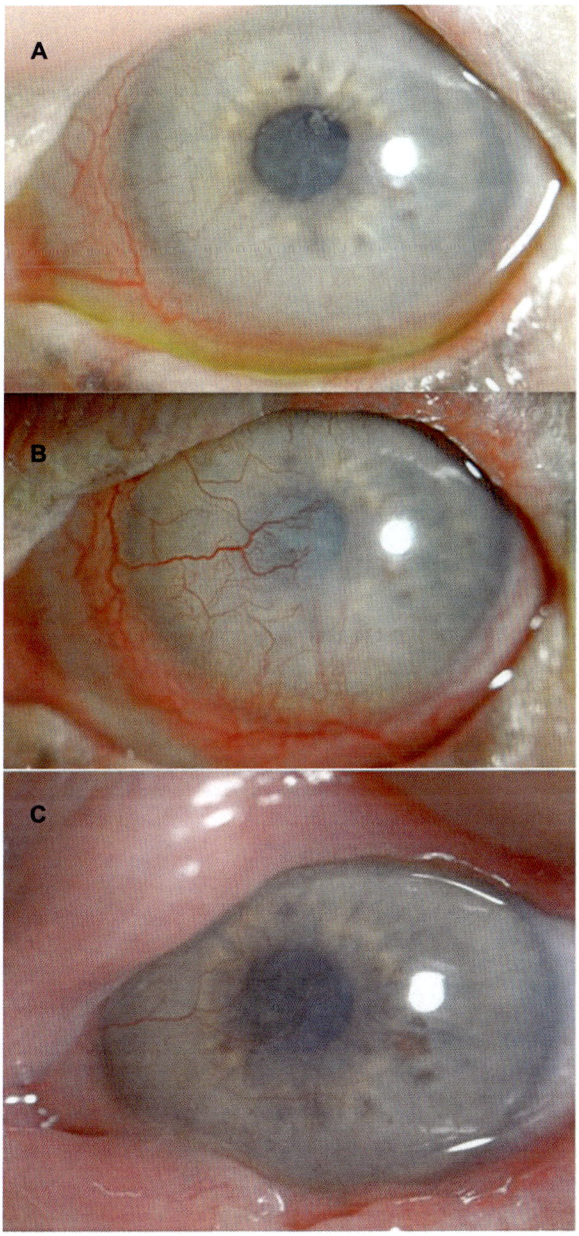

Fig. (7). SJS patient treated with a scleral lens in 2005 (A). Progressive corneal neovascularization noted in 2009 without response to steroids or Avastin® (bevacizumab) (B). Examination of fit revealed insufficient clearance at the limbus with touch and compression. Increasing limbal clearance (C) led to ghosting of blood vessels and inactivation of progressive corneal neovascularization. Images courtesy of Karen Carrasquillo.

Problem Solving Neovascularization

- Reduce center thickness in high plus powered lenses.
- Change to hyper Dk materials in the presence of neovascularization.
- Rule out extended wear of lenses.
- Neovascularization may require medical intervention such as
  - Topical corticosteroids
  - Topical cyclosporine
  - Topical vitamin A
  - Oral doxycycline
  - Punctal occlusion
  - Or a combination of the above
- Monitor the patient in frequent intervals.
- If the lens is tight, loosen the peripheral curves and reduce the amount of peripheral toricity to ensure fluorescein exchange and no resistance upon removal.
- Increase limbal clearance.

Limbal Bearing

Complications as a result of the weight of the scleral lens bearing on the limbus contribute to corneal compromise (Fig. **8**). Practitioners should reduce harsh bearing of the scleral lens on the limbus to avoid significant corneal complications such as corneal edema, neovascularization, keratitis, and prevent lens induced limbal stem cell deficiency.

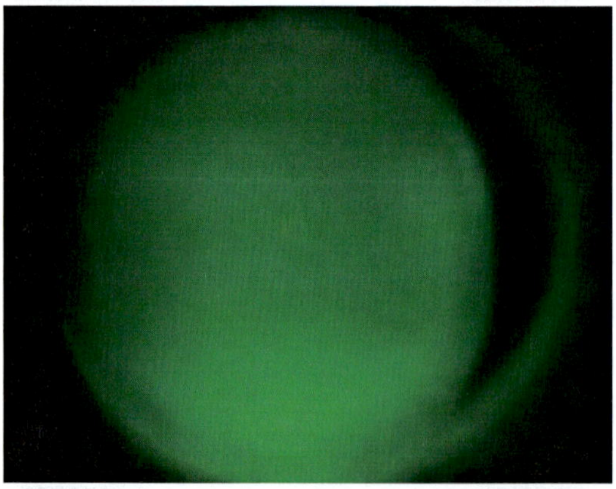

Fig. (8). Limbal bearing of scleral lens. Image courtesy of Lynette Johns.

If limbal bearing is observed, adjust the design to avoid complications. In some designs, a larger diameter scleral lens may increase clearance at the limbus. If working with a lens design that has an adjustable independent limbal curve feature, follow the manufacturers' recommendation or discuss with laboratory consultants. Manipulating optic zone diameter or mid-peripheral curve widths may allow for successful clearance of the limbus.

Complications as a result of the weight of the scleral lens bearing on the limbus contribute to corneal compromise. Practitioners should reduce harsh bearing of the scleral lens on the limbus to avoid significant corneal complications such as corneal edema, neovascularization, keratitis, and prevent lens induced limbal stem cell deficiency.

Problem Solving Limbal Bearing

- Increase the scleral lens diameter to increase limbal clearance.
- Increase the sagittal depth at the limbal zone of the lens.
- Adjust optic zone and/or mid peripheral curve widths to alleviate limbal contact.
- Contact the lens manufacturer consultants to aid in changing the lens.

Corneal and Conjunctival Staining/Excessive Hyperemia

With scleral lens wear, hyperemia/injection/redness is the easiest sign to observe by both practitioners and patients. Some patients have a natural predilection for hyperemia. Over time with an optimal scleral lens fit, patients show improvement in corneal health and hyperemia with continuous use of scleral lenses. Baseline corneal staining can be significantly reduced with the use of scleral lenses (Fig. **9**). Various changes in lens parameters and/or lens care products can minimize or eliminate redness.

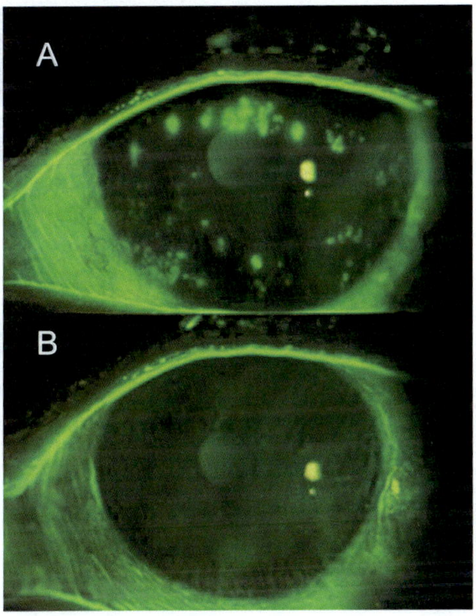

Fig. (9). Baseline corneal staining in a patient with GvHD (A). Corneal appearance of same patient after 6 hours of lens wear (B). Image courtesy of Lynette Johns.

Hyperemia may occur due to solution incompatibility related to preservatives, buffers or pH. Chemical toxicity from solutions and metabolic build up under the scleral lens can also cause superficial punctate keratitis. Revising the care system to ensure that preservative free saline is used to fill the lens, as well as changing to a preservative free disinfection system can reduce chemical toxicity. Patients may confuse preservative free with saline made for sensitive eyes. Those products with preservatives under a scleral lens can cause significant toxicity and symptomatology. Practitioners should recommend preservative free solutions for application. If a patient is highly sensitive, consider a buffer free formulation.

A scleral lens with excessive corneal bearing can cause superficial punctate keratitis. An increase in the sagittal depth will overcome this issue. A scleral lens with corneal peripheral contact can elicit corneal staining and adjacent limbal injection. Increasing the limbal clearance and avoiding contact will reverse corneal staining and limbal injection by clearing the peripheral cornea.

Excessive hyperperfusion of corneal neovascularization and conjunctival hyperemia can be attributed to many factors. If hyperemia is associated with the lens fit, there is likely compression or impingement in the landing area. The hallmark of compression is blanching of vessels under the scleral landing zone. Hyperemia will be observed adjacent to the compression, either at the limbus or outside the edge of the lens (Fig. **10**). Impingement does not cause vascular blanching; hyperemia will occur bordering the impinging edge. After lens removal, rebound hyperemia will occur in the area of compression or blanching. If the compression is significant, the entire eye may be hyperemic after lens removal. If the peripheral curve of a scleral lens is too steep, a flatter peripheral curve of a scleral lens will resolve this injection. To eliminate compression or impingement, flatten the periphery or specify toric peripheries if the compression or impingement is meridional [10 - 12].

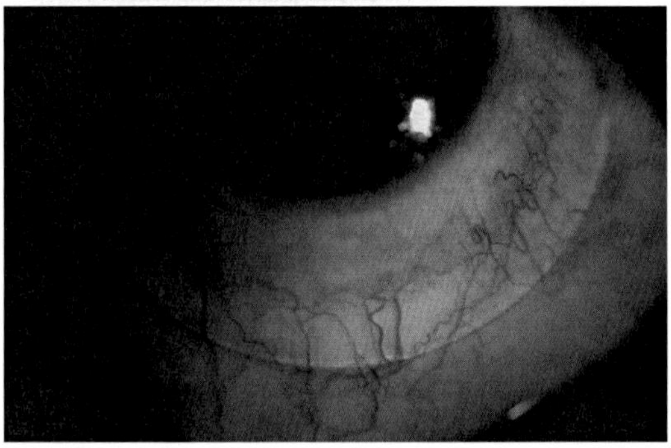

Fig. (10). Compression of the peripheral landing zone with limbal hyperemia and peripheral hyperemia outside of the lens edge. Image courtesy of Lynette Johns.

If hyperemia is caused by impingement on a conjunctival elevation such as a pinguecula, bleb or glaucoma drainage device, design the lens with a localized area of vaulting over the elevation. In addition, a notch can be incorporated at the lens edge to avoid contacting the elevation (Fig. **11**). To resolve hyperemia due to compression or impingement, flatten the periphery or specify toric peripheries.

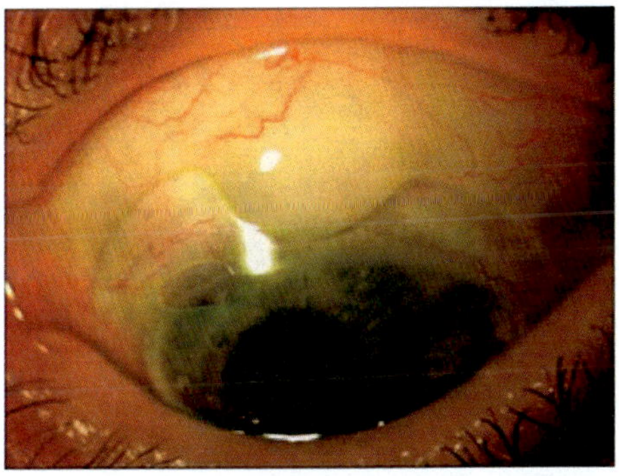

Fig. (11). Notched scleral lens to accommodate a conjunctival bleb. Image courtesy of Greg DeNaeyer.

Conjunctival staining is often seen on initial evaluation in patients with severe anterior surface disease such as Graft *vs*. Host Disease (GvHD), Sjögren's disease and ocular cicatricial pemphigoid. In these cases, the level of conjunctival staining is significantly reduced with scleral lens wear. Staining outside the scleral lens edge will persist. It may not be possible to completely eliminate conjunctival staining (Fig. **12**).

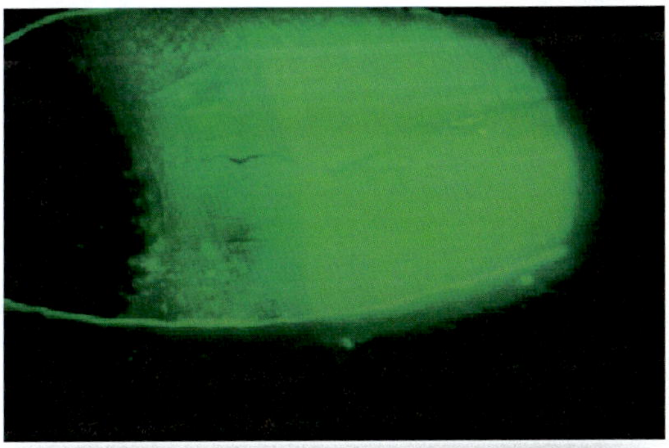

Fig. (12). Conjunctival staining improved underneath the landing zone of the scleral lens but persists outside of the edge. Image courtesy of Lynette Johns, I-Site e-newsletter (June 2014).

A patient having lens-induced conjunctival staining may or may not be symptomatic, usually this depends on the degree of impingement. In general, impingement associated with conjunctival staining (Fig. **13**) should be avoided. As described previously, complications from impingement can arise in the form of hypertrophic nodules, keratinized nodules and/or lead to scleral lens intolerance and drop out.

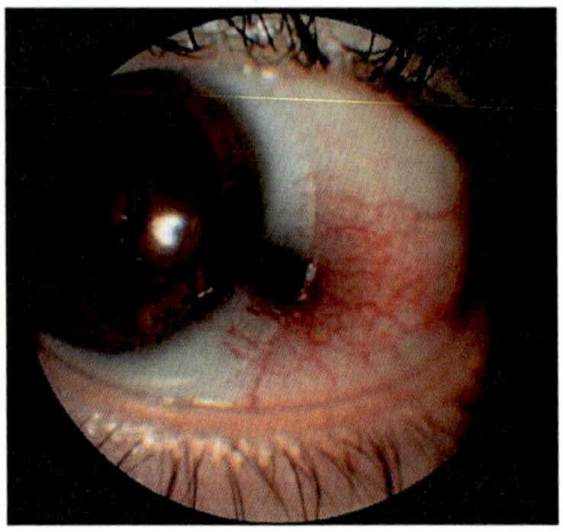

Fig. (13). Significant impingement and associated conjunctival injection in patient with keratoconus. Image courtesy of Damon Ezekiel.

Conjunctival staining is useful to evaluate both dry eye patients and scleral lens wearers. In scleral lens patients, circumlimbal staining observed with lissamine green may be an indicator of lens induced conjunctival staining. This may indicate that the scleral lens is too tight, impinging at the edge or has a sharp edge design.

Excessive impingement and landing zone compression could also lead to significant conjunctival injection. Prolonged wearing time and chronic insult could lead to sensitivity and discomfort, which may result in lens intolerance and/or reduced wearing time. Flattening the periphery or landing zone of the scleral lens will increase alignment. This will eliminate vessel impingement and also increase tear exchange. If working with a spherical design, it is likely that toric peripheries are warranted in order to properly align the sclera. If the current design does not offer toric peripheries, changing the diameter or working with a different design may be indicated.

Problem Solving Corneal and Conjunctival Staining/Hyperemia

- Eliminate use of preservatives by using preservative free filling solutions.
- Consider a preservative free disinfection system.
- Increase sagittal depth of lens if there is excessive corneal bearing.
- Increase limbal clearance (see above) if there is limbal staining.
- Loosen peripheral curves if there is compression from the landing zone or impingement of the scleral lens edge.
- Consider toric peripheral curves if findings are meridional.
- Reduce the diameter of the scleral lens to avoid a conjunctival elevation.
- Notch the edge to avoid a conjunctival elevation.
- If available in the design, regionally vault over the elevation.
- Flatten the landing zone to rest gently on an elevation. Toric peripheral curves may be required to compensate for the opposing meridian.

Conjunctival Impression Ring

When a scleral lens is too tight, the mechanical force of the scleral landing zone may cause an indentation or impression ring in the conjunctiva (Fig. **14**), which may be observed by pooling of sodium fluorescein or lissamine green. This complication can be observed while the scleral lens is being worn but is often more apparent immediately after lens removal. It is usually a result the landing area of the lens being too tight, creating marked bearing on the conjunctiva and sclera. An impression ring may occur in some patients with unusually soft conjunctival tissue regardless of parameter changes.

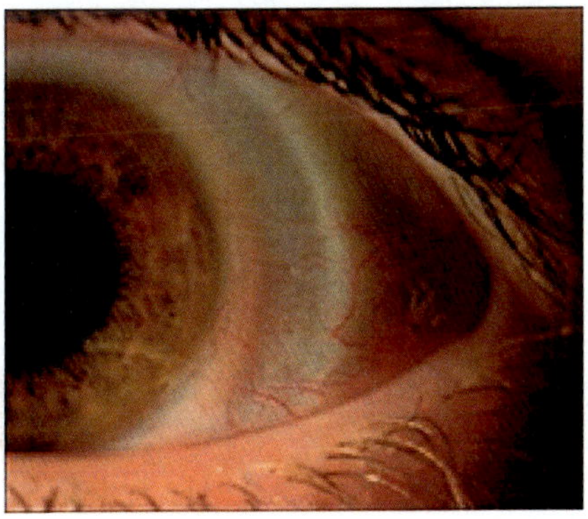

Fig. (14). Impression ring with impingement ridge. Image courtesy of Greg DeNaeyer (Contact Lens Spectrum, March 2014).

To improve or resolve an impression ring, modify the lens with a higher edge lift or flatter peripheral curve or increase the landing zone surface area to distribute the weight of the lens.

Problem Solving Impression Ring

- Flatten the scleral landing zone periphery or increase the edge lift.
- Increase the overall diameter of the lens to bear the weight more evenly on the conjunctival surface.
- Monitor if patient being asymptomatic (no soreness or aching after removal).
  - If monitoring, proceed with extreme caution in:
    - Cases of Neurotrophic Keratopathy (as the patient will have decreased or no sensation)
    - Cases of patients prone to keratinization
      - Even if asymptomatic, the risk of hypertrophic ridges or nodules are higher
    - Cases of profound impression rings, as these may ultimately lead to hypertrophic ridges or nodules, despite being asymptomatic

Conjunctival Hypertrophy

In the context of scleral lenses, tight and impinging lenses could lead to the formation of hypertrophic nodules and elevated ridges (Fig. **15**) that if chronic, could become keratinized. This is the reason why scleral landing zone alignment is imperative when fitting scleral lenses. In cases where chronic corneal and conjunctival desiccation is already present, chronic or acute significant impingement could lead to complications from scleral lens wear.

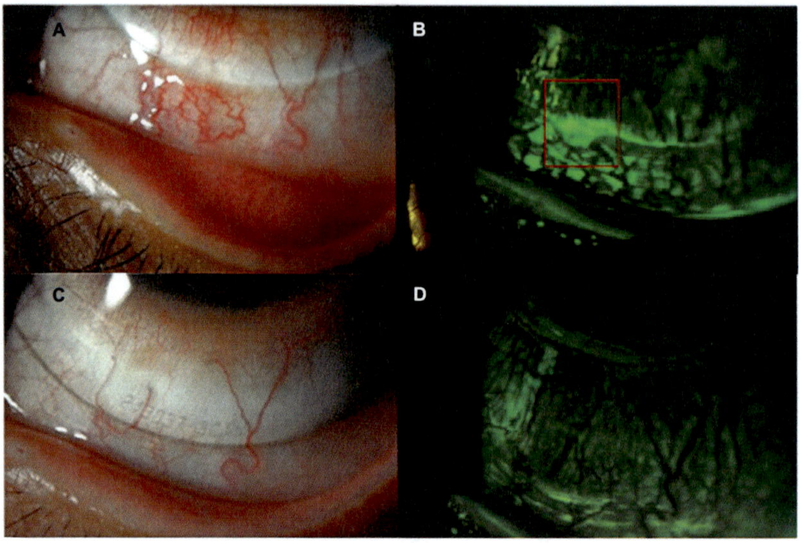

Fig. (15). Hypertrophic nodule (B) as a result of an impinging edge in a small diameter scleral lens fit (A) and resolution of nodule by fitting with a larger diameter lens and achieving scleral haptic alignment. Image courtesy of Karen Carrasquillo.

Relieving edge impingement and/or fitting with a larger diameter lens to cover a larger surface area and protect the conjunctiva from exposure will improve clinical manifestations. Ultimately, the goal to avoid edge impingement is to prevent hypertrophic nodules or ridges from becoming keratinized. A clinical pearl is to always apply sodium fluorescein after removing a scleral lens that has settled in the eye after at least three hours of wear. If there is no visible staining of the conjunctival surface, then the likelihood of this complication to manifest is minimal.

Problem Solving Conjunctival Hypertrophy

- Flatten the scleral landing zone periphery or increase the edge lift.
- Increase the overall diameter of the lens to bear the weight more evenly on the conjunctival surface.

Conjunctival Keratinization

There are a number of clinical scenarios where the tarsal (Fig. **16**) and bulbar conjunctiva may produce keratinized cells and become keratinized. Some of the most common scenarios or etiologies are chronic exposure and/or desiccation [13]. Vitamin A deficiency, scar formation after trachoma, SJS or irradiation of the lids are also other contributing factors. Another source of keratinization is hypertrophic nodules. Scleral lens induced hypertrophic nodules may be subject to keratinization. In cases of complete corneal keratinization, fitting may be contraindicated (Fig. **17**).

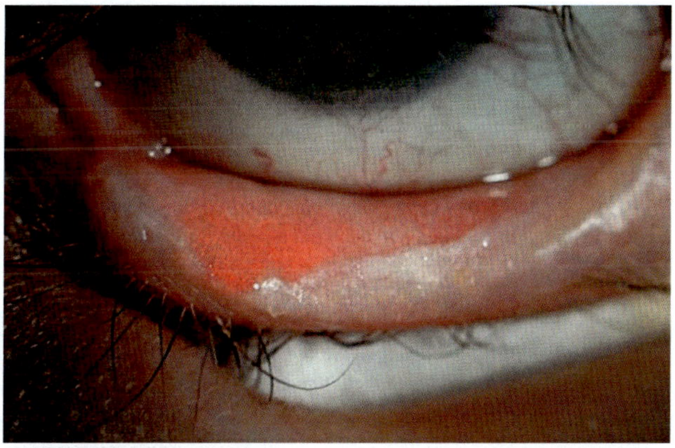

Fig. (16). Keratinization of palpebral conjunctiva. Note associated corneal pannus in the location of eyelid apposition. Image courtesy of Lynette Johns.

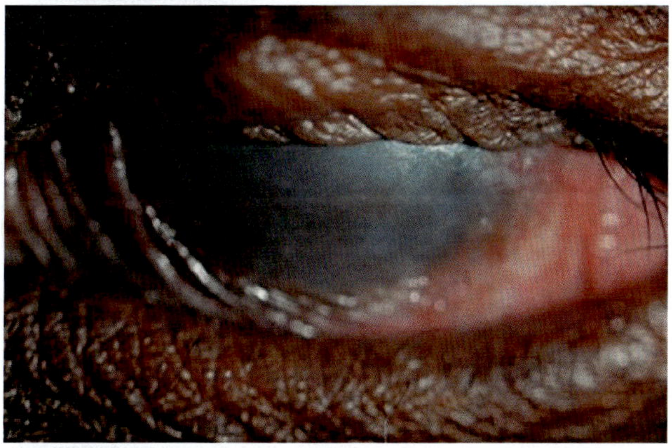

Fig. (17). Complete conjunctivalization and keratinization of the cornea. Image courtesy of Lynette Johns.

Problem Solving Conjunctival Keratinization

- Medical management of keratinzed tissues may be required.
  - Topical lubricants
  - Vitamin A
- Lubrication over the lens during wearing time.
- Reduce any conjunctival impingement of lens (see above).
- Consider overnight bandage contact lens wear. If using scleral lenses overnight, closely monitor for signs of hypoxia.

Conjunctival Prolapse

With age, there are minor changes and alterations in the conjunctiva that include conjunctival thinning and a loss of tissue transparency. The conjunctival vessels become more prominent, tortuous and dilated.

When fitting scleral lenses with complete corneal and limbal clearance, occasionally the conjunctival tissue is drawn beneath the lens at the limbus, otherwise known as conjunctival prolapse. This condition is most frequently seen in elderly patients, those who have undergone multiple ocular surgeries, such as strabismus or retinal procedures or those with loose conjunctival tissue and/or dermatochalasis.

While mostly thought to be a benign event, conjunctival prolapse has a disconcerting look to patients and practitioners alike. In most cases, it does not have long-term ramifications, but there are exceptions.

If observed during the course of fitting, document, and if possible, photo document areas of the cornea covered by conjunctival tissue (Fig. **18**). In some patients, corneal neovascularization develops at the leading edge of the conjunctival prolapse. The amount of neovascularization depends on how tight or snug of a fitting relationship is in that area.

Revising the fit to either change corneal clearance or minimize adjacent landing zone compression may allow for the conjunctival tissue to recede and allow for improved oxygen permeability at the limbus. It is unknown which patients are predisposed to corneal neovascularization with conjunctival prolapse. Patients with LSCD may be more vulnerable and should be closely monitored.

Adherence of conjunctival prolapse to the cornea creates a pseudopterygium. In most cases after lens removal, the prolapsed tissue recedes. However, in these cases, with digital manipulation, the conjunctival prolapse remains adherent. Adherent prolapse has been observed in patients predisposed to atopy and inflammation.

Problem Solving Conjunctival Prolapse

- Reduce excessive central clearance.
- Reduce excessive limbal clearance.
- Adjust the peripheral curves to align more closely to the sclera.
- Monitor the cornea for neovascularization underneath unresolvable prolapse.
- Consider surgical resection if the patient has neovascularization or is symptomatic for dry eye without the lens.

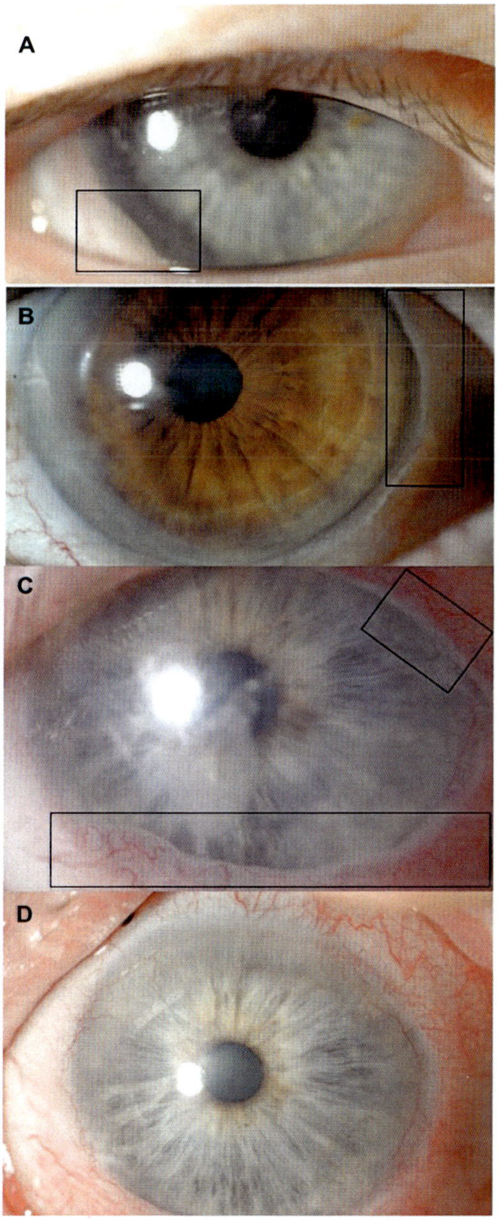

Fig. (18). Different scenarios of mild conjunctival prolapse (A) and (B) – where monitoring is completely adequate. C) Case of pronounced conjunctival prolapse (hooding) in a SJS patient with limbal stem cell deficiency. D) The patient was refit as a precaution for further risk of neovascularization. Images courtesy of Karen Carrasquillo.

Midday Fogging

Fogging of vision while wearing scleral lenses is one of the most frustrating and challenging problems for practitioners and patients alike. When encountered, there may be no apparent cause and no single solution. Even with ideal fitting characteristics and lens care regimen, fogging may still occur. Reservoir fogging occurs when debris accumulates between the lens and cornea after minutes to hours of lens wear [14, 15].

Causes of scleral lens fogging may be increased tear exchange and accumulation of tear debris in the lens reservoir, increased mucin production from rubbing of the conjunctival tissue, accumulation of protein and lipid deposits on the front surface of the lens and corneal edema. Typically fogging is associated with particulate debris either on the front surface or in the post-lens tear reservoir. However, symptoms of fogging are similar despite the cause. Corneal edema should be ruled out immediately. If the patient experiences rainbows around lights, it is critical to evaluate the cornea for MCE. If the patient has corneal edema, removing and reinserting the scleral lens will not resolve the symptoms.

This is frustrating for the patient and practitioner because typically the visual quality is excellent immediately after lens application and then degrades over time. In clinical practice, practitioners have encountered what they think are three types of debris. Many times, these three types can occur in combination. Depending on the type, they are managed differently.

Mucus Debris

Mucin debris is typically, white, opaque, fluffy, small debris that floats in the post-lens fluid reservoir (Fig. **19**). In some extreme cases of larger debris, it can settle in the inferior reservoir with increased wearing time. Two situations are considered when this type of debris is observed. First, it is important to evert the eyelid and evaluate for any signs of giant papillary conjunctivitis (GPC). Even in mild cases, if the palpebral conjunctiva is injected, this may contribute to the debris. To manage this situation, wearing time is reduced, the lens is deep cleaned with a sodium hypochlorite-potassium bromide-based system, and an enzymatic cleaner is introduced to the care regimen. It is also critical to evaluate the fit of the scleral lens. If there is edge lift superiorly confirmed by fluorescein, the lens edge-eyelid interaction may be the source of the papillary reaction, and edge lift is reduced either by tightening the peripheral curves or adding toric peripheries. A second source of this debris may be from a reaction to preservatives in the cleaning or soaking solution. The bulbar conjunctiva may be mildly injected; however, the reaction to the preservative is not significant enough to induce corneal staining. Eliminating the preservative can have a dramatic effect on reducing the particulate white reservoir debris.

Fig. (19). White fluffy particulate debris thought to be mucus in the tear reservoir. Image courtesy of Lynette Johns.

Fogging Associated with Atopic Disease

Some patients have both atopic disease and keratoconus; there is a known association between these conditions [16]. A unique type of fogging under the lens in patients with atopy appears as much-diluted milk (Fig. **20**). Efforts to reduce tear exchange by improving the alignment of the fitting with tighter peripheral curves or toric peripheries are not always effective. In these patients, topical mast cell stabilizers are introduced, and in extreme cases, a topical steroid of low penetrance (commonly referred to as a "soft steroid") is added. As a reminder, careful monitoring of patients using a steroid should include evaluation of intraocular pressure and ruling out infection with contact lenses is strongly advised.

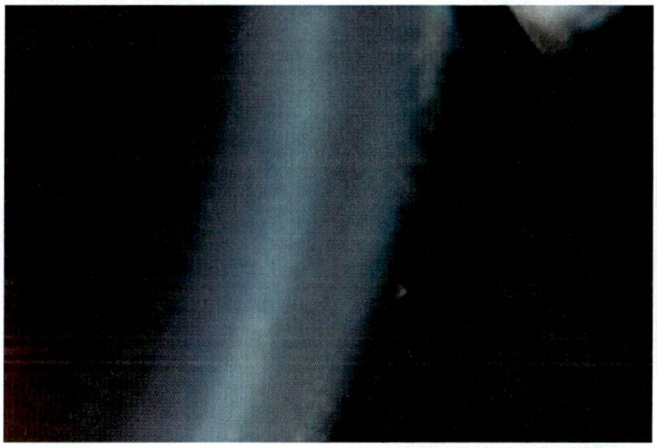

Fig. (20). Milky tear reservoir found often with active atopic disease. Image courtesy of Lynette Johns.

Meibomian Debris

The third and last type of debris observed is an oil droplet/semi-transparent form of debris that looks like olive oil floating on water (Fig. **21**). It can be a yellowish color, and is sometimes refractile in nature. When this type of debris is observed, it is critical to carefully re-examine the eyelids for any signs of meibomian gland dysfunction or blepharitis. Aggressively treating the eyelids can minimize this debris. In addition, reducing excessive tear exchange by manipulating the peripheral curves can be quite helpful in managing this debris.

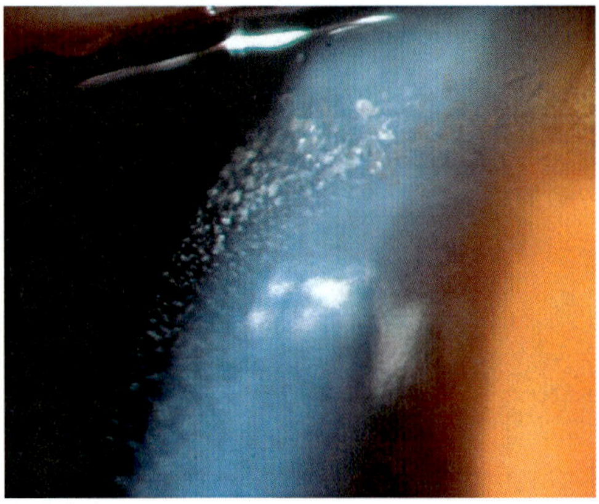

Fig. (21). Semitransparent oil-like debris, thought to be meibomian debris. Image courtesy of Lynette Johns.

Clinically, variations of these three types of debris can occur together. Laboratory analysis of clouding has demonstrated tear film proteins and predominately lipids are found in turbid reservoir samples [17]. Since patients with a variety of conditions are fit with scleral lenses, reservoir samples of these patients with different diagnoses needs to be further evaluated [17].

Managing Reservoir Debris

At times, it is necessary for patients to remove the lens and refresh the filling solution. Patients can use a more viscous solution in the bowl of the lens when applying, reapplying or wearing a scleral lens. Patients are encouraged to experiment with the ideal amount of preservative free solution with a higher viscosity relative to the preservative free saline in order to achieve the optimal result. The scleral lens fit could be modified to reduce excessive tear exchange (Fig. **22**) with the addition of toric peripheries, decreasing the central vault or reducing the diameter.

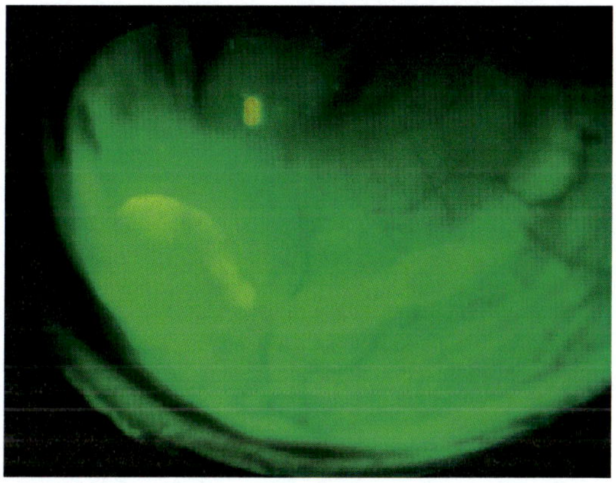

Fig. (22). Excessive tear exchange in an oblique quadrant. Image courtesy of Lynette Johns.

Optimizing the Tear Reservoir

An assessment of the tear reservoir beneath the scleral lens is valuable. Ideally the tear reservoir thickness should be equally distributed. This would be a sign of a stable and centered lens supported by an aligned scleral landing zone. It is preferred to evaluate the tear reservoir after at least six hours of lens wear.

Poor Anterior Surface Wettability

Similar to fogging is the observation of an uneven anterior lens surface tear film that does not improve after blinking (Fig. **23**). Again, this can be created by atypical tear chemistry, oily substances entering the tear film, inconsistent lipid layer (Fig. **24**) solutions that are incompatible with the lens material or solutions not mixing well with the patient's tears.

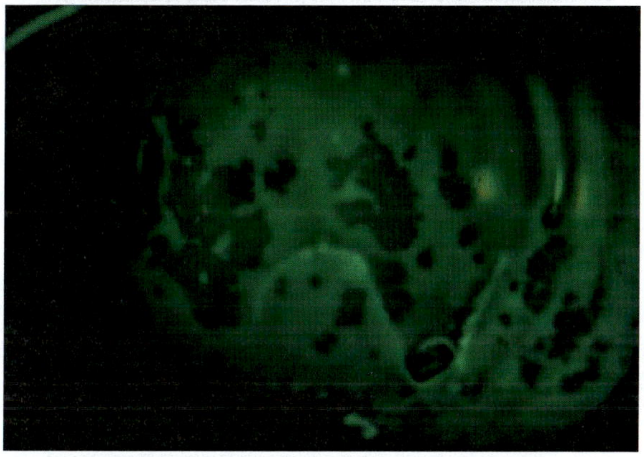

Fig. (23). Poor anterior surface wetting. Image courtesy of Lynette Johns.

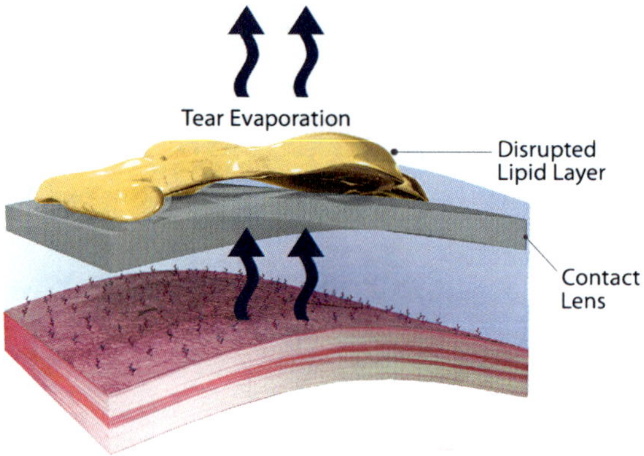

Fig. (24). Disrupted tear layer on surface of contact lens. Image courtesy of Tangible Science.

Front Surface Debris

Fogging may also be due to front surface debris accumulation. Possible causes include tear abnormalities, especially in patients with severe dry eyes from conditions such as: GvHD, Stevens-Johnson syndrome (SJS), severe meibomian gland dysfunction, blepharitis, rosacea and atopic conditions.

It is important to treat ocular surface disease aggressively. Despite changes in lens material and designs, the lens surface may continue to be compromised with resultant poor vision if ocular surface disease is not managed.

There are a variety of options to manage front surface debris depending on the cause. Fogging may also be related to external sources such as oil-based lotions, makeup and soaps. Ask patients about hand soap and change soap to contact lens hand soap or acne treatment hand soap to avoid surface debris. Makeup can contaminate the front surface of the lens causing cloudy vision and decreasing the wettability of the lens. Contamination may occur because a scleral lens is two to five times thicker than other lens designs and can protrude from the front surface of the eye due to the amount of apical clearance under the lens. Remove the lens, clean and reinsert the lens if makeup adheres to the front surface of the lens. It is recommended to apply creams and makeup after scleral lens application. Some cosmetics, creams, and removal products are specifically indicated as contact lens compatible. Similarly, residue left on plungers can compromise the lens surface. Instead of disinfecting the surface of the plunger with alcohol, which may disrupt the hydrophilic surface, soak it in gas permeable contact lens conditioner.

A material with a low wetting angle may improve the wettability of the lens and reduce hydrophobic areas that can attract deposits. Plasma treatment can also help optimize wettability.

Plasma surface treatment is the removal of hydrophobic and hydrophilic elements from the surface of a lens through electrostatic discharge. Plasma treatment to the surface is used to remove any remaining residue from the lens after the manufacturing process, increase comfort and decrease lens awareness by creating a very clean lens, maximize wettability of the lens and provide possible resistance of protein and bacterial deposits and create crisp vision through the lens. Avoid plasma treatment on crazed lenses (Fig. **25**).

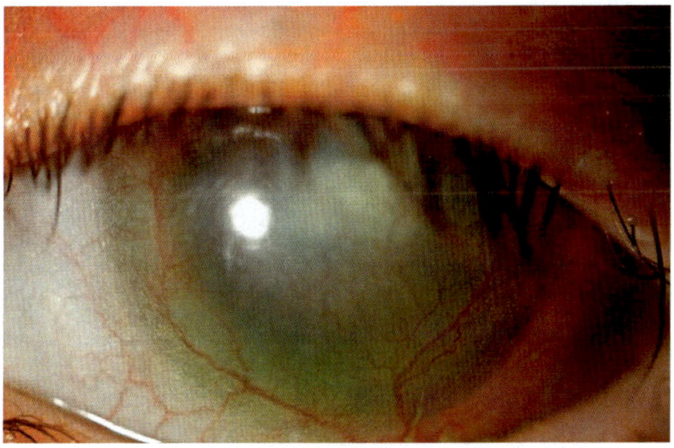

Fig. (25). Example of an old crazed lens. Plasma treatment is contraindicated on this lens. Image courtesy of Lynette Johns.

Consider Hydra-PEG, a biocompatible polymer mixture that is covalently (permanently) bound to lens surface. Hydra-PEG improves wettability, minimizes protein and lipid deposition and increases lubricity to reduce friction between the eyelid and lens (Fig. **26**).

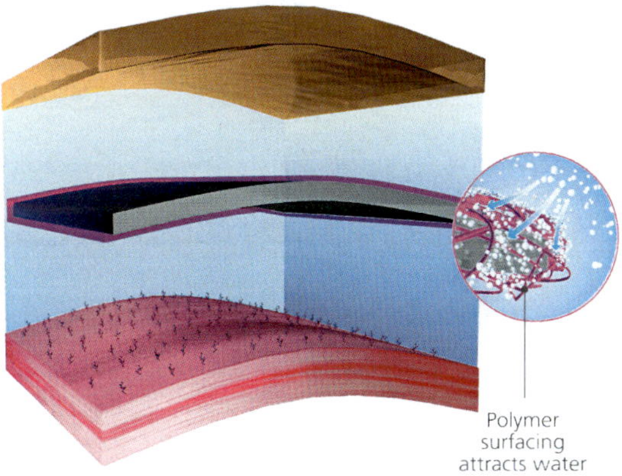

Fig. (26). Hydra-PEG surface encapsulates lens to create a mucin-like surface. Image courtesy of Tangible Science.

At times, it is necessary for patients to remove and clean the front surface of the lens to eliminate deposits. To eliminate non-wetting or deposits, it is beneficial to manually polish the surface with an approved gas permeable polishing solution or an alcohol based daily cleaner, then rinse and rub the surface with soft multipurpose contact lens solution. Gas permeable laboratory lens cleaner for in-office use only is used to remove pitch, wax and other solvents used in the manufacturing process. This cleaner also removes lipids, body oils, and other contaminants. Switching to a peroxide based disinfection solution is also helpful to eradicate surface deposits. An additional cleaner such as Menicon Progent may be used one to two times per week. This is a two-component cleaner with sodium hypochlorite and potassium bromide that removes deposits, bacteria, fungus, molds and yeasts.

On-eye surface cleaning using a saline moistened cotton swab or eye shadow applicator or wet DMV applicator can be used to remove surface debris (Fig. **27**). In addition, increased lubrication over the lens throughout the day may be beneficial.

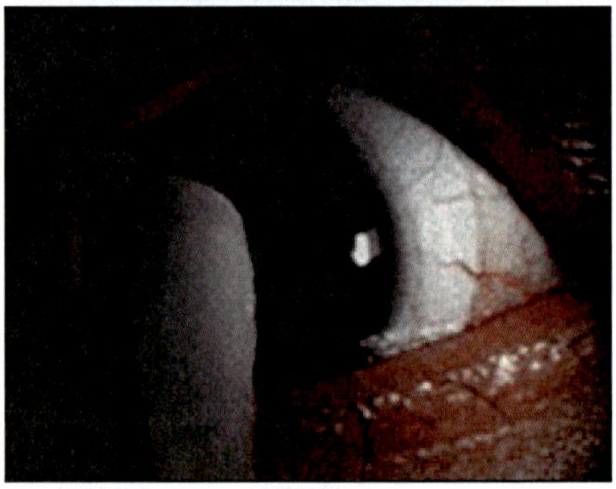

Fig. (27). On-eye surface cleaning with moistened cotton swab. Image courtesy of Chistine Snidt.

Alternative Strategies

Aggressive treatment and management of the eyelids including treatment of meibomian gland dysfunction with mechanical, topical, and oral methods has been beneficial. Recommending dietary changes such as taking omega-3 supplements and reducing fried and fatty food can be helpful.

Other management strategies for reservoir debris, front surface debris and fogging from corneal edema can include mid-day breaks from scleral lens wear. Although not popular with patients, this option can lessen the effect of mid-day fogging from all sources. Patients should be cautioned against excessive manipulation as it may induce an unintentional mucous fishing syndrome response.

Some practitioners prescribe inhalation saline, which is also preservative-free and comes in a unit-dose package. This solution is non-buffered and the pH often tends to be acidic and varies ampule to ampule. This may cause stinging and/or superficial keratitis. Patients fit with scleral lenses for ocular surface disease should continue preservative free topical lubrication.

Punctal plugs are a useful treatment option for dry eye disease. In some cases where there is excessive reservoir debris, removing the punctal plug is beneficial. The patient requires additional topical lubrication in lieu of the punctal plugs. Conversely, in patients with front surface debris, punctal occlusion can increase residual lubrication of the front surface.

Problem Solving Midday Fogging

- Rule out corneal edema.
  - No rainbows around lights.
  - No microcysts in epithelium.
- Determine if fogging is in post-lens tear reservoir *versus* front surface.

Mucus Debris

- Reduce scleral lens wearing time.
- Clean the lens with sodium hypochlorite and potassium bromide cleaner.
- Use enzymatic cleaner.
- Remove lens and refresh filling solution, then reapply lens.
- Evaluate the fitting relationship of lens and reduce excessive edge lift.
- Consider toric peripheries if edge lift is meridional.
- Evaluate superior tarsus for giant papillary conjunctivitis.
- Eliminate preservatives from care system.

Atopic Debris

- Remove lens and refresh filling solution, then reapply lens.
- Evaluate the fitting relationship of lens and reduce excessive edge lift.
- Consider toric peripheries if edge lift is meridional.
- Consider topical mast cell stabilizers or "soft" steroid.

Meibomian Debris

- Remove lens and refresh filling solution, then reapply lens.
- Evaluate the fitting relationship of lens and reduce excessive edge lift.
- Consider toric peripheries if edge lift is meridional.
- Evaluate the eyelids for meibomitis and blepharitis. Treat underlying eyelid disease if present.

General Management of Reservoir Debris

- Remove lens and refresh filling solution, then reapply lens.
- Evaluate the fitting relationship of lens and reduce excessive edge lift and/or tear exchange.
- Consider toric peripheries if edge lift/tear exchange is meridional.
- Reduce central clearance.
- Reduce the overall diameter of the lens.
- Use a preservative free viscous artificial tear in the reservoir with preservative free saline.
- Ensure that there is an even relationship of the clearance with the corneal topographical profile. For example using a reverse geometry lens on a cornea with a plateau profile.

Poor Anterior Surface Wettability/Front Surface Debris
• Remove lens and clean surfaces with an alcohol based cleaner or laboratory cleaner.
• Consider plasma treatment or retreatment of lens.
• Treat ocular surface disease aggressively.
• Ask patients about hand soaps, lotions, makeup and eye creams.
• Change hand soap to either contact lens hand soap or acne treatment hand soap without lotion additives.
• Explain to patients to apply makeup, facial moisturizers after lenses are applied.
• Remove and clean the surfaces of the lenses if makeup or other products adhere to the surface of the lens.
• Disinfect the application and removal devices (plungers) in gas permeable contact lens solutions.
• Consider a material with a low wetting angle.
• Consider Hydra-PEG treatment where available.
• Manually polish the surface with an approved gas permeable polishing solution.
• Moisten a cotton swab or removal plunger with solution and clean the surface on-eye.
• Consider the pH of filling solution by either using solutions with buffers or without.
• Schedule midday breaks of lens wear.
• Avoid multiple mechanical manipulations (applications/removals) because it may stimulate mucus production.
• Consider removing the punctal plug in the presence of excessive chamber debris.
• Consider punctal occlusion in the presence of front surface debris.

Poor Vision

Many different aspects can contribute to poor visual acuity. As previously discussed, front surface debris can reduce visual acuity due to lipids/ proteins/mucins or make-up and moisturizers resulting in a non-wetting scleral lens surface. Tear debris under the scleral lens may potentially compromise vision.

Correction of refractive error with rigid scleral lenses is usually excellent. Practitioners are familiar with the visual advantages using rigid optics to correct refractive astigmatism, particularly corneal astigmatism. Correction of astigmatism and other corneal irregularities with a rigid lens is accomplished due to a combination of factors. First, the lens creates a smooth front surface to refract light evenly. The tear lens is formed between the back surface of the scleral lens and the cornea. This tear layer is the critical component of rigid optics that corrects regular astigmatism, irregular astigmatism, corneal surface irregularities and other corneal distortions.

In many cases, lenses that have a spherical front surface and a spherical back surface will provide excellent visual acuity. Often a spherical over-refraction will provide very good acuity. Poor visual acuity can be caused by uncorrected refractive error. A pinhole test can provide insight to the patient's potential optimal visual acuity. If the patient does not achieve optimal visual acuity with a spherical over-refraction, it may be due to residual astigmatism. In this case, perform a careful sphero-cylindrical over-refraction. If there is an improvement in one or more lines of acuity or ≥ 0.75D, include the astigmatic correction in the lens. Ensure that the lens is stabilized with dual thin zones, prism ballast, double slab off or toric peripheries to minimize rotation.

Visual acuity can be compromised due to poor optics, which includes flexure or warpage of a scleral lens. Scleral lens flexure can cause a decrease in the patient's potential visual acuity with a spherical over-refraction. Visual acuity can be corrected with a sphero-cylindrical over-refraction. Flexure can easily be differentiated from residual astigmatism by performing over-keratometry or over-topography measurements. Any finding of cylinder suggests flexure as the scleral lens anterior curve is often spherical. To resolve flexure, either increase lens center thickness and/or add toric peripheries. After the lens is removed, the lens will resume its normal shape.

Scleral lens warpage can decrease visual acuity. As opposed to a lens with flexure, the optics of a warped lens will demonstrate atypical results. After removing a lens demonstrating flexure, the optical measurements of that lens are spherical. However, a warped lens can demonstrate atypical cylinder with differing radii of curvature when measured with a radiuscope. If in doubt, send the lens back to lab for measurement and analysis. In the office, refract the patient with a non-warped diagnostic lens. If visual acuity is improved with the diagnostic lens, the patient's lens is likely warped.

When scleral lens flexure and warpage have been ruled out, and visual acuity does not meet pinhole acuity, higher order aberrations (HOA) are the likely cause. Currently, there are aspheric options to improve visual acuity. Custom HOA correction is limited in availability at this time.

Problem Solving Poor Vision

- Double check the over-refraction and correct appropriately.
- Correct astigmatism if cylinder ≥ 0.75D.
- If there is no improvement in pinhole acuity or with over-refraction, rule out ocular pathology.
- Ensure that the lenses are worn on the appropriate eyes.
- Evaluate the lens for front surface or reservoir debris (see above).
- Rule out corneal edema.
  - No rainbows around lights.
  - No microcysts in epithelium.
- Perform over-topography/over-keratometry to rule out lens flexure. If cylinder is detected on a spherical lens, either increase center thickness of the lens or add toric peripheral curves.
- Check for warpage by comparing power and base curve to ordered parameters.
- If pinhole acuity cannot be achieved, add aspheric optics, or attempt to improve vision with different base curve and over-refraction combinations.
- Employ higher order aberration correction (limited availability).

Asthenopia and Visual Adaptation

Patients may have complaints of asthenopia for a variety of reasons. First, ensure that an over-refraction is not required. In many cases patients are being fit with scleral lenses because of poor vision with unaided or habitual correction; it may take time to adapt to their new optimized visual acuity. Patients who have suffered from poor visual acuity for a long time may have trouble adapting to regaining binocularity. If only one eye is fit with a scleral lens, a patient may struggle with asthenopia and/or adaptation. Scleral lenses are known to decenter infero-temporally, thus creating a prismatic effect. In these cases, fitting the other eye with a scleral lens will improve or resolve this problem, even if the opposite eye does not require a scleral lens. Alternatively, improving scleral lens centration, often achieved with the use of toric peripheral curves, will help minimize prismatic effect.

Spectacle blur theoretically should not occur with a well-fit scleral lens. However, one study demonstrated 1.10D of central corneal flattening [18]. Another study showed 0.08mm of peripheral corneal flattening [19]. Mechanical limbal bearing can induce spectacle blur and should be ruled out. If the sagittal depth is too deep, and the limbus is compressed, corneal edema can occur. Decreasing the sagittal depth may resolve corneal edema, thus improving vision.

With a history of corneal gas permeable lens wear, patients may undergo corneal unmolding with a scleral lens (Fig. **28**). Spectacle blur has been observed clinically in some post radial keratotomy patients, although this finding is anecdotal and needs to be investigated more thoroughly. Since most patients are disabled without scleral lenses, they infrequently require spectacles and remove their lenses before bedtime. A practitioner should rule out mechanical effects of the lens bearing on the cornea and corneal edema as discussed previously. Corneal edema will decrease the visual acuity and this can be due to the sagittal depth being too great, and lower sagittal depth is required.

Anterior segment pathology will also cause a decrease in the patient's visual acuity, whether it is a corneal scar, striae, or epithelial disruption. Corneal edema, corneal dystrophy or cataracts could also compromise the patient's vision. Posterior segment pathology will also hinder the potential visual outcome that a patient can achieve. Examples are glaucoma, vitreous degeneration, retinal or optic nerve diseases.

Halos around lights can be caused by a lack of oxygen to the cornea, causing corneal edema. An increase in Dk/t will improve the health of the cornea. Sleeping/napping with scleral lenses may induce edema and cause halos. A small optical zone on scleral lenses can cause halos as well.

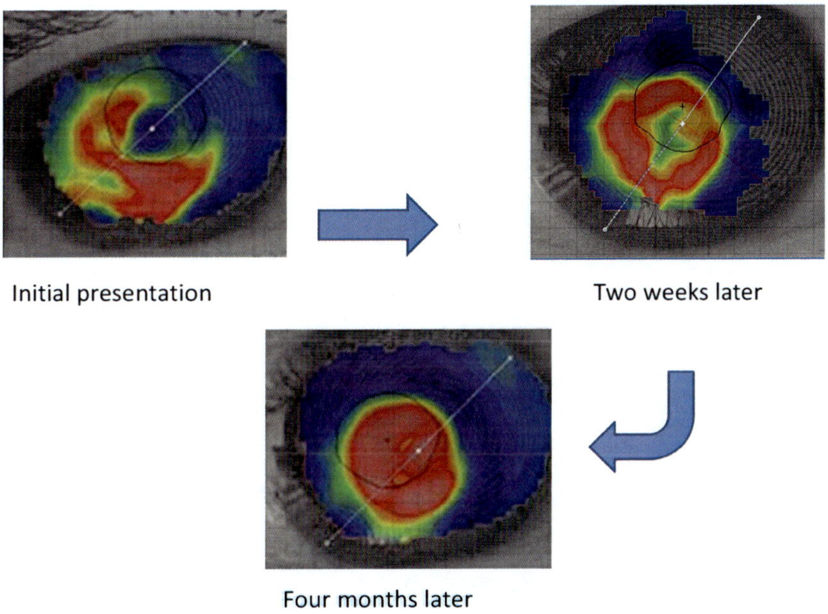

Fig. (28). Corneal unmolding of a patient with keratoconus who was wearing a flat fitting corneal GP lens. Images courtesy of Lynette Johns.

Steep peripheral curves can create a seal-off effect, potentially leading to edema and can cause poor visual acuities. In these cases, flatter peripheral curves are required to the scleral lens design. Debris trapped under the scleral lenses can also reduce visual acuity.

Problem Solving Asthenopia and Visual Adaptation

- Over-refract to optimize visual acuity.
- Ensure adequate time for visual adaptation.
- Consider fitting both eyes with a scleral lens if there is decentration and induced prism.
- Monitor topography of the patient to determine if unmolding has occurred.
- Rule out corneal touch or bearing.
- Rule out ocular pathology.
- Increase optic zone if patient observes halos.
- Rule out corneal edema if patient complains of halos by making sure that their complaint is halos and not rainbows.
- Consider changing the base curve of the lens to improve vision.
- Steepen or flatten the base curve to create a plano power if there is induced prism from lens decentration.
- Add toric peripheral curves if the lens is decentered and is inducing prism.

Comfort

As contact lens practitioners are acutely aware, comfort is very subjective. Although a well-fit scleral lens is usually quite comfortable, there will inevitably be patients who complain of lens awareness or frank discomfort. There are numerous lens fitting parameters to maximize comfort during scleral lens wear. While obtaining a thorough history, patient subjective complaints can provide clues to necessary parameter changes to achieve comfortable wear.

In general, scleral lenses are very comfortable. Either during the fitting process or after lenses have been worn for some time, lens awareness or discomfort can develop. Symptoms of discomfort immediately after lens application differ from those at the end of the day after hours of wear.

Lens awareness may be caused by an application bubble under the lens during the fitting process. Symptoms will increase with time and the patient will report irritation. To alleviate symptoms, remove and reapply the lens without a bubble.

During the fitting process, the most common reason for discomfort with scleral lenses is excessive edge lift/standoff. The patient will report that the lens feels tight, when it fact it is too loose. Patients can easily locate the area and describe the area of discomfort. Edge lift can be confirmed with the addition of fluorescein. Comfort can usually be improved by reducing the edge lift, in other words, a steeper peripheral curve.

However, if the edge profile is too tight, scleral compression or impingement may occur. This will lead to discomfort with scleral lenses after hours of wear. Symptoms include eye ache, discomfort, tightness or sensation of a bruise. Sometimes patients complain that their eyes are tired. To alleviate scleral compression or impingement, increase the edge lift, flatten peripheries, or increase the overall diameter to create a larger landing zone.

Irritation may occur after hours of wear due to limbal or corneal contact. It will be particularly pronounced after lens removal due to epithelial erosions from lens adherence. The patient may report a foreign body sensation and excessive tearing in extreme cases after the lens is removed. When evaluating the lens, verify adequate central and limbal clearance. Ensure that there is no touch or bearing. If central or limbal clearance is difficult to visualize, anterior segment OCT imaging is quite helpful if available.

To alleviate central bearing, increase the overall sagittal depth or steepen the base curve in order to increase apical clearance. To eliminate limbal bearing, increase the limbal zone depth, increase the overall sagittal depth of the lens, increase the optical zone and/or increase the overall lens diameter.

Bubbles trapped in the lens fluid reservoir may also contribute to discomfort. There are a variety of sources where bubbles occur. Bubbles may be caused by incorrect application techniques or if an aerated solution is used to fill the bowl of the scleral lens. Misalignment of the scleral landing zone may result in bubbles. For example, edge lift in one or more quadrants or a lens with excessive movement may allow bubbles to enter.

Peripheral bubbles in a fenestrated scleral lens are acceptable, especially if they are mobile. However, in a fluid-ventilated (semi-sealed) scleral lens, bubbles may contribute to discomfort, desiccation and potential dellen formation. Practitioners can differentiate the source of the bubble from application errors or the need to revise the fit.

If a bubble is observed immediately after application, the source is likely a handling issue. However, if a bubble appears subsequently, the practitioner should evaluate scleral landing zone alignment. The path of the bubble can be determined by excessive fluorescein exchange.

Problem Solving Comfort

- Take a detailed history of symptoms.
- Rule out bubbles in the post lens tear reservoir.
- Evaluate the scleral lens periphery with fluorescein. Fluorescein will highlight edge lift.
- Steepen the scleral lens periphery if there is edge lift is causing the symptom.
- If symptoms worsen or increase with wearing time, evaluate the scleral landing zone for compression and impingement.
- If compression or impingement are present, flatten the scleral lens periphery.
- Add toric peripheral curves if scleral landing zone findings are meridional.
- Change the lens diameter to improve symptoms. This may require trial and error.
- Rule out corneal or limbal contact/bearing. Increase sagittal depth, limbal depth, or diameter if there is corneal or limbal contact.
- If bubbles enter after the lens was applied bubble-free, suspect excessive edge lift and tear exchange. Add toric peripheral curves to improve scleral lens alignment.
- If the lens is fenestrated, make sure that the bubbles are mobile to prevent long term desiccation. Change the base curve and peripheral corneal curves to reduce bubble size.

Handling Complications

Complications are not limited to disease process or the scleral lens fit. Sometimes complications can occur with improper handling of the lenses. Proper education and reinforcement of application and removal is important at each visit.

Application

Patients should be closely supervised during the application and removal training process. It is important that they center the scleral lens directly over the cornea. If a patient is misaligned, the rigid edge of the scleral lens can cause harm to the cornea (Fig. **29**). In particular, patients with neurotrophic corneas require close supervision since they cannot feel the lens when it is applied to their eyes (Fig. **30**).

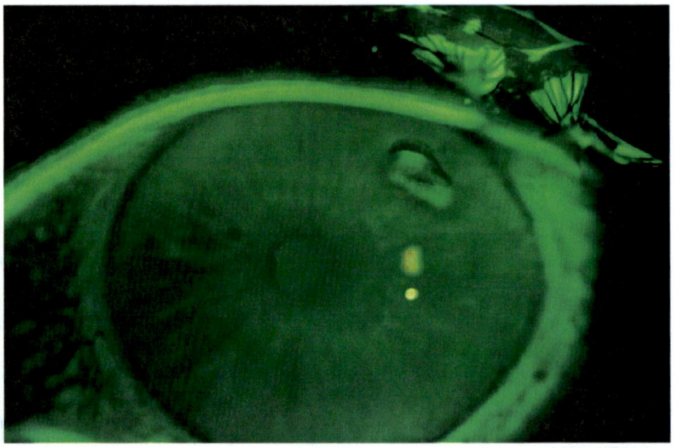

Fig. (29). Application error where the patient attempted to apply the lens while the eye rolled upwards during Bell's phenomenon. The edge dug into the epithelium rolling it, but not abrading it. Image courtesy of Lynette Johns I-Site e-newsletter (January, 2013).

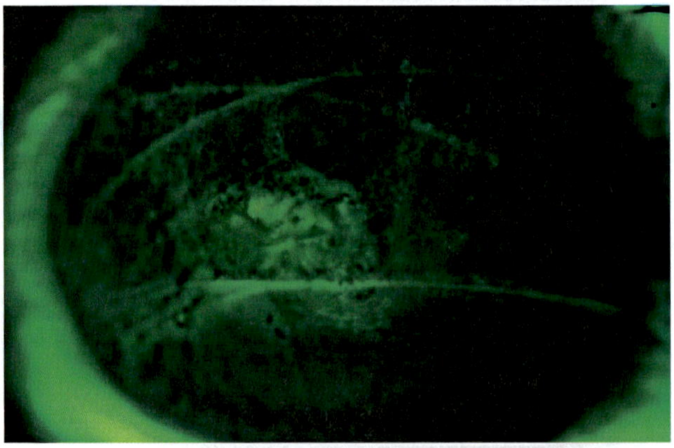

Fig. (30). Multiple improperly aligned application attempts on a neurotrophic cornea. Image courtesy of Lynette Johns I-Site e-newsletter (January, 2013).

Air bubbles should be avoided with scleral lens wear. A bubble may form due to insufficient filling or flawed application technique (Fig. **31**). In addition, a bubble may exist with excessive scleral lens vault, movement and an insufficient scleral landing zone. Air bubbles may cause discomfort, blurriness and dry eye. Corneal tissue can become desiccated beneath a bubble relatively quickly. If a bubble is present, it is recommended to remove and reapply the lens.

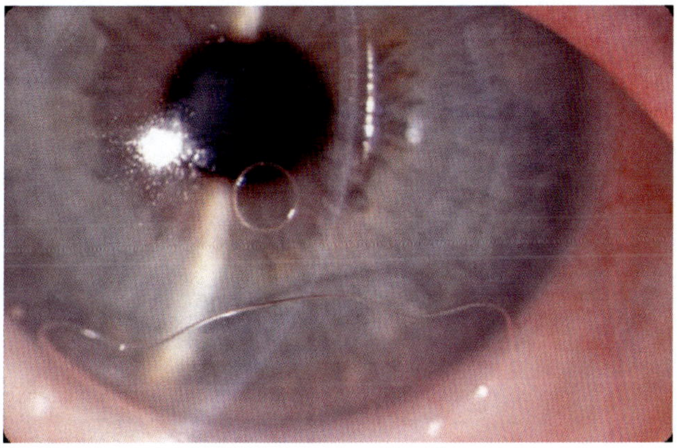

Fig. (31). Small and large application bubbles trapped in the post lens tear reservoir. Image courtesy of Muriel Schornack.

Removal

There are numerous plungers available to aid with insertion and removal of scleral lenses. The most common problem is applying the lens removal device too close to the center of the lens creating too much surface tension force to pull the lens straight out. Even a well fit scleral lens that demonstrates tear exchange (proving that the fit is not sealed off) can exhibit extreme suction on the eye if the plunger is placed in the center during removal (Fig. **32**). Instruction on peripheral placement and angled removal usually makes this an easy process to master. Proper instruction and education is necessary for successful removal. In patients with corneal transplants, it is crucial to observe the patients with removal and reinforce proper technique to prevent graft dehiscence.

A drop of preservative free saline or artificial tears is instilled in the eye to loosen the lens prior to removal. With the manual two-finger method, the lens is removed by combining pressure into the globe with the eyelid and prying the edge with the fingertip.

One of the most common reasons for an after-hours emergency phone call is that the patient "cannot get the lens out." There may be a variety of reasons that this occurs. The first is that the lens is already out of the eye and the patient continues to use the plunger directly on the ocular tissue. At each follow-up visit, it is helpful to ensure that the dots are dark enough for the patient to see if the lens manufacturer utilizes dots. The dots allow for confirmation of the lens in the eye, in case the patient is having difficulty with removal. Sometimes a material can be ordered with a handling tint to aid in identification of the lens on the eye. Another reason for the emergency call is if the patient is having difficulty with removal and the lens is confirmed to be in the eye, the lens may have suctioned or sealed itself to the eye. When a patient makes multiple removal attempts, the eye becomes hyperemic and swollen. As a result, the fit becomes tighter. The patient should take a break from all removal attempts and relax. Often, they are panicked when this occurs. Applying cool compresses can reduce the swelling and aid in removal.

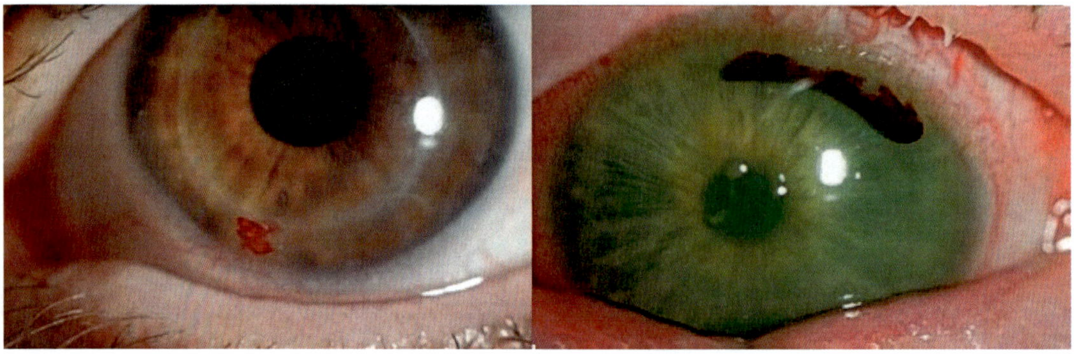

Fig. (32). Examples of subepithelial hemorrhages from improper removal techniques. Images courtesy of Lynette Johns I-Site e-newsletter (August, 2013).

Problem Solving Handling Complications

- Closely supervise all patients with application and removal.
- Provide a handout with instructions for patients to review at home.
- Ask if there are any handling problems at each visit.

Application

- Ensure proper centration of the lens during training for smooth application.
- Chill filling solution in the refrigerator if the patient requires help with centration. The cool sensation provides a cue for lens centration.
- Use application aids like the See Green Lens Inserter by Dalsey Adaptives (http://dalseyadaptives.net/store/), EZi Scleral Lens Applicator by Q-Case Inc. (http://ezibyqcase.com/), or a #8 O ring that is available at any hardware store.
- If the patient has a tremor, prop their application arm on a phonebook to raise their hand and steady their arm.
- Use viscous preservative free solution to help prevent liquid spilling during application that can cause a bubble.
- Evaluate the lens immediately after application to rule out a bubble. If a bubble is present, the lens should be removed and reapplied.
- If a lens is fenestrated, educate the patient that a bubble will likely be present.

Removal

- Educate the patient that the removal plunger should never be applied to the center of a semi-sealed scleral lens for removal.
- If, and only if the lens is fenestrated, then the plunger can be applied to the center of the lens for easy removal.
- Reinforce and supervise proper removal technique of every patient with a corneal transplant.
- Differentiate the lenses with either dots or handling tints to aid the patient in identifying whether the lens is on the eye.
- If the eye is injected and swollen, take a break from attempting to remove the lens. Cold compresses can be helpful in reducing swelling.

SUMMARY

Although not every problem encountered during scleral lens fitting can be solved, most complications can be resolved with a combination of lens modifications and lens care routines. Practitioners must continuously educate themselves on potential complications from scleral lens wear and proactively address atypical findings prior to initiating the fit or early in the scleral lens fitting process. When problems occur despite preventative measures, specific scleral lens design modifications will likely minimize or eliminate the issue.

If struggling with design modifications, manufacturer consultants are valuable to assist with lens design modification and troubleshooting. With experience, practitioners will be able to identify potential complication sources earlier in the fitting process. Even without experience, most complications can be resolved with lens design changes and time. Even when complications arise, most do not necessitate discontinuation of lens wear during the troubleshooting process.

In addition, new designs, materials, solutions and fitting techniques are always evolving. Continual education is necessary by following the literature, attending lectures, webinars or workshops to stay up to date with the latest developments to keep improving problem-solving skills.

Proper scleral lens care, technique and handling are essential. Practitioners must have a continual dialogue with the patient that reinforces proper scleral lens cleaning, storing, rinsing and handling and maintenance at each visit. Open-ended questions will provide insight to ensure scleral lens success.

Proper understanding of the disease process and its limitations are important to avoid scleral lens induced complications. Appropriate follow up and adequate collaboration with specialists are also essential to ensure successful treatment with scleral lenses. From the care and handling aspect, as well as disease management strategies, patient communication and involvement can improve compliance and favorable outcomes.

CONFLICT OF INTEREST

The authors declare no conflict of interest, financial or otherwise.

ACKNOWLEDGEMENTS

None Declared.

REFERENCES

[1] Dohlman CH. The function of the corneal epithelium in health and disease. The Jonas S. Friedenwald Memorial Lecture. Invest Ophthalmol 1971; 10(6): 383-407.
[PMID: 4325305]

[2] Waring GO, Bourne WM, Edelhauser HF, *et al.* (1082) The corneal endothelium: Normal and pathologic structure and function. Ophthalmology (89): 531.

[3] Lim P, Ridges R, Jacobs DS, Rosenthal P. Treatment of persistent corneal epithelial defect with overnight wear of a prosthetic device for the ocular surface. Am J Ophthalmol 2013; 156(6): 1095-101.
[http://dx.doi.org/10.1016/j.ajo.2013.06.006] [PMID: 24075432]

[4] Rosenthal P, Cotter JM, Baum J. Treatment of persistent corneal epithelial defect with extended wear of a fluid-ventilated gas-permeable scleral contact lens. Am J Ophthalmol 2000; 130(1): 33-41.
[http://dx.doi.org/10.1016/S0002-9394(00)00379-2] [PMID: 11004257]

[5] Morrison S, Walker M, Caroline P, *et al.* Tear exchange beneath scleral lenses. Global Specialty Lens Symposium.

[6] Lim P, Fuchsluger TA, Jurkunas UV. Limbal stem cell deficiency and corneal neovascularization. Semin Ophthalmol 2009; 24(3): 139-48.
[http://dx.doi.org/10.1080/08820530902801478] [PMID: 19437349]

[7] Chan CC, Holland EJ. Severe limbal stem cell deficiency from contact lens wear: patient clinical features. Am J Ophthalmol 2013; 155(3): 544-549.e2.
[http://dx.doi.org/10.1016/j.ajo.2012.09.013] [PMID: 23218703]

[8] Shovlin JP. LCSD-It may be the lenses. Review of Cornea and Contact Lenses 2014.

[9] Kim BY, Riaz KM, Bakhtiari P, *et al.* Medically reversible limbal stem cell disease: clinical features and management strategies. Ophthalmology 2014; 121(10): 2053-8.
[http://dx.doi.org/10.1016/j.ophtha.2014.04.025] [PMID: 24908203]

[10] Schornack M. Toric haptics in scleral lens design: a case series. Poster Present Glob Spec Lens Symp. Las Vegas, Nevada. 2013.

[11] Visser ES, Visser R, Van Lier HJ. Advantages of toric scleral lenses. Optom Vis Sci 2006; 83(4): 233-6.
[http://dx.doi.org/10.1097/01.opx.0000214297.38421.15] [PMID: 16614579]

[12] Visser ES, Van der Linden BJ, Otten HM, Van der Lelij A, Visser R. Medical applications and outcomes of bitangential scleral lenses. Optom Vis Sci 2013; 90(10): 1078-85.
[http://dx.doi.org/10.1097/OPX.0000000000000018] [PMID: 23974663]

[13] Maumenee AE. Keratinization of the conjunctiva. Trans Am Ophthalmol Soc 1979; 77: 133-43.
[PMID: 94716]

[14] McKinney A, Miller W, Leach N, Polizzi C, van der Worp E, Bergmanson J. The cause of midday visual fogging in scleral gas permeable lens wearers. Invest Ophthalmol Vis Sci 2013. ARVO E-Abstract 5483

[15] Walker M. Scleral lenses, clearing the fog. ISITE Online J 2014.

[16] Harrison RJ, Klouda PT, Easty DL, Manku M, Charles J, Stewart CM. Association between keratoconus and atopy. Br J Ophthalmol 1989; 73(10): 816-22.
[http://dx.doi.org/10.1136/bjo.73.10.816] [PMID: 2818991]

[17] Walker M, Morrison S, Caroline P, *et al.* Laboratory analysis of scleral lens tear reservoir. Poster GSLS 2014.

[18] Soeters N, Visser ES, Imhof SM, Tahzib NG. Scleral lens influence on corneal curvature and pachymetry in keratoconus patients. Cont Lens Anterior Eye 2015; 38(4): 294-7.

[http://dx.doi.org/10.1016/j.clae.2015.03.006] [PMID: 25865408]

[19] Vincent SJ, Alonso-Caneiro D, Collins MJ. Miniscleral lens wear influences corneal curvature and optics. Ophthalmic Physiol Opt 2016; 36(2): 100-11.
[http://dx.doi.org/10.1111/opo.12270] [PMID: 26690831]

CHAPTER 13

Scleral Lens Handling

Melissa Barnett[1,*] and **Mindy Toabe**[2]

[1] *University of California, Davis, Sacramento, CA, USA*

[2] *MetroHealth Medical Center, Cleveland, OH, USA*

Abstract: Scleral lenses have become more of a mainstream option for the treatment of distorted corneas and ocular surface disease. Well-fitted scleral lenses vault the cornea and are supported entirely by the sclera. They create a tear layer reservoir which helps neutralize an irregular, damaged or diseased cornea while creating constant lubrication and necessary oxygen supply. They provide optics comparable to corneal gas permeable lenses, with equivalent comfort to soft contact lenses. Like any type of medical treatment, there has to be first and foremost an understanding of the disease process and pathology being treated when fitting scleral lenses. Without true understanding of the disease process and its limitations, practitioners may inadvertently induce complications. A comprehensive understanding of the intended scleral lens design and fitting parameters is paramount. Equally important is establishing a close relationship with the lens manufacturing laboratory and their consultants. This is particularly critical when troubleshooting challenging cases. Establishing appropriate scleral lens follow up and close communication with the referring corneal or medical specialist is very important. Proper understanding of the disease process and its limitations are important to avoid scleral lens induced complications. Appropriate follow up and adequate collaboration with specialists is also essential to ensure successful treatment with scleral lenses. From the care and handling aspect as well as disease management strategies, patient communication and involvement can improve compliance and favorable outcomes.

Keywords: Application, Cleaning, Disinfection, Enzymatic cleaner, Hand washing, Handling, Hydrogen peroxide, Inhalation, Lens replacement, Microbial keratitis, Multipurpose, Patient education, Plasma treatment, Plunger, Preservative free, Removal, Rinse, Solutions, Storage case, Surfactant.

INTRODUCTION

More and more practitioners are realizing the benefits that scleral lenses have to offer including protection of the ocular surface and visual acuity correction. By

* **Corresponding author Melissa Barnett:** University of California, Davis, Sacramento, CA, USA; Tel: 916-734-4641; Fax: 916-565-1640; E-mail: drbarnett@ucdavis.edu

definition, a scleral lens is one whose bearing is supported entirely by the sclera and does not contact the cornea [1]. With a fluid-filled reservoir and choice of gas permeable materials, these lenses allow the cornea to be submerged in an artificial pool of non-preserved saline solution (Fig. **1**).

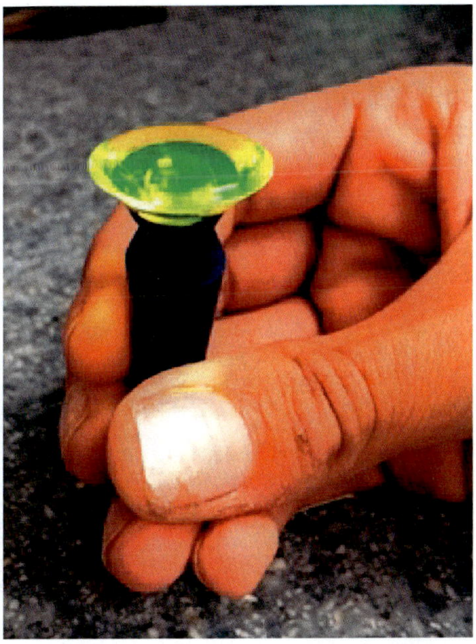

Fig. (1). Scleral lens prior to insertion on large plunger filled with saline and sodium fluorescein.

Scleral lenses differ from corneal gas permeable (corneal GP) designs primarily in size, thickness and weight. A scleral lens can be as large as 24.00 mm and can weigh about 10-15 mg with an approximate center thickness between 0.25-0.50 mm. The center thickness can increase up to 0.30 mm or more in aphakic designs. Lens material is similar to a corneal GP lens and is made with a large polymer button in a hyper Dk material including, but not limited to, the following arranged in order of increasing Dk:

- Boston Equalens II (Bausch & Lomb, Dk 85)
- Tyro 97 (Lagado, Dk 97)
- Boston XO (Bausch & Lomb, Dk 100)
- Optimum Extra (Contamac, Dk 100)
- Paragon HDS 100 (Paragon, Dk 101)
- Optimum Extreme (Contamac, Dk 125)
- Boston XO2 (Bausch & Lomb, Dk 141)
- Menicon Z (Menicon, Dk 163)

Replacement of a scleral lens is similar to a corneal lens made of the same material. These materials will scratch over time and generally will need to be replaced every one to two years, or as needed.

Scleral lenses assist in the management of anterior segment disorders. A large diameter lens can vault irregular surfaces such as keratoconus, pellucid marginal degeneration, penetrating keratoplasty, ocular trauma and post-refractive surgery complications. In addition, scleral lenses are useful in diseases that affect the ocular ecosystem such as severe dry eye due to Sjögren's disease, Graft *versus* Host disease (GvHD), Stevens Johnson syndrome (SJS), chemical burns, and neurotrophic keratopathy. Large diameter scleral lens designs are handled and cared for differently than corneal GP lenses or soft contact lenses. Scleral lenses offer patients many advantages but they come with a unique set of problems, including:

Minimal Tear Exchange

The application solution stays in contact with the cornea throughout the duration of wear and therefore should be preservative free. Unlike corneal lenses that rest on the cornea and tear film and are continually replenished with fresh tears, scleral lenses have a large fluid reservoir in a semi-sealed state. Most scleral lenses are designed as a fluid-ventilated system with minimal tear exchange [2].

Tear Reservoir

The tear reservoir between the cornea and the posterior lens surface consists of protein, lipids and mucin that can accumulate over time causing foggy vision. In 2016, Walker *et al.* demonstrated that this opaque film consists of a high concentration of lipids [3]. The researchers proposed that minimal limbal clearance may enhance lipids, leading to foggy vision. Since patients with a variety of conditions are fit with scleral lenses, reservoir samples of these patients with different diagnoses need to be further evaluated [3].

Air Bubbles

Air bubbles should be avoided with scleral lens wear. A bubble may form due to insufficient filling or flawed application technique. In addition, a bubble may exist with excessive scleral lens vault, movement and an insufficient scleral landing zone. Air bubbles may cause discomfort, blurriness and corneal staining. Corneal tissue can become desiccated beneath a bubble relatively quickly.

Insertion Challenges

The large size of the lens leads to difficulty with application and the need for special insertion devices.

Wetting Issues

Wetting issues may be present with severe ocular surface disease. This may occur anywhere from initial lens insertion to several weeks or months later. Surface deposits can adversely affect scleral lens wetting over time.

Removal Challenges

The large lens design can rub against the cornea upon removal and could cause a corneal abrasion.

Interaction with Makeup and Moisturizers

A scleral lens can protrude from the eye and may come into contact with makeup or hair products causing debris to adhere to the front surface of the lens.

Handling Challenges

A large diameter lens design can be intimidating to patients who are accustomed to smaller diameter GP designs. Decreased vision without a scleral lens increases the risk of mixing up cleaning agents, insertion solutions and disinfecting systems while inserting or removing a lens. Hand tremors, disfigured appendages or paresthesia of the extremities can cause difficulty with lens handling.

Risk of Noncompliance

Zimmerman and Marks in 2014 reported a case of microbial keratitis with scleral lens wear due to poor lens care [4]. Another report by Bruce and Nguyen in 2013 documented a case of non-ulcerative keratitis with mini-scleral lens wear due to poor lens hygiene [5]. There have been a total of eleven cases of infectious conditions as summarized by Walker *et al.*, 2016 [3]. Furthermore, over-wear or extended wear of scleral lenses may be detrimental to ocular health, especially in corneas with reduced endothelial cell count.

Practitioner Education

Scleral lenses are fit and assessed differently than corneal lenses requiring a new skill set for the practitioners to learn and utilize in patient care. Some manufacturers offer an on-line or live training program prior to fitting different scleral lens designs. The Scleral Lens Education Society is committed to teaching practitioners how to fit scleral lenses and provides the public with a listing of qualified scleral lens practitioners who have completed fellowship with the society.

This chapter will cover scleral lens handling. There are four steps to caring for scleral lenses: cleaning, disinfection, storage and application. The products that are traditionally used for scleral lens care are the same as those approved for corneal GP lenses as they are made out of the same materials. Gas permeable conditioners and multipurpose solutions can be quite viscous and coat the inside of the scleral lens; this can induce a solution sensitivity, likely due to preservatives. Ultimately, the products used for scleral lens care should be corneal GP lens care systems approved by the United States Food and Drug Administration (FDA).

Handwashing

Prior to handling scleral lenses, proper handwashing is critical. Washing hands with soap and water, rather than just water or not at all, decreases the risk of contamination. Hands must be completely dry using a clean towel to avoid contamination. Using a soiled towel may also be a risk for contamination. Mechanical friction does remove contaminants, however rubbing the case without washing hands with soap and water causes increased contamination compared to not rubbing lens cases. Dirty fingers can transfer contaminants to the lens case [6].

The current care systems for corneal rigid gas permeable lenses are listed in Table **1**. It is important to cater the care system regimen to the needs of the patient. Many of these patients are poorly sighted without scleral lenses and can easily mix up the care system regimen causing chemical toxicity to the eye.

Table 1. Scleral Lens Solution.

Non-Generic Contact Lens Solutions						
Multipurpose Disinfecting Solutions (Rinse, Clean, Disinfect, Store, and Remove Protein)	**Multipurpose Disinfecting Solutions** (Clean, Disinfect, Store)	**Multipurpose Disinfecting Solutions** (Disinfect, Store)	**Daily Cleaners**	**Extra Strength Cleaners**	**Enzyme / Chemical Cleaners** (Remove Protein)	**Hydrogen Peroxide Disinfection System**

(Table 1) contd.....

Non-Generic Contact Lens Solutions						
Naturalens RDS Solution (Advance Vision Technologies)	Optimum CDS (Lobob Laboratories)	Bausch + Lomb Boston Advance Comfort Formula Conditioning Solution	Naturalens GP Daily Cleaner (Advanced Vision Technologies)	Sereine Extra Strength Daily Cleaner (Optikem International)	Boston One-Step Liquid Enzymatic (Bausch+Lomb)	Clear Care Cleaning and Disinfection Solution (Alcon)
Boston Simplus Multi-Action Solution (Bausch + Lomb)	Menicon GP CDS (Menicon)	Bausch + Lomb Boston Conditioning Solution	Original Formula Boston Cleaner (Bausch + Lomb)	Polish Brite/Super Cleaner (Contex) Weekly (can be used as an in-office cleaner)	Ultrazyme Enzymatic Cleaner (Abbott Medical Optics)	Sauflon One-Step Cleaning & Disinfection Solution (Sauflon Pharmaceuticals)
	Unique PH Multipurpose Solution (Menicon)	Optikem International Sereine Wetting & Soaking Solution	Boston Advance Cleaner (Bausch + Lomb)	Boston® Laboratory Lens Cleaner (in-office use only. Not approved for patient use)	Progent (Menicon) Bi-weekly (removes protein, deposits, bacteria, fungus, molds and yeasts)	PeroxiClear Cleaning and Disinfection Solution (Bausch & Lomb)
			Optimum by Lobob Extra Strength Cleaner (Lobob Laboratories)			Oxysept Ultracare Disinfecting/Neutralizer Solution (Abbott Medical Optics)
			Sereine Cleaner (Optikem International)			Clear Care Plus Cleaning and Disinfection Solution (Alcon)
			Opti-Free Daily Cleaner (Alcon)			

The very first solution specifically approved for scleral lenses in 2015 by the FDA was Menicon's Saline Rinse Solution, LacriPure, as "an insertion solution for large diameter (scleral) lenses [7]." In 2017, ScleralFil was introduced by Bausch + Lomb Specialty Vision Products for use as an insertion solution for scleral, soft and gas permeable lenses. These solutions will be discussed later in this chapter.

Cleaning

Cleaning daily in the palm of the hand or between the thumb and index finger with a lens cleaner that contains a surfactant prepares the lens surface for disinfection. This also helps to remove debris that gets trapped under the lens due to the slow tear exchange process. Cho *et al.* demonstrated that rubbing contact lenses for cleaning is more effective in order to remove deposits [8]. Butcko *et al.* reviewed the literature on whether rubbing of the lens prior to use of a multipurpose disinfection system was necessary and found evidence supporting rubbing in conjunction with care systems [9]. Rubbing corneal GP lenses did not lead to lens warpage based on Cho's study in 2004 [10]. However, no study to date has shown handling induced warpage with scleral lenses. Anecdotally it has been observed with scleral lenses.

Plasma Treatment

Plasma treatment is essentially the removal of hydrophobic elements from the surface of a lens through electrostatic discharge. This reaction may be affected by the surrounding atmosphere. However, manually rubbing a lens may alter the superficial lens surface to expose hydrophobic elements, altering plasma treatment, and thus affecting lens surface wettability. Scleral lenses that are plasma treated are usually more comfortable and have better wettability than non-plasma treated lenses. Cleaning agents that can safely be used with plasma treated scleral lenses are listed in Table **2**. Things to consider regarding plasma treatment include:

Table 2. Plasma Treated Lens: Cleaning Agents.

Plasma Treated Lens: Cleaning Agents		
Type	**Product**	**Notes**
Non-Abrasive	Optimum Extra-Strength Cleaner (Lobob Laboratories)	May be used with plasma treated lenses
Mildly Abrasive	· Bausch + Lomb Boston Advance Cleaner · Alcon Opti-Free Daily Cleaner · Walgreens Extra Strength Daily Cleaner	· Use with care on high Dk lenses · Can scratch the surface and could increase minus power by decreasing center thickness of the lens.[32]
Abrasive	Bausch + Lomb Original Formula Boston Cleaner	· Use with low Dk materials · Should not be used on plasma treated lenses

- Plasma treated lenses are shipped in solution and should not be handled until lenses are dispensed.
- Aggressive manual rubbing of a plasma treated scleral lens may alter the superficial lens surface to expose hydrophobic elements, thus affecting lens surface wettability.
- Plasma treatment wears off over time.
- Abrasive cleaners may affect plasma treated lenses.
- Plasma treated scleral lenses should be cleaned and disinfected with either a multipurpose solution with a surfactant such as Boston Simplus (Bausch + Lomb) or Unique pH (Menicon) or with a hydrogen peroxide solution.

Rinsing Scleral Lenses after Cleaning

Rinsing the scleral lens with a multipurpose conditioning solution or saline solution after rubbing the lens to remove the cleaning agent will enhance disinfection and avoid risk of chemical toxicity of the anterior surface. It is important not to use tap water to rinse lenses. The FDA states "do not expose contact lenses to tap, bottled, distilled, lake or ocean water [11]." Bonilla-Lemus *et al.* (2010) and Legarreta *et al.* (2013) warned against the use of tap or distilled water for cleaning contact lenses or their storage cases due to the association of Acanthamoeba keratitis with tap water [12, 13].

Enzymatic Cleaners

Enzymatic cleaners to remove proteins and other deposits can be added to the cleaning system regime on a daily or weekly basis depending on the product. Menicon Progent®, a chemical biweekly cleaner, contains a 2-component cleaner with sodium hypochlorite and potassium bromide, which loosens and removes surface protein, deposits, bacteria, fungus, molds and yeasts after a 30-minute soak without manual rubbing (www.meniconamerica.com). Ultrasonic cleaning is not recommended for scleral lens use.

Disinfection

Scleral lenses worn on a daily basis require overnight storage in a disinfecting solution that kills pathogens associated with eye infections. Disinfecting solutions should be stored at room temperature and not in a refrigerator since this action reduces the disinfecting capacity at a quicker rate.

There are two types of daily use disinfection systems for corneal GP lenses, multipurpose disinfecting care systems or hydrogen peroxide disinfection systems. Multipurpose disinfecting solutions provide two steps of care with one bottle: cleaning and disinfecting. Hydrogen peroxide disinfecting solutions require the patient to clean the lens prior to disinfection. The disinfection process occurs over a period of 4-6 hours *via* a platinum disc. A surfactant cleaner can be added to both care systems to improve the cleaning process for scleral lenses. Boost *et al.* studied the efficacy of multipurpose solutions for corneal GP lenses and found that open bottles of disinfecting solutions should be replaced every three months as they lose activity over time against fungal and bacterial species as a result of daily contamination [14]. Risk of contamination with opened care system bottles increases the longer the bottle has been opened with organisms detected as soon as five days after use [15].

Hydrogen peroxide solutions are effective for all scleral lenses, especially for those patients sensitive to chemicals and preservatives in multipurpose solutions. Hydrogen peroxide solutions neutralize into saline within 4 to 6 hours via a platinum disc. An incorporated surfactant loosens dirt, debris, protein and deposits. Several different brands of hydrogen peroxide systems are available in the United States at this time. Practitioners should caution patients using the cases of hydrogen peroxide systems, as they were not designed for use with scleral lenses. There is a risk of chipping, cracking or breaking the scleral lens while inserting or removing the scleral lens from the basket case.

Disinfecting solutions should not be stored in a refrigerator since this action reduces the disinfecting capacity more quickly. Kuzman *et al.* compared the antimicrobial activity of various corneal GP multipurpose contact lens solutions and determined that the disinfection process works well with more variability in antifungal activity than in removal of bacteria [16]. It is critical to not reuse disinfecting solution. In 2006, Chang *et al.* found an association with increased fungal contamination and "topping off" solution [17].

Microbial keratitis has been associated with contamination in lens care system bottles. The organisms are primarily located at the rim of the opening of the bottle or the cap covering the tip of the bottle. Bottles can transfer microbes that could contaminate contact lenses and storage cases [15].

Storage

Scleral lenses are stored in cases overnight during the disinfection process. Microbes can be transferred to these storage cases which were found to have the highest rate of microbial contamination followed by lenses, tip of solution bottles and lens care solutions [18]. The primary contaminants were *Staphylococcus aureus* in lens cases, bottles and lens care solutions. *Pseudomonas,* associated with microbial keratitis, was found as the primary contaminant on lenses and accessories due to poor storage case care and infrequent case replacement [19]. Wu *et al.* found 66% of lens cases were contaminated with primarily gram-negative bacteria [6]. Multiple species of microorganisms were found in 37% of the contaminated cases. Only 1% of the contaminated cases had *Pseudomonas aeruginosa*. Gram-negative bacteria may build a pathway for more pathogenic bacteria. Fungal contamination was observed in both multipurpose and hydrogen peroxide lens storage cases according to a study done by Mela *et al.* [19]. Biofilm can shed and adhere to a contact lens transferring the pathogen from the lens case to the lens surface and to the eye [15, 20]. Biofilm can also be transferred directly from the hands. The case itself is a poor environment for organisms to survive and grow, except that there are areas such as corners, cracks, ridges, and baskets that can protect the organism and aid in biofilm development [15].

Microbial bioburden in storage cases has been reported to be greater than 50% in most studies [15]. Risk factors include smoking and clerical work with the bioburden transferring from the patient's own hands. Computer users should disinfect computer keyboards on a regular basis to reduce contamination [20]. Tilia *et al.* (2014) notes that when tap water is used to rinse cases after overnight storage, there is increased biofilm formation [21]. Eliminating tap water and discarding cases on a monthly basis resulted in a very low bacterial count creating a low risk of biofilm and microbial contamination [22]. Cases and solutions should be replaced every 90 days [23].

How to Clean a Storage Case

The most effective way to clean a storage case and remove biofilm with a multipurpose solution is to rub the case, rinse the case using a multipurpose solution, wipe the case with a tissue and then air-dry the case face down [21, 23]. This process removes excess moisture and decreases the risk of microbial keratitis and airborne contamination [6, 24]. Placing a case on a clean tissue prevents it from coming into contact with a contaminated surface. Lens cases should not be stored in the bathroom or near the toilet to reduce contamination. Keeping the cases wet rather than air-drying increases the risk for contamination. It is critical to not boil cases in water as this can distort the case and increase risk of contamination [24].

Hiti *et al.* investigated microwaving cases and found that three minutes in the microwave removed *Acanthamoeba* trophozoites and cysts without distorting the cases [25]. Further investigation needs to be done to determine if this option would be adequate for case disinfection. Additionally, case contamination is increased in part time wear where the solution is not replaced on a regular basis.

Lens storage depends on the disinfection system. A multipurpose disinfection system maintains disinfection over time and requires a case that is large enough for the solution to cover the lens completely [22]. Matching the lens case to the solution by manufacturer decreased the risk of contamination [6].

A hydrogen peroxide solution needs either a large disinfection case or two smaller cases (one for each lens). A basket case increases the risk of chipping or breaking a scleral lens when inserting or removing the lens. A large basket case, the PROSE disinfection case, is available from dryeyezone.com. This case does not have a neutralizing disc attached to the bottom of the basket. Thus, a neutralizing disc needs to be taken off of a hydrogen peroxide basket case and placed in the bottom of the case.

Seal *et al.* demonstrated that hydrogen peroxide cases have a higher contamination rate of bacteria than multipurpose disinfecting solution cases [22]. Hydrogen peroxide systems work quickly to disinfect lenses creating a saline solution in the case without any disinfecting properties. This process may lead to increased risk of contamination within the case where bacteria can survive and multiply. Part time wearers should also use this disinfection method on a daily basis.

There was less case contamination with participants that had worn contact lenses for less than two years. Long-time lens wearers tend to become less observant with lens care practices as the perception of harm decreases over time [6].

Boost *et al.* described that patient understanding of the risk of infection and implementing case cleaning on a regular basis decreased overall risks of infection. The key to decreasing the risk of infection due to contaminated cases is patient understanding and implementing case cleaning on a regular basis [14]. Using verbal and written instructions, supplemented by practical demonstrations as suggested by Tilia, improves patient compliance [21]. Reinforcing lens care and handling should be a priority at each patient visit as suggested by Hickson-Curran *et al.* [26].

Insertion Solution

Scleral lens application solution has a longer contact time with the cornea compared to corneal gas permeable (GP) lenses. Therefore, it is important to prevent exposing the cornea to preservatives or buffers to enhance performance and maintain corneal health. As previously stated, gas permeable conditioners and multipurpose solutions can be quite viscous and coat the inside of the scleral lens; this can induce a solution sensitivity, likely due to preservatives. These solutions should be rinsed off the lens with preservative free saline prior to insertion. In 2015, the FDA approved Menicon's saline rinse solution, LacriPure, for use as an insertion solution for scleral lenses after proper disinfection [7]. This solution can also be used to rinse lenses prior to insertion, to remove debris and bacteria after the disinfection process and to rinse lens cases or lenses as needed during the day. This solution is a 5 mL sterile unit dose single use non-preserved, 0.9% sodium chloride (normal saline) solution.

In 2017, ScleralFil was introduced by Bausch + Lomb Speciality Vision Products for use as an insertion solution for scleral, soft and gas permeable lenses. ScleralFil is available in 10mL vials that stand up for single use. Thirty vials are available in a carton. The solution is buffered in order to maintain a pH from 7.2 to 7.8.

Prior to the FDA approval of LacriPure, the standard of care in the United States was non-FDA approved non-preserved 0.9% sodium chloride inhalation solution in a single use vial. This solution is not buffered and does not have any preservatives or active ingredients, which is beneficial due to minimal tear exchange with scleral lenses. This solution may be obtained with a prescription from a pharmacy in the United States and may be covered by a patient's medical pharmaceutical insurance program. Alternatively, sodium chloride 0.9% inhalation solution vials may be purchased without a prescription through the internet.

Saline with preservatives are associated with an increased risk of chemical sensitivities. Non-preserved saline has a greater risk of microbial contamination. According to two studies by Sweeney (1992 and 1999), during normal use, multi-use unpreserved saline bottles became significantly contaminated with Gram-negative and Gram-positive bacteria [27, 28]. This may be due to contamination from the skin or ocular flora of a patient. In a study of continuous wear silicone hydrogel contact lenses, daily irrigation with sterile saline solution did not mitigate increases in corneal epithelial permeability or decrease the risk of adverse events [29].

Unisol 4 is a buffered solution, which can be used for insertion up to 48 hours after the bottle has been opened. At the time of publication, Unisol 4 is no longer available but was widely incorporated into scleral lens care and used almost exclusively during the formative years of the re-emergence of scleral lenses. Buffers in contact lens care systems maintain the pH to match the ocular tears of the eye. However, the buffer in Unisol 4 may have contributed to irritation of the ocular surface and increased post lens tear debris when used longer than 48 hours. Unisol 4 was used for rinsing lenses for up to two weeks. It was recommended to mark the date on the bottle once the bottle was opened. Non-preserved or preserved saline may be used for rinsing prior to insertion as an alternative to Unisol 4.

Purilens plus preservative free saline is a sterile solution buffered with boric acid and sodium borate approved for use with GP lenses. Purilens Saline is available in 4 ounce bottles and is used for rinsing lenses for up to fifteen days or for lens application. Similar to Unisol 4, it is recommended to mark the date on the bottle once the bottle has been opened.

There are other non-preserved single use options to fill scleral lenses. According to the Scleral Lens Education Society, more viscous artificial tears may be used in combination with non-preserved application solution or may be used alone. Ingredients in these artificial tears include carboxymethylcellulose glycerin and hyaluronic acid. The increased thickness of the combination solution prevents debris from migrating underneath the lens. The combination solutions also help increase comfort, prevent loss of fluid with scleral lens application and thereby reduce the risk of air bubbles.

Insertion of Scleral Lenses

Prior to handling scleral lenses, as with any contact lens modality, meticulous hand washing is essential. It is critical to use soap without perfumes or oils to wash hands prior to lens handling to reduce the risk of normal flora contaminating the lens or the case. Hand cream should be used after lens application since it can leave a residue on the front or back surface of the lens.

Insertion of a scleral lens can be challenging due to the large size of the lens compared with the palpebral fissure. The center of gravity of the lens makes it hard to balance on the fingers causing the lens to tip and fall off the fingers. Therefore, a rubber device called a plunger, commercially sold as a scleral cup, is used to stabilize the scleral lens and prepare the lens for application.

There are numerous plungers available to aid with insertion and removal of scleral lenses. The DMV scleral cup is a large plunger with a hole in the center (Fig. **2** left). A DMV vented plunger, with a hole on the top and bottom of the plunger is used to prevent suction (Fig. **3**). Both plunger designs can be used with a scleral lens; preference is practitioner dependent. The DMV vented plunger allows the lens to balance in the cup without suction.

Since suction is not employed, the lens could tip or be displaced if the lens is bumped during the application process. A non-ventilated DMV plunger maintains lens stability; however it is necessary to squeeze the plunger when applying the lens. Pinching the plunger at the junction between the cup and the handle will remove the plunger from the scleral lens in the event of the plunger remaining on the scleral lens upon insertion.

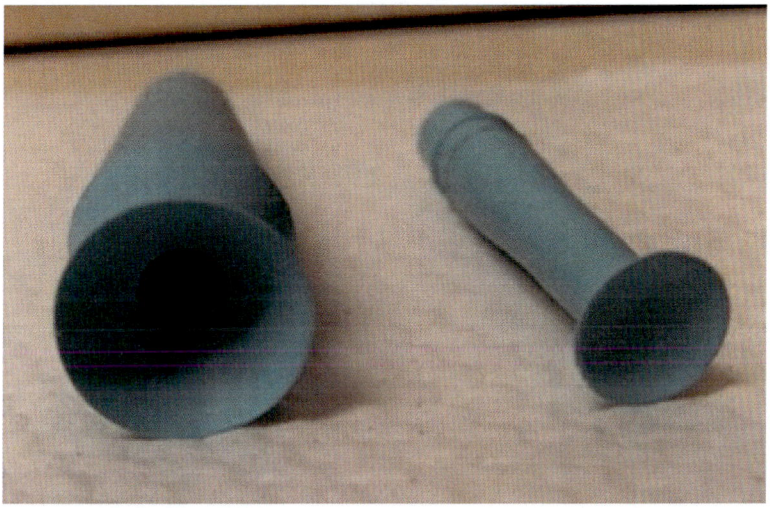

Fig. (2). DMV Scleral Cup (left) and DMV Ultra Remover (right) plungers. The large plunger is used for insertion and a small plunger is used for removal.

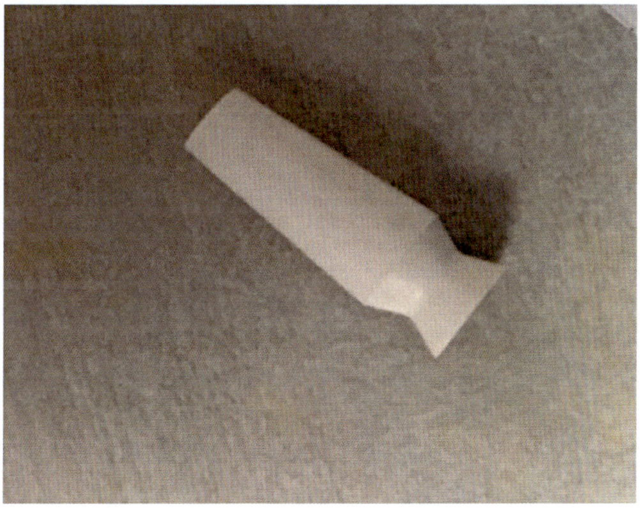

Fig. (3). DMV Vented Scleral Cup.

There are two methods for scleral lens application: the three-finger approach or the plunger (also known as inserter) method. It is advised to sit in a chair and place a clean towel on a flat table. A mirror lying flat on the table is helpful when applying the lens. With the three-finger method, the thumb, index, and middle fingers are used to create a tripod stand for scleral lens application (Fig. **4**). The lens is filled with sterile non-preserved saline solution, the eyelids are held open, and the scleral lens is placed on the eye.

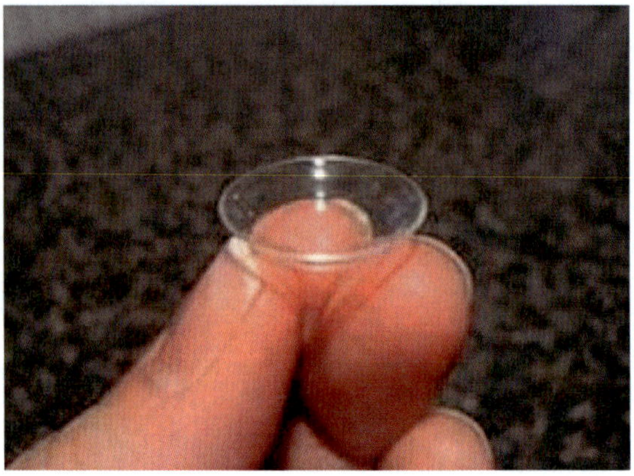

Fig. (4). Example of holding the scleral lens with three fingers for optimal balancing of the lens.

With the large plunger method, the ventilated and non-ventilated DMV plungers are prepared by wetting the plunger's surface with one to two drops of sterile preservative free saline solution. When using the non-ventilated plunger, it should be squeezed and the patient should hold the outside edge of the lens and place it on the plunger. When the squeeze is released, the lens is tightly secured to the non-ventilated plunger (Fig. **5**). With the ventilated plunger, the patient should hold the outside edge of the lens and place it on the plunger. Next, the patient overfills the bowl of the lens with sterile preservative free saline so that the saline appears as a convex or round surface above the lens.

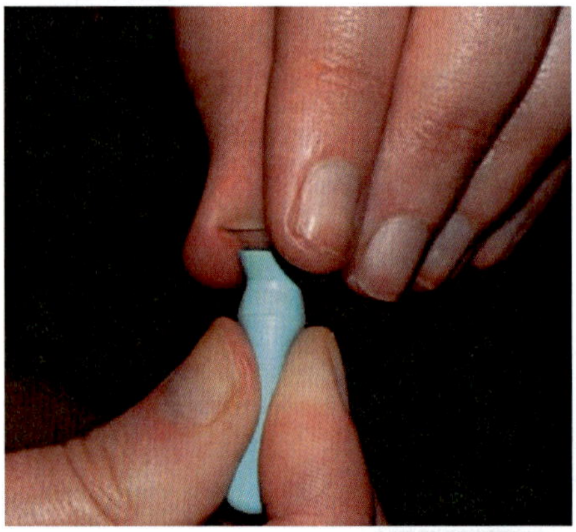

Fig. (5). Applying the lens to a non-ventilated plunger. Note that the plunger is squeezed during lens placement.

The lens is held with the dominant hand. The patient leans forward sitting with the chin towards the chest and eyes facing the mirror on the table. The head is parallel to the ground. The eyelids are held wide open with the index finger on the upper eyelid and middle finger or thumb on the lower eyelid with the non-dominant hand. While holding the eye open, the lens is steadily moved closer to the eye (Fig. **6**).

The patient is instructed to look straight down toward the mirror on the table and then at the plunger or the hole of the plunger while inserting the lens. To visualize the hole, the patient may want to close the opposite eye, which may impede application. It is actually beneficial to have both eyes open with scleral lens application. The goal of lens placement is to be perfectly centered over the cornea. If the lens is placed in the lower cul de sac when applied, the lens should be moved superiorly to center the lens. Some patients may pull back from the lens or squeeze their lids as the lens approaches their eye.

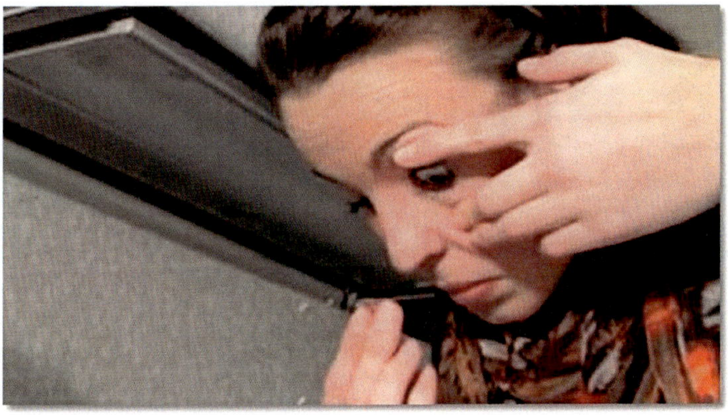

Fig. (6). Patient applying scleral lens with head almost parallel to the floor separating both eyelids. (Image courtesy of Scleral Lens Education Society)

As the solution touches the eye, the lens is inserted gently. Here again patients may squeeze their eyes and pull back once they feel the fluid sensation. Reassure the patient that the sensation of fluid on the eye prior to the lens touching the eye is part of the insertion process. The eyelids are released once the lens is on the eye. If using the DMV ventilated eyecup, the plunger is removed from the lens gently. If using the DMV non-ventilated eyecup, the plunger is gently squeezed in order to release suction and the lens. The plunger is cleaned with alcohol or peroxide after each use and then is allowed to air dry.

Next, patients should look in the mirror after insertion and inspect the eye for air bubbles that can cause discomfort and decrease vision if the air bubble is in front of the pupil. An air bubble creates a dry area underneath the lens and can cause corneal desiccation over time. Air bubbles may appear upon insertion if the head pulls back and is not parallel to the ground causing the lens to tilt upon insertion and allowing air between the solution and the eyeball. If an air bubble is present, the lens should be removed and reinserted. To avoid air bubbles, use 1-2 drops of a thicker, more viscous preservative free artificial tear such as carboxy-methylcellulose combined with preservative free saline solution to fill the bowl of the scleral lens. If an air bubble occurs after insertion, this could be due to an asymmetrical scleral surface allowing air to flow underneath the lens over time or eye movement during insertion.

Poor wetting of the front surface of the lens may be observed after scleral lens insertion. During the scleral lens manufacturing process, the over use of diamond cutting arbor feeds or the incomplete removal of blocking material can result in compromised surface wetting. To eliminate non-wetting or deposits, a practitioner can have the lens polished. A gas permeable laboratory lens cleaner or alcohol based daily cleaner is used to remove pitch, wax and other solvents used in the manufacturing process. This cleaner also removes lipids, body oils, and other contaminants. Another option may be to rub the GP multipurpose conditioning solution on the front surface of the scleral lens to enhance wettability. It is useful to rinse the solution to avoid solution toxicity and sensitivity under the lens.

Makeup and hair products can contaminate the front surface of the lens causing cloudy vision and decreasing the wettability of the lens. Contamination occurs because a scleral lens is two to five times thicker than other lens designs and can protrude from the front surface of the eye due to the amount of apical clearance under the lens. Remove the lens, clean and reinsert the lens if makeup adheres to the front surface of the lens.

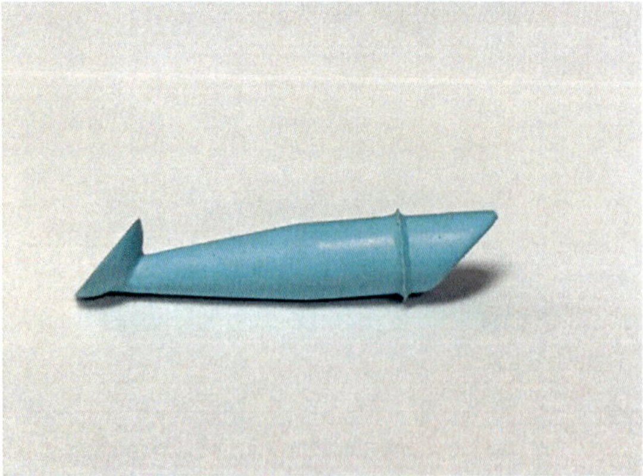

Fig. (7). The DMV 45 angled lens remover.

Scleral Lens Removal

The most efficient tool for the removal of scleral lenses is the DMV Ultra remover (Fig. **2** right). This is a small plunger with suction capabilities to hold on to the large lens during the removal process. The DMV Classic without suction can also be used for removal. The DMV 45 angled lens remover is angled at 45 degrees to eliminate the hand from interfering with vision during scleral lens removal with a mirror (Fig. **7**). Generally speaking, the large plunger is used for insertion and the small plunger is used for removal.

In addition to DMV plungers and accessories, a latex free plunger is also available from Amcon, called the Royal Remover/Inserter (Fig. **8**). The suction cup is mounted perpendicular to the handle. In addition, the Magic Touch by Amcon has a 20 degree angled suction cup with a hole for ventilation, allowing increased suction (Fig. **9**).

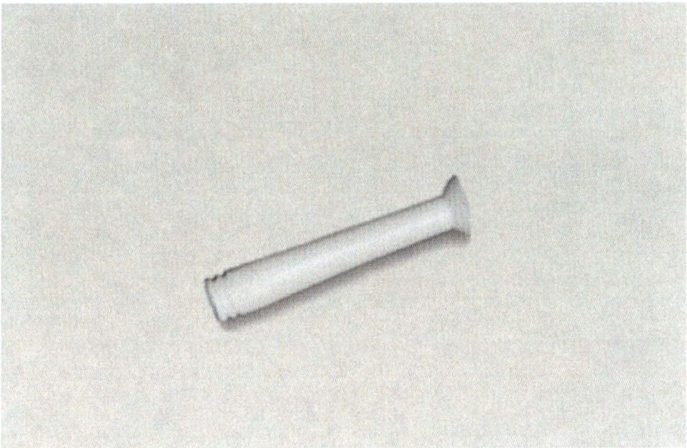

Fig. (8). The Amcon Royal remover/inserter

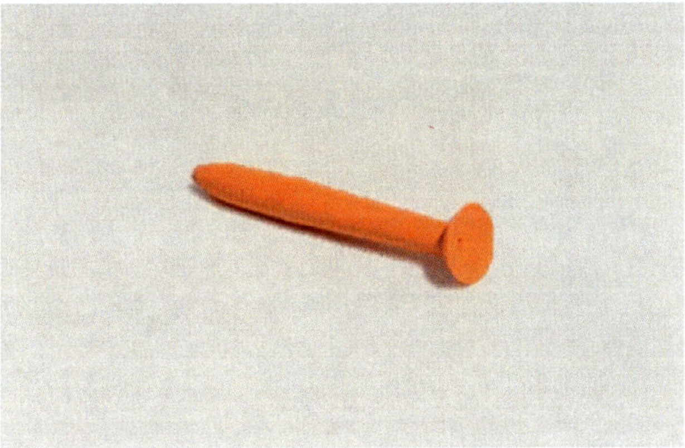

Fig. (9). The Amcon Magic Touch vented inserter/remover.

A drop of preservative free saline or artificial tears is instilled in the eye to loosen the lens prior to removal. With the manual two-finger method, the lens is removed by combining pressure into the globe with the eyelid and prying the edge with the fingertip (Fig. **10**). To begin, the patient first looks up and pressure is applied to the middle of the lower eyelid below the lashes. The lid is manipulated underneath the inferior edge of the lens. Pressure is then applied to the globe and the lens is lifted. Next the lower eyelid and finger are used together to nudge the lower edge of the lens off the eye and the lens is removed. Stabilize and anchor the upper edge of the lens with the upper lid.

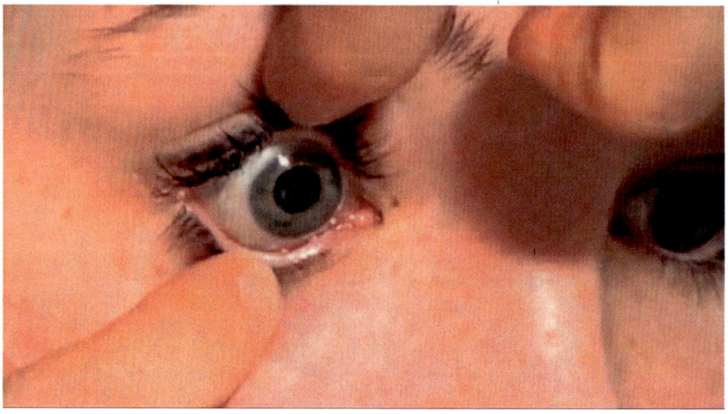

Fig. (10). Removal of a scleral lens without a plunger using two fingers. (Image courtesy of Scleral Lens Education Society).

With the small plunger method, have the patient sit in a chair and place a clean towel on a flat table. Next, a mirror is placed on the table to view when removing the lens. Wet the plunger's surface with one to two drops of sterile preservative free saline solution. The patient then looks into the mirror. While holding the eye open, the plunger is applied to the lens in the peripheral inferior or superior quadrant by the limbus. The lens is removed by releasing suction of the lens on the eye with the plunger (Fig. **11**).

Pressing just below the lens at the edge of the lens with the plunger may be needed to break the seal of the lens and allow for a bubble under the lens to loosen the lens prior to removal. As the lens is being removed, it is advised to be cautious not to rub the lens against the cornea, to risk causing a corneal abrasion. If the plunger is centered on the lens, pinch the plunger to remove it from the lens and re-apply the plunger in the peripheral lower or upper quadrant of the lens. The patient holds the outside edge of the lens while squeezing the base of the plunger to remove the plunger from the lens. After removal, disinfect and store the lenses. The plunger should be cleaned with alcohol and left to air dry after each use.

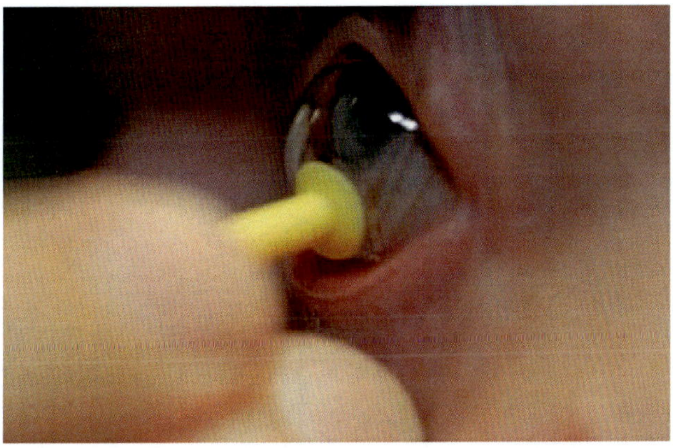

Fig. (11). Removal of the scleral lens with a small plunger aligned with the periphery of the scleral lens. Note that the plunger should never be applied to the center of the lens.

Cleaning the plunger is critical as an old plunger can become cracked, leave residue on the lens surface, and not provide good suction on the scleral lens. Some practitioners recommend that plungers should be replaced every 3-6 months, or sooner if the edges become rough, uneven, or if suction is not sufficient. Plungers may not be readily obtainable at the local pharmacy. An on-line resource for plungers is the dryeyeshop.com.

The Scleral Lens Education Society video titled Scleral Contact Lens Insertion, Removal, Troubleshooting and Lens Care (www.sclerallens.org/how-use-scleral-lenses) is a useful resource for both practitioners and patients alike.

Additional Options for Scleral Lens Handling

Understanding scleral lens handling is critical to succeed with scleral lenses. Scleral lens dropout rates vary in the literature and range from approximately 25% to 49% [30, 31]. Handling is the most common reason for dropout [32]. Additional tools may be used to succeed with scleral lens handling.

Certain patients may have difficultly seeing the lens for application. These include an older patient, a patient that lives alone, has a high refractive error, aphakia, or a patient who has dexterity hand issues due to arthritis or missing digits.

There are several tools that are beneficial for such patients. One is the See Green Lens Inserter by Dalsey Adaptives (http://dalseyadaptives.net/store/), which is available with and without a stand (Fig. **12**). The lighted plunger helps center the device for application. The stand holds the plunger and lens in place prior to application. This is helpful for patients who have unsteady hands or for those who need both hands to hold their eyelids open.

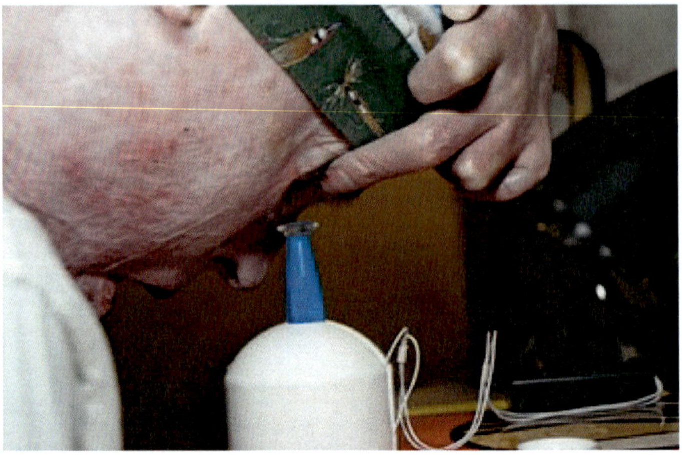

Fig. (12). See Green Lens Inserter by Dalsey Adaptives.

Another tool is the EZi Scleral Lens Applicator by Q-Case Inc. (http://ezibyqcase.com/) (Fig. **13**). This device is placed on the finger like a ring and has a base for scleral lens application. This design provides stability and allows patients to apply scleral devices with one finger.

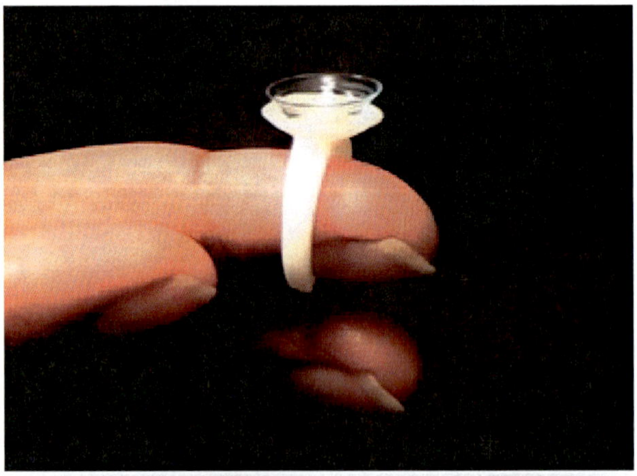

Fig. (13). EZi Scleral Lens Applicator by Q-Case Inc.

A third option is a #8 O ring that is available at any hardware store (Fig. **14**). O ring dimensions are 3/8" x 9/16" x 3/32". The scleral lens rests on the O ring on a patient's finger, which can allow for stable application.

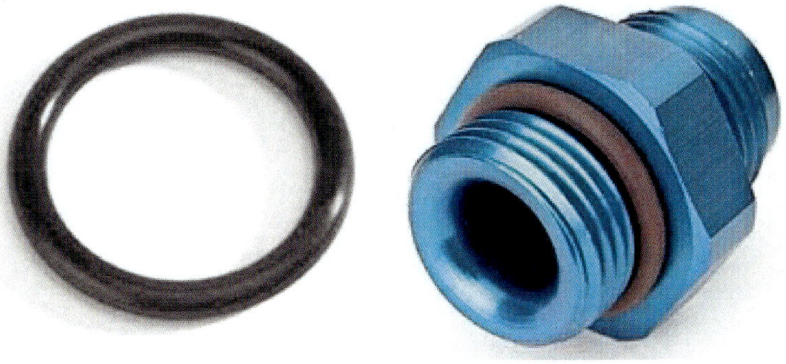

Fig. (14). O-ring used for lens insertion.

An additional option for scleral lens insertion is a sterile orthodontic ring placed on a patient's hand (Fig. **15**). These come in packages of 100 and may be used for single use insertion of scleral lenses.

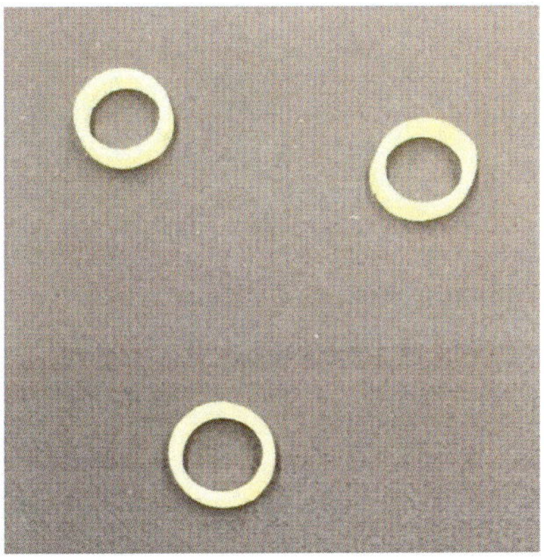

Fig. (15). Examples of orthodontic rubber bands.

CONCLUSION

No matter how well a scleral lens is fit, the patient needs to understand proper application and removal for success. It is the responsibility of practitioners to help patients with the scleral lens care and handling process in order to achieve optimal results with scleral lenses. Healthy habits should be reviewed at each visit. Patients should be supplied with an after-hours contact number in case of an emergency. As the resurgence of scleral lenses is relatively new, there is more research that needs to be performed on best practices including the most effective method of cleaning and disinfection for scleral lenses. Furthermore, additional knowledge on the ideal solution to fill the bowl of the scleral lens is needed.

CONFLICT OF INTEREST

The authors declare no conflict of interest, financial or otherwise.

ACKNOWLEDGEMENTS

None Declared.

REFERENCES

[1] Scleral Lens Education Society Website. http://www.sclerallens.org. 2015.

[2] Caroline P, Andre M. How much tear exchange occurs beneath scleral lenses? Contact Lens Spectr 2014.

[3] Walker MK, Bergmanson JP, Miller WL, Marsack JD, Johnson LA. Complications and fitting challenges associated with scleral contact lenses: A review. Cont Lens Anterior Eye 2016; 39(2): 88-96.
[http://dx.doi.org/10.1016/j.clae.2015.08.003] [PMID: 26341076]

[4] Zimmerman AB, Marks A. Microbial keratitis secondary to unintended poor compliance with scleral gas-permeable contact lenses. Eye Contact Lens 2014; 40(1): e1-4.
[http://dx.doi.org/10.1097/ICL.0b013e318273420f] [PMID: 23392303]

[5] Bruce AS, Nguyen LM. Acute red eye (non-ulcerative keratitis) associated with mini-scleral contact lens wear for keratoconus. Clin Exp Optom 2013; 96(2): 245-8.
[http://dx.doi.org/10.1111/cxo.12033] [PMID: 23387325]

[6] Wu YT, Willcox MD, Stapleton F. The effect of contact lens hygiene behavior on lens case contamination. Optom Vis Sci 2015; 92(2): 167-74.
[http://dx.doi.org/10.1097/OPX.0000000000000477] [PMID: 25951478]

[7] 2015. 510(k) Number K151768, Trade/Device Name: Menicon Saline Rinse Solution. Regulation Number: 21 CFR 886.5928, Regulation Name: Soft (Hydrophilic) Contact Lens Care Products; Regulatory Class: Class II; Product Code: LPN, MRC

[8] Cho P, Cheng SY, Chan WY, Yip WK. Soft contact lens cleaning: rub or no-rub? Ophthalmic Physiol Opt 2009; 29(1): 49-57.
[http://dx.doi.org/10.1111/j.1475-1313.2008.00606.x] [PMID: 19154280]

[9] Butcko V, McMahon TT, Joslin CE, Jones L. Microbial keratitis and the role of rub and rinsing. Eye Contact Lens 2007; 33(6 Pt 2): 421-3.
[http://dx.doi.org/10.1097/ICL.0b013e318157f3df] [PMID: 17975438]

[10] Cho P, Ng H, Chan I, Law J, Tsang J. Effect of two different cleaning methods on the back optic zone radii and surface smoothness of menicon rigid gas-permeable lenses. Optom Vis Sci 2004; 81(6): 461-7.
[http://dx.doi.org/10.1097/01.opx.0000135101.86416.09] [PMID: 15201720]

[11] http://www.fda.gov/MedicalDevices/ProductsandMedicalProcedures/HomeHealthandConsumer/ConsumerProducts/ContactLenses/ucm062589.htm2015.

[12] Bonilla-Lemus P, Ramerirez-Bautista GA, Zamora-Munoz C, *et al.* Acanthamoeba spp. In domestic tap water in houses of contact lens wearers in the metropolitan area of Mexico City. Exp Parasitol 2010; 126(1): 54-8.

[13] Legarreta JE, Nau AC, Dhaliwal DK. Acanthamoeba keratitis associated with tap water use during contact lens cleaning: manufacturer guidelines need to change. Eye Contact Lens 2013; 39(2): 158-61.
[http://dx.doi.org/10.1097/ICL.0b013e31827a79ee] [PMID: 23392300]

[14] Boost M, Cho P, Lai S. Efficacy of multipurpose solutions for rigid gas permeable lenses. Ophthalmic Physiol Opt 2006; 26(5): 468-75.
[http://dx.doi.org/10.1111/j.1475-1313.2006.00398.x] [PMID: 16918771]

[15] Szczotka-Flynn LB, Pearlman E, Ghannoum M. Microbial contamination of contact lenses, lens care solutions, and their accessories: a literature review. Eye Contact Lens 2010; 36(2): 116-29.
[http://dx.doi.org/10.1097/ICL.0b013e3181d20cae] [PMID: 20168237]

[16] Kuzman T, Kutija MB. Comparative study of antibacterial and antifungal effects of rigid gas permeable contact lens disinfecting solutions. Coll Anthropol 2013; 37(Suppl 1): 127-31.
[PMID: 25297366]

[17] Chang DC, Grant GB, O'Donnell K, *et al.* Fusarium Keratitis Investigation Team. Multistate outbreak of Fusarium keratitis associated with use of a contact lens solution. JAMA 2006; 296(8): 953-63.
[http://dx.doi.org/10.1001/jama.296.8.953] [PMID: 16926355]

[18] Thakur DV, Gaikwad UN. Microbial contamination of soft contact lenses & accessories in asymptomatic contact lens users. Indian J Med Res 2014; 140(2): 307-9.
[PMID: 25297366]

[19] Mela EK, Anastassiou ED, Gartaganis SP, Christofidou M. Fungal isolation from disinfectant solutions of contact lens storage cases among asymptomatic users. Eye Contact Lens 2015; 41(2): 87-90.
[http://dx.doi.org/10.1097/ICL.0000000000000069] [PMID: 25503912]

[20] Jiang Y, Jacobs M, Bajaksouzian S, *et al.* Risk factors for microbial bioburden during daily wear of silicone hydrogel contact lenses. Eye Contact Lens 2014; 40(3): 148-56.
[http://dx.doi.org/10.1097/ICL.0000000000000026] [PMID: 24756119]

[21] Tilia D, Lazon de la Jara P, Zhu H, Naduvilath TJ, Holden BA. The effect of compliance on contact lens case contamination. Optom Vis Sci 2014; 91(3): 262-71.
[PMID: 24413272]

[22] Seal DV, Dalton A, Doris D. Disinfection of contact lenses without tap water rinsing: is it effective? Eye (Lond) 1999; 13(Pt 2): 226-30.
[http://dx.doi.org/10.1038/eye.1999.56] [PMID: 10450387]

[23] Vijay A, Willcox M, Zhu H, *et al.* Contact Lens Storage Case Hygiene Practice and Storage Case Contamination. Eye Contact Lens 2014.
[PMID: 25230082]

[24] Hall BJ, Jones L. Contact lens cases: the missing link in contact lens safety? Eye Contact Lens 2010; 36(2): 101-5.
[http://dx.doi.org/10.1097/ICL.0b013e3181d05555] [PMID: 20090542]

[25] Hiti K, Walochnik J, Faschinger C, Haller-Schober EM, Aspöck H. Microwave treatment of contact lens cases contaminated with acanthamoeba. Cornea 2001; 20(5): 467-70.
[http://dx.doi.org/10.1097/00003226-200107000-00005] [PMID: 11413399]

[26] Hickson-Curran S, Chalmers RL, Riley C. Patient attitudes and behavior regarding hygiene and replacement of soft contact lenses and storage cases. Cont Lens Anterior Eye 2011; 34(5): 207-15.
[http://dx.doi.org/10.1016/j.clae.2010.12.005] [PMID: 21227735]

[27] Sweeney DF. Corneal exhaustion syndrome with long-term wear of contact lenses. Optom Vis Sci 1992; 69(8): 601-8.
[http://dx.doi.org/10.1097/00006324-199208000-00002] [PMID: 1513555]

[28] Sweeney DF, Willcox MD, Sansey N, *et al.* Incidence of contamination of preserved saline solutions during normal use. CLAO J 1999; 25(3): 167-75.
[PMID: 10444054]

[29] Lin MC, French HM, Graham AD, Sanders TL. Effects of daily irrigation on corneal epithelial

permeability and adverse events with silicone hydrogel contact lens continuous wear. Invest Ophthalmol Vis Sci 2014; 55(2): 776-83.
[http://dx.doi.org/10.1167/iovs.13-13508] [PMID: 24425854]

[30] Pullum KW, Whiting MA, Buckley RJ. Scleral contact lenses: the expanding role. Cornea 2005; 24(3): 269-77.
[http://dx.doi.org/10.1097/01.ico.0000148311.94180.6b] [PMID: 15778597]

[31] Ensley R, Miller H. Good Chemistry: Are you up to date on pairing GP lenses and solutions? Here's a look at what makes a perfect match. Review of Cornea and Contact Lenses 2016.

[32] Pecego M, Barnett M, Mannis MJ, Durbin-Johnson B. Jupiter Scleral Lenses: the UC Davis Eye Center experience. Eye Contact Lens 2012; 38(3): 179-82.
[http://dx.doi.org/10.1097/ICL.0b013e31824daa5e] [PMID: 22543730]

CHAPTER 14

Scleral Lens Challenges

Melissa Barnett[1], Karen G. Carrasquillo[2], Gregory DeNaeyer[3], S. Barry Eiden[4], Karolien Elving-Kokke[5], Jason Jedlicka[6], Carina Koppen[7], Michael J. Lipson[8], Jason Marsack[9], Jennifer Anne McMahon[10], Henny M. Otten[5], Young Kee Park[11], Perry Rosenthal[12], Esther-Simone Visser[5], Lynette K. Johns[13,*], Maria K. Walker[9] and **Geunyoung Yoon[14]**

[1] *University of California, Davis, Sacramento, CA, USA*

[2] *BostonSight, Needham Heights, MA, USA*

[3] *Arena Eye Surgeons, Columbus, OH, USA*

[4] *North Suburban Vision Consultants, Ltd, Keratoconus Specialists of Illinois, Deerfield, IL, USA*

[5] *Visser Contactlenzenpraktijk B.V., EJ Nijmegen, The Netherlands*

[6] *School of Optometry, Indiana University, Bloomington, IN, USA*

[7] *Faculty of Medicine and Health Sciences, University of Antwerp, Antwerp, Belgium*

[8] *Department of Ophthalmology and Visual Science, University of Michigan, Northville Health Center, Northville, MI, USA*

[9] *College of Optometry, University of Houston, Houston, TX, USA*

[10] *Great Western Hospitals NHS FT, Swindon, UK*

[11] *YK Eye Clinic, Seoul, South Korea*

[12] *Harvard Medical School, Boston, MA, USA*

[13] *The New England College of Optometry, Boston, Massachusetts, USA*

[14] *Flaum Eye Institute, Institute of Optics, Center for Visual Science, Biomedical Engineering, University of Rochester, Rochester, NY, USA*

Abstract: Despite a recent resurgence in popularity of scleral lenses, the literature to date is quite limited regarding challenges faced by practitioners. Practitioners may manage one or multiple challenges daily. This chapter explores different topics from the contributors' personal perspectives. Authors were asked to write about their unique experiences and fitting philosophies for a variety of situations that scleral lens practitioners may encounter. Common topics are included, however not every possible challenge is covered.

* **Corresponding author Lynette K. Johns:** The New England College of Optometry, Boston, Massachusetts, USA; Tel: 617-262-2020; Fax: 617-236-6323; E-mails: johnsl@neco.edu; lynettekjohns@gmail.com

Melissa Barnett & Lynette K. Johns (Eds.)

Keywords: Asian, Conjunctival hypertrophy, Corneo-scleral topography, Elevations, Fuchs', Graft rejection, Handling, Impingement, Impression molded, Modify, Molded, Neovascularization, Notch, Nystagmus, Pain, Pediatric, Pinguecula, Pterygium, Symblepharon, Wavefront.

INTRODUCTION

Despite a recent resurgence in popularity of scleral lenses, the literature to date is quite limited regarding challenges faced by practitioners. This chapter explores different topics from the contributors' personal perspectives. Authors were asked to write about their unique experiences and fitting philosophies for a variety of situations that scleral lens practitioners may encounter. Common topics are included, however not every possible challenge is covered.

CONJUNCTIVAL AND SCLERAL ELEVATIONS: "LUMPS AND BUMPS"

Elevations on the scleral and conjunctival surface can be significant challenges to scleral lens fitting. After all, the scleral lens is rigid and will not "drape" over the scleral surface. Modifications to the fit are required to properly align to the scleral surface. If the lens overly compresses or impinges the tissue, complications may occur. Pingueculae, pterygia, nodules, hypertrophy from scleral lenses, glaucoma drainage devices and symblephara will all be covered in this section. Sometimes conjunctival irregularities are too challenging for the most custom scleral lens, and the eye may require impression molded scleral lenses.

Pinguecula and Pterygium (Michael Lipson, OD, FAAO, FSLS)

Pingueculae are seen very commonly in a variety of patients. Pre-existing pingueculae should be carefully noted during the evaluation for fitting scleral lenses. Due to variations in size and location, they may or may not create issues for scleral lens fitting. Large pingueculae must be addressed with lens modifications.

The presence of a pterygium is also a challenge but not a contraindication for scleral lens fitting. Pterygia can also create unique fitting challenges. They vary in height (sometimes raised and other times very flat). They overlap anteriorly beyond the limbus onto the cornea. As with pingueculae, heavy bearing on the pterygium and adjacent tissue should be avoided or minimized. Fitting a scleral lens that bears on a pterygium can aggravate the inflamed tissue and can alter the fitting characteristics of the lens to cause lens decentration. An inflamed pterygium has the potential to advance. Since pterygia vary individually in width and height, the ideal approach is to fit lenses with higher sagittal depth to clear the pterygium.

When fitting scleral lenses, the presence of either a pinguecula or pterygium presents a scleral fitting challenge for three reasons. First is the location, second is the effect on the fit/landing and third is the cosmetic appearance (redness) when the lens is worn.

For a pinguecula, I have found four fitting modifications that may help resolve these issues. They include:

- Fitting a smaller lens
- Fitting a larger lens
- Notching the lens
- Specifying a local area of increased clearance (microvault)

Similarly, for a pterygium, fitting modifications include:

- Increase sagittal depth/clearance in combination with a larger lens diameter
- Notching the lens
- Specifying a local area of increased clearance (microvault)

These may be done independently or in combination.

Fitting a smaller lens – If the pinguecula is more than 2 mm beyond the limbus, a smaller diameter scleral lens can be fit such that it does not impinge upon the pinguecula. For a patient with an average corneal diameter of 11.8 mm, this would require the use of lens diameter of 15.5 mm or less.

Fitting a larger lens – If the pinguecula is very close to the limbus (within 2 mm) or is not highly elevated, fitting a larger lens with a larger landing zone may allow the lens to land more gently on the pinguecula or even vault over it. The increase in diameter may be in the range of 1-4 mm. When using these larger diameters, it is also helpful to design the lens with a flatter periphery (higher edge lift).

Notching the lens – To avoid touching the pinguecula or pterygium while maintaining the same lens diameter, a notch can be contoured in the edge of the lens. This method necessitates the use of a lens that is rotationally stable. Initially, a scleral lens should be fit to assure the rotational stability with using toricity in the landing zone or double thin zone design. Once stability is established, the location and depth of the notch can be marked or described to the laboratory consultant with the axis and depth.

Specifying a localized area of increased clearance (microvault) – this process involves lathing a vaulted hemispherical portion of the lens edge overlying the location of the pinguecula. As a result, there is reduced bearing over the pinguecula. As described above, a rotationally stable lens is required to keep the lens oriented over the area of interest. Unlike notches which are typically done by hand, these microvaults are manufactured by a lathe and are reproducible.

In rare instances, all efforts to avoid the pinguecula are not totally successful. Usually, even with a pinguecula, the modifications to scleral lenses described above can make both the practitioner and patient happy with vision, comfort and cosmetic appearance.

Increase Clearance – Increasing the sagittal depth is accomplished by fitting a larger lens that is designed to fit with higher corneal and limbal clearance. This allows the lens to avoid bearing and totally clear the pterygium. The diameter used for this purpose is usually 5-8 mm larger than the corneal diameter (16.5 mm or larger).

Even with a pterygium, the modifications to scleral lenses described above can allow for a successful fit. On occasion, I have recommended that patients have the pterygium surgically removed and re-fit the scleral lens after surgery.

Pinguecula (Greg DeNaeyer, OD, FAAO, FSLS)

Pingueculae are a common clinical finding that typically do not impact general contact lens fitting. Soft lenses or hybrid lenses often can drape over these scleral obstacles without issue. Corneal GP, intralimbal lenses or smaller, are out of range for the typical nasal or temporal positioned pinguecula. However, scleral lenses have a large enough diameter that pingueculae have the potential to complicate fitting, especially because the rigid surface is not able to conform to these isolated bumps. With that said, most of the time mild pingueculae do not negatively impact the patient's comfort or health with scleral lens wear. In my experience, scleral lenses that land on pingueculae with a relatively low elevation profile rarely cause issues, which allows the practitioner to fit standard scleral lenses without special design considerations. For relatively elevated pingueculae (Fig. **1**) or when the edge of the scleral lens digs into the pinguecula (Fig. **2**), modifications might be necessary to ensure that the scleral lens is comfortable and doesn't lead to irritation and redness.

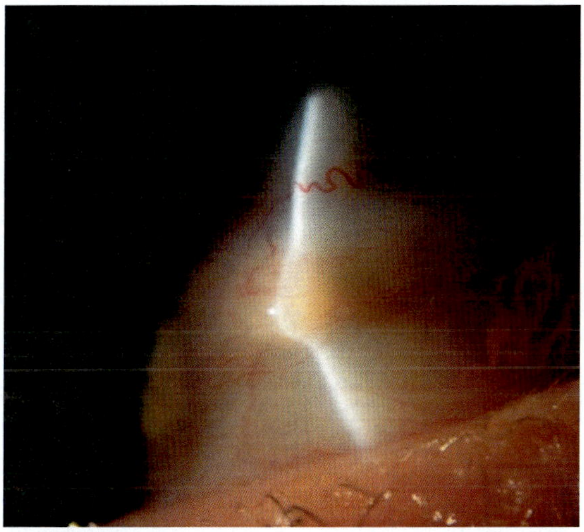

Fig. (1). Example of a highly elevated pinguecula as demonstrated with an optic section. Image courtesy of Greg DeNaeyer.

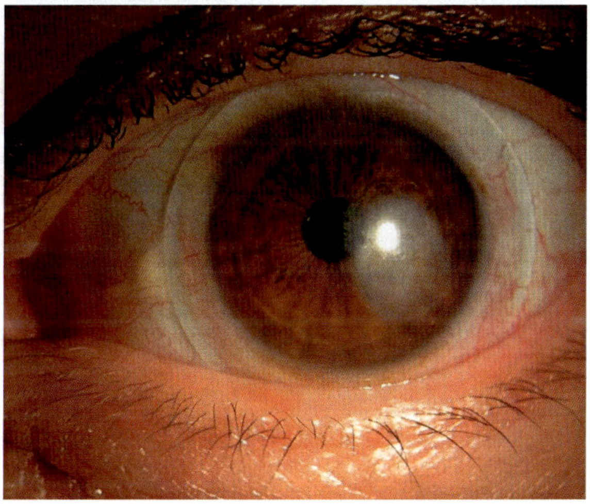

Fig. (2). Example of impingement and compression of the nasal pinguecula. Image courtesy of Greg DeNaeyer.

I carefully examine an initial diagnostic scleral lens on a patient's eye. If the haptic section of the lens doesn't contact the pinguecula or if it rests on the surface of the elevation without any apparent edge lift, then I proceed with the standard fitting process. If the haptic edge of the scleral lens imbeds into the pinguecula or it cause edge lift, then I consider modifying the approach. The easiest modification is to decrease the diameter of the lens design. Decreasing the lens diameter by 1mm or 2mm is sometimes enough to avoid the pinguecula but hopefully won't impact the lenses vaulting capability. For pinguecula that reside relatively close to the limbus or where reducing the diameter isn't a good option, then you can add a design modification to bypass the pinguecula. Asymmetric lens vaults or microvaults can be used to vault over the region of the pinguecula. The lens must be stabilized with ballasting or back surface toric haptics. The axis and amount of peripheral vault should be communicated to the fitting consultant. Photographs of a diagnostic lens can be helpful. A measurement can also be made from corneo-scleral topography (Fig. **3**). The consultant can use these measurements to exactly create a vault over the pinguecula while simultaneously designing the rest of the lens including customized back surface toricity. Alternatively, a notch can be beveled out of the lens edge to literally allow the lens to bypass the pinguecula. A notched lens may rotationally stabilize on its own or stabilizing techniques such as a ballast or back toric might be needed. A notched diagnostic lens is helpful for measurement. In addition, measurements can be utilized from corneo-scleral topography. Of note, the patient must apply the scleral lens with the notch in the direction of the pinguecula.

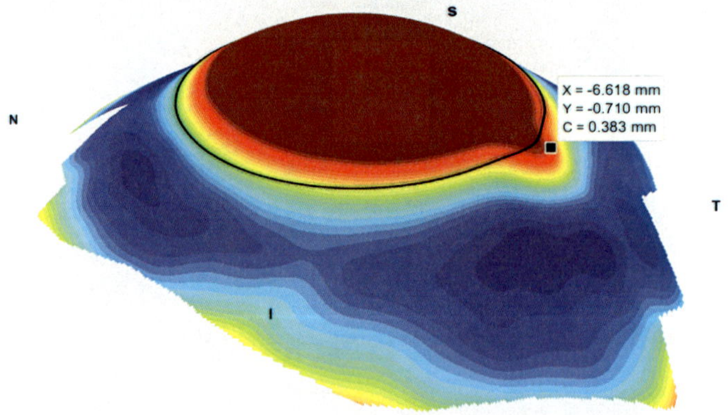

Fig. (3). Corneo-scleral topography map demonstrating elevation in red and a recession of the tissue in blue. Image courtesy of Greg DeNaeyer.

Conjunctival Hypertrophy and Nodules (Esther-Simone Visser PhD)

A conjunctival nodule is a relatively common condition characterized by a localized elevated area on the bulbar conjunctiva (Fig. **4**). Although treatment is generally not indicated, its presence can complicate scleral lens wear, as illustrated in Fig. (**5**). Moreover, early conjunctival hypertrophy (a precursor to the development of a conjunctival nodule) can arise as the result of scleral lens impingement [1].

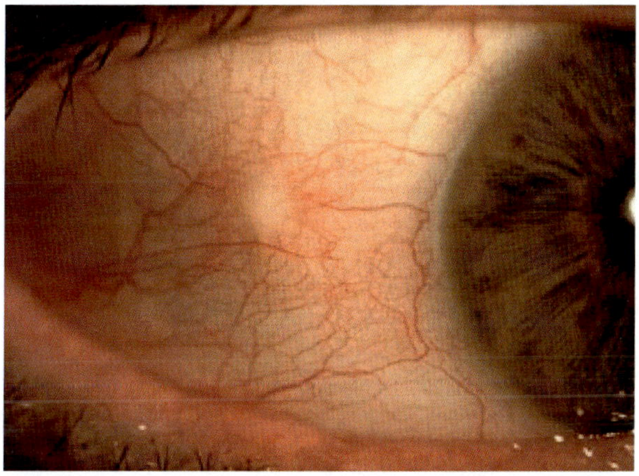

Fig. (4). A conjunctival nodule (arrow). Image courtesy of H.M. Otten.

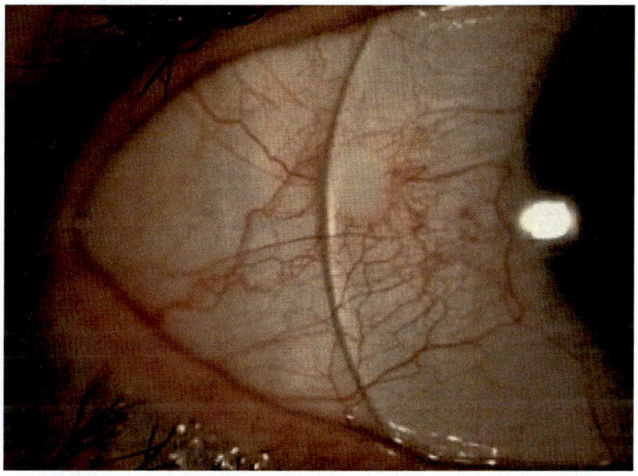

Fig. (5). The presence of a conjunctival nodule can complicate scleral lens wear. Image courtesy of H.M. Otten.

Soft contact lenses can usually adapt to fit the shape of most bulbar surface irregularities; however, because of their rigid nature, scleral lenses cannot adapt to these irregularities [2]. As a result, the elevated nodule can become compressed by the scleral zone and/or edge of the scleral lens. This compression can have a significant impact on local ocular physiology causing increased swelling and redness of the nodule and can reduce the lens user's tolerance by increasing awareness of the lens and causing discomfort and/or pain. Therefore, this compression should be minimized as much as possible.

Correctly fitting a scleral lens requires achieving properly balanced bearing of the scleral zone without causing impingement or excessive compression. In this respect, focal elevations such as conjunctival nodules can pose a challenge in achieving a proper fit.

To overcome this challenge, several strategies can be used to optimize lens fit and reduce mechanical pressure from the scleral lens on the nodule. These strategies include:

- Modifying the lens fit by improving scleral zone alignment. Because the scleral surface is often asymmetrical [3], toric (or quadrant-specific) scleral lens designs can improve lens fit [4]. The degree of back-surface toricity should be optimized to minimize localized conjunctival impingement.
- If the nodule is located in the periphery, a smaller diameter scleral lens that does not interfere with the nodule can be used (Fig. **6**).
- In the event of a mid-peripheral nodule, a larger diameter scleral lens can be used. In this case, the scleral radius should be as steep as possible (while avoiding a steep edge fit) to vault the elevation and avoid compressing the nodule.
- Some practitioners have instructed the lens manufacturer to create a small "notch" in the lens to avoid contacting the nodule [2, 5]. However, if the notch is too large, air bubbles can be introduced beneath the lens [2]. This strategy also has the disadvantage of leading to unpredictable lens performance, particularly regarding the interaction between the edge of the lens and the anterior scleral surface, leading to poor reproducibility.

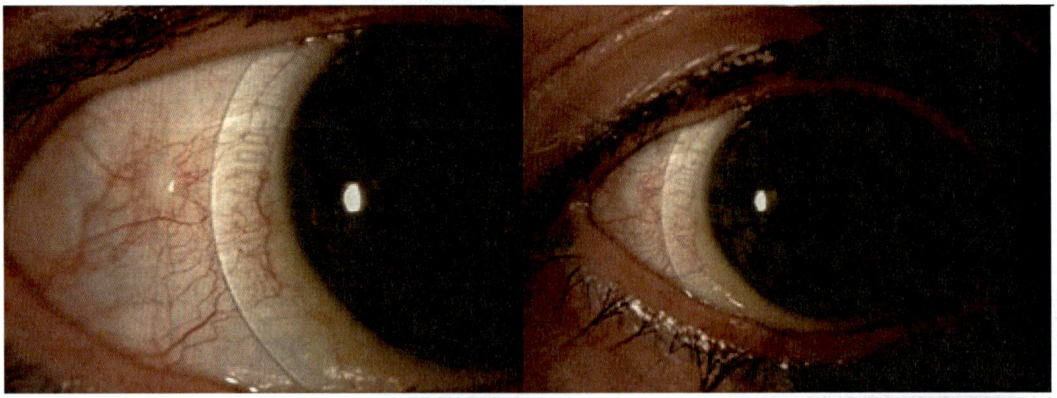

Fig. (6). A smaller diameter scleral lens can prevent interference between a peripheral nodule and the lens. Images courtesy of H.M. Otten.

During fitting, the scleral zone should be assessed circumferentially as the patients move their eyes in all directions. However, the fit should also be evaluated with the lens in the primary position (or as close to the primary position as possible), as the interaction between the lens and the nodule can have a false appearance due to lens decentration induced by eye movements.

If the aforementioned strategies and suggestions do not provide a suitable fit and mechanical pressure from the lens on the nodule remains, the steps provided below may help improve the patient's comfort and tolerance. These steps can also be used in patients with early conjunctival hypertrophy; however, it is important to monitor the patient closely and adjust the lens fit if the condition progresses.

- Apply a few drops of a non-preserved lubricant containing hyaluronic acid (if available) in the lens and eye just before inserting the lens and reapply regularly during lens wear.
- Decrease lens wearing time, and periodically remove the lenses combined with the previous tip.
- If the nodule is located close to the lens edge, care should be used when removing the lens. After applying rewetting drops, a plunger can be placed just inside the lens edge adjacent to the nodule and used to lift the lens without applying pressure to the nodule.

In patients who are susceptible to developing conjunctival hypertrophy and/or conjunctival nodules, the use of eye drops containing hyaluronic acid can help prevent these conditions by providing a "cushion" effect between the lens and the ocular surface. In advanced and/or active cases, it may become necessary to temporarily stop scleral lens wear; in these cases, the practitioner may consider prescribing a corneal rigid gas-permeable (RGP) lens, a specialty soft lens, or a hybrid lens [2].

Conjunctival Hypertrophy and Scleral Lenses (Jason Jedlicka, OD, FAAO, FSLS)

Conjunctival hypertrophy is an enlargement of the conjunctival cells, typically due to chronic, low-grade trauma or damage to the cells. Scleral lens edges, when poorly fit, can lead to conjunctival hypertrophy.

The human sclera is rarely symmetric in its shape. This irregularity of shape adds to the challenge of fitting scleral lenses in some cases. When scleral lens edges are focally tight, they can impinge on the sclera and "pinch" the overlying conjunctival tissue. When left in this state without modification for weeks or months, the conjunctiva will undergo hypertrophy of the cells external to the lens edge. Often the tight lens edge will cause mild discomfort or awareness, but as conjunctival hypertrophy increases, patient symptoms will often increase as well, reaching a point where adjustments will need to be made to the lens design. Fluorescein application will typically demonstrate that the area of hypertrophy stains. Modifying a scleral lens to lessen conjunctival hypertrophy can take the form of a diameter change or localized adjustment to the lens edge profile. Changing the diameter is the most straightforward approach. This can include either decreasing the diameter to pull the lens edge away from the area of hypertrophy, or increasing the diameter to cover the area of hypertrophy.

Scleral shape tends to be more regular as you approach the limbus, and increasingly more toric / asymmetric moving away from the limbus. If the area of impingement is due to a highly asymmetric scleral shape, decreasing the diameter may be of benefit. This will only be possible if decreasing the diameter is possible without altering the lens fit in an otherwise adverse way. Increasing the diameter is another option. By making the lens larger, the edge profile can often be flattened to reduce the impingement while still allowing for a wide enough landing area to avoid loose edge related problems. Changes in diameter will need to be significant in order to impact the fit with a change of at least 1 mm smaller or larger have an impact. Over time, and with the offending stimulus taken away, conjunctival hypertrophy will resolve.

Glaucoma Drainage Device (Michael Lipson, OD, FAAO, FSLS)

Some patients have complicated cases of glaucoma and have previously been treated with a surgical placement of a bleb or a glaucoma drainage device (GDD). The placement of these devices varies by surgeon and ocular anatomy.

The presence of a GDD is not necessarily a contraindication for scleral lens fitting. However, its presence can create a problem if the scleral lens abuts the GDD. This may alter the intended function of the device and potentially compromise it.

A GDD presents a scleral fitting challenge for three reasons. First is the location, second is the effect on the fit/landing and third is the cosmetic appearance (redness) when the lens is worn. I have found three fitting modifications that may help resolve these issues. Generally, efforts are made to avoid the lens edge from touching the GDD. These include using a smaller lens diameter, lens notching and specifying a local area of increased clearance (microvault). These may be done independently or in combination.

First, verify with the glaucoma specialist that the eye is healed and can sustain scleral lens wear.

Smaller Lens – Decreasing the diameter is a simple modification that can avoid contact with the GDD. Depending on the corneal diameter and the location of the device, this could involve lenses in the range of 14.0 to 15.0 mm. As a reminder, when using smaller scleral lenses, there is a smaller landing area of lens to bear on the sclera.

Notching the lens – To avoid touching the GDD while maintaining the same lens diameter, a notch can be contoured in the edge of the lens. This method necessitates the use of a lens that is rotationally stable. Initially, a scleral lens should be fit to ensure the rotational stability with using toricity in the landing zone, prism ballast or a double thin zone design. Once stability is established, the location and depth of the notch can be marked or described to the laboratory consultant with a specified axis and depth.

Specifying a localized area of increased clearance (microvaulting)–This process involves lathing a vaulted hemispherical portion of the lens edge overlying the location of the GDD. As a result, there is reduced bearing over the GDD. As described above, a rotationally stable lens is required to keep the lens oriented over the area of interest.

Even with a GDD, the modifications to scleral lenses described above can allow for a successful fit. At follow-up visits in these cases, in addition to evaluating the corneal health and scleral lens fitting characteristics, intraocular pressure should be monitored regularly.

Conjunctival Blebs (Greg DeNaeyer, OD, FAAO, FSLS)

Conjunctival blebs result as a secondary consequence of glaucoma surgery and are typically located superiorly above the cornea. The bulbar conjunctiva is elevated secondary to aqueous that has been directed into the subconjunctival space. The elevation and location of a bleb can vary dramatically depending on the type of surgery and particularities of the patient's case. Typically, blebs secondary to trabeculectomies reside closer to the limbus than those that form secondary to tube shunt procedures. These elevated scleral obstacles can interfere with scleral lens fitting if the patient requires a GP contact lens for high ametropia or corneal irregularity. If a patient has a conjunctival bleb I consider starting with a corneal GP lens to completely avoid the bleb. The corneal GP needs to be fit as an interpalpebral design to avoid mechanical insult of the bleb from the lens edge that can occur if the corneal GP rides high, such as the case with a lid attachment fit. If a corneal GP won't center or spontaneously dislodges, a scleral lens can be fit to improve stability. For blebs that are proximal to the limbus, mechanical interaction between the bleb and the scleral lens can cause tissue erosion, which can lead to a bleb leak. Additionally, a scleral lens may compress a bleb reducing its functionality. To avoid these complications, the practitioner should design a scleral lens that avoids physical interaction with the conjunctival bleb. One way to avoid interaction between the scleral lens and the bleb is to design a scleral lens that incorporates a beveled notch within the haptic that will allow the lens to bypass the bleb (Fig. **7**).

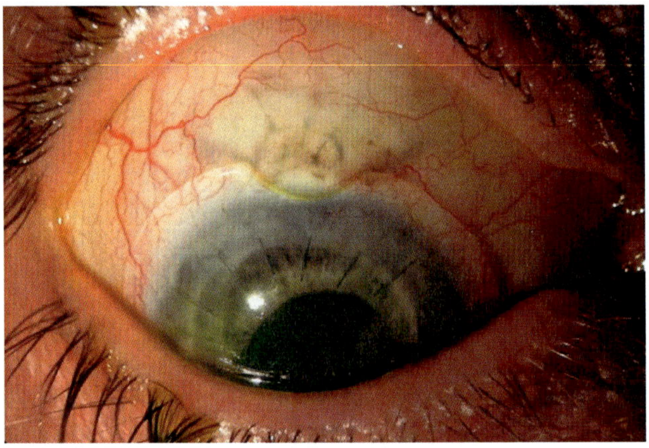

Fig. (7). Example of a scleral lens with a superior beveled notch to accommodate the elevation. Image courtesy of Greg DeNaeyer.

Measurement and photographs will aid the laboratory consultant to estimate the size of the notch required for a successful fit. A pre-notched diagnostic scleral lens that the practitioner can keep in their fitting set can be helpful for diagnostic evaluation. Corneo-scleral topography can be used for measurement of the bleb size and location, which allow consultants to more accurately bevel the amount of haptic for adequate clearance (Fig. **8**).

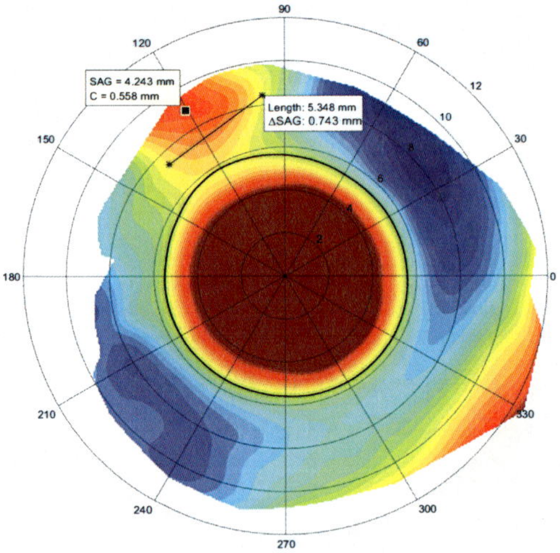

Fig. (8). Example of corneo-scleral topography measuring the superior elevation length, depth and angle. Image courtesy of Greg DeNaeyer.

Mini-scleral lenses are recommended because they will require relatively smaller notches. Deeper notches for larger scleral lenses may induce bubble formation within the liquid reservoir. Once successfully fit, the patient is directed to apply the scleral lens so the notch matches with the bleb. Alternatively, a microvault can be used to avoid scleral lens interaction with a conjunctival bleb. Measurement and photographs or corneo-scleral topography can be sent to the manufacturing laboratory for assessment and design. Scleral lens designs with microvaults need to be stabilized with ballast, double slab off prisms, or toric back surface haptics. The conjunctival bleb of a tube shunt may be far enough from the limbus that a standard scleral lens can be used without complication (Fig. **9**). Monitor these patients for mechanically related injury to the bleb secondary to the lens. Injuries could result in bleb leak or increased intraocular pressure secondary to bleb compression.

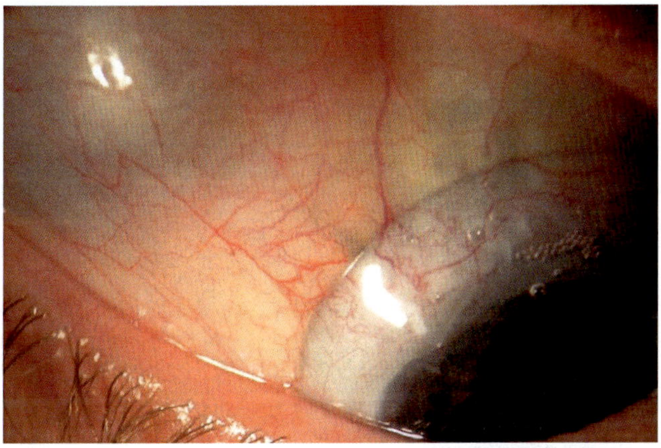

Fig. (9). A mini-scleral lens avoids touching or landing on the elevated conjunctival bleb. Image courtesy of Greg DeNaeyer.

Scleral Lenses Following Glaucoma Surgery (Henny M. Otten, BOptom, FAAO, FSLS)

Glaucoma surgery is generally indicated when medical therapy is unable to maintain stable intraocular pressure (IOP) or fails to treat the underlying condition. Moreover, patients with a specific condition such as penetrating keratoplasty are more likely to develop secondary glaucoma [6], thereby requiring glaucoma surgery. Several surgical approaches are currently available for reducing IOP, including trabeculectomy, placement of a glaucoma drain implant (GDI) such as a Baerveldt GDI or Ahmed GDI with a valve and placement of a glaucoma filtration device (Ex-PRESS). Following glaucoma surgery, if the cornea is irregular and contact lens correction is needed, several contact lens options are available. When selecting a suitable lens, it is important that the lens does not interfere with IOP. Moreover, when present, a glaucoma drainage device or glaucoma filtration bleb should not be irritated by the contact lens or scleral lens. Rigid gas-permeable lenses and a piggyback system can be used; if these are not tolerated, scleral lenses can be used, albeit with certain caveats. The possibilities with respect to scleral lenses include:

1. A mini-scleral lens with a toric periphery in the smallest diameter.
2. A mini-scleral lens with or without truncation.
3. A large scleral lens with a notch [7, 8]; a proper fit can be achieved after notching (*i.e.*, truncation-placing a flat part in the edge of the lens), but this approach can have disadvantages, including:
   a. Difficulty making a suitable notch to prevent irritation of the conjunctiva and the filtration bleb or GDI, and
   b. The formation of a bubble behind the lens.
4. A large scleral lens with truncation; the same advantages and disadvantages noted above for notching apply.

Trabeculectomy

Trabeculectomy is a suitable procedure for lowering IOP and for providing long-term maintenance of normal IOP. The complications associated with trabeculectomy include leakage of the filtration bleb and the risk of infection, particularly with a thin bleb [9]. If a lens is prescribed, it must be fitted properly in order to minimize irritation. Currently available options include a large scleral lens with a notch [7, 8] and a mini-scleral lens or a toric mini scleral lens with a flat periphery (Fig. **10**), which may not rest entirely on the filtration bleb, thereby minimizing pressure on the bleb itself (Fig. **11**). If maintaining good vision requires the use of a scleral lens, a fornix-based conjunctival flap is preferred [10].

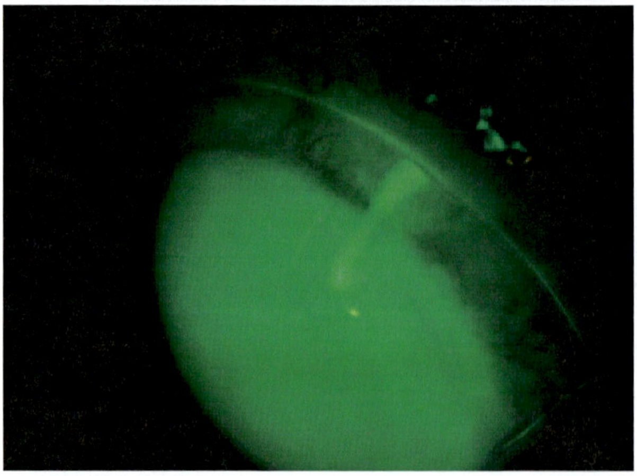

Fig. (10). A toric mini-scleral lens with a flat periphery; the flat axis is stabilizing in the direction of the conjunctival bleb. Image courtesy of H. M. Otten.

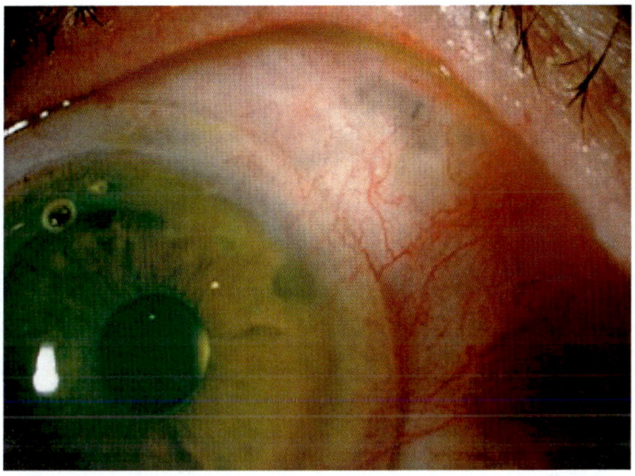

Fig. (11). A toric mini-scleral lens with a flat periphery overlying a small part of the conjunctival bleb. Image courtesy of H. M. Otten.

In cases in which a large, soft lens fails, a temporary, large scleral lens can be used to restore the anterior chamber, particularly in cases with extremely low IOP and/or when hypotony maculopathy occurs [11].

Glaucoma Drain Implants

A Baerveldt or Ahmed valve can be placed on the ocular bulbus, with a small tube shunt placed in the anterior chamber. The Baerveldt implant has a large capacity, whereas the Ahmed implant has a relatively small capacity but includes a valve for regulation. The implant can be based either in the limbal area or in the fornix; however, fitting of a scleral lens is generally easier if the valve is fornix-based (Fig. **12**).

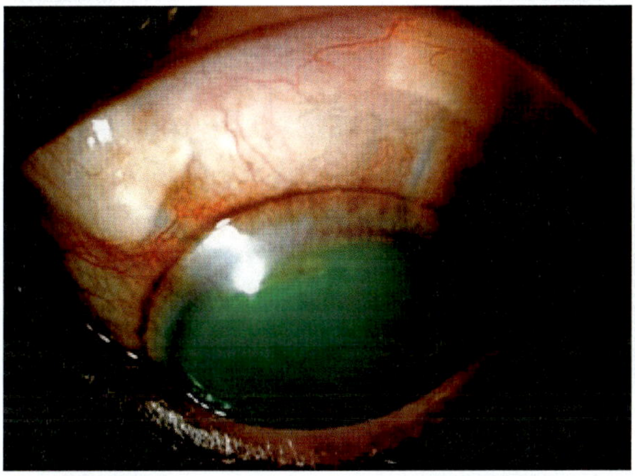

Fig. (12). A toric mini-scleral lens with two Baerveldt implants; one of the scleral patches is placed in the fornix area. Image courtesy of H. M. Otten.

The risk associated with wearing a scleral lens is blockage of the underlying tube shunt; to minimize this risk, a large scleral lens with a notch or a mini-scleral lens with the smallest diameter can be used. A toric mini-scleral lens with a flat edge lift in the horizontal axis is a good approach for minimizing pressure on the tube shunt. When a scleral lens is indicated, the preference is to place the GDI in the fornix and the scleral patch (Fig. **13**) at least 3-4 mm from the limbal area [12].

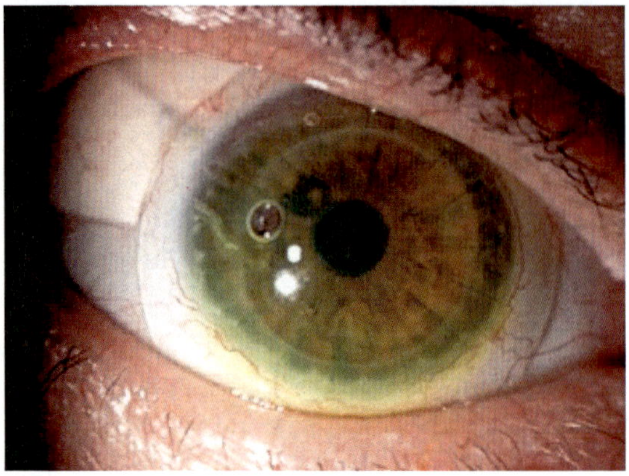

Fig. (13). A toric mini -scleral lens fitted with the scleral patch placed outside of the limbal area. Image courtesy of H. M. Otten.

Glaucoma Filtration Device (*e.g.*, the Ex-PRESS Miniature Glaucoma Shunt)

The Ex-PRESS glaucoma filtration device is placed directly in the limbal area, with an overlying small filtration bleb [13]. Both full scleral lenses and mini-scleral lenses can be used, provided there is no compression on the small filtration bleb and provided that the bleb can function normally without affecting IOP (Fig. **14**).

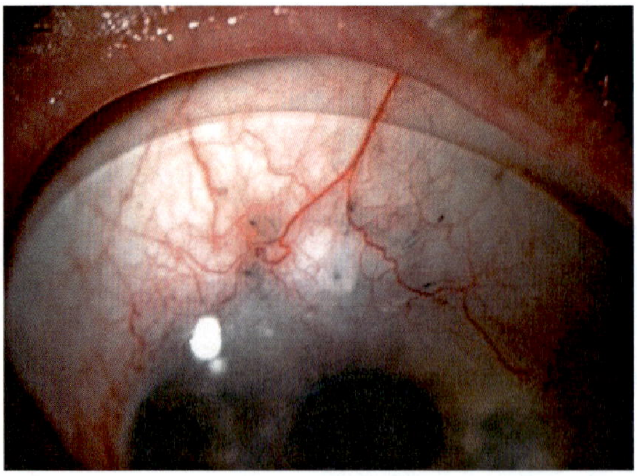

Fig. (14). A large toric scleral lens placed over a flat scleral flap with an underlying glaucoma filtration device. Image courtesy of H. M. Otten.

In summary, scleral lenses can be helpful for correcting irregular astigmatism after keratoplasty following glaucoma surgery. However, the lens should be designed in such a way that it does not disturb the function of a filtration bleb or drain implant.

Symblepharon and Scleral Lenses (Jason Jedlicka, OD, FAAO, FSLS)

Symblepharon can be a significant added challenge to scleral lens fitting, while being an indication for scleral lenses at the same time. Symblepharon is a partial or complete adhesion of the palpebral conjunctiva to the bulbar conjunctiva, resulting from trauma or a disease process. Causative conditions include Stevens-Johnson syndrome, ocular cicatricial pemphigoid, chemical injury, erythema multiforme, and severe conjunctival infection. These diseases can cause symptoms of pain, irritation, and blurred vision due to damage to the ocular surface beyond the symblepharon. In order to manage these symptoms, scleral lenses can be fitted to improve quality of life.

If a symblepharon is not present at the time of fitting, scleral lens fitting can proceed as planned. However, in chronic conditions, symblepharon can still form and the eye should be monitored for signs of new adhesions, as they may alter the fit or patient satisfaction with the lens over time. In addition, in rare cases, a scleral lens that is poorly fitted may exacerbate the conjunctiva and pose a potential added risk for symblepharon formation through added inflammation. However, more frequently, a scleral lens can act as a barrier to reduce the risk of adhesion formation [14].

When fitting a scleral lens to an eye with a symblepharon that is already present, there are considerations to be made to optimize the outcome. Location of the symblepharon is crucial to lens fitting. When symblepharon are located far enough away from the cornea, a scleral lens can be fitted without significant modification in many cases. Choosing a lens diameter as large as possible while avoiding significant interaction with an area of adhesion is helpful in mitigating the advancement of the symblepharon. However, changes in the shape of the ocular surface as a result of the adhesions can complicate scleral lens fitting. Balancing the ability to obtain an optimal fit and maximize lens diameter will need to be determined by the practitioner.

When the area of symblepharon approaches the cornea, the lens may require significant customization to achieve an optimal fit. This can be done through notching a lens corresponding to the adhesion, creating a localized vault in the lens edge to accommodate an adhesion, or creating a completely freeform lens design to align the lens to even the most irregularly shaped conjunctiva. The decision how to best manage these situations will depend upon the specific case, but all options should be considered to achieve a best-fit situation.

IMPRESSION BASED SCLERAL LENSES

Scleral impression molding was the original technique for fitting scleral lenses. Its benefits allow close alignment of the scleral lens to the anatomy of the scleral surface. This classic technique is still being practiced in several parts of the world. Current advancements in technology allow 3D scanning of molds to create new scleral lens designs. The authors will describe their experience with either the classic technique or the latest impression based technology in the form of EyePrintPRO™.

Impression Molded Scleral Lenses (Jennifer McMahon, BOptom, MCOptom, FBDO)

There are some clinical situations where a scleral lens is clearly indicated however, the fitting process proves to be difficult using preformed diagnostic lenses. In such cases, scleral lenses can be custom made from an eye impression or mold of the eye.

Indications

The main are two main indications for taking an eye impression:

1. Insufficient Alignment of the Scleral Landing Zone

Asymmetry or localised irregularity of the ocular surface sometimes cannot be catered for sufficiently by modifying the peripheral configuration or changing the diameter of preformed scleral lens designs. This may cause failure to seal or, conversely, unacceptable compression of the underlying tissue. Examples of irregularities include pingueculae, pterygia and glaucoma drainage tubes.

2. Atypical Corneal Profile

Eccentric corneal apices can encroach the transition zone of a scleral lens making it difficult to vault the area with preformed designs. In other, more symmetrical, cases there may be a big difference between the flattest and steepest zones of the cornea such as proud plateau grafts or advanced nipple cones. Both situations can create very irregular corneal clearance patterns – excessive in some areas and minimal in others. This can result in failure to seal, decentration, poor visual acuity or difficulty inserting without bubbles.

It could be considered that impression scleral lenses are required less frequently than perhaps ten years ago since currently there is much greater potential for modifications to preformed designs due to advances in lens design and manufacturing capabilities. The back surface peripheral configuration of many designs can now be modified circumferentially, to a toric or even a quadrant specific specification. Conversely, it could be argued that with the increasing use of scleral lenses for a wider range of pathologies, the need for impression lenses may well come to the fore once more.

Molding Materials

Historically, alginates were used as the primary molding material; however, practice in the UK has largely changed to the use of polyvinyl siloxane (PVS) as it causes less post-impression corneal staining and the molds do not appear to degrade as quickly.

PVS is dispensed into the impression tray *via* a mixing device. The silicone based monomer and the initiator come from separate cartridges and are combined in the mixing tip where the polymerization process begins.

Procedure

- Instill local anesthetic
- Give patient a fixation target
- Deliver the impression material into an impression tray
- Wait 20-30 seconds
- Ask the patient to look down
- Retract the upper lid and slide the upper edge of the tray onto the superior globe under the upper lid
- Ask the patient to look straight ahead
- Support the impression tray and retract lower lid to bring over the bottom edge
- Gently rotate the tray *in situ* and move gently to spread impression material
- Hold in position until impression material appears to be set on the outside of tray
- Retract the upper lid and slowly ease impression tray from the globe

Manufacture

Once the eye impression has been taken, a cast is acquired of the mold using dental stone and is sent to the lab.

The cast is scanned, and a CAD program is used to create a representative three-dimensional model. This can then be manipulated in terms of its z coordinates to elevate the optic zone to allow for corneal clearance.

This information is inverted and sent to a lathe to cut the back surface of the required lens.

Fitting Process

Usually a first stage fitting shell is produced in PMMA material from the modified file. This is examined on eye to check for optimum fitting characteristics and can be modified by hand if necessary using appropriate tools to increase clearance, alter the edge profile or reduce diameter.

Once the lens fit is considered optimum, the shell can be cast, scanned and then reproduced in RGP material.

Conclusion

Impression scleral lenses are a significant clinical undertaking not least because of the underlying pathology where molding is required. However, advances in manufacturing have made the process of impression scleral lens production more predictable and reproducible. Impression scleral lenses remain a vital tool in the armory for the serious scleral lens practitioner.

Impression Molded Scleral Lenses with EyePrintPRO™ (S. Barry Eiden, OD, FAAO)

In the management of irregular corneas with contact lenses, the challenge is always to provide optimized visual performance along with comfort in lens wear and, of course, appropriate physiological response. However, there are many cases where the degree of ocular surface irregularity is so great that even with conventional scleral lenses, we can't achieve the required lens to ocular surface fitting relationships. In these cases, we are privileged to be able to provide totally customized fitting of a scleral prosthetic with the use of EyePrintPRO™.

The ability to take an impression of the ocular surface and design a virtually "3-D printed" prosthetic lens has allowed us to address the needs of the most advanced cases of ocular surface irregularity. When all else has failed, the EyePrintPRO™ has given us an option to help the most desperate of cases. A wonderful example among others, we have treated is of a middle-aged gentleman with highly, advanced keratoconus. He failed numerous attempts in the past with corneal gas permeable lenses. He could not tolerate conventional scleral lenses due to complications of either bearing over the most anteriorly displaced portions of his cornea or excessive vaulting over the less involved areas of his cornea. His only option provided by prior eye care practitioners was to have a penetrating keratoplasty. He wanted to avoid a corneal transplant if at all possible. We proceeded with the utilization of EyePrintPRO™ and were able to provide an excellent physical fit along with very good vision (acuity of 20/30 and significant reduction of high order aberrations). The patient has been wearing the EyePrintPRO™ now for over 2 years without any evidence of physiological compromise.

We appreciate additional technological developments available now and some still in development with EyePrintPRO™ including the correction of residual high order aberrations, as well as the use of toric and prism correction as well as presbyopic correction, thus making the EyePrintPRO™ an even more powerful tool in our armamentarium for the management of ocular surface disease and irregularity.

CORNEAL CHALLENGES

Whether fitting a scleral lens over an irregular cornea, a diseased cornea, or a normal cornea, the physiology of the cornea needs to be supported and optimized. As with any type of contact lens wear, infiltrates, edema and neovascularization can occur. If these findings are present prior to initiating the scleral lens fitting, they should be well-documented, and efforts to reduce or eliminate these abnormalities should be made. The authors describe the challenges of subepithelial infiltrates, corneal edema and neovascularization with respect to scleral lenses. Since corneal transplants are also a main indication for scleral lens fitting, the contributors will also discuss graft rejection.

Corneal Infiltrates (Michael Lipson, OD, FAAO, FSLS)

In my experience, infiltrates (Fig. **15**) are rarely observed with scleral lens wear. In general, infiltrates are an inflammatory reaction to a bacterial, viral or chemical presence. Diagnosing and eliminating the source of an offending entity can be challenging. A careful history of lens care products, eye drops, solution, soaps, skin care products and other potential chemical exposure is critical.

If infiltrates are present, I ensure that only preservative free saline is used for filling the bowl of the lens and single use vials are discarded after one use. When treating infiltrates, preservative free topical medications should be substituted if possible. Lubricating drops should be preservative free. The patients should make sure that hand soap is thoroughly rinsed from their hands prior to handling their lenses. Skin or hand creams should be avoided prior to lens application. After lens application, patients should avoid use of facial creams near eyes and eyelids. Lastly, patients should avoid exposure to highly vaporous cleaning agents (bleach, acids).

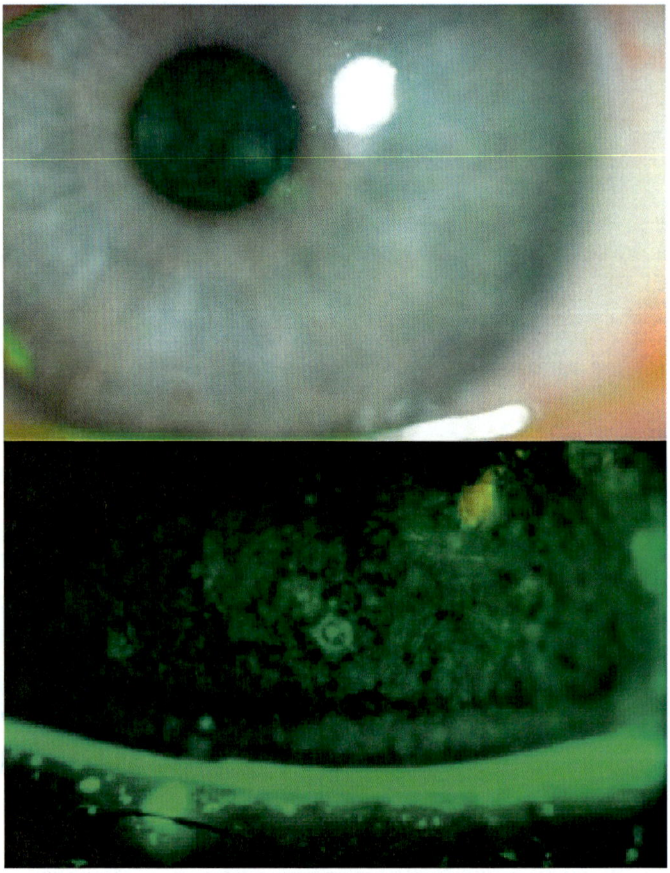

Fig. (15). Atypical paracentral infiltrates in patient with a history of chronic graft *versus* host disease. Infiltrates resolved with topical corticosteroids and temporary cessation of scleral lenses. The bottom image is the same patient featured in the top image. Images courtesy of Lynette Johns.

Corneal Infiltrates (Maria K. Walker, OD, MS, FAAO, FSLS)

Subepithelial corneal infiltrates (SEI) are the accumulation of immune cells in the corneal stroma, most often appearing in the peripheral cornea due to the proximity of limbal vasculature to this area. Bacteria or bacterial byproducts and endotoxins are the most common cause, but other infectious and non-infectious agents can also be the culprits. There has been limited research on the risk factors of SEIs or their incidence during scleral lens wear; however, in my experience, infiltrates are not a particularly common complication that I see in my scleral lens patients. I do not consider patients in scleral lenses to be at specific risk for SEIs. However, when SEIs present in a scleral lens wearer, I regard them as a potentially serious condition.

First of all, if I see an infiltrate, or several infiltrates, I always consider the underlying state of the corneal health of the patient. I expect to see these types of events more commonly in an ocular surface disease patient, but do not expect it as readily in a keratoconus patient. It is important to meticulously evaluate the cornea prior to initiating scleral lens wear, since many corneas that are candidates for scleral lenses demonstrate scarring, neovascularization, and perhaps infiltrates. This baseline data is important to be able to properly follow and manage the scleral lens treatment, especially on diseased eyes. As with all treatments, we need to carefully consider the specific cause of the infiltrative event on each individual patient. Below are the main causes that I consider when evaluating SEIs on a scleral lens patient, and the courses of action to mitigate them. Keep in mind that the causes of SEIs are often multifactorial, and often a combination of these factors collectively creates an infiltrative event.

1. ***Infection*** - If the cause is due to an active infectious invasion, there is going to be an epithelial break, and probably a much bigger overall reaction within the cornea and surrounding tissue. The state of the rest of the eye and adnexa are also big factors in determining whether or not the infiltrates are sterile or infectious. I look carefully at the anterior chamber, adjacent conjunctiva, and surrounding corneal stroma for edema to determine if the cause seems to be an active infection. These cases need to be treated like other contact lens related infections – with strong and aggressive anti-infective medications. Lens wear is discontinued until the infection clears, and I often use steroids to reduce the infiltrates once the infective agent is controlled.
2. ***Tear Reservoir contamination*** – This is a new and unique avenue for noxious agents to linger and provoke inflammation during scleral lens wear. Fortunately, we don't see a high rate of microbial keratitis in scleral lens wearers, but we do see patients who have non-specific inflammation with scleral lenses. I always look closely at the cornea when I see patients with other inflammatory signs during scleral lens wear, and don't often see infiltrates. If there are infiltrates and there does not appear to be adequate replenishment of the tear film reservoir, different application solutions such as preservative free artificial tears can be explored, or lens changes can be made to maximize tear exchange.
3. ***Lens contamination*** – bacterial adhesions to contact lenses are classic inducers of corneal infiltrates. All my patients with SEIs are instructed to use a peroxide cleaning system to reduce the buildup of bacteria and other contaminants on the surface of the lens.
4. ***Blepharitis*** – Patients with SEIs during scleral lens wear should be treated to reduce the bacterial buildup on the lashes and eyelid margins. SEIs can be precipitated by the sloughing of bacteria and endotoxins on the lids/lashes into the tear film.

5. ***Lens solutions*** – contact lens cleaning and application solutions can interact negatively with the lens and the ocular surface to create inflammation and SEIs. Some patients with sensitive eyes have to develop a very specific and meticulous routine with scleral lens care in order to mitigate inflammation, so I work with each on an individual basis to determine what system works best for each patient. The specific regimen for each patient is often unique to them, but certainly the most common recommendation I give is to use a peroxide cleaning system and all preservative-free application products to reduce solution-induced SEIs.

Other than reducing all these underlying causes for an infiltrative event, I usually acutely treat with an antibiotic/steroid combination drop to reduce the inflammatory response as well as the bacterial load on the ocular surface. I try to reduce or discontinue lens wear during treatment, specifically if the patient is symptomatic. If the patient is asymptomatic and the reaction is mild, I do not necessarily discontinue lens wear in the sclera lens population. Overall, I regard infiltrative events as potentially serious, but don't see them as especially problematic or with frequency in my scleral lens patients.

Corneal Edema (Maria K. Walker, OD, MS, FAAO, FSLS)

I consider corneal edema to be a significant factor to consider when fitting and managing scleral lens wear. This topic continues to be hotly debated between many practitioners and researchers who question whether or not there is corneal swelling during scleral lens wear, and whether or not we should be concerned about it.

At this point, most experts will agree that there is a degree of corneal swelling that occurs during scleral lens wear, but there is still some debate about its potential detriments. In our clinic, corneal edema during scleral lens wear typically occurs in the range of 5-6%, and in some individuals, it is more concerning. During an examination, there are a few questions that I ask myself in order to determine my management of scleral lens wear in regard to corneal swelling.

1. **How much swelling occurs during lens wear?** Baseline pachymetry measurements should be taken prior to initiating scleral lens wear. Pachymetry should be measured at follow-up appointments to determine changes in thickness. However, it may be complicated. There are many factors to consider when looking at the change in corneal thickness throughout scleral lens wear. Are the measurements being taken at the same time during the day? How long have the lenses been worn prior to measuring (1 hour, 8 hours)? How long has it been since lens removal prior to the measurements (5 minutes or 30 minutes)? Are the thickness measurements being confounded by disease

progression? These are all questions to consider before determining how much swelling is truly occurring in an individual patient.

2. **How much corneal swelling is there?** Different practitioners have varying comfort levels regarding the amount of corneal swelling. Depending on individual disease states, the amount of corneal swelling should be somewhat variable for each patient. In my average patients (which aren't in reality so average), I start to have concerns with more than 40 µm swelling, and definitely if there is greater than 50 µm (40-50 is the danger zone). I try not to go by percent swelling, since we are often dealing with corneas that are very thin or thick relative to normal corneas and may appear as more or less severe if measured by percent of swelling.
3. **What should be done when we see corneal swelling that is outside of our comfort zone?** If corneal swelling is occurring at an amount which is determined to be too great (40-50 µm in most patients), there are a few steps I take to maximize oxygen availability to the cornea.
   a. Tear Reservoir Thickness – I try to reduce the tear reservoir thickness to about 75 µm in the shallowest location. I also manipulate the limbal clearance to reduce excessive limbal clearance.
   b. Tear Exchange – Maximizing tear exchange can help deliver more oxygen to the cornea. To evaluate tear exchange, I apply fluorescein over the top of the scleral lens after the lens has settled to evaluate the presence of tear exchange. If tear exchange is not present, I will alter the haptic zone toricity and/or increase lens diameter to help to encourage exchange.
   c. Lens Changes – The Dk should be changed to be at least 125, and maximized to 163 if needed. Lens thickness can also be reduced to maximize oxygen availability.

If these changes do not reduce corneal edema to an acceptable level, wearing time should be adjusted to maintain the health of their eye. A close look at the underlying disease should be taken in these cases, as excessive corneal edema usually occurs in patients with predisposing disease.

Corneal Edema in Transplant Corneas (Carina Koppen, MD, Ph.D., FEBO)

Corneal edema can be a major concern when using scleral lenses in a post-keratoplasty setting. We do not have data yet about tear exchange, oxygen availability and corneal swelling under a scleral lens in normal corneas. Thus, we will have to watch the health of these more fragile corneas extra carefully.

Before setting out to fit a scleral lens, endothelial microscopy is routinely performed; more importantly, I recommend obtaining a pachymetry map. You can use Scheimpflug imaging or OCT, either of which appropriate for follow-up. I find the endothelial cell count a less important parameter: the endothelial cell count after grafting will go down by more than 30% in the first year regardless of scleral lens fitting. Repeated pachymetry maps, however, will reflect endothelial function and they will detect corneal swelling before it is detectable at the slit lamp.

Some patients are fit with scleral lenses a few months after PK or DALK in order to obtain maximal visual rehabilitation. Typically, these patients are young, active and require fast visual recovery. Some are fortunate and have simple myopia; I correct these patients as soon as possible with a soft lens. In those eyes with astigmatism, I try a corneal RGP lens first but if I don't like the way the lens bears on the cornea, my threshold is low to switch to scleral lenses. In my experience, scleral lens wear without impact on corneal swelling can be possible from three months post-keratoplasty. These patients should come to the cornea department for regular postoperative check-ups anyway, so they can be closely monitored for any side-effects with scleral lens wear.

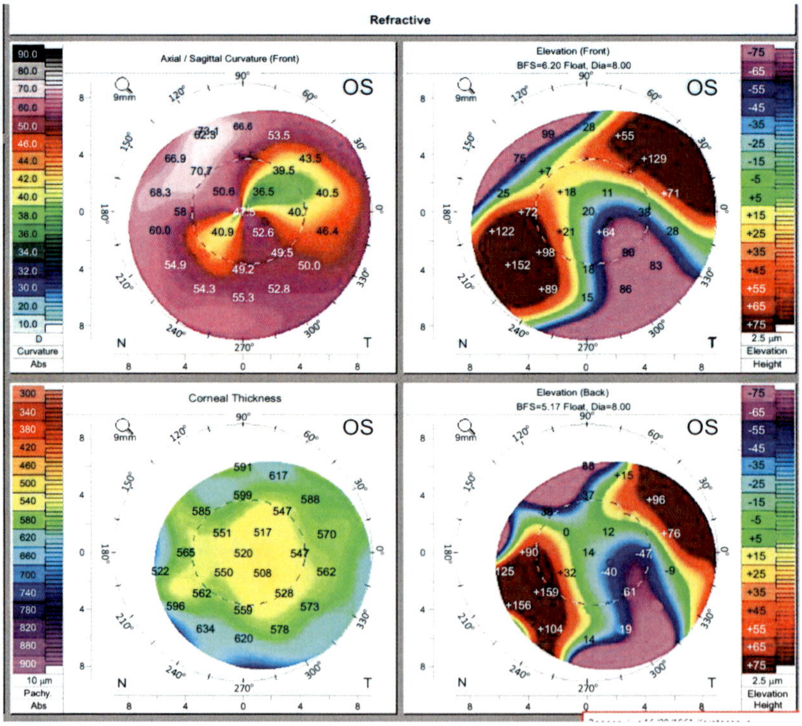

Fig. (16). Pentacam images of a post-keratoplasty patient. Note the high astigmatism on the anterior curvature and anterior and posterior elevation maps with a relatively normal pachymetry distribution. Image courtesy of Carina Koppen.

Obviously, patients hope that the final refractive result will be good after suture removal and/or additional laser correction. For those eyes that need to continue with scleral lens correction, we can reassure them that wearing scleral lenses does not have to interfere with graft survival. Fig. (**16** and **17**) represent a penetrating keratoplasty that is still going strong 19 years after grafting and 13 years of scleral lens wear.

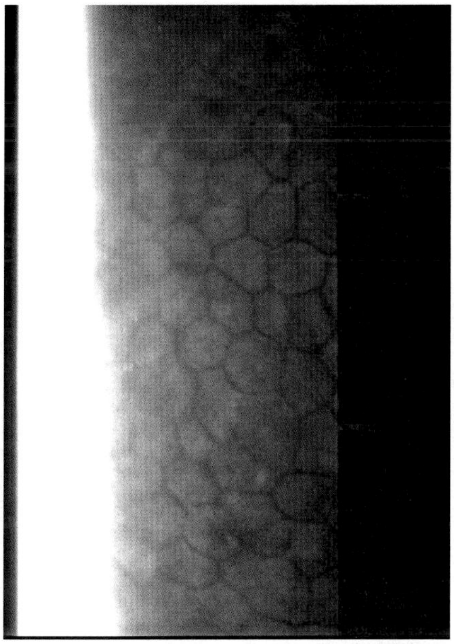

Fig. (17). Specular microscopy of endothelium 19 years after PK; cell count 559 cells/mm^2. Image courtesy of Carina Koppen.

Corneal Neovascularization (Greg DeNaeyer, OD, FAAO, FSLS)

Neovascularization of the cornea can result from wearing various types of contact lenses, including scleral lenses. One of the primary triggers of neovascularization is hypoxia. For soft contact lenses this complication has mostly been resolved with the use of silicone hydrogel lenses. Although modern scleral lenses are mostly manufactured with hyper Dk material, with values of 100 or greater, hypoxic related neovascularization can still occur secondary to fitting conditions and ocular health status. Scleral lenses are generally manufactured with relatively thicker center thicknesses compared to corneal GP lenses in order to avoid flexure. Scleral lens thickness can range from 0.2mm to 0.5mm depending on the design, power, and requested customization. However, it is well known that increasing thickness of a scleral lens decreases oxygen permeability. Oxygen permeability may be impacted by the thickness of the liquid reservoir. The liquid may act as a potential barrier to oxygen and therefore oxygen permeability is reduced with increasing lens vault. With this in mind, the practitioner should be mindful of the scleral lens design and fit to reduce complications such as hypoxia and secondary neovascularization. Unless the case requires a high plus power, I try to keep center thickness to around 0.3mm and keep post-settled central corneal clearances to 200 microns or less, if possible. This can be difficult when fitting keratoconus patients because the central and superior cornea can have increased vault when a scleral lens is fit to adequately clear a low apex (Fig. **18**).

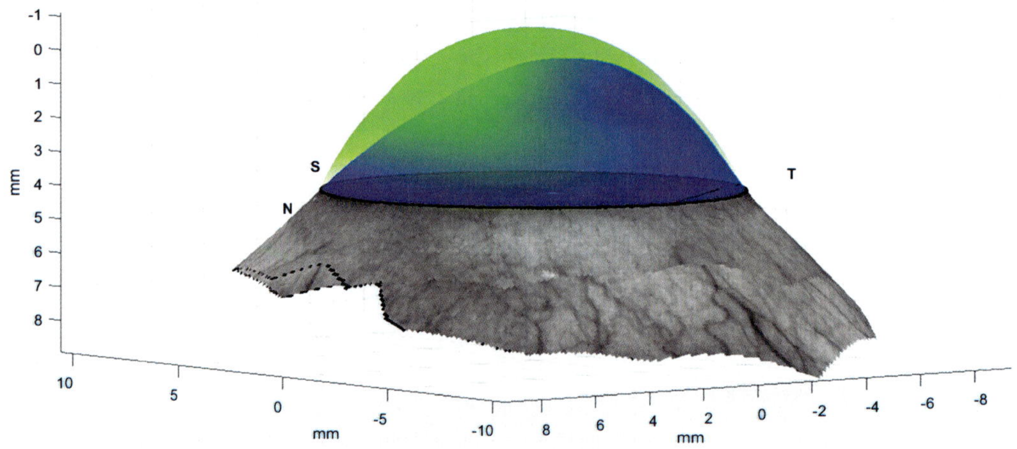

Fig. (18). Example of increased vault (green area) in a keratoconus patient with a low apex (blue area). Image courtesy of Greg DeNaeyer.

In addition, make sure to avoid localized bearing of the scleral lens because chronic irritation or trauma can also initiate a neovascular response. Some corneas are more susceptible to neovascularization, such as patients with full thickness corneal transplants, so extra care and follow-up should be considered for these patients. Patients may have pre-existing neovascularization prior to scleral lens fitting secondary to previous contact lens wear (Fig. **19**). A rest period before fitting may help to initiate recession of the vessels. Some patients require a specialty lens for functional vision and those patients may need to transition directly to a scleral lens. If a scleral lens is the best option, make sure to maximize transmissibility by using hyper Dk materials, reducing center thickness, and minimizing vault.

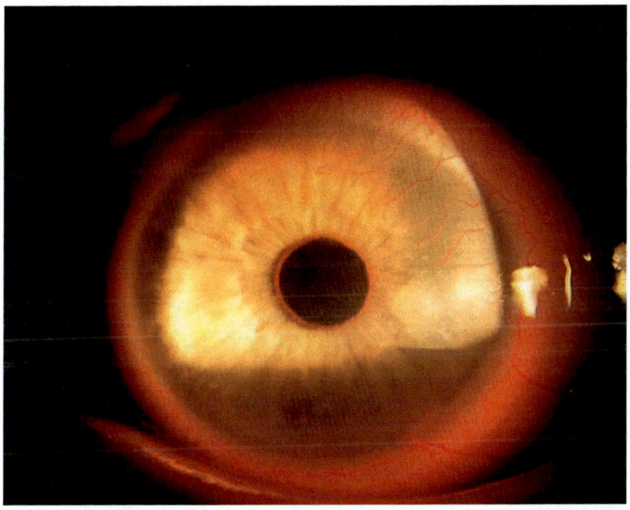

Fig. (19). Patient presents with pre-existing neovascularization prior to scleral lens fitting. Image courtesy of Greg DeNaeyer.

Corneal Neovascularization (Maria K. Walker, OD, MS, FAAO, FSLS)

Corneal neovascularization is a relatively simple complication of scleral lens wear. It is easy to diagnose and the cause is generally straightforward. It occurs when there is a need for nutrients, usually oxygen but sometimes other vascular components, in the avascular corneal tissue. The primary goal in patients who present with neovascularization is to maximize the amount of oxygen available for corneal metabolism. Corneal neovascularization can also grow in response to an insult to the cornea, such as an injury or infectious invasion, which if applicable will need appropriate management. Most commonly, neovascularization of the cornea indicates a chronic state of hypoxia.

Neovascularization should be approached differently in patients with various conditions. I generally group patients into two major classes – those who are post-transplant and those who are not. There could even be a third class designated as ocular surface disease/injury patients who have severe corneal states that may be predisposed to neovascularization, but usually my mentality is post-transplant or not.

Transplant patients in scleral lenses must be regarded with special care, due to the implications of invading blood vessels on the survival of the transplant. Many post-transplant patients will have some degree of neovascularization, especially on the host rim, even prior to being fit into a contact lens. Mild host rim neovascularization is normal, but when it grows inward toward the graft/host interface and onto the graft, or begins to extend deep (below the upper third) into the cornea, it is cause for concern (Fig. **20**).

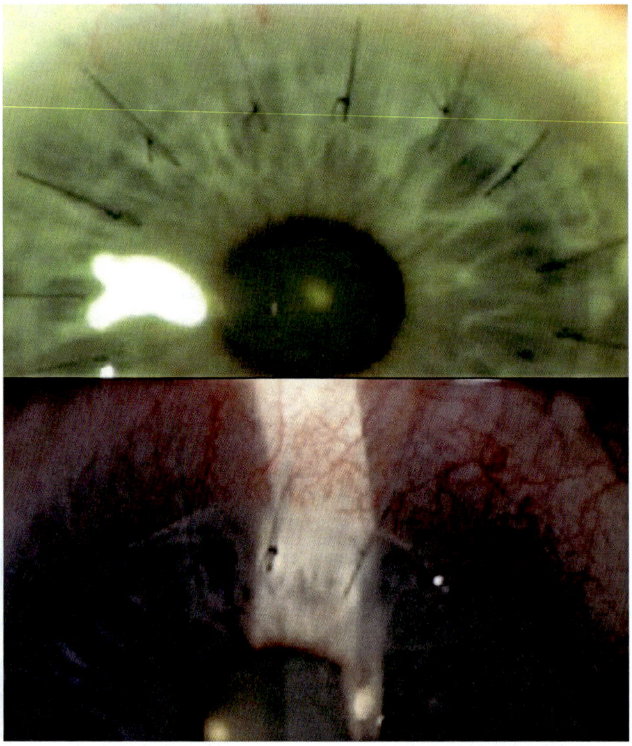

Fig. (20). Small amounts of neovascularization are expected on the host tissue of a post-transplant patient (top). However, when there are numerous vessels and dilated (bottom), steroids are necessary to quiet the reaction. Images courtesy of Maria Walker.

When I fit a transplant patient, I always fit with a priority of maximizing oxygen availability to the cornea (low tear reservoir, high Dk lens, optimized tear exchange). When monitoring the neovascularization on post-transplant patients, we should remember that about 35% of penetrating keratoplasty (PK) transplants will have some type of rejection episode in which steroids must be used to intervene, regardless of scleral lens wear. If corneal neovascularization becomes uncontrolled in a transplant patient, I treat with steroids in consultation with their corneal surgeon, and lenses may or may not need to be discontinued. If scleral wear is continued, I take steps to maximize oxygen availability if not already done, and often have patients restrict their wearing time. Full rejection episodes in the presence of dense neovascularization and other signs of rejection require an immediate referral back to the surgeon and discontinuation of lens wear.

I generally approach patients with ocular surface disease or irregular corneas who present with neovascularization with less urgency, keeping in mind that each case should be individually evaluated for severity. In my experience, patients with ocular surface disease will often show a "*regression*" of neovascularization during scleral lens treatment, so I can enjoy watching the blood vessels gradually ghost as the surface is restoring. Scleral lens treatment is intended to be restorative in these patients, but I certainly monitor closely. I do not often see a concerning amount of neovascularization on irregular cornea patients who wear scleral lenses. When I do see neovascularization, I take all aforementioned steps to maximizing the amount of oxygen getting beneath the scleral lens. In all patients, it is critical to document (and photograph!) the presence of neovascularization on the cornea at baseline so that it can be monitored for changes over time.

Don't Be Afraid of Corneal Neovascularization (Carina Koppen, MD, PhD, FEBO)

Ideally an eye with corneal neovascularization is fit with scleral lenses only after inflammation has subsided and corneal vessels have regressed. Typical examples are irregular and scarred corneas after infectious keratitis or trauma. In practice, we see that these ghost vessels are easily reactivated. From soft contact lens practice we know that oxygen is a driving force for neovascularization: with the advent of silicone hydrogel materials the typical limbal vascularization has almost disappeared. For scleral lenses, highly oxygen permeable materials need to be used. Mechanical forces bearing down on the limbal and conjunctival vessels can also be a trigger for vascular growth. In Fig. (**21**), you can see corneal neovascularization in a keratoconus patient that was caused by adherence of a corneal RGP lens over the inferior limbus.

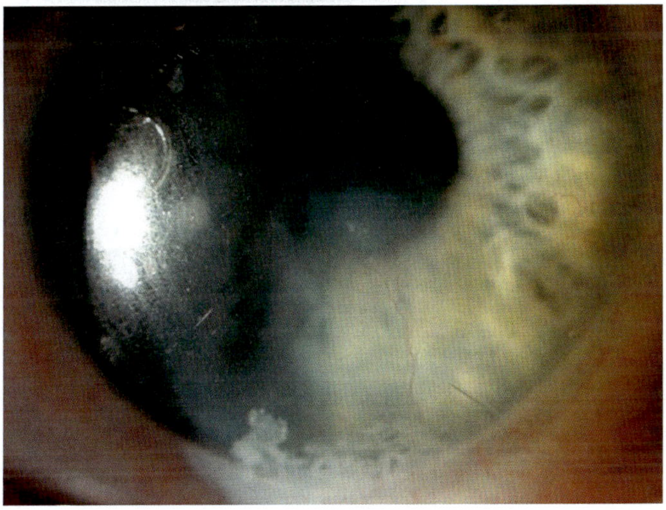

Fig. (21). Inferior neovascularization from an adherent corneal gas permeable lens. Image courtesy of Carina Koppen.

The patient was refit with a scleral lens three years ago. In Fig. (**22**), you can see the result, regression of the corneal vessels and infiltration. When fitting scleral lenses, a good limbal clearance is always essential. If the lens is bearing down on the limbus or fitting too tightly over the conjunctiva, corneal neovascularization at the limbus can be seen even in corneas that previously were free of vessels. Excessive settling of the lens leading to suction cannot be accepted. Extra attention should be given in eyes with corneal transplants in which progression of neovascularization can develop at a surprisingly quick pace.

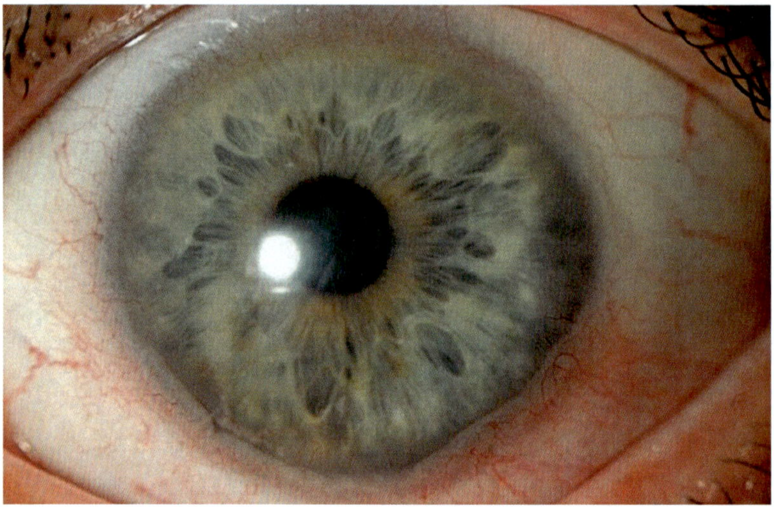

Fig. (22). Neovascularization and infiltration regressed after wearing a scleral lens. Image courtesy of Carina Koppen.

Cicatrizing conjunctivitis is a very different situation with corneal neovascularization in that the disease is progressive. The application of scleral lenses in these cases carefully weighs pros and cons. Treatment of this type of vascularized corneas should be referred to dedicated cornea centers. Topical medication, usually corticosteroids, are essential to control low grade inflammation and further scarring and neovascularization, making management of theses corneas even more complex. Regular photographic documentation is essential to make correct and objective evaluations of the corneal vessels.

Graft Rejection (Michael Lipson, OD, FAAO, FSLS)

Scleral lenses are commonly used in patients who have had a corneal transplant. Prior to fitting with scleral lenses, make sure post-operative healing is stable, and consult with the corneal surgeon to confirm that the eye is ready for scleral lens wear. Graft rejection can occur at any time after a corneal transplant, with or without the use of contact lenses or scleral lenses. After initiating scleral lens fitting, careful follow-up and observation for signs of graft rejection is crucial. Watch for these signs and discontinue wear of scleral lenses if a rejection or reaction occurs. Signs of graft rejection include some or all of the following: an epithelial rejection line (rare), corneal edema (Fig. **23**), subepithelial and/or stromal infiltrates, corneal neovascularization, keratic precipitates on the graft (but not on the peripheral host cornea), and a Khodadoust line (deposition of killer lymphocytes) on the endothelium (Fig. **24**). In general, treatment and management for graft rejection should be prescribed and monitored by the surgeon or a corneal specialist. Topical steroids, antibiotics and/or oral immune-suppressants may all be utilized.

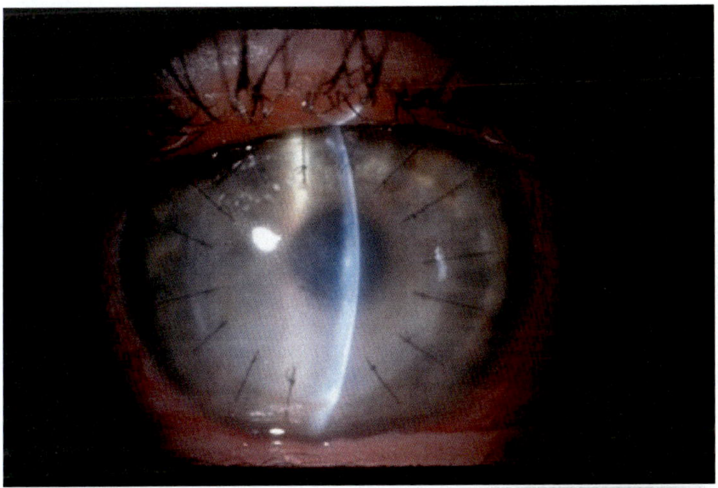

Fig. (23). Example of an acute graft rejection. Image courtesy of Mark Mannis.

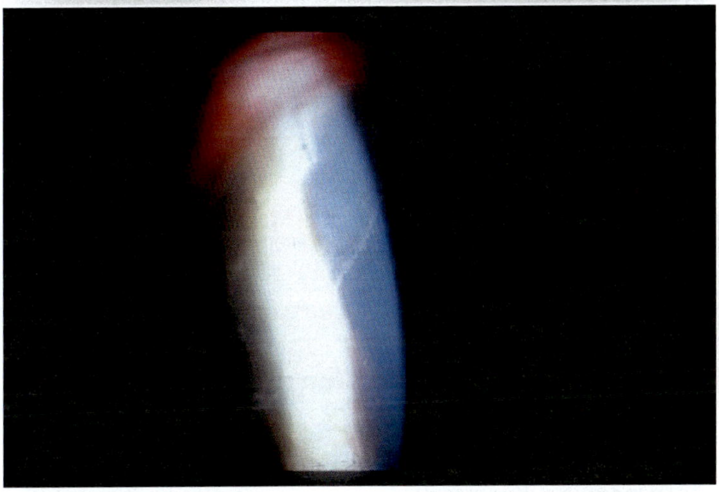

Fig. (24). Example of a Khodadoust line of an active graft rejection. Image courtesy of Mark Mannis.

Graft Rejection (Carina Koppen, MD, Ph.D., FEBO)

Typically, patients who have undergone penetrating keratoplasty instill topical corticosteroid drops for about a year to prevent graft rejection. Although all layers of the cornea can undergo rejection, endothelial rejection is the most common type of graft rejection. An episode of endothelial rejection will lead to endothelial cell loss and will shorten the survival span of the graft. Patients need to be regularly reminded of the symptoms of rejection: redness, photophobia and decreased visual acuity. Signs at the slit lamp rarely include the typical Khodadoust line. Much more often there is ciliary redness, cells in the anterior chamber and keratic precipitates on the endothelium. Treatment of corneal rejection is a medical emergency. Usually one episode of endothelial rejection is not fatal for the graft if managed appropriately. Corticosteroids will be tapered as the signs of rejection clear; most corneal surgeons will decide to continue cortisone drops indefinitely at a low dosage.

For patients wearing scleral lenses, lens wear should be interrupted during the rejection episode. The endothelium is attacked by the immune rejection and we need to avoid any additional metabolic stress for the endothelium caused by scleral lens wear. Furthermore, the dosage of cortisone drops is quite high, often starting at once per hour; this is not compatible with lens wear. When dosing with ocular medications, the tear exchange under the scleral lens is so limited, that the medication may not exchange beneath the scleral lens. Scleral lenses should be removed for ocular medications. Once the rejection is over and the cortisone drops are being tapered, scleral lens wear can resume. We recommend patients to use the drops before inserting the scleral lens or after lens removal – or take an extra break during the day; this way the accessibility to the ocular surface is not impeded by the presence of the lens. Eventually many patients are kept on a low dose of corticosteroids (fluorometholone, loteprednol) indefinitely. I recommend patients to take their once a day drop at the end of the day: this way it can be beneficial to calm down any ocular irritation that developed during the day.

It is important to remember that there is no evidence that lens wear can trigger graft rejection. Any lens, however, that encourages corneal neovascularization can indirectly increase the risk of rejection. As DALK is slowly becoming more popular as treatment for stromal disease, there is no evidence that it is superior in visual and refractive outcome over penetrating keratoplasty. The main benefit at this time is that endothelial rejection is no longer a threat.

Graft Rejection and Scleral Lenses (Jason Jedlicka, OD, FAAO, FSLS)

Graft Rejection, whether epithelial, subepithelial, or endothelial, is a potential complication of scleral lens wear due to mechanical, inflammatory, and hypoxic influences. Rarely, if ever, is graft rejection present and active at the initiation of fitting; this needs to be resolved prior to fitting an eye in a scleral lens. However, it can absolutely occur at any time in the life of a scleral lens wearer with a corneal graft.

Potential causes of graft rejection that may be induced by scleral lens wear include corneal vascularization, active inflammation, and trauma. Corneal vascularization can arise from hypoxia due to lack of oxygen through the scleral lens when tear exchange is absent, the lens is too thick or not oxygen permeable enough, or when vault over any aspect of the cornea or limbus is excessive. Scleral lens wear can contribute to inflammation if the lens fit is too tight or "suctioned" to the eye, or if the filling solutions are incompatible with the ocular surface. Corneal trauma can be induced by a lens that does not vault adequately. Any of these scenarios can, over time, induce or contribute to corneal graft rejection, and care should be taken to initiate a scleral lens fit on a corneal graft to ensure that the eye is not already at significant risk of rejection. Significant neovascularization of the host tissue, low endothelial cell count, or a history of an inflammatory-based ocular condition that lead to the graft as in the case of herpes simplex virus (HSV), are all high-risk characteristics that should lead to careful consideration of whether a scleral lens is the best approach to correcting vision. In these cases, a corneal GP lens may be more appropriate for vision correction.

When rejection does occur, whether epithelial, subepithelial, or endothelial, managing the rejection is the first step, and scleral lens wear may need to be discontinued for a period to allow the rejection to subside. Once the episode has resolved, scleral lens wear may be carefully resumed, but if the lens was a contributing factor, it will likely need to be refit. Attention to the aspect of scleral lens wear that may have been contributory, whether hypoxia, trauma, or inflammation based in the process of refitting will hopefully reduce the likelihood of recurrence. Although in some cases, scleral lens wear may be incompatible with a highly risky corneal graft.

SCLERAL LENSES AND PAINFUL EYES

Scleral lenses are an effective treatment for dry eye disease and severe ocular surface disease. Patients with dry eye symptoms often seek scleral lenses as a treatment option. Typically, patients who are suffering are their own advocates and perform extensive therapy searches on the internet. However, there is a subset of patients who have symptoms that far exceed ocular signs and findings. These patients are seeking relief of their symptoms with scleral lenses and may refer themselves to scleral lens practitioners. However, these patients sometimes have an exacerbated response and discomfort with scleral lenses. Dr. Rosenthal will describe his experience with this unique group of patients.

Oculofacial Pain (Perry Rosenthal, M.D.)

Maintaining the integrity of the mirror-smooth corneal tear layer was critical to our remote ancestors' transition from water to land and drove the evolution of our complex, sensitive and powerful dry eye alarm system. Its role, in concert with the lacrimal glands, is to prevent the breakup of the optical tear film and consequent sudden impairment of functional vision.

Dry eye symptoms are a unique type of corneal pain that alerts us to the immanent or actual breakup of the tear film. Moreover, I have proposed that otherwise poorly explained chronic dry eye symptoms are consequences of increased corneal sensitivity to tear evaporation caused by unidentified malfunctions in the dry eye alarm system [15 - 18]. Anecdotal observations have suggested that patients with chronic dry eye symptoms characterized by the disparity between symptoms and signs suffer from consequences of an as yet undiscovered disorder of the trigeminal sensory system and represents neuropathic pain, a disease in its own right. Nevertheless, while orofacial pain has been recognized as a sensory trigeminal neuropathic disease typically characterized by a paucity of causal signs, that involving the eyes and orbits, which I have named oculofacial pain, has been overlooked or dismissed by ophthalmic professions for that very reason -- the paucity of causal signs. On the other hand, surface body pain in the absence of supportive causal signs is characteristic of projected pain. Moreover, studies point to the trigeminal brainstem as the likely source of oculofacial pain [19].

Because non-fenestrated scleral lenses completely block tear evaporation, chronic dry eye symptoms are completely suppressed on their insertion. On the other hand, I believe that those symptoms caused by hypersensitivity of the tear thickness sensors such as TRMP8 cold sensors [16] located in many corneal interepithelial nerves terminals are the underlying cause of symptoms in oculofacial pain disease. Moreover, many of these eyes appear to be hypersensitive to mechanical stimuli, a phenomenon known as secondary hyperalgesia. Consequences include scleral lens intolerance that can be an unsurmountable challenge to fitting them with these devices.

SCLERAL LENSES AND THE ASIAN EYE

It has long been speculated that the Asian eye anatomy differs from Caucasian anatomy. In routine eye care, the differences in anatomy are inconsequential. However, when fitting scleral lenses, the anatomy is important for improved scleral lens centration and alignment for Asian eyes. Dr. Park will describe his experiences fitting scleral lenses on a Korean population.

Scleral Lens Challenges in Korea (Young Kee Park, MD, PhD)

While scleral lenses are very new in Korea, I have fit the lens on more than 600 Korean eyes during the last three years. Scleral lenses have been prescribed for severely compromised eyes when existing corneal gas permeable lenses dislodge, or for eyes that are intolerant to corneal gas permeable lenses. Even though scleral lenses have brought astonishing results to provide solutions to these patients, lenses designed for Caucasian eyes demonstrate limitations on Korean eyes. Patients with severely damaged eyes were able to tolerate scleral lenses despite some discomfort when the lens improved visual acuity. Tinted or presbyopic lenses for normal eyes require much more careful prescriptions. Additionally, comfortable wearing without side effects is the key factor for choosing a specific scleral lens. Based on my 30-year expertise with various RGP lenses, I will highlight some findings and explain necessities to customize scleral lenses for Asians. I will first identify issues from the different eye structures and then explain actual circumstances in Korea.

The structural differences between Asian and Caucasian eyes reported in studies include: 1) Smaller HVID of Asian eye of both sexes: Asian (average 11.63mm) *vs*. Caucasian (average 11.79mm); 2) Asians have a more prolate cornea with much more flattening to the periphery; 3) Asians have a smaller palpebral fissure; 4) Asians have greater eyelid tension. Based on these anatomic differences, guidelines to design a lens that fits better to Korean eyes are summarized below.

The average diameter of the first scleral lens introduced in Korea was 15.8mm, but the lens occasionally seemed to be larger due to relatively smaller corneal size of Koreans compared to Caucasians. Additionally, this lens had fitting limitations due to lack of variable parameters. My patients have a wide range of corneal sizes: those larger than 13.0mm, especially among young patients and those smaller than 10.5mm. Based on my experience, the diameter of the scleral lens needed ranges widely from 14.0mm to 16.0mm to fit Koreans. As demand to fit scleral lenses on normal eyes is expected to increase, smaller diameter lenses will be preferable for pricing, easier prescription and handling. On the other hand, diseased eyes require much larger diameter lenses for a full coverage on the irregular cornea.

Currently, a 14.7 mm scleral lens for Asian eyes was the standard and first tried for Korean patients. This design provided more clearance at the limbus, a constant haptic zone width (0.95mm), with various edge clearances and various options (oblate, front toric, PC toric and multifocal). These advanced smaller size lenses with a variety of parameters and options provide a range of choices according to the patient's condition and easier insertion and removal handling. Ongoing and continuous improvement in the design is required to optimize the fit for Asian eyes.

As the pressure on the sclera by the lens is proportional to the size and depth of the lens, a slight increase in width of the haptic zone and increase in diameter of the corneal vaulting zone is necessary to disperse pressure on the sclera. Larger diameter lenses (above 15.8mm) are also available when necessary in Korea. The Asian cornea flattens rapidly peripherally (prolate), and the limbal clearance is insufficient, especially on the nasal side. Therefore, curves at the limbus need to create greater clearance, and an Asian design has this parameter design. Fitting findings of the Asian type show that central clearance is sufficient, but the peripheral clearance may exert higher limbal compression compared to the Caucasian design. Based on my experience, the transition between vaulting and haptic zone should be designed sigmoidally or junctionless for a smooth landing on the conjunctiva overlying the sclera.

In my opinion, due to the narrow lid fissure of an Asian eye, the size of the scleral lens needs to be as small as the width of the lid fissure because it is difficult to apply and remove a scleral lens over 18.0mm in diameter. When applying the lens to a Korean patient, the bottom of the lens is inserted first, and the upper lid is lifted slightly before inserting the remaining part of the lens. It is easier to remove the lens when it is lifted slightly to insert air and create space. Also, it is better to place a suction cup on the periphery of the lens than the center for scleral lens removal.

Some Koreans have oval corneas (wider horizontal width) probably due to uneven lid compression. For these patients, the scleral lens is frequently decentered inferiorly, and thus the upper part of the lens has shallow clearance yet the lower part has relatively higher clearance. To solve this problem, a toric design of the haptic is frequently prescribed. When the lens is not centered over the cornea and a good scleral alignment is not achieved even with maximum toricity, post-fabrication polishing is done to enable more toricity. As the sclera near the limbus has lower toricity than further from the limbus, toric haptics are used less frequently with smaller overall diameter scleral lenses.

Due to the stronger lid tension of an Asian eye, the eyelid presses and pushes the lens strongly to the sclera resulting in a lens mark after removal. Tears may not be circulated appropriately and conjunctival hyperemia is induced even with proper initial lens fitting. Size reduction decreases the pressure from the lid, while the landing zone portion must be widened to disperse the pressure applied to the sclera. In addition, the landing zone should not simply be one tangent but should be divided into several parts in tangents or curves.

Koreans also have tight lids that I suspect make the haptic edge irritate the meibomian gland orifices resulting in turbid tears; therefore, the anterior edge of the haptic must be polished smoothly.

While my above analysis was driven by rather general characteristics of an Asian eye, there are some perspectives considering actual circumstances more specific to the Korean culture.

Koreans with wide and protruded cheekbones usually have wide orbital sockets, and the sclera near the limbus is very flat making the junction of the vaulting/corneal clearance zone and the haptic zone very tight as well. Lens design for this type of population needs to make the junction of the vaulting zone and haptic part much flatter. Because this lens design is not available, the flattest haptic is initially selected, and the vaulting zone and the nearby haptic part are polished heavily to match the contour of the very flat sclera adjacent to the limbus.

Refractive surgeries are common in Korea, therefore, methods of correcting residual myopia and regular or irregular astigmatism after surgeries are required. A normally designed smaller diameter scleral lens is preferable for this patient, but sometimes an oblate design is needed for the cornea with high myopia. When designing an oblate lens, the vaulting zone curve is determined first on the corneal parameters before surgery. Next the sagittal depth of the lens is lowered. In my experience, if the designing process is in reverse, the junction of the vaulting zone can compress the sclera more than a normally designed lens. I have had some difficulties when deciding whether to use a normal design with high clearance or an oblate design with compression on the sclera.

With the approval by the Ministry of Food & Drug Safety in Korea, tinted scleral lenses are expected to be prescribed frequently. Because they are mostly prescribed for normal eyes, practitioners feel greater pressure to provide perfect prescriptions than for diseased eyes. When fitting a tinted lens to an eye with a very small cornea, a small diameter lens is first fit and prescribed, and the color print is applied afterwards. The purpose of wearing a tinted lens is cosmetic and makes the cornea look larger. Since the lens is much larger than a typical Korean patient's small corneal size, here are frequent demands for a much larger tinted lens than the cornea. When I work with these normal cornea cases, pressure applied to the sclera can be reduced by maintaining the vaulting zone size and only widening the haptic size.

A presbyopic scleral lens is now approved by the Korean Ministry of Food & Drug Safety and will be frequently prescribed to the presbyopic population. With age, the conjunctiva gets thin and loose, resulting in easy entrapment of the conjunctiva by the lens. Because prescriptions for presbyopia are needed after LASIK and LASEK surgeries as well, the oblate design is required for an optimal fit.

Since keratoplasty is not common in Korea and very severe keratoconus is frequently fit with scleral lenses, a specialized design is required. The vaulting zone is divided into several parts; the central part is steeper with a higher sagittal depth. It flattens to the periphery, and the end of the vaulting zone junction should not apply too much pressure on the sclera. The eyelid may apply great pressure since the center of the lens is steep and protrudes forward. Thus, the haptic must be relatively wider to support the increased sagittal depth of the lens.

To cover a severely protruding cornea after the keratoplasty, the lens must be designed similar to the case of severe keratoconus described above.

Scleral lenses now available now in Korea have improvements in design, successfully solve problems and provide many successful outcomes. While I have relatively short clinical experience on a limited number of patients, I conclude that customized scleral lens designs will overcome scleral lens complexities in order to enhance the quality of prescriptions and compatibility for Korean eyes.

PEDIATRICS

Fitting scleral lenses is challenging in general, but there are special considerations when working with children. Establishing trust is crucial for applying and removing these large diameter lenses which can be a very scary experience for children to comprehend. There are many indications for scleral lens wear in children.

Similar to adults, some children have conditions that have painful eyes and others have completely anesthetic eyes. Dr. Carrasquillo describes her experiences in approaching scleral lens fitting and management in different pediatric populations.

Pediatric Scleral Lenses (Karen Carrasquillo, OD, PhD, FAAO, FSLS)

Conditions

In general, there are two situations when I use scleral lenses in the pediatric population. Either I use them to strictly rehabilitate vision in cases of corneal irregularity or to treat ocular surface disease. Within these two subsets lie the most important category distinction when approaching pediatric patients: corneal sensation *versus* diminished sensation or the lack thereof.

Decreased or Absent Corneal Sensation

Among the conditions in the decreased or anesthetic category, we have familial dysautonomia, Möbius syndrome, hereditary sensory autonomic neuropathy (HSAN), and unspecified neurotrophic keratopathy, among others.

The lack or decreased sensation will enable the clinician to manipulate the eye, lids and proceed with application/removal with more ease. This makes managing these patients with the above conditions easier to approach with scleral lens fitting.

Corneal Sensation

Conditions where corneal sensation is retained but require scleral lenses include irregular cornea from trauma, scarring, irregular astigmatism, aphakia and ectasia among others. Pediatric patients may also suffer from various types of ocular surface disease: Stevens-Johnson syndrome, graft-*versus*-host disease, lacrimal gland dysfunction, among others.

When working with a child that has corneal sensation, the challenge is greater but not impossible. Pediatric ocular examinations can be quite difficult; in particular, having to apply and remove a large diameter scleral lens can increase the challenge.

Setting Up for Success

In order to prepare for success with managing this special population, the first step is to allow adequate time in the schedule. Allow for sufficient time for the first evaluation/consultation – which would ideally include a successful diagnostic lens application and removal. In my experience, when managing this population, the minimum time allowed for consultation is two hours. If the child is an appropriate candidate for scleral lenses, schedule their follow up evaluations and assessments with sufficient time.

It is important to develop a quick rapport with the patient and parents or caretakers in order to establish trust. In my opinion, building that trust and empathy is crucial for success. It's important for the patient to overcome the fear of something new, especially the fear of a big piece of plastic coming to the eye. For children suffering from severe ocular surface disease and are extremely symptomatic, it is important for them to overcome the fear of the lens being a source or contributor to more pain.

Visual Acuity/Slit Lamp Examination – Key Take-Aways

- Methods for visual acuity determination at baseline and while wearing scleral lenses include Fix and Follow, Lea Cards, Preferential Looking, and Snellen –determine best approach based on the patient's ability.
- For proper baseline and post slit lamp examination, if the patient isn't able to be positioned in the slit lamp, seat the child in the parent's lap.
- Use an ophthalmoscope at high plus magnification to aid with gross examination of the cornea in white light (search for corneal opacities, neovascularization) and also with cobalt blue light and a yellow Wratten filter (search for epithelial defects, staining patterns).
- If the patient is photophobic, topical anesthetic may be useful.
- Confirm the presence of a red-reflex with retinoscopy. Depending on the age of the patient, a cycloplegic over-refraction with retinoscopy will determine the prescription of the scleral lens.

First Application of Diagnostic Lens

"Eye Dunks" – If Symptomatic

For many, preservative free saline coming in contact with the cornea is associated with a cold sensation. This sensation often leads the pediatric patient to be surprised, potentially even more fearful, trigger a stronger eye reflex, and defense mechanism – making it even more challenging to properly apply lenses. This can be particularly a concern in the very young pediatric population with corneal sensation. It is helpful to approach the application process with caution and not try to force the application. The patient may become even more frightened. There is an increased chance of an application bubble. In cases of fidgety patients, there is a risk of scratching the cornea. It is important to take appropriate time and break down the process in a step by step manner to gain trust of the child during lens application.

It helps to slowly de-sensitize the cornea by performing what we have coined at BostonSight as "eye dunks". These consists in filling the lens with saline and place the lens inside the lower lid (by pulling lower lid down – not exerting pressure down on the lower lid with the lens) and having the child's cornea be exposed to the saline solution by having the patient look down as you approach the eye slowly, but not fully applying the lens. This helps the patient get used to the "cold" sensation and also get use to the eye getting wet. The sensation of wetness is soothing; the pediatric patient will start to realize, slowly but surely, the benefits of the lens – enabling the transition to successfully apply the lens.

Lid Spreads

Once the "eye dunks" have been performed, then move onto perfecting the lid spreads. Ultimately, the key to success for a proper application is the lid spread! The parent/caregiver can act as an extension of the practitioner by properly holding the upper lid by the eyelashes. This allows the practitioner to focus on the lower lid and secure it by the eyelashes. The key in this situation is to focus on maximizing the extent that both eyelids are secured. Many patients or those assisting the patient pull down the skin around cheekbone area; this may lead to an unsuccessful application.

Once the eyelids are spread widely and secured, steadily hold the lens in an upright position with the other hand for the first application attempt. In order to minimize spilling of fluid, and ultimately an application bubble, I overfill the lens and hold it in an upright position until I'm convinced I have a proper lid spread and have a good "shot." Once I do, I move in as quickly and swiftly as I can, centering the lens over the cornea.

If the child is less than one year old and has no corneal sensation, I like to lay the patient across the parent's lap, facing down, with head pointed in my direction. This allows the parent to hold the head steady and provide adequate support. While the parent holds and supports child's head with one hand by the chin and the other hand by the forehead, it enables the parent to retract the upper lid at the same time. I am then able to hold the bottom lid open with my left hand, while I hold the lens in the plunger in the right hand. You can also use one hand to open both lids and have the parent support the child's head, while you approach application with your other hand (Fig. **25**).

It is advisable to overfill the lens in order to minimize bubble formation upon application (Fig. **26**). Sometimes, I have to demonstrate for the parents different aspects of lens application, so they are ready to participate in their role. These are practice attempts, mainly to ensure a wide lid spread, but the lens is not applied. When I am ready, I apply sodium fluorescein in the reservoir, as this allows a quick assessment of corneal touch both centrally and in the periphery with the use of an ophthalmoscope, blue light and a #12 yellow Wratten filter.

To remove the lens, the patient can be seated in the parent's lap. The key again is the lid spreads. In my experience, it's easier to remove lenses by breaking the suction and withdrawing the lens from superior or lateral edge using a removal plunger – depending on which is easier and will allow you to remove the lens without risk of scratching the cornea. Once application/removal is mastered for each pediatric patient, proceed to cycloplege the patient.

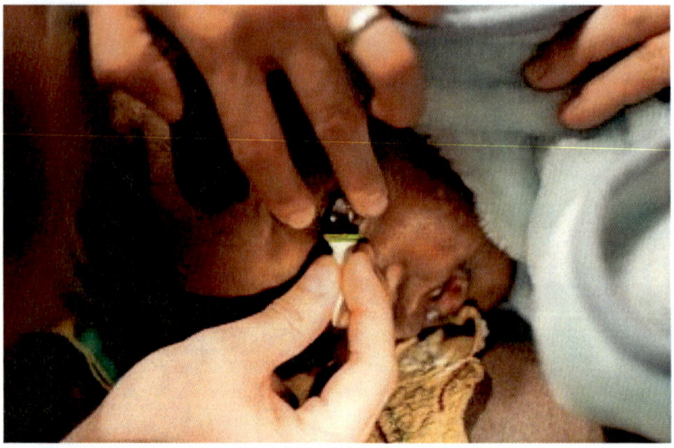

Fig. (25). Scleral lens application in a pediatric patient while patient is laid across in parent's lap. Image courtesy of *BostonSight.*

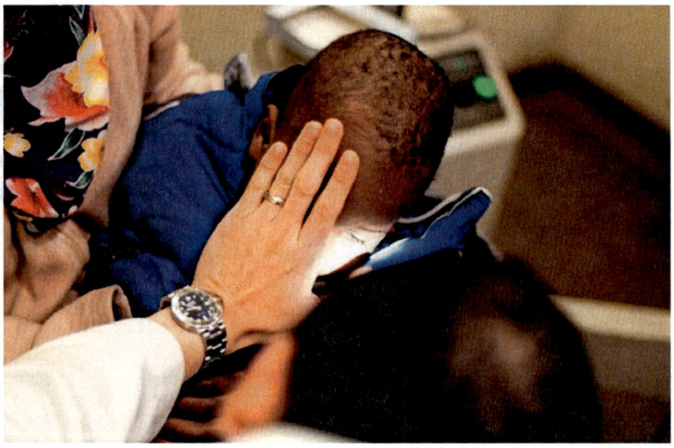

Fig. (26). Evaluating the scleral lens for a bubble in a pediatric patient. Image courtesy of *BostonSight.*

Assessing and Finalizing Fit

Determine visual acuity at baseline without over-refraction by the method best suited for the patient. Perform cycloplegic over-refraction using retinoscopy. Work closely with patient's pediatric ophthalmologist to determine the best prescription.

If the patient cannot be positioned behind a slit lamp, and a handheld slit lamp is unavailable I, again, use my ophthalmoscope at a high plus magnification and assess with white light and blue light/fluorescein.

My approach is to always assess the fit after 3 hours of wearing time. I assess with white light to identify obvious impingement areas and blanching patterns or conversely, any edge lift patterns. I then use blue light to again assess corneal clearance (as fluorescein was already applied). I then re-apply fluorescein and remove the lens. I assess with blue light in all four quadrants in the eye to identify conjunctival staining patterns that would be indicative of tight fitting peripheries. Based on the conjunctival staining patterns, I determine how much flattening, if any, the lens will need in any given quadrant.

In my opinion, it is imperative to photo document as much as possible, especially if there's an epithelial defect. It is possible to use a hand-held camera and place a #12 yellow Wratten filter in front of the lens to better document extent of epithelial defects.

After ordering the first lens, I approach scleral lens fitting in this special population in an iterative fashion – performing three and six hour fit assessments each time, refining prescription endpoint and fitting parameters, until there's no evidence of physiological compromise.

1. Endpoint cycloplegic over-refraction: Determine the prescription in conjunction with the referring pediatric ophthalmologist.
2. Ensure good peripheral corneal clearance 360°: increase limbal clearance or increase sagittal height (depending on the lens design) if clearance is insufficient.
3. Rule out corneal staining: increase the sagittal height.
4. Rule out conjunctival staining in any quadrant: flatten the haptic/landing zone in the meridian of staining. Employ back surface toricity, or quadrant specific changes if available.
5. Rule out significant hyperemia upon lens removal: If there was no impingement (conjunctival staining), rebound hyperemia may result from significant haptic/landing zone compression. Loosen the periphery of the lens. When hyperemia is meridional, then flatten one meridian of the periphery, thus making a toric lens periphery.
6. Rule out post-application (intrusional) air bubbles. If the lens did not have any air bubbles immediately after application, and then one is present, that is a sign of a loose lens in one meridian or all around.

Apply fluorescein and monitor areas of quick fluorescein intake, the path for bubble entry will likely be revealed. A toric or quadrant specific lens design may be helpful when tightening the meridian of excessive fluorescein intake. Steepen the lens in a particular quadrant or all around, based on the findings.

Post-Scleral Lens Fitting

With pediatric patients, it is very important to co-manage closely with the referring ophthalmologist. The best way to guarantee success is for the parents, referring doctors, and the practitioner to be in synch. Adequate follow-up and monitoring is very important.

I typically see patients every 3-4 months after fitting for at least 1.5 years. If there are no complications compromising the physiological function of the eye with the scleral lenses, then I see patients in a 6-month interval for the next 2-3 years. Once I determine that the eye is stable, then I recommend is that the patient is seen twice a year, alternating between the referring ophthalmologist and myself. In my opinion, one can't be too conservative when dealing with pediatric patients.

Fuchs' Corneal Dystrophy (Melissa Barnett, OD, FAAO, FSLS, FBCLA and Lynette K. Johns, OD, FAAO, FSLS, FBCLA)

Fuchs' corneal dystrophy is a degeneration of the corneal endothelium. It is associated with the thickening of Descemet's membrane and the loss of endothelial cells (Fig. **27-29**). Both the pump function of the endothelium and the barrier function of Descemet's membrane are compromised, resulting in stromal and epithelial edema. Fuchs' dystrophy is a bilateral, asymmetric condition that presents most commonly age 50-60 [20, 21]. An early sign of Fuchs' dystrophy is pigment dusting around the age 30-40. Patients who inherit Fuchs' have a 50% chance of passing it onto their children [22].

Typically, scleral lens wear is contraindicated with any evidence of baseline corneal edema. Exogenous fluid present in the scleral lens reservoir can exacerbate pre-existing corneal edema, further compromising the cornea and visual acuity. While Fuchs' corneal dystrophy is a contraindication to scleral lens wear, a patient who has had a corneal transplant is a candidate for scleral lenses. When managing these patients with scleral lens wear, it is important to have a baseline endothelial cell count and global pachymetry in order to monitor the cornea carefully.

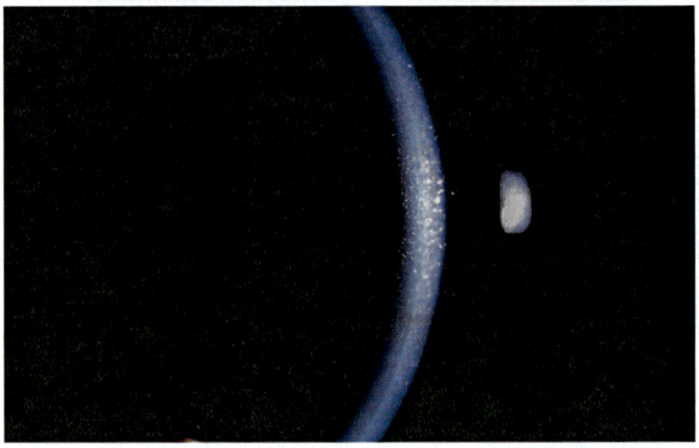

Fig. (27). A cornea exhibiting guttata in Fuchs' corneal dystrophy. Image courtesy of Mark Mannis.

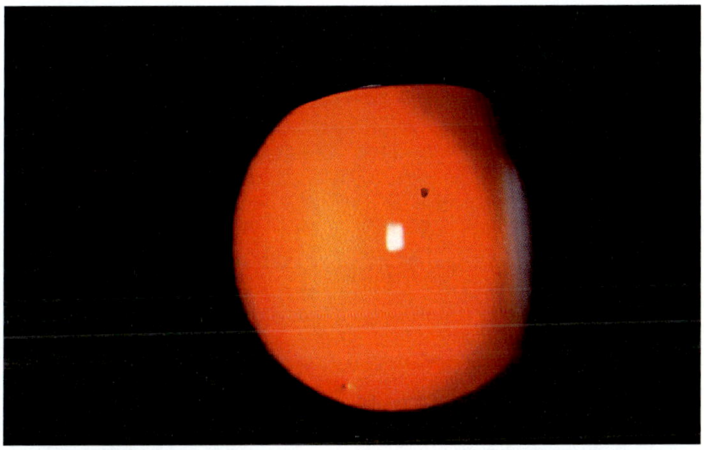

Fig. (28). Retroillumination of a cornea with Fuchs' corneal dystrophy. Image courtesy of Mark Mannis.

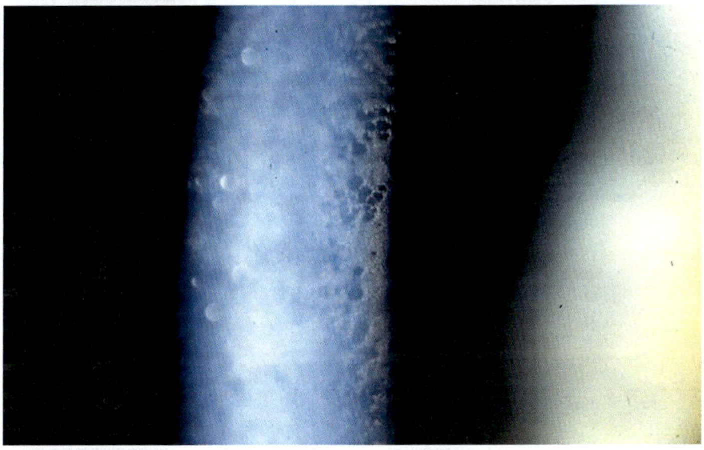

Fig. (29). A magnified view of advanced Fuchs' corneal dystrophy with guttata, stromal haze and epithelial microcysts. Image courtesy of Mark Mannis.

It is not uncommon to see corneal edema in the host tissue surrounding the transplant. Documentation and photo-documentation of existing edema prior to commencing scleral lens fitting is pertinent.

Some practitioners have used a hypertonic solution in the bowl of the lens. In our experience, the hypertonic solution does not provide adequate management of corneal edema. Practitioners who do fit scleral lenses in patients with Fuchs' tend to fit lenses that have a reduced center thickness, smaller diameter and minimal reservoir. However, it is our opinion that fitting scleral lenses for these patients could exacerbate the Fuchs' process including corneal edema (Fig. **27**).

Nystagmus (Melissa Barnett, OD, FAAO, FSLS, FBCLA and Lynette K. Johns, OD, FAAO, FSLS, FBCLA)

There are many different types of nystagmus; all have a rhythmic, involuntary oscillation of one or both eyes [23]. The clear image obtained by gas permeable contact lenses has been used in nystagmus to improve foveation time and the decrease nystagmus intensity [24]. In a recent study, nystagmus was not decreased when soft contact lenses, gas permeable contact lenses and spectacles were compared [25].

Nystagmus can be quite a challenge for the scleral lens practitioner. When applying a scleral lens to an eye with nystagmus, the patient's gaze and head posture should be optimized at the null point of nystagmus. Sometimes a larger scleral lens can reduce the occurrence of an application bubble because exact alignment is not necessarily required for the cornea to be completely submerged in the reservoir of a larger diameter scleral lens.

An advantage of scleral lens is their stability. Since scleral lenses have a larger diameter, they are less likely to dislodge compared to small diameter gas permeable contact lenses. Scleral lenses are a very effective management option for patients with nystagmus.

However, scleral lens evaluation is very challenging in patients with nystagmus due to rapid eye movements. Careful evaluation of the central and limbal clearance as well as the landing zone may be suboptimal due to the brief views in each quadrant. Attempts to observe the fit when the patient is at their null point may be impossible due to head and eye positioning behind the slit lamp. If evidence of central or peripheral staining is observed after the lens is removed, an automatic increase in sagittal depth should be considered if the view of the clearance was limited during the fitting.

HIGHER ORDER ABERRATIONS

Rigid gas permeable optics are considered the best among all forms of contact lens optical correction. Unfortunately, there are still limitations in the form of higher order aberrations (HOA). Since scleral lenses are stable, they are the ideal platform for HOA correction. The authors will describe the measurements of HOAs though a scleral lens and the results of applying HOAs into scleral lenses.

Advanced Vision Correction with Wavefront-Guided Scleral Lenses (Professor Geunyoung Yoon, PhD)

It has long been known that the human eye suffers from both lower and higher order aberrations. Lower order aberrations include defocus and astigmatism, or sphero-cylindrical refractive errors that can be corrected by conventional spectacles or contact lenses. Higher order aberrations refer to irregular astigmatism that cannot be corrected with the conventional optical aids. For more than two decades, advances in ocular wavefront sensing technology, such as Shack-Hartmann aberrometry, have enabled us to quantify the ocular aberrations objectively and rapidly. This development has revolutionized the way we understand the optics of the eye and how it affects our vision. Several studies have demonstrated that the visual performance of normal eyes with best conventional correction can still be limited by uncorrected higher order aberrations and that correcting these aberrations can further improve visual performance, especially when the eye's pupil is relatively large under dim light conditions. This visual benefit of correcting higher order aberrations is even more substantial in highly aberrated eyes, such as eyes with keratoconus.

Keratoconus affects approximately 1 in 2,000 people and, in this disease, the corneal stroma progressively thins and assumes a conical shape that preferentially forms on the inferior half of the cornea. An increase in surface irregularity of the anterior cornea causes decreased levels of visual acuity. As the disease advances, large amounts of the higher order aberrations develop, such that penetrating keratoplasty eventually becomes necessary. Unfortunately, the outcome of this corneal transplant procedure is variable and graft rejection often occurs, requiring additional transplants. Even with a successful transplant, an irregular corneal shape often remains problematic. The lack of reliable and non-invasive therapeutic interventions for keratoconus leaves patients with debilitating, life-long visual deficits.

Rigid contact lenses have effectively managed higher order aberrations induced by irregular corneal surfaces when a spherical surface of the lens and an underlying layer of fluid are placed on top of the front surface of the irregular cornea. However, these lenses have a limited tolerance because they rest primarily on the distorted surface of the cornea and the fact that successful wear is dependent on a well lubricated interface, a healthy corneal epithelium, and a compatible corneal shape. Most importantly, these lenses cannot correct the higher order aberrations of the posterior corneal surface, which have significant impact on retinal image quality in keratoconus.

Recently, my laboratory demonstrated that wavefront-guided spectacles and soft contact lenses can significantly reduce the higher order aberrations in keratoconic eyes. They resulted in significant improvements of visual performance in comparison to the results obtained with conventional soft toric lenses and even with rigid lenses. However, the spectacles effectively corrected the aberrations only when the subject's gaze angle was fixed - *i.e.* when centration of the spectacles with respect to the pupil center is within specific limits. Although wavefront-guided soft contact lenses have largely overcome this limitation, the residual uncorrected higher order aberrations with the lens were still larger than is commonly present in normal eyes. The instability of lens position and rotational orientation after blinks explain why the visual acuity of abnormal eyes with wavefront-guided soft contact lenses is still worse than typical normal visual acuity. Therefore, eliminating unpredictable lens movements is critical for patients with abnormal corneal surfaces to achieve 20/20 or better visual acuity.

The PROSE device (prosthetic replacement of the ocular surface ecosystem, BostonSight), is custom spline-based scleral lens that has a large diameter (17-23 mm) that enables the lens to rest entirely on the relatively insensitive sclera and vault above the sensitive cornea to create a fluid-filled space between the back surface of the lens and the front corneal surface. The internal optic zone of the lenses that were used was 12 mm and is surrounded by an approximate 2 mm wide transitional zone designed to vault the limbus and merge seamlessly into the posterior haptic surface. The posterior haptic surface of the lens was designed to create channels at its interface with the scleral surface to permit tears (but not air) to be aspirated into the post-lens fluid reservoir and prevent the development of fluid-ventilated lens suction. Since the PROSE is fabricated from the Boston Equalens II (oprifocon A) with a high oxygen permeability (Dk = 85×10^{-11} units), patients can wear these lenses during all waking hours. However, similar to rigid contact lenses, the uncorrected aberrations from the posterior corneal surface could prevent a large vision improvement especially in advanced keratoconus. These findings suggest that correcting the residual aberrations is the next essential step to further improve the optical quality of the eye. The fact that the stability of the scleral lens in position and rotational orientation is superior to conventional rigid contact lenses makes it almost an ideal candidate to apply the wavefront-guided optical design. Recent advances in high-precision lathe technology make it possible to precisely create surface perturbations at submicron accuracy on the lens, which is necessary to correct higher order aberrations.

My laboratory in collaboration with BostonSight has developed the wavefront-guided PROSE device to correct higher order aberrations. Advanced KC subjects (11 eyes) were first fit with conventional PROSE, which was followed by measurements of aberrations, as well as static decentration and rotation with respect to the pupil. A submicron-precision lathe was then used to create computed irregular lens surface profiles designed to neutralize the measured aberration. These lenses effectively corrected most of higher order aberrations with higher order RMS wavefront error reduced ~3.1 times to 0.37±0.19 μm for a 6mm pupil. This is similar to a level of higher order wavefront RMS wavefront error observed in typical normal eyes. This correction resulted in a significant VA improvement (~1.9 lines), however, the average logMAR VA was 0.21 - significantly worse than normal logMAR acuity. Importantly, this finding may suggest that prolonged exposure to poor optics (as in keratoconus) limits the benefits that can be obtained by optical correction, indicating a key role of neural adaptation processes. In other words, attempts to improve visual performance by correcting the optics of the eye will only work if the brain is capable of processing the increased sharpness and contrast of the retinal image.

Our previous studies, in which neural functions were investigated by bypassing optical factors with adaptive optics technology, found significant neural deficits in keratoconic eyes compared to the normal control group. This cannot be explained by optical factors, since aberrations in both groups were well corrected with adaptive optics. This could be attributed to the effects of long-term neural adaptation to their own aberrations. Neural adaptation to image blur is known to occur even in normal eyes and a plausible extension of this phenomenon is that neural adaptation to the large magnitude of keratoconus aberrations may have a substantial effect on visual performance with advanced correction. Thus, it is critical to understand how long-term visual deprivation caused by defects in ocular optics affects quality of vision and to evaluate the short- and long-term visual benefits of correcting these defects. The knowledge gained from this study will enhance not only our understanding of the optical and neural contribution to visual performance, but also our ability to provide patients with an optimal vision correction protocol.

Scleral Lenses – Reducing Compromise for the Individual with Keratoconus (Jason Marsack, PhD, FAAO)

Scleral Lenses Work… Period

For individuals with highly aberrated ocular optics, such as is the case of keratoconus, pellucid marginal degeneration and post-LASIK ectasia, scleral lenses are, as I have heard one prominent contact lens fitter proclaim, “nothing short of a miracle.” The miracle that scleral lenses are most often associated with performing is providing good on-eye comfort while, at the same time, providing good visual performance. Very plainly, scleral lenses do these two things well at the same time, which until the resurgence in scleral contact lens technology, had previously not always been possible. This meant that an individual with one of these conditions might on some level be required to make a compromise between better vision and better comfort. As scleral lenses can do both of these things, they have, to a degree, eliminated the need to make this choice. That said, they have not eliminated all compromises associated with patient satisfaction, and many challenges remain to be solved.

Evolving Technology for the Highly Aberrated Eye

As someone that spends the vast majority of my time in the laboratory, I see part of my role related to the evolution of contact lens technology for the highly aberrated eye as developing methods that may eliminate compromise. Most of the time, the solutions we hypothesize in the laboratory are accurately defined as small evolutions of existing technologies in order to make that technology more efficacious on one or more dimensions for the individual. If performance can be improved on several dimensions with a single improvement in technology, this reduces the need for both the patient and practitioner to compromise. Work on wavefront-guided scleral lenses is an example of this evolutionary approach to moving technology forward, using the comfortable scleral platform to improve comfort (something scleral lenses already do well), while tailoring the optics to the individual subject (the need for this aspect of the correction depending on the severity of the disease in the eye being treated). However, comfort and optics are only two of the areas that are important to the individual with keratoconus. As I have previously discussed in several forums, I feel comfort and performance are two of the three aspects most important to patients, the third being cost. In my opinion, these are the three areas that are of most importance to the patient. My opinion is formed from three points of view: 1) interfacing with expert clinicians that fit these lenses on a daily basis 2) interfacing with subjects that participate in our laboratory research projects and 3) my own experience as an individual with keratoconus. I accept that others may consider different dimensions equally, if not more important. For instance, I understand the practitioner demands that ocular health rightfully be considered paramount to all other factors.

An Observation about Corrections for the Highly Aberrated Eye

When I look at the treatment modalities associated with the typical eye, and those associated with highly aberrated eye, I believe the main difference is that those associated with the typical eye require much less of this patient/practitioner compromise that we have discussed above. Good comfort, performance and cost are achievable for the individual with typical eyes through a host of correction modalities (spectacles, contact lenses, orthokeratology, refractive surgery… the list is long). In fact, the number of correction modalities available to this individual is, in my opinion, almost an embarrassment of riches when contrasted against the number of efficacious modalities available to individuals with highly aberrated eyes. As a simple example, a 2.0 D myope may achieve equivalent visual performance and overall comfort with a pair of glasses or a pair of soft contact lenses. The patient is not forced to compromise on these dimensions, meaning one correction method is not vastly superior to the other. In the end, the choice between spectacles and contact lenses is often made based on lifestyle needs. Simply put: the correction is chosen based on the subject's goals for using their time.

Certainly, from this perspective, one of the corrections may be seen as more beneficial for a particular activity (*e.g.*: soft contact lens to exercise). But, from the point of view of comfort and performance, they may be relatively equal. Now, contrast this with the situation associated with the highly aberrated eye. In my opinion, the correction chosen for the highly aberrated eye is driven more by "what works for this individual given their disease severity?" than the lifestyle needs of the individual. What this means is that the patient and practitioner are being forced to make a compromise in one of several dimensions, and this compromise may negatively impact the patient's quality of life.

Where the Rubber Hits the Road

A real-world example that has always resonated with me came during one of our early research studies where we enrolled habitual gas permeable contact lens wearers. During the history intake, a question about how one of the subjects daily wore their GP lenses, the reply was "it depends on what I plan to do the next day." The explanation of this statement was that if the patient needed to stay up late, this resulted in a delay in GP lens wear for several hours after waking the following day due to lingering discomfort. If the patient needed to be up early, then GP lenses needed to be out by mid-evening the night before. This rather extreme example is a demonstration of a compromise that an individual with typical eyes would simply not have to consider.

A Long-term Goal - Reducing Compromise

One long term goal for the development of novel corrections for the individual with highly aberrated optics is, in my opinion, to reduce compromise. Scleral lenses are an excellent example of a technology that reduces some of the compromise that is associated with these conditions. Or, perhaps, to think about it more rigorously, the dimensionality of the compromise has been reduced. That said, scleral lenses do not reduce all compromise. As some concerns are addressed, new ones take their place. Cost, complexity of the wear/care systems and a need for improved optical performance in some patients are areas where I feel we should continue to focus effort to reduce compromise with this technology. More generally, as a community, we will work to continue to reduce compromise across all correction modalities for this patient population, thus in turn increasing the choices available to every patient.

Summary

The work that the entire field is doing today will create more efficacious choices and less compromise in the future. This will manifest most meaningfully, in my opinion, in the following way.... Somewhere out there, right now, there is a 7-year-old child that will eventually develop keratoconus. The signs and symptoms are not manifesting yet, but they will.... I would personally like to see technology (scleral lenses and others) move forward such that this child's experience later in life when they are being diagnosed with keratoconus is accompanied by increased clinical options for treating the disease and therefore less compromise. If we as a community of clinicians, researchers, industry partners and advocates succeed in continually moving technology forward, the result will reduce the impact of keratoconus on this individual, and promote this child reaching their full potential.

NEUROTROPHIC CORNEAS (Lynette K. Johns, OD, FAAO, FSLS, FBCLA)

Scleral lenses are effective at providing hydration and protection in patients who suffer from neurotrophic or hypesthetic corneas. Since these corneas have little to no sensation, there are a variety of risks for these patients in general. Without a pain response, a patient can be unaware of a potentially blinding ulcer. Therefore, the category of neurotrophic corneas poses a challenge for scleral lens fitting, training and overall management.

Scleral lens landing zones should be optimally aligned for long term success in all patients; however, in this group, it is crucial. As stated before, there are no pain cues, so the only signal of a potential ocular emergency for the patient is hyperemia. Therefore, care must be taken to prevent any excessive compression that may result in peripheral and limbal hyperemia as well as rebound hyperemia after lens removal. Edge impingement may also induce hyperemia and should be avoided during the fitting process.

Training patients who have neurotrophic corneas with application and removal can be challenging. Any misaligned application attempt can potentially result in a corneal abrasion or epithelial defect (Fig. **30**). Teaching a patient to center the lens over the cornea reduces the risk of "misfires." If the patient uses an application cup/plunger, they can view the hole in the center for proper alignment. In cases where the patient still struggles, a lighted plunger can be incorporated into the training. If the patient loses visualization of the LED light, the lens is not properly aligned for application. Over time, patients can "wean off" of these training aids.

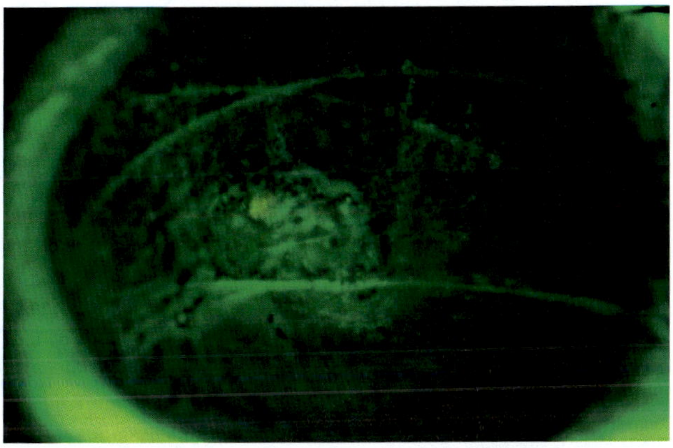

Fig. (30). Example of poorly aligned application attempts on a neurotrophic cornea. This patient is at risk for a corneal abrasion. Image courtesy of Lynette Johns and I-Site newsletter.

Once fit, these patients should be monitored more frequently. Any patient complaints of "redness" should be taken seriously and the patient should be evaluated immediately to rule out any infectious or inflammatory process. Often these patients have concurrent exposure or lagophthalmos, so proper lubrication and protection measures require implementation into their nightly routine.

Despite the significant challenge that a neurotrophic cornea poses, the reward for the patient far exceeds the risk. If a practitioner is new to scleral lens fitting, patients should be monitored more frequently for fitting complications. With proper patient education and setting of expectations, patients appreciate the close care and monitoring to ensure proper ocular health and long term success.

HANDLING CHALLENGES (Melissa Barnett, OD, FAAO, FSLS, FBCLA and Lynette K. Johns, OD, FAAO, FSLS, FBCLA)

An in-depth understanding of scleral lens handling is critical to succeed with scleral lenses. Handling is the most common reason for scleral lens dropout. For patients with missing digits or hand dexterity issues due to arthritis or tremors, scleral lens handing may be particularly problematic.

Careful observation of the patient and creativity will enable the practitioner to customize the application and removal technique for each patient's needs. Proper bracing of the hand in patients who have tremors using dictionaries or large books to provide an arm rest to stabilize the arm and reduce the overall tremor. In addition, the use of a more viscous solution in the bowl of the lens is helpful to prevent spilling when the lens is tipped.

In patients that have strong reaction or blepharospasm to liquid on the cornea, the patient can practice opening their eye in the saline using an eyecup in order to acclimate the patient to the sensation. Saline can be heated or cooled based on the patient's preference.

Additional tools may be used to succeed with scleral lens handling to benefit patients. One is the See Green Lens Inserter by Dalsey Adaptives (http://dalseyadaptives.net/store/), which is available with and without a stand (Fig. **31**). The lighted plunger helps center the device for application. The stand holds the plunger and lens in place prior to application. This is helpful for patients who have unsteady hands or for those who need both hands to hold their eyelids open.

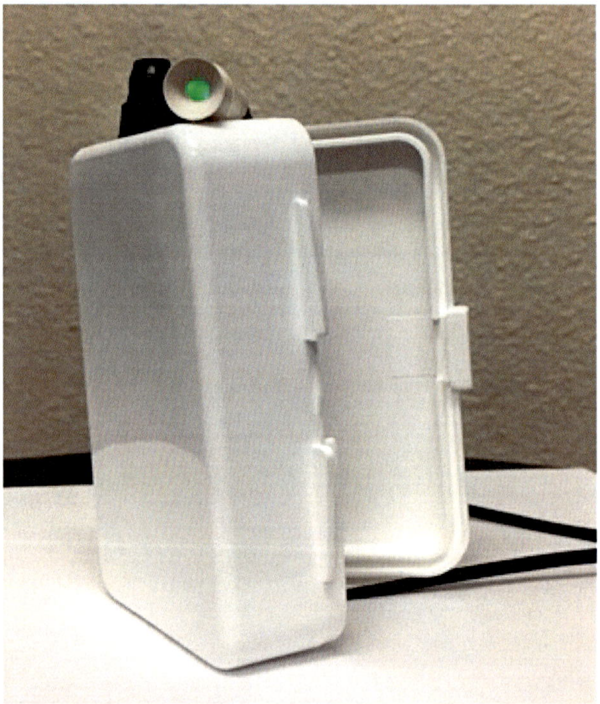

Fig. (31). See Green Lens Inserter. Image courtesy of Melissa Barnett.

Another tool is the EZI Scleral Lens Applicator by Q-Case Inc. (http://ezibyqcase.com/) (Fig. **32**). This device is placed on the finger like a ring and has a base for scleral lens application. This design provides stability and allows patients to apply scleral devices with one finger.

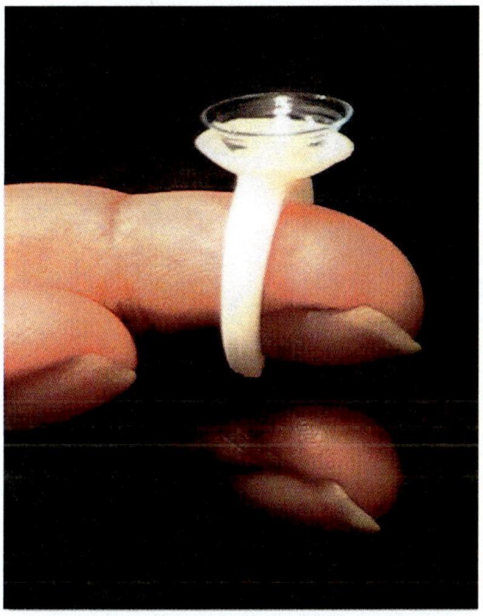

Fig. (32). Example of the EZI scleral lens applicator. Image courtesy of Melissa Barnett.

A third option is a #8 O ring that is available at any hardware store. O ring dimensions are 3/8" x 9/16" x 3/32". The scleral lens rests on the O ring on a patient's finger, which can allow for stable application.

An additional option for scleral lens insertion is a sterile orthodontic ring placed on a patient's hand. These come in packages of 100 and may be used for single use insertion of scleral lenses.

It is the responsibility of practitioners and their staff to help patients with the scleral lens care and handling process in order to achieve optimal results with scleral lenses.

MANAGEMENT OF PERSISTENT EPITHELIAL DEFECTS WITH SCLERAL LENSES (Lynette K. Johns, OD, FAAO, FSLS, FBCLA)

In cases of ocular surface disease such as limbal stem cell deficiencies and neurotrophic corneas, the epithelium is prone to breakdown. A longstanding epithelial breakdown is known as a persistent epithelial defect (PED) (Fig. **33**). Treatments for PEDs include patching, intensive lubrication, bandage contact lens, and amniotic membrane grafts. Tarsorrhaphy is used in extreme cases. A scleral lens can be an ideal treatment modality from the patient's perspective. They are not disfigured by having a tarsorrhaphy and have the ability to see with scleral lenses. It is important to evaluate the anterior ocular health carefully and rule out microbial keratitis.

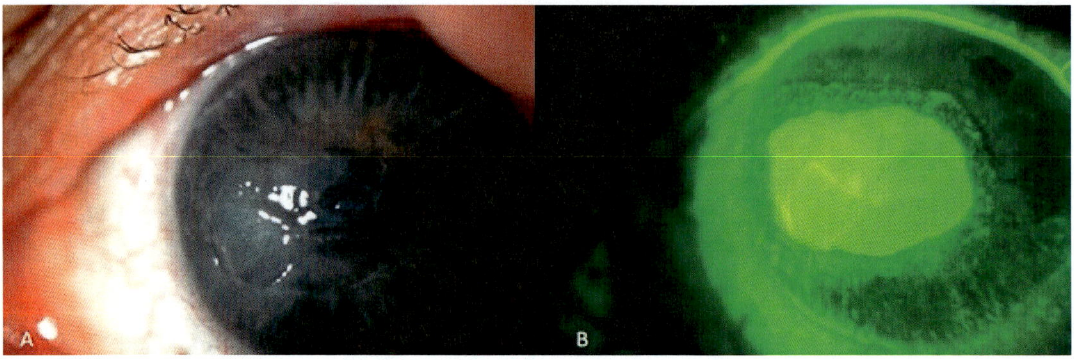

Fig. (33). Example of a persistent epithelial defect prior to scleral lens wear. In A, the white light appearance of the longstanding PED without a hyperemic response. In B, the size of the PED is easily viewed with cobalt blue light and a Wratten filter. Images courtesy of Lynette Johns.

When managing a PED with a scleral lens, the scleral lens is worn on an extended wear basis. Therefore, it is important to optimize oxygen delivery by selecting a material with the highest Dk, reducing the center thickness of the lens and reducing the clearance while avoiding corneal or limbal contact. Tear exchange is also important so the landing zone should not be perfectly aligned 360 degrees. If there is evidence of meridional edge lift, it can be reduced a little, but maintaining some edge lift will allow tear exchange. Ideally, there should be no evidence of suction. The presence of tear exchange signifies that the lens is not suctioned.

The lens is filled with preservative free saline and one drop of a preservative free antibiotic acting as prophylaxis. Each day, the practitioner removes the scleral lens to check the defect. The scleral lens is cleaned with an alcohol based gas permeable lens cleaner. I disinfect the lens briefly with hydrogen peroxide while the lens is out of the patient's eye and soak the lens in preservative free saline afterward to prevent peroxide corneal toxicity. Fresh preservative free saline and one drop of preservative free antibiotic are placed in the reservoir of the lens. The patient is seen daily until the defect has resurfaced. In my experience, resuming daily wear immediately after the defect resurfaces may cause the PED to return. The patient continues one more night of extended wear after the defect has resurfaced to strengthen the epithelium. The first night after daily wear of the lens, the patient is instructed to aggressively lubricate the eye with ointment and use a tape tarsorrhaphy in the presence of lagophthalmos.

Since the lens is worn on an extended wear basis, it is not uncommon to see microcysts or bullae (Fig. **34**). Here, the immediate risk of the PED is greater than the short-term risk of edema, so the patient can resume extended wear of the lens until the PED is resurfaced. In some patients with defects that are slow to resurface, the patient is taught how to apply and remove lenses independently.

They are dispensed two lenses. While one lens is disinfecting, the second lens is being worn, and the patient is instructed to switch lenses in the morning upon waking and in the evening prior to bedtime. The patient is seen every 3-4 days or once a week as long as they are carefully instructed about signs and symptoms of complications like redness, pain, discharge, vision changes, and photophobia. If the patient has neurotrophic or hypesthetic cornea, then redness is the important finding that requires immediate assessment.

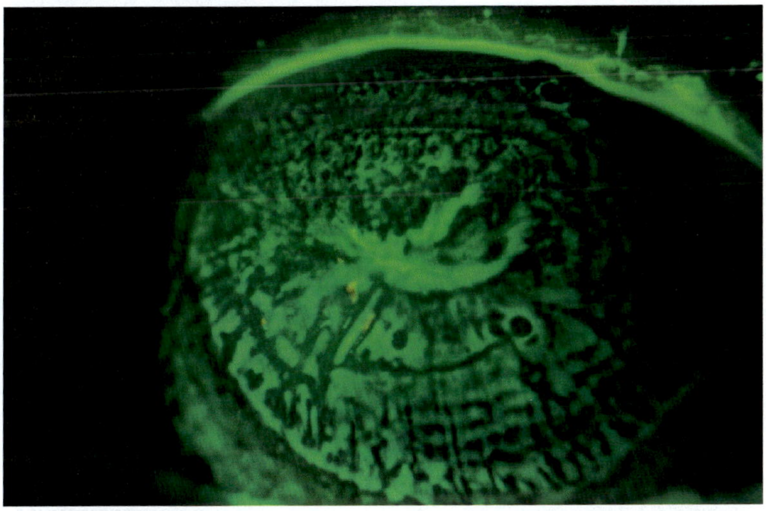

Fig. (34). The PED from Fig. (**18**) healed in five days of extended wear with a scleral lens and prophylactic antibiotic. The lens was removed, disinfected and refilled with preservative free saline and antibiotic daily. Note there are a few epithelial bullae present. Image courtesy of Lynette Johns.

In many cases, a scleral lens is required for daily wear after the PED has resurfaced. Patients with a history of a PED should be monitored closely. Patients with nighttime lagophthalmos or exposure require supplemental support in the form of lubrication and protection to prevent a recurrence of PED.

SCUBA AND DEEP SEA DIVING WITH SCLERAL LENSES (Karoline Elving-Kokkee, BOPTOM, MSC)

Some scleral lens wearers like to test the limits of wearing their lenses in extreme conditions. For example, some patients want to be able to wear their scleral lenses while scuba diving. However, several factors should be considered when determining whether scleral lenses can be worn safely while diving. These factors include the possibility of losing a lens while swimming and/or diving, increased risk of microbial infection and the effect of changing pressure on the lens-eye interface.

Successful use of a scleral lens requires a proper fit. When assessing the lens fit, the scleral landing zone should be aligned properly with the anterior ocular surface. Small uneven areas in the scleral surface underneath the lens can allow air bubbles to enter the landing zone during wear and affect the lens clearance (see Fig. **35**).

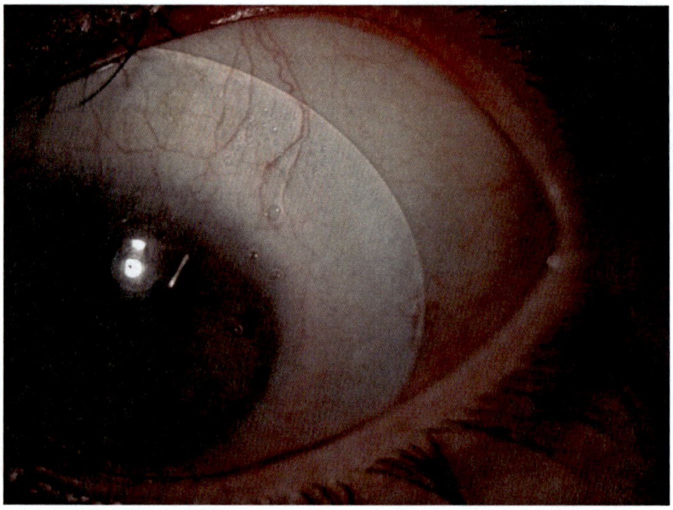

Fig. (35). Air bubbles drawn in underneath the landing zone to the lens clearance. Image courtesy of Karolien Elving-Kokke.

Given that scleral shape is usually asymmetric, back-surface scleral lenses can provide a better fit, improved comfort, and increased wearing time [26 - 28]. Before diving, the scleral lens wearer should confirm that the lens is inserted correctly without air bubbles under the lens.

Although lens loss can be a worry when swimming or diving with a scleral lens, the actual risk of this happening is extremely low, as a non-fenestrated scleral lens creates a seal when worn, and this seal can grow tighter with prolonged wear time. In addition, this seal can increase slightly when diving, further decreasing the risk of losing the lens. Finally, because a mask is worn when diving, the lens can only be lost when water enters the mask; therefore, the mask must fit well, and the wearer should close his/her eyes when clearing the mask [29].

When we dive, our body is subjected to changes in external pressure. This pressure increases while descending and decreases upon ascending to the surface. During descent, inert gases accumulate in the tissues, and these gases are released from the tissues upon ascent.

Therefore, ascending too rapidly can cause these inert gases to leave the tissues too quickly; in extreme cases, this can cause a condition commonly known as "the bends" or decompression sickness. Although all divers should take steps to prevent this condition, wearers of rigid contact lenses—including scleral lens wearers—can also develop painful eyes and/or blurry vision after diving. The most likely cause of these complications is the formation of air bubbles due to the escape of inert gases from the tear film or cornea during ascent, which can be easily prevented by performing a well-regulated ascent, which allows any accumulated gases to disperse harmlessly [30].

Wearing contact lenses also reduces oxygen transmission to the eyes. Because the mask covers the nose, oxygen exhaled through the nose can remain trapped in the mask. During an average length dive of 45 minutes, approximately 3.200 µl of O_2 can accumulate in the mask, which is ample oxygen to meet the cornea's requirements in that space of time [31]. Although patients have not complained of blurred vision either during or after a dive, exactly how oxygen permeability through a scleral lens is affected while diving is currently unknown.

Given the increased risk of infection associated with wearing any form of contact lens in the water, after diving and—if conditions allow—between dives, the scleral lens should be removed, cleaned, and reapplied using preservative-free saline [32, 33]. Special care should be used when removing the lens, and the wearer should wait 15-30 minutes after the dive before removing the lens. In case of increased lens tightness when attempting to remove the lens, the seal can be released by gently lifting the lens edge or by moving the lens around with a plunger placed near the lens edge after instilling rewetting drops.

Research is currently underway to document the experiences of divers who wear scleral lenses, and such studies will likely provide valuable insight into the effect of wearing scleral lenses while diving. Nevertheless, practical experience has shown that scleral lenses appear to be compatible with diving, provided that appropriate care is taken before, during and after the dive.

SUMMARY

It is evident that with all the indications and features of scleral lenses that are known, there remains a large amount of information about scleral lenses that still requires investigation. Worldwide experts in scleral lens fitting shared their experiences and challenges that they encounter daily when fitting these large diameter gas permeable lenses. Hopefully, there will be less challenges in years to come with the amount of research and investigation that the resurgence of scleral lenses has inspired.

CONFLICT OF INTEREST

Dr. Yoon: Johnson & Johnson (research grant), Bausch and Lomb (research grant), Coopervision (research grant), TearLab (Research grant), Ovitz (consultant), Bausch and Lomb (consultant), Allotex (consultant)

ACKNOWLEDGEMENTS

Dr. Yoon would like to acknowledge his grant support: NIH/NEI EY014999 and Research to Prevent Blindness and personally: Ramkumar Sabesan, Perry Rosenthal, Lynette Johns, Olga Tomashevskaya, Debbie Jacobs.

REFERENCES

[1] Ensley R, Miller H. Happy Landings. Review of Cornea & Contact Lenses 2016; 10-1.

[2] DeNaeyer GW. Improve your scleral lens fitting success. Contact Lens Spectr 2014; 29: 22-5.

[3] Van der Worp E, Graf T, Caroline P. Exploring beyond the corneal borders. Contact Lens Spectr 2010; 6: 26-32.

[4] Visser E-S, Van der Linden BJ, Otten HM, Van der Lelij A, Visser R. Medical applications and outcomes of bitangential scleral lenses. Optom Vis Sci 2013; 90(10): 1078-85. [http://dx.doi.org/10.1097/OPX.0000000000000018] [PMID: 23974663]

[5] Morrison SD. The importance of scleral shape. Contact Lens Spectr 2016; 31: 40-4.

[6] Yildrim N, Gursov H, Sahin A, Ozer A, Colak E. Glaucoma after penetrating keratoplasty: Incidence, risk factors, and management. J Ophthalmology 2011; 95129.

[7] DeNaeyer GW. Contact lenses after trabeculectomy. Contact Lens Spectr 2010; (Jan): 36.

[8] Carrasquillo KG, Barnett M. Scleral lens applications in unique populations. Contact Lens Spectr 2014; (April): 29.

[9] Vijaya L, Manish P, Ronnie G, Shantha B. Management of complications in glaucoma surgery. Indian J Ophthalmol 2011; 59 (Suppl.): S131-40. [http://dx.doi.org/10.4103/0301-4738.73689] [PMID: 21150025]

[10] Nguyen AH, Dastiridou AI, Chiu GB, Francis BA, Lee OL. Glaucoma surgical considerations for PROSE lens use in patients with ocular surface disease. Contact Lens and Anterior eye 2016; 39: 257-61. [http://dx.doi.org/10.1016/j.clae.2016.02.002]

[11] De Beer F, Visser ES, J, De Boer J. Behandeling van een opgeheven voorste oogkamer door middel van een sclera lens. Visus 2012; 21-3.

[12] Ghazafari R, Libassi D. Notching a scleral lens to avoid pressure on glaucoma shunts: A case study, SUNY college of optometry. Scientific and Clinical Poster at GSLS congress 2016.

[13] Sarkisian SR. The ex-press mini glaucoma shunt: technique and experience. Middle East Afr j Ophthalmol 2009; 16(3): 134-7.

[14] Schornack MM, Baratz KH. Ocular cicatricial pemphigoid: the role of scleral lenses in disease management. Cornea 2009; 28(10): 1170-2. [http://dx.doi.org/10.1097/ICO.0b013e318199fa56] [PMID: 19770718]

[15] Rosenthal P, Bradley J. Dry eye-like symptoms without dry eyes is a neurological disease. Invest Ophthalmol Vis Sci 2011; 52(6): 3855.

[16] Rosenthal P, Borsook D. The corneal pain system. Part I: the missing piece of the dry eye puzzle. Ocul Surf 2012; 10(1): 2-14.
[http://dx.doi.org/10.1016/j.jtos.2012.01.002] [PMID: 22330055]

[17] Rosenthal P, Baran I, Jacobs DS. Corneal pain without stain: is it real? Ocul Surf 2009; 7(1): 28-40.
[http://dx.doi.org/10.1016/S1542-0124(12)70290-2] [PMID: 19214350]

[18] Rosenthal P, Borsook D. Ocular neuropathic pain. Br J Ophthalmol 2016; 100(1): 128-34.
[http://dx.doi.org/10.1136/bjophthalmol-2014-306280] [PMID: 25943558]

[19] Hirata H, Okamoto K, Tashiro A, Bereiter DA. A novel class of neurons at the trigeminal subnucleus interpolaris/caudalis transition region monitors ocular surface fluid status and modulates tear production. J Neurosci 2004; 24(17): 4224-32.
[http://dx.doi.org/10.1523/JNEUROSCI.0381-04.2004] [PMID: 15115818]

[20] Wilson SE, Bourne WM. Fuchs' dystrophy. Cornea 1988; 7(1): 2-18.
[http://dx.doi.org/10.1097/00003226-198801000-00002] [PMID: 3280235]

[21] Adamis AP, Filatov V, Tripathi BJ, Tripathi RC. Fuchs' endothelial dystrophy of the cornea. Surv Ophthalmol 1993; 38(2): 149-68.
[http://dx.doi.org/10.1016/0039-6257(93)90099-S] [PMID: 8235998]

[22] Weiss JS, Møller HU, Lisch W, *et al.* The IC3D classification of the corneal dystrophies. Cornea 2008; 27 (Suppl. 2): S1-S83.
[http://dx.doi.org/10.1097/ICO.0b013e31817780fb] [PMID: 19337156]

[23] Papageorgiou E, McLean RJ, Gottlob I. Nystagmus in childhood. Pediatr Neonatol 2014; 55(5): 341-51.
[http://dx.doi.org/10.1016/j.pedneo.2014.02.007] [PMID: 25086850]

[24] Penix K, Swanson MW, DeCarlo DK. Nystagmus in pediatric patients: interventions and patient-focused perspectives. Clin Ophthalmol 2015; 9: 1527-36.
[PMID: 26345377]

[25] Jayaramachandran P, Proudlock FA, Odedra N, Gottlob I, McLean RJ. A randomized controlled trial comparing soft contact lens and rigid gas-permeable lens wearing in infantile nystagmus. Ophthalmology 2014; 121(9): 1827-36.
[http://dx.doi.org/10.1016/j.ophtha.2014.03.007] [PMID: 24811959]

[26] Visser ES, Visser R, van Lier HJ, Otten HM. Modern scleral lenses part I: clinical features. Eye Contact Lens 2007; 33(1): 13-20. a
[http://dx.doi.org/10.1097/01.icl.0000233217.68379.d5] [PMID: 17224674]

[27] Visser ES, Visser R, van Lier HJ, Otten HM. Modern scleral lenses part II: patient satisfaction. Eye Contact Lens 2007; 33(1): 21-5. b
[http://dx.doi.org/10.1097/01.icl.0000228964.74647.25] [PMID: 17224675]

[28] Van der Worp E. A guide to scleral lens fitting. 2nd ed., Pacific University 2015.http://commons.pacificu.edu/mono/10/

[29] Elving-Kokke K. Diving with scleral lenses. I-site 2016.http://netherlens.com/october_2016

[30] Divers Alert Network Europe. www.daneurope.org

[31] Brown MS, Siegel IM. Cornea-contact lens interaction in the aquatic environment. CLAO J 1997; 23(4): 237-42.
[PMID: 9348447]

[32] Stapleton F, Keay L, Edwards K, Holden B. The epidemiology of microbial keratitis with silicone hydrogel contact lenses. Eye Contact Lens 2013; 39(1): 79-85.

[http://dx.doi.org/10.1097/ICL.0b013e3182713919] [PMID: 23172318]

[33] Lindsay RG, Watters G, Johnson R, Ormonde SE, Snibson GR. Acanthamoeba keratitis and contact lens wear. Clin Exp Optom 2007; 90(5): 351-60. [http://dx.doi.org/10.1111/j.1444-0938.2007.00172.x] [PMID: 17697181]

CHAPTER 15

Scleral Lens Patient Recruitment

Damon J. Ezekiel*

Ezekiel Eyes, Nedlands WA 6009, Australia

Abstract: The establishment of a specialty scleral lens practice can be a time-consuming but worthwhile process. The practice can be both financially and personally rewarding. Expending the necessary resources to develop the practice can result in a loyal and long-term patient base. According to some specialist practitioners, they attract patients who have consulted numerous other eye care practitioners with little success. Once these patients realize the quality of life improvement that can be achieved with properly fit scleral lenses, they become patients for life who recommend the practice to others. By making the patient a top priority, business will be successful. Patients wearing specialized contact lenses will return on an annual basis and refer their family and friends. Successful practitioners are very talented at building value into every aspect of their practice and therefore building a contact lens specialty niche. In order to continue to grow the practice, an investment in advertising and networking can aid in referrals. Staying up to date with scleral lens and equipment technology can streamline the scleral lens fitting process, thus saving time for the practitioner and patient. Establishing relationships with contact lens laboratories is critical to a thriving scleral lens practice.

Keywords: Advertise, Continuing education, Disposition, Enthusiasm, Equipment, Experience, Indications, Laboratory consultants, Loyalty, Marketing, Mentorship, Multifocal, Ocular surface, Passion, Patient, Practice builder, Relationship, Social media, Technology, Time.

INTRODUCTION

The establishment of a specialty scleral contact lens practice can be a worthwhile and strategic professional endeavor, with the potential to assist many patients.

Expending the necessary resources to develop the practice can result in a loyal, long-term patient base. According to some specialist practitioners, they attract patients who have consulted numerous other eye care practitioners with little success. Once these patients realize the quality of life improvement that can be

* **Corresponding author Damon J. Ezekiel:** Ezekiel Eyes, Nedlands WA 6009, Australia; Tel: +61893863620; Fax: +61893896124; E-mail: damon@ezekieleyes.com

Melissa Barnett & Lynette K. Johns (Eds.)

achieved with properly fit scleral lenses, they become patients for life who recommend the practice to others.

INVESTMENT IN THE PRACTICE

When developing a specialty contact lens practice, it is highly important that eye care practitioners are prepared to invest in the practice. Investments can include equipment and technology, training of staff, marketing and business development, and ongoing professional development.

Equipment and Technology

The field of contact lenses is continually evolving with technological advancements of contact lenses, equipment and knowledge. In order for a specialty contact lens practice to succeed, at a minimum, a practice requires a corneal topographer, a wide range of diagnostic fitting sets, and an anterior segment camera or imaging device. Additionally, anterior segment optical coherence tomography (OCT) can be a valuable tool.

Staff Training

Staff should be trained to recognize that every single patient is a potential contact lens candidate. During preliminary testing, staff should ask every non-contact lens wearer if they have ever considered contact lenses. Contact lens opportunities can be discussed with the eye care practitioner. Some patients have been told previously that they are not candidates for contact lenses, and they therefore might not re-visit the option without prompting.

Business Development

Referrals should be cultivated. Satisfied patients will help the practice grow from within the patient base. In order to grow the practice from the outside, referrals are necessary. Referrals might come from ophthalmology, corneal specialists or from other eye care practitioners who do not specialize in contact lenses.

Professional Development

Eye care practitioners must understand how to fit specialty contact lenses. This includes understanding indications, candidacy, lens designs and fitting techniques that may require additional training and certifications. Additional contact lens modalities can be offered to improve visual outcomes. Practitioners must ensure that they stay up to date with changes in the industry and technical advances. Advances in specialty contact lenses are continually being made, with contact lenses in general growing in popularity. From keratoconus to myopia control, it is important to stay current with the newest technologies available for eye conditions. Being comfortable with multiple contact lens designs and their uses may open a practice to a new group of contact lens wearers [1].

ADVANTAGES OF PRACTICE INVESTMENT

Patient Loyalty and Recurring Appointments

Loyalty is defined by patients entrusting the care of their eyes to an eye care practitioner or practice, over the long term, and continually returning to have their vision and ocular health monitored and managed. Fostering loyalty can be as simple as taking a moment to provide an explanation that helps to gain a patient's trust. Case studies have shown that when this occurs, not only does a patient order new contact lenses; he or she schedules family members for an appointment [2].

A successful, sustainable practice generally employs strategies to retain loyal patients and attract new ones. Contact lenses are a key ingredient because the satisfaction with the product is registered every day that contact lenses are worn. This significantly impacts their satisfaction with their eye care professional and practice. Patients might quietly slip away and find another eye care provider if solutions are not found to improve their visual acuity or comfort. A satisfied patient becomes the practice advocate thus retaining their business as well as opening up opportunities to attract new patients [3].

Practice Identification as a Niche Office Promotes Growth

Establishing the reputation of the practice as a niche office and cultivating its growth can occur through being current, innovative and technologically savvy in the provision of scleral lenses. An eye care practice with a strong and positive reputation in the community as being a leading service provider usually finds it easy to grow its patient base. Kelly Kerksick, OD (private eye care practitioner in Columbia, IL) described the importance of reputation in the following way:

"If there's a new lens, I want it in my practice because I want to be out there ahead of everyone else. People seem to have a perception — perhaps related to some of the articles I've written — that I am the go-to eye care practitioner for new technology, and I promote myself that way." She explained that reputation went beyond the latest contact lens technology; most important was making patients happy. *"If I can make a patient happy, they will go to work or tell friends how great the experience is, and I get four or five new patients from referral. I am known as the eye care practitioner with specialty contact lenses, and this reputation differentiates me from other practices. If a patient is looking for a*

certain contact lens, like a bifocal or something he can't get elsewhere, I'm the eye care practitioner to see [4]."

Disadvantages

A disadvantage of building a scleral lens niche is that it can be time consuming due to the greater than usual amount of chair time required to ensure the correct fit for the patient. However, this perceived downside must be viewed in the context that specialty contact lenses have the potential to be profitable for a practice. Since they are unique, specialty lenses require higher fees for contact lens fitting and materials. Once an eye care practitioner gains familiarity with a particular lens, he or she will spend less time troubleshooting it.

Patient Types

There are three major groups of patients who can benefit from scleral lenses: those with dry eye and ocular surface disease, those requiring visual rehabilitation and patients with refractive error. Specialty contact lenses provide several key growth opportunities, particularly in certain niches such as dry eye, pediatrics, keratoconus, low vision and cosmetic correction.

Dry Eye Syndrome and Ocular Surface Disease

Eye care practitioners are increasingly seeing patients with dry eye syndrome, and there are many opportunities to offer solutions for these patients.

Over 14% of adults over 48 years of age have some form of dry eye, according to the Beaver Dam Eye study [5].

Further, the incidence of dry eye is much higher among contact lens wearers (64%) than among those who wear glasses only (39%) or those who don't require vision correction (28%) [6].

Dry eye is underdiagnosed and undertreated. It is important to take a proactive approach in diagnosing and treating dry eye rather than waiting for a patient to complain of symptoms. Many practitioners are missing out on opportunities to assist patients, and generate practice benefits, as they wait for patients to complain of dry eye instead of taking a proactive approach in promoting their ability to diagnose and manage the condition [7]. Patients rarely report dry eye until it is moderate to severe, and even then, they might not tell their eye care practitioner about their symptoms.

There are several avenues that practitioners can take in order to identify dry eye in patients and assist in improving their quality of life, with the central theme being patient awareness and education:

1. **Train Staff:** Employees are the outward face of the practice. It is imperative that they are trained in educating patients, so that they become firm advocates for the practice.
2. **Use a Questionnaire:** An ocular surface disease (OSD) questionnaire can provide clues about a patient's dry eye status. Currently, the International Dry Eye Workshop [DEWS] cites 13 existing symptom questionnaires [8].
3. **Be Proactive in Inquiring about Dry Eye:** In the examination chair, the patient should be questioned about whether the OSD questionnaire has been filled out, and if any questions arise about the dry eye brochures. Some patients might not realize that the symptoms to which they've grown accustomed are related to dry eye disease, a serious condition that requires eye care practitioner intervention.
4. **Patient Education:** At the patient's dry eye evaluation, an eye care practitioner should explain the different types of dry eye, their causes, and risk factors. An eye care practitioner should also describe the testing that will be conducted and the purpose for each test. Finally, the patient should have the management options explained to them [9].

The management of ocular surface rehabilitation falls to the eye care practitioner who has developed a niche eye care practice. The deterioration of the ocular surface is a complex phenomenon and needs to be carefully managed to an end point of the patient regaining their quality of vision. Scleral lenses are just the therapeutic devices to heal these patients. Scleral lenses by nature of their size will restore a patient's health, visual acuities and comfort. The delicate balancing of the scleral lenses on the sclera and vaulting the cornea with a large tear reservoir promote corneal healing.

Visual Rehabilitation

Irregular corneas require specialty contact lenses almost exclusively. The eye care practitioner should be well educated not only on contact lens options but also disease management strategies. In some cases, patients require co-management, and that, too, can generate referrals. Each patient has a unique history, which is often multifaceted with multiple visits and sometimes multiple practitioners. Patient and family education is critical for long term success. There are multiple resources that are available to educate patients and their families about keratoconus and irregular corneas.

Refractive Error

Scleral lenses are also becoming more common for treatment of refractive error such as myopia, hyperopia and presbyopia. The advantage of scleral lenses for patients with high astigmatism is that lenses can rotate while retaining excellent vision. Patients with residual refractive error post LASIK surgery are particularly pleased with scleral lenses as dry eye may be more prevalent in this population. Multifocal contact lenses require the expertise that niche contact lens practitioners can add to the extensive range of contact lens options. Patience and time is certainly an important aspect to aid in the fitting of these lenses.

Practitioner Traits for Success

Passion and Enthusiasm

A successful scleral lens specialist is generally someone who has passion and enthusiasm to truly make a difference for their patients. For many eye care practitioners, the personal and professional rewards can be great, particularly when they experience the satisfaction of assisting patients who have had past difficulties, or "tough to fit" corneas, and have not known where to turn. Specialty contact lens practice also enables a practitioner to follow areas of passion or interest, and capitalize on unique skills. The enthusiasm and outcomes that can result from this can set an eye care practitioner apart from others. "Push yourself outside your comfort zone," says Dori Carlson (American Optometric Association past president, Park River, ND) "You never know where you'll end up [10]."

A critical practice management rule is to do whatever is in the best interest of the patient. When that mindset for clinical decision making is employed, the stage is set for healthy, loyal contact lens wearers. By carefully reviewing patient encounters, clinical assessments, and contact lens materials and designs to improve patient outcomes, practitioners will be assured of meeting patient expectations and creating a profitable practice with a highly loyal patient base [11].

For many eye care practices, a change in attitude about contact lenses along with strategic changes in marketing and clinical operations can generate an increase in practice profitability.

Practitioners could consider the following changes to the contact lens fitting process:

- **Recommend contact lenses enthusiastically:** Instead of starting a discussion with patients about the potential problems of contact lenses, eye care practitioners should present them in a positive way. Patients should be educated about new contact lens technology and that the vast majority of patients can wear contacts with ease, even if they have had difficulty in the past. They should understand that presbyopia and astigmatism are now easily corrected, and new lens modalities and materials have helped many people with dry eyes and allergies. Bring up the idea of contact lens wear to patients, rather than waiting for them to ask about it.

- **Put trial (diagnostic) lenses on more people:** Free trial lens inventory already sitting in practices is a vastly underutilized resource. Most patients, if asked to try the newest and greatest lenses in the practice, agree to do so. This trial process should be considered a part of a practice's marketing program. Trial a scleral lens on a mild or moderate dry eye patient, and have the patient experience the benefits of a scleral lens firsthand. If the free trial takes place in the eye care practice while frames are also being tried on, many patients will purchase contact lenses, eyeglasses and sunglasses!
- **Set fees appropriately:** Many eye care professionals charge too little for their services. It is pointless to try to match fees or product prices with optical chains, discount stores or internet providers. Patients are generally loyal to an eye care practice because they trust the products and services they are receiving; as a result, they may purchase solely from the practice. Patients value the expertise of their regular eye care professional, and find it convenient to get everything they need in one place.
- **Use advanced instrumentation and build the fee into the evaluation or fitting:** A practice should be positioned according to the quality of its services and products, not according to price. The provision of a high level of service, and the use of technology such as corneal topography or specular microscopy performed on an annual basis, will assure patients that they are receiving the best possible care.
- **Don't make contact lens fitting more complex than it should be:** Some eye care practitioners have developed their contact lens procedures to appear complex, as a strategy to impress patients. Patients are more impressed when contact lenses are easy and convenient [12].

Empathy

Patients who require specialty contact lenses often include those who suffer with irregular corneas and severe ocular surface disease. Scleral lenses have long been viewed as a last resort, and practitioners must be mindful that patients view scleral lenses as their last hope. Practitioners should be aware of the fragile and sometimes challenging nature of these patients. Many of these ocular conditions can be debilitating and affect many aspects of the patient's life. Some patients may be anxious, depressed or suicidal and great care, active listening, and careful observation may provide clues to direct the patient to the proper medical care they require. Empathy experienced by the patient can lead to improved outcomes and loyalty to the practitioner.

Education, Training and Mentorship

There are various forms of education, training and mentorship within the eye care world. A few are mentioned below. The Gas Permeable Lens Institute is dedicated to educating eye care practitioners. The institute provides information for all types of rigid lenses and custom speciality soft contact lenses for practitioners and patients (www.gpli.info). The Scleral Lens Education Society is an excellent resource dedicated to scleral lens related topics. The mission of the Scleral Lens Education Society is to "Teach contact lens practitioners the science and art of prescribing scleral contact lenses. SLS supports public education that highlights the benefits and availability of scleral contact lenses." The website, (www.sclerallens.org), contains information about sponsors, scleral lens fitting, scientific articles and publications, videos on scleral lens handling, as well as a forum for scleral lens practitioners to exchange information and advice.

The Association of Optometric Contact Lens Educators (AOCLE) is a non-profit organization that brings together contact lens educators from schools and colleges of optometry throughout North America. Their mission statement is, "The Association of Optometric Contact Lens Educators is committed to fostering the highest levels of education in the areas of cornea and contact lenses and supporting the faculty in these areas at each of the North American schools and colleges of optometry." The AOCLE, supported by the contact lens industry, creates educational materials for patients and students that can be useful for all eye care practitioners. The website, (www.aocle.org), has downloadable resources about healthy contact lens habits as well as a pocket guide with an overview of all contact lens products.

The mission of the American Optometric Association Contact Lens and Cornea Section (www.aoa.org) states that they are to "serve its members by providing leadership, education, advice and guidance in contact lenses, anterior segment management, and refractive technologies, thus promoting quality and professional patient care." They provide an online anterior segment catalogue of various conditions.

Similarly, the Cornea, Contact Lenses, and Refractive Technologies Section of the American Academy of Optometry fosters professional growth and advocates excellence in patient care through education and research according to their mission (www.aaopt.org).

The British Contact Lens Association "provides a wide range of benefits to help members at all stages of their educational and professional career access a range of high quality resources" (www.bcla.org.uk), while the International Society of Contact Lens Specialists (www.iscls.net) offers similar benefits to its members.

Mentoring is a good way to transfer skills and knowledge across generations and geographic boundaries, and mentorships can provide students and interns with solid training and knowledge. Mentoring can also exist in practitioner-patient relationships, as well as practitioner-staff relationships [13]. While mentoring is typically viewed as a one-to-one relationship, it can also exist among organizations. Since the contact lens market evolves at a fast pace, industry partners are valuable to keep practitioners abreast of new developments in a timely manner. All of the organizations described above have unique relationships with industry.

Continuing Education

Specific meetings about contact lenses can help practitioners stay informed with developments in contact lenses and contact lens technology. Meetings such as the Global Specialty Lens Symposium (GSLS, www.gslsymposium.com), held in January each year in Las Vegas, USA, and Contact Lens Society meetings are ideal for professional development, helping practitioners to keep up to date with lens designs as well as networking with other specialists in the field. The British Contact Lens Association (BCLA) and the Cornea & Contact Lens Society of Australia (CCLSA, www.cclsa.org.au) are also great sources of education. Conferences are necessary for the contact lens practitioner who is specializing in contact lenses and looking at growing their niche practice. The Nederlands Contactlens Congress (NCC, www.ncc2016.com) is the largest contact lens meeting in the world held biannually. The American Optometric Association has a complete list of meetings on its website, and meetings are also advertised in optometric journals.

Practitioners can align with specialty organizations, such as the National Keratoconus Foundation (www.nkcf.org) or the Sjögren's Syndrome Foundation (www.sjogrens.org) and can also become a fellow of the Scleral Lens Education Society [14].

Networking

Establishing networks with peers is an important part of practice building. Good communication is essential, particularly in managing referrals. After seeing a patient who was referred, an eye care practitioner must always correspond with the referring practitioner. The communication should include an explanation of the findings, the recommendations for the patient, time frame for follow up, as well as when the patient will return to the referring practitioner. Correspondence, preferably in the form of a letter, should be succinct and to the point. Status updates are not just important in ensuring information is shared and patient care optimized, but can help to grow referrals.

Advertising

Successful contact lens advertising requires a strategic approach. It must have a theme, be appropriate to target patients and have a call-to-action. The ten key guidelines for developing a powerful contact lens advertising campaign:

1. **Only focus on your target audience:** Any advertising campaign needs to be geared at your niche market. It is a mistake to produce generic advertising that does not effectively communicate or grab the attention of your audience. Decide what sort of patients to engage, and ensure your adverts connect with them on the correct level.
2. **Highlight your competitive advantage:** The bedrock of your advertising campaign is to emphasize the benefits of your expertise; those factors that give your practice its competitive edge. Too many advertisements are clever but fail to focus on the unique benefits of the promoted offering. Unless the focus is on the benefits, the advertising delivers no value for possible patients.
3. **Establish your contact lens business image:** Image is crucial when it comes to advertising and promoting your contact lens business. Far too many advertisers do not work to form a consistent image, and they are missing the opportunity to influence likely patients.
4. **Invest in advertising to make money:** There is no point in having an amazing idea if no one finds out about it. There are many ways to reduce your costs, but advertising is obviously not the place to cut corners. Doing so will affect your revenue and damage your bottom line. Powerful advertising for your contact lens business may be costly; however, it can add value to your practice especially when it is effective.
5. **Advertise in the right place:** Your favored magazine, radio station, or even television show might not be a favorite of your target patients. Examine your target market to understand who they are and determine what they read, watch, and tune into. Your practice can place its advertisements in the relevant media to ensure that you are seen by the target market of your contact lens practice.
6. **Do not let your budget run your contact lens businesses advertising campaign:** If you budget $1,000 per month for advertising, you will make it easy from an administrative perspective. However, you will have cyclical highs and lows that mean you might be spending too much money advertising during slow times and not enough when you need to attract new business. Far too many contact lens business owners do not plan according to their seasonal advertising needs.
7. **Diversify:** It is all too common for contact lens practice owners to pick the best way to advertise based on price and the potential rate of returns, and little else. As with investing your savings, you do not want to place all of your eggs

in one basket. Spread your advertising money by choosing a cross section of suitable media for your targeted audience and your budget.

8. **Do not try to sell everything to everyone:** Not every product or service will appeal to everyone. Most contact lens business owners spend a lot of time and money thinking of various methods to reach all markets. Typically, this simply does not work and it can spell disaster for new contact lens practices that do not have the time and money and will spread themselves too thin. Accordingly, you should identify your ideal patients and provide paramount care.
9. **Test your advertisements:** If you have the time and money, consider focus groups and evaluate your advertisements on non-partisan patient groups as well. Do they understand and recognize the message you are communicating? If not, you will not gain insight into how you might effectively broadcast your message.
10. **Monitor your contact lens practice advertisements:** It is very easy to ask patients where they heard about your practice. As easy as this is, many contact lens business owners do not take the time to do so. It is beneficial to know which features of your advertising are the most effective and which method provides the greatest advertising opportunities for your practice [15].

Methods of Advertising

Deciding on which method of advertising to use involves the assessment of the target patient group and creating messaging that is most relevant to them. The main advertising channels are print (newspapers, magazines and journals), electronic (radio and television), public (billboards and posters) and social media (websites, blogs, Facebook, Twitter and other platforms). There are different costs associated with all of these avenues, and investment decisions need to be made in accordance with predicted returns.

The content of the message a practice is seeking to express also influences the advertising method. For example, new technologies or innovations in contact lenses can be particularly relevant to social media platforms. Messaging (the theme of the advertisement) can be related to:

- A new or enhanced product
- A new technology or innovation in contact lenses
- Eye health and disease topics
- Health check "reminders"
- The expertise and offerings of the practice

Internal marketing should be considered part of the overall advertising approach. Trained staff can discuss products and services that complement point-o-

-purchase materials within the practice such as brochures, posters or videos. Staff members who are fit with contact lenses can also be enthusiastic ambassadors for your practice. Even if they are not fit with contact lenses, they mirror your excitement with the unique technologies and expertise your practice offers.

Recruitment of Patient Advocates

Patient testimonials are a long-standing marketing technique, and can be one of the best and often least expensive forms of advertising. People are usually interested in hearing about how others have experienced the practice, products or services.

Experts recommend asking patients who have voiced their satisfaction whether they would be willing to share their experience in a short (30-60 second) video, which can be shot in the practice alongside relevant "props" such as any technology that was used to treat the patient. Videos, with patients' permission, can be used on the practice's website and social media platforms, and played in a loop in waiting rooms. Prospective patients can be directed to view these videos [16].

Strategies and Approaches to Challenging Patients

Niche practices should be able to meet a variety of challenges, including the management of ocular surface disease and irregular corneas with different types of complicated contact lenses. Regardless of the circumstance, patients need to feel assured that their practitioner will evaluate, diagnose, and manage their unique ocular condition.

Don't forget about corneal gas permeable lenses. If a patient can be successfully fitted with corneal gas permeable contact lenses and achieve good all day comfort and excellent visual acuity, they are receiving the best possible outcome. Corneal gas permeable contact lenses are easier to fit and the costs are more manageable for both the patient and the eye care practitioner than other options.

If the outcome is not satisfactory for the patient - whether the issue is poor comfort or unacceptable visual acuity, then the practitioner should trial fit the patient with a mini scleral or scleral lens. If this provides the patient with the desired outcomes in visual acuity and comfort, then the practitioner can re-fit the patient with that type of scleral lens.

Scleral Lens Fitting

Fitting scleral lenses can be a very time-consuming process compared with the fitting of other modalities. However, it can be a niche for many contact lens practices. For these practices, it is important that the costs and chair time are explained to patients in detail, and that the patient understands why they are being fit with a particular lens to obtain the ultimate outcome. It is essential to explain chair time, as scleral lenses do require more aftercare visits than fitting other modalities. Communication is an essential part of a specialty contact lens practice. The process of fitting, the number of aftercare follow ups, review appointments, and scleral lens adjustments prepare the patient for the investment in time of this process. Patients also need to be educated about scleral lens maintenance and scleral lens complications. A scleral lens patient is usually desperate for knowledge and education about their condition, management and prognosis.

Always Put Your Patients First

Your patient's time is valuable and so is the time they spend with their practitioner. By making the patient a top priority, business will be successful. Patients wearing specialized contact lenses will return on an annual basis and refer their family and friends. Successful eye care practitioners are very talented at building value into every aspect of their practice and therefore building a contact lens specialty niche.

Setting Up the Office

Investing in state of the art technology in the office will yield benefits. There are several considerations:

Basic Equipment and Advanced Technology

Slit Lamp

Used to view the ocular health and contact lens-cornea relationship.

Corneal Topographer

Used to diagnose, view, and evaluate the shape and elevation of the cornea to help determine the correct fit for the lens or progression of the condition. In multifocal lenses, the practitioner can determine if the lens optical center lines up with the visual axis; this may help troubleshoot and optimize a contact lens fitting.

Aberrometry

Used to determine higher order aberrations of the visual system. Useful for irregular corneas and multifocal fittings and may help to determine why a lens may not provide adequate vision.

Optical Coherence Tomography (OCT)

Anterior segment OCT greatly assists in evaluating the fitting relationship of any contact lens on the cornea. It is very useful in determining clearances in scleral designs and the overall fitting relationship.

Specular Microscope

Photographs the endothelial cell layer to determine overall cell count, morphology, and endotheliopathies.

Tomography

Provides true elevation data of the anterior and posterior surfaces and three-dimensional model of the anterior segment based on calculated elevation data. Corneal thickness of the entire cornea can be mapped as well as densitometry of media opacities.

Meibomography

Used to evaluate the state of meibomian glands. This is useful to diagnose one of the most common reasons for contact lens dropout [17].

Non-invasive Anterior Segment Imaging

Useful in diagnosing ocular surface disease, monitoring disease progression, and complementary to other diagnostic testing.

Diagnostic Trial Sets

Having accessibility to a variety of specialty lens sets to address any patient who has not been able to find solutions elsewhere will help a practitioner differentiate the practice [18].

Diagnostic corneal and scleral trial sets need to cover a broad range to fit myopes, hyperopes, astigmats, presbyopes, post-surgical, keratoconus, and orthokeratology.

Establishing Relationships with Contact Lens Laboratories

Contact lens company representatives and consultants can be valuable sources of information and advice, because they have deep knowledge of their particular designs and product portfolio. Laboratory consultants provide assistance with managing changes to a particular fit and troubleshooting when suboptimal results occur either with comfort or vision. Consultants may also educate the practitioner about the limits of their proprietary lens designs.

In summary, the establishment of a scleral lens practice can be a time-consuming but worthwhile process. A specialty practice can be financially and personally rewarding with the development of a loyal and long-term patient base. In order to continue to grow the practice, an investment in advertising and networking can aid in referrals. Staying up to date with contact lens and equipment technology can streamline the fitting process while impressing the patient.

CONFLICT OF INTEREST

The author declares no conflict of interest, financial or otherwise.

ACKNOWLEDGEMENTS

None Declared.

REFERENCES

[1] Miller J. Contact lens practice pearls: How to make specialty lenses your contact lens niche. Contact Lens Spectrum, Volume 2015; 30(September): 41.

[2] Nixon G. Contact lens practice pearls: Communication can build patient loyalty. Contact Lens Spectrum, Volume 2012; 27(November): 47.

[3] Schnider C. Patient perceptions drive referrals. Contact Lens Spectrum 2013; 28(May): 41-4.

[4] Ritson M. Build lifetime relationships. Contact Lens Spectrum 2006.

[5] Paulsen AJ, Cruickshanks KJ, Fischer ME, *et al.* Dry eye in the beaver dam offspring study: prevalence, risk factors, and health-related quality of life. Am J Ophthalmol 2014; 157(4): 799-806. [http://dx.doi.org/10.1016/j.ajo.2013.12.023] [PMID: 24388838]

[6] The Gallup Organization, Inc.. The 2008 gallup study of dry eye sufferers. Princeton, NJ: Multi-Sponsor Surveys, Inc 2008.

[7] The definition and classification of dry eye disease: report of the definition and classification subcommittee of the international dry eye workShop (2007). Ocul Surf 2007; 5(2): 75-92. [http://dx.doi.org/10.1016/S1542-0124(12)70081-2] [PMID: 17508116]

[8] Paulsen AJ, Cruickshanks KJ, Fischer ME, *et al.* Dry eye in the beaver dam offspring study: prevalence, risk factors, and health-related quality of life. Am J Ophthalmol 2014; 157(4): 799-806. [http://dx.doi.org/10.1016/j.ajo.2013.12.023] [PMID: 24388838]

[9] Morris M, Rogers T. Create a dry-eye niche. Optometric Management 2008.

[10] Hunt K. Finding your optometric niche. Optometric Management 2012; (September): 58-9.

[11] Brujic M. Contact lenses: A tool for building patient loyalty. Optometric Management, Volume 2012; 47(September): 52-4.

[12] Gailmard N. Contact lens practice: Your key to profitability. Optometric Management Tip of the Week 2012.

[13] Bitton E, Littlefield J. Mentorship is both a role and a skill. Contact Lens Spectrum 2010.

[14] Barnett M. Creating a specialty contact lens niche. Optometric Management 2013; 48(January): 57-9.

[15] www.advertising-4-you.com2016.

[16] Gerber G. The business of contact lenses. Using testimonials in marketing dry eye treatments. Contact Lens Spectrum, Volume 2015; 30(Issue: July): 46.

[17] Geffen D. How to create a high-tech, high-value CL exam. Review of Optometric Business 2016.

[18] Cole J. How to build a dry eye center of excellence. Review of Optometry 2014.

CHAPTER 16

Collaborative Care of the Scleral Lens Patient: Working with Referring Doctors

Jennifer Y. Li[1,*] and **Deborah S. Jacobs**[2]

[1] *University of California, Davis, Sacramento, CA, USA*

[2] *BostonSight, Needham Heights, MA 02494, USA*

Abstract: As technological advances in scleral lenses have improved the comfort and function of these lenses for patients, there has been increasing acceptance and use of scleral lenses by ophthalmologists. Historically, scleral lenses were most frequently used for visual rehabilitation of patients with corneal ectasias such as keratoconus, pellucid marginal degeneration and keratoglobus. Scleral lenses are also indicated for other patients with high or irregular astigmatism such as in post-keratoplasty patients or after complications of LASIK vision correction. Increasingly, scleral lenses are used in patients with severe ocular surface disease such as Stevens-Johnson syndrome (SJS), graft *versus* host disease (GvHD), and ocular cicatricial pemphigoid. Few ophthalmologists have expertise in fitting contact lenses, much less specialty lenses including scleral lenses. When patients are referred for scleral lenses by a comprehensive ophthalmologist, or more often, a corneal specialist, the patient is best served if the fitting practitioner understands the purpose of the referral. Scleral lenses have altered how corneal specialists manage patients with a variety of diseases. They have helped to decrease the progression to corneal transplantation in patients with corneal ectasia and irregular astigmatism. Scleral lenses have also helped to improve the quality of life for patients with severe ocular surface diseases. It is important for all eye care providers to be aware of the utility of these lenses for even the most complex eyes.

Keywords: Astigmatism, Collaborative, Complex, Conjunctiva, Consultation, Edema, Graft, Graft *vs*. host disease (GvHD), Intra-ocular lenses, Keratoconus, Oncology, Ophthalmologist, Patient, Pellucid marginal degeneration, Quality of life, Referral, Scleral lens, Suture, Symptoms, Tumor.

INTRODUCTION

As technological advances in scleral lenses have improved the comfort and function of these lenses for patients, there has been increasing acceptance and use

* **Corresponding author Jennifer Y. Li:** University of California, Davis, Sacramento, CA, USA; Tel: 916-734-4641; Fax: 916-565-1640; E-mail: jyli@ucdavis.edu

Melissa Barnett & Lynette K. Johns (Eds.)

of scleral lenses by ophthalmologists. Historically, scleral lenses were most frequently used for visual rehabilitation of patients with corneal ectasias such as keratoconus, pellucid marginal degeneration and keratoglobus [1 - 3]. Scleral lenses are also used for other patients with high or irregular astigmatism such as in post-keratoplasty patients or after complications of LASIK vision correction. Increasingly, scleral lenses are used in patients with severe ocular surface disease such as Stevens-Johnson syndrome (SJS), graft *versus* host disease (GvHD), and ocular cicatricial pemphigoid [4 - 6].

Few ophthalmologists have expertise in fitting contact lenses, much less specialty lenses including scleral lenses. When patients are referred for scleral lenses by a comprehensive ophthalmologist, or more often, a corneal specialist, the patient is best served if the fitting practitioner understands the purpose of the referral.

In the context of a patient with keratoconus or significant irregular astigmatism, the referring physician most likely wants to know the patient's best-corrected visual acuity as well as lens tolerance in contrast to any other sort of contact lens correction. The visual acuity, visual function, and tolerance of a scleral lens may help determine next steps in surgical intervention. For patients with severe ocular surface disease, the purpose for the referral may not be to achieve improved visual acuity, but rather, to improve patient comfort or support the ocular surface; improvement in visual acuity may be an incidental "side effect." Ideally, the scleral lens practitioner will be in contact with the referring doctor to determine if scleral lenses can achieve the intended goals. Referring ophthalmologists may not be aware of technical advances and/or limitations related to newer designs which may need to be explained. Open pathways for communication, whether by letter, fax, telephone or shared notes on routine, borderline or complex patients are helpful. In this situation, the scleral lens practitioner and referring doctor may develop a consensus to determine if fitting, training, and dispensing is worth undertaking. Once a practitioner has successfully fit a patient and succeeded in application and removal training, the lenses are dispensed and appropriate follow up occurs. Once the fitting is deemed complete, communication with the referring doctor should include outcomes pertaining to the original goals.

With advances in scleral lens designs, availability and increased expertise in fitting lenses for healthy eyes and eyes with disease, scleral lenses are no longer a historical oddity. Good communication with referring doctors and collaborative care of challenging patients is imperative to improve patient outcomes. This can also increase appreciation of scleral lenses as an alternative to other medical and surgical interventions.

Cataract Surgery in the Scleral Lens Patient

Patients who wear scleral lenses for irregular astigmatism or ocular surface disease may develop age related or secondary cataracts that limit vision and require surgical intervention. A patient may wish to resume scleral lens wear as soon after surgery as possible for comfort, vision or support of the ocular surface. For this reason, we recommend that a scleral tunnel or near-clear corneal wound be considered, and a suture used, even if the wound appears to be self-sealing. If there is no evidence of endophthalmitis or wound problems at the one-week post-operative visit, then the patient may resume daily application and removal of a scleral lens. The surgeon, contact lens specialist and patient may feel more confident if the first attempt at application and removal is done under clinician's supervision to confirm that there is no disruption of the wound or anterior chamber. In the authors' experience, the suture should be left in and removed if and when it loosens, or in the event of vascular in-growth after one month has elapsed.

Toric intra-ocular lenses are ill-advised in scleral lens patients, unless the lens is worn solely for correction of astigmatism and if the full cylindrical error can be corrected with an IOL. If a toric IOL does not correct all astigmatism, this will create residual astigmatism with a scleral lens. Any residual astigmatism with the scleral lens will require neutralization with either spectacles over the scleral lens or the fitting of a new stabilized/non-rotating lens that includes a front surface cylindrical correction. The patient may not be happy with either option.

Corneal Transplantation in the Scleral Lens Patient

Patients who wear scleral lenses for support of the ocular surface in the setting of neurotrophic keratoconjunctivitis or limbal stem cell deficiency (LSCD) may require penetrating keratoplasty for visual rehabilitation of corneal scarring. These patients may benefit from prompt resumption of scleral lens wear after keratoplasty. The authors recommend the use of interrupted sutures (Fig. **1**) rather than continuous running sutures (Fig. **2**) in these cases as such patients are more prone to loosening of sutures (Fig. **3**). The authors advise a temporary tarsorrhaphy and use of ointment until one to two weeks after surgery at which time daily wear of scleral lens can be resumed. The patient may find it reassuring to do the first application and removal under a clinician's supervision. Patients who would benefit from scleral lenses immediately after corneal transplantation should be trained in application and removal of a scleral lens prior to surgery to minimize manipulation postoperatively with its associated discomfort and potential for post-operative mechanical complications. In the authors' experience, scleral lenses for visual rehabilitation after penetrating keratoplasty can be considered earlier than rigid gas permeable corneal lenses, because there is no need to wait for reshaping and smoothing of the graft-host interface to assure stability of the lens. It is critical that adequate fluid ventilation/tear exchange is established so that the scleral lens does not add hypoxic stress to the recovering graft.

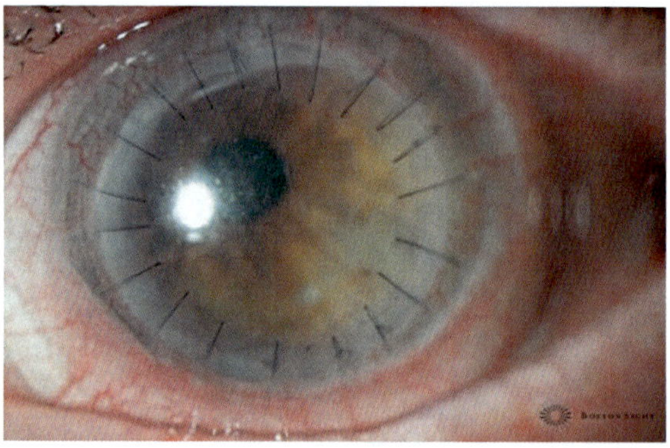

Fig. (1). Corneal transplant with interrupted sutures. Image courtesy of BostonSight.

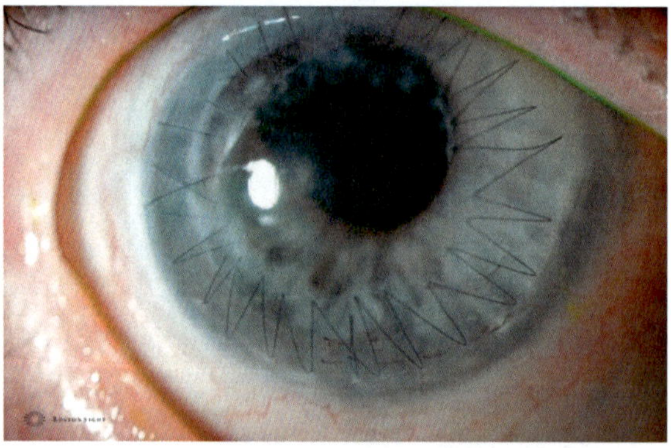

Fig. (2). Corneal transplant with continuous running sutures. Image courtesy of BostonSight.

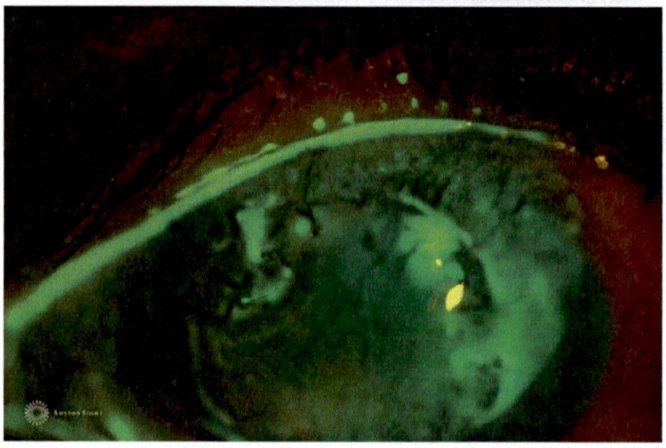

Fig. (3). Broken and vascularized sutures. Image courtesy of BostonSight.

Scleral Lenses for Corneal Diseases

The most common reason why patients are referred for scleral lenses is for the management of corneal ectasias such as keratoconus and pellucid marginal degeneration [7, 8]. Although these lenses do not mitigate the natural progression of these disease processes, it may often provide a viable alternative to corneal transplantation for these patients with superior outcomes [9, 10].

The second most common reason why patients are referred for scleral lenses is astigmatism or corneal irregularity after corneal transplantation. Scleral lenses can provide excellent vision in eyes with significant post-keratoplasty astigmatism [8].

Although complications of scleral lenses are uncommon [8, 11], bacterial keratitis has been reported with daily-wear of scleral lenses [8]. Additionally, patients with pre-existing corneal edema will have worsening of their edema with scleral lens use [8]. Patients should be screened for endothelial disease and corneal edema prior to scleral lens fitting, and all eye care providers should be aware of this side effect of scleral lenses. Proceeding with a scleral lens fitting in the presence of corneal edema, for example in bullous keratopathy or Fuchs' endothelial dystrophy, is ill-advised and may be contraindicated.

Scleral Lenses in the Oncology Patient

Another indication for the use of scleral lenses is for patients with ocular GvHD. GvHD is the most frequent and serious complication of allogeneic hematopoietic stem cell transplantation (HSCT) [12]. Ocular involvement of GvHD occurs in 60-90% of patients and can have potentially devastating ocular symptoms [12]. Patients may have signs and symptoms of severe keratoconjunctivitis sicca or cicatrizing conjunctivitis which can lead to corneal involvement and loss of vision.

Management of patients in both the acute and chronic stages of GvHD is dependent on close cooperation between the patient's hematologist/oncologist and ophthalmologist. Severity of the disease varies from patient to patient, and systemic immunosuppression is a mainstay for both prevention and treatment of GvHD. Ocular management consists of supportive care with topical lubricants in addition to topical steroids, topical cyclosporine, topical lifitegrast, and autologous serum eye drops [13 - 16].

Scleral lenses should also be considered for patients with moderate to severe chronic GvHD who are unresponsive to conventional therapy. Several studies have demonstrated efficacy in this patient population [17]. Takahide *et al.* and

Jacobs *et al.* reviewed results of the Boston Scleral Lens Prosthetic Device used in prosthetic replacement of the ocular surface ecosystem treatment (PROSE) on chronic GvHD patients [18, 19]. Takahide *et al.* looked at 9 patients with chronic GvHD and found improvement in ocular symptoms in all cases [18]. Similarly, in their larger study of 33 patients, Jacobs *et al.* found that 97% of surveyed patients reported a reduction in eye pain and an improvement in their quality of life [19]. Ninety-four percent of patients had improvement in photophobia [19]. In addition to symptomatic relief, scleral lenses have also been demonstrated to help improve vision in patients with chronic GvHD. Theophanous *et al.* performed a retrospective analysis of 79 eyes with chronic GvHD and found that 90% had improved visual acuity with scleral lens use [20]. In addition to the use of the PROSE device, the Jupiter scleral lens has also demonstrated efficacy in improving ocular comfort and visual acuity in this patient population [21]. It is important for both oncologists and eye care providers to be aware of the benefits of scleral lenses for chronic GvHD ocular symptoms in order for patients to benefit from early referral for scleral lens fitting.

An additional subset of oncology patients who should be considered for scleral lenses are those with neurotrophic keratopathy or exposure keratopathy related to head and neck tumors and the treatments used to address these tumors [5, 7, 22, 23].

Glaucoma in the Scleral Lens Patient

Glaucoma and corneal diseases often co-exist. Corneal transplantation can lead to the development of glaucoma [24, 25], and multiple glaucoma medications can lead to corneal toxicity/epitheliopathy or corneal decompensation [26, 27]. Given these factors, it is not an uncommon situation to find a patient with both severe corneal disease and advanced glaucoma in need of a scleral lens for both visual and therapeutic reasons.

If a patient on glaucoma drops develops transient increase in corneal epithelial edema with scleral lens wear, consideration should be given to loosening of the scleral lens fit to reduce any challenge to epithelial tight junctions created by suction. Additionally, the clinician treating the glaucoma and the scleral lens practitioner might jointly consider substituting preservative free drops or agents with less direct toxicity.

Fitting scleral lenses in a patient with prior glaucoma surgery can be more challenging, but advances in scleral lens technology have made these lenses a viable option for patients with advanced glaucoma. There are several ways to address elevations of the limbal conjunctiva associated with prior glaucoma surgery with a scleral lens. To start, simply increasing or decreasing the diameter of the lens may avoid the area of concern. However, in some cases, it may be necessary and advantageous to create a notch in the scleral lens to go around the glaucoma drainage device or the bleb from a trabeculectomy surgery. This has been successfully performed with various styles of scleral lenses, and these patients should not be precluded from consideration for scleral lenses [28, 29]. Close monitoring of these patients cannot be over-emphasized. It is possible for there to be erosion of the conjunctiva overlying a glaucoma drainage tube adjacent to the edge of an initially well-fitting scleral lens.

CONCLUSION

Scleral lenses have altered how corneal specialists manage patients with a variety of diseases. They have helped to decrease the progression to corneal transplantation in patients with corneal ectasia and irregular astigmatism. Scleral lenses have also helped to improve the quality of life for patients with severe ocular surface diseases. It is important for all eye care providers to be aware of the utility of these lenses for even the most complex eyes.

QUESTIONS OF CORNEAL SPECIALISTS

1. We realize that each corneal specialist has a different approach. How soon after the scleral lens fitting is complete should we recommend the patient return to your office and why?

Dr. Jacobs: I think it's useful for the cornea specialist to have opportunity to examine the patient with the scleral lens on the eye within a month or two after the fit is completed to record vision in the device, document the state of the ocular surface and monitor for any factors that might lead to complications from device wear. This is particularly true for eyes with corneal grafts or prior glaucoma surgery.

Dr. Li: For my patients, I typically see them within two to three months after their scleral lens fitting is complete. The purpose of this visit is not only to monitor the state of their ocular surface and their cornea, but to follow-up with the patient to make sure that their visual and functional needs are being met with the scleral lenses.

2. When would you not recommend a scleral lens fit and why?

Dr. Jacobs: Any eye with corneal endothelial dysfunction (to the point that there is diurnal fluctuation in the vision) or any microcystic edema is not likely to do well with a scleral lens. Also, if a patient and caretakers cannot manage daily application and removal, then a scleral lens is not an option.

Dr. Li: Patients with corneal edema may have a tendency towards worsening edema with scleral lens wear. Patients with dense central corneal scarring would also likely not benefit from lenses of any sort. Otherwise, for patients who I think will benefit from scleral lenses, I encourage them to at least attempt a fitting even if they may be reticent initially. They may have had prior failed attempts at rigid contact lenses or concerns about learning to insert and remove lenses daily, but many of these patients can still be successfully fit in a scleral lens with appropriate training.

3. When do you decide between a cornea transplant and a scleral lens fitting referral for advanced keratoconus?

Dr. Jacobs: I think that a referral for a scleral lens trial is warranted for any patient with advanced keratoconus prior to consideration of keratoplasty. Failure of other lens types does not mean scleral lenses will fail, although patients who've suffered adherent lens syndrome with hybrid, corneal or mini-scleral lenses may be reluctant to try yet another lens.

Dr. Li: I certainly agree with Dr. Jacobs. Even patients with advanced keratoconus with significant apical steepening and thinning can do quite well with a scleral lens and corneal transplantation should always be last resort. That being said, patients with significant corneal scarring particularly after an episode of acute hydrops, may not achieve their desired visual acuity in a scleral lens and elect to pursue corneal transplantation at that time.

4. When do you remove sutures after corneal transplantation and is it any different for a scleral lens patient?

Dr. Jacobs: My practice is to use only interrupted sutures and to remove sutures only if they loosen or break in the first 6 months. After that, sutures are removed selectively in the steep axis to reduce high or irregular astigmatism, or if there is vascular ingrowth (Fig. **4**). I would not change this practice in a scleral lens patient. If the lens is being worn for ocular surface disease, then the only basis for removal is loosening, breakage, or vascular ingrowth.

Dr. Li: Timing of suture removal is not affected by scleral lenses. After corneal transplantation, I begin suture removal at approximately 3 months for a graft that has both a running suture and interrupted sutures and at 6 months for a graft with all interrupted sutures. Once suture removal commences, they are selectively removed every 4-6 weeks from the steep axis in order to decrease the overall amount of astigmatism. The exceptions are sutures that become vascularized, loosened, or broken – these sutures are removed immediately upon recognition.

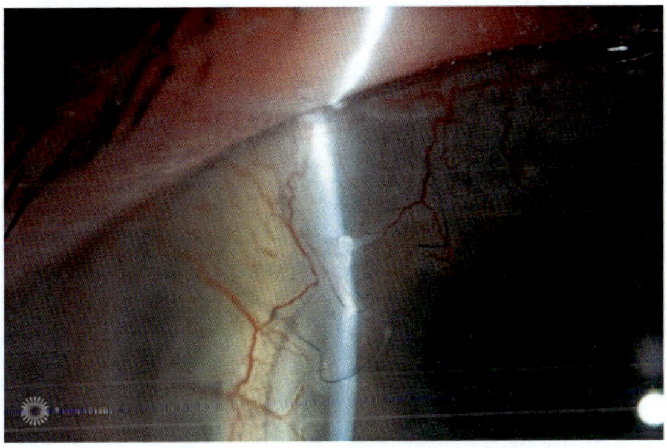

Fig. (4). Vascular ingrowth along a suture. Image courtesy of BostonSight.

5. In your experience, what is the most common indication for scleral lenses?

Dr. Jacobs: My practice has always had a large component of ocular surface disease, with underlying medical disease such as GvHD and Sjögren's, so I would say my referrals have been equally split between keratoconus/pellucid marginal degeneration and ocular surface disease.

Dr. Li: The two most common indications for referral for scleral lenses amongst my patients are corneal ectasia and severe ocular surface disease that has failed typical medical management.

6. In your experience, what have you seen as the most common complication of scleral lens wear?

Dr. Jacobs: Fortunately, serious complications such as infection or triggering of rejection or graft failure are very rare in daily wear of scleral lenses. As with any contact lens wear, patients are at risk of corneal neovascularization, and there is likely higher risk if there is underlying disease. Scleral lens patients with underlying disease must be monitored more closely than typical contact lens patients. I think semi-annual evaluation is worthwhile, although these visits might be split and coordinated between the scleral lens practitioner and the ophthalmologist so that each is seeing the patient yearly, but the patient is being seen at 6 month intervals by one clinician or the other.

Dr. Li: The side effect that my patients complain about most often is the development of mucous/debris that can cause vision to fluctuate during daily lens wear. Although this does not affect their underlying disease process or the health of their corneas, they complain of the inconvenience of having the remove and clean the lens throughout the day.

CONFLICT OF INTEREST

The author declares no conflict of interest, financial or otherwise.

ACKNOWLEDGEMENTS

None Declared.

REFERENCES

[1] Tan DT, Pullum KW, Buckley RJ. Medical applications of scleral contact lenses: 1. A retrospective analysis of 343 cases. Cornea 1995; 14(2): 121-9. [http://dx.doi.org/10.1097/00003226-199503000-00001] [PMID: 7743792]

[2] Tan DT, Pullum KW, Buckley RJ. Medical applications of scleral contact lenses: 2. Gas-permeable scleral contact lenses. Cornea 1995; 14(2): 130-7. [http://dx.doi.org/10.1097/00003226-199503000-00001] [PMID: 7743793]

[3] Rathi VM, Mandathara PS, Taneja M, Dumpati S, Sangwan VS. Scleral lens for keratoconus: technology update. Clin Ophthalmol 2015; 9: 2013-8. [http://dx.doi.org/10.2147/OPTH.S52483] [PMID: 26604671]

[4] Jacobs DS. Update on scleral lenses. Curr Opin Ophthalmol 2008; 19(4): 298-301. [http://dx.doi.org/10.1097/ICU.0b013e328302cc4f] [PMID: 18545010]

[5] Schornack MM. Scleral lenses: a literature review. Eye Contact Lens 2015; 41(1): 3-11. [http://dx.doi.org/10.1097/ICL.0000000000000083] [PMID: 25536528]

[6] van der Worp E, Bornman D, Ferreira DL, Faria-Ribeiro M, Garcia-Porta N, González-Meijome JM. Modern scleral contact lenses: A review. Cont Lens Anterior Eye 2014; 37(4): 240-50. [http://dx.doi.org/10.1016/j.clae.2014.02.002] [PMID: 24631015]

[7] Dimit R, Gire A, Pflugfelder SC, Bergmanson JP. Patient ocular conditions and clinical outcomes using a PROSE scleral device. Cont Lens Anterior Eye 2013; 36(4): 159-63. [http://dx.doi.org/10.1016/j.clae.2013.02.004] [PMID: 23499361]

[8] Rosenthal P, Croteau A. Fluid-ventilated, gas-permeable scleral contact lens is an effective option for managing severe ocular surface disease and many corneal disorders that would otherwise require penetrating keratoplasty. Eye Contact Lens 2005; 31(3): 130-4. [http://dx.doi.org/10.1097/01.ICL.0000152492.98553.8D] [PMID: 15894881]

[9] Baran I, Bradley JA, Alipour F, Rosenthal P, Le HG, Jacobs DS. PROSE treatment of corneal ectasia. Cont Lens Anterior Eye 2012; 35(5): 222-7. [http://dx.doi.org/10.1016/j.clae.2012.04.003] [PMID: 22633003]

[10] DeLoss KS, Fatteh NH, Hood CT. Prosthetic Replacement of the Ocular Surface Ecosystem (PROSE) scleral device compared to keratoplasty for the treatment of corneal ectasia. Am J Ophthalmol 2014; 158(5): 974-82. [http://dx.doi.org/10.1016/j.ajo.2014.07.016] [PMID: 25058902]

[11] Schornack MM, Pyle J, Patel SV. Scleral lenses in the management of ocular surface disease. Ophthalmology 2014; 121(7): 1398-405. [http://dx.doi.org/10.1016/j.ophtha.2014.01.028] [PMID: 24630687]

[12] Espana EM, Shah S, Santhiago MR, Singh AD. Graft *versus* host disease: clinical evaluation, diagnosis and management. Graefes Arch Clin Exp Ophthalmol 2013; 251(5): 1257-66. [http://dx.doi.org/10.1007/s00417-013-2301-z] [PMID: 23504086]

[13] Robinson MR, Lee SS, Rubin BI, *et al.* Topical corticosteroid therapy for cicatricial conjunctivitis associated with chronic graft-*versus*-host disease. Bone Marrow Transplant 2004; 33(10): 1031-5.

[http://dx.doi.org/10.1038/sj.bmt.1704453] [PMID: 15048138]

[14] Rao SN, Rao RD. Efficacy of topical cyclosporine 0.05% in the treatment of dry eye associated with graft *versus* host disease. Cornea 2006; 25(6): 674-8.
[http://dx.doi.org/10.1097/01.ico.0000208813.17367.0c] [PMID: 17077659]

[15] Malta JB, Soong HK, Shtein RM, *et al.* Treatment of ocular graft-*versus*-host disease with topical cyclosporine 0.05%. Cornea 2010; 29(12): 1392-6.
[http://dx.doi.org/10.1097/ICO.0b013e3181e456f0] [PMID: 20847658]

[16] Ogawa Y, Okamoto S, Mori T, *et al.* Autologous serum eye drops for the treatment of severe dry eye in patients with chronic graft-*versus*-host disease. Bone Marrow Transplant 2003; 31(7): 579-83.
[http://dx.doi.org/10.1038/sj.bmt.1703862] [PMID: 12692625]

[17] Balasubramaniam SC, Raja H, Nau CB, Shen JF, Schornack MM. Ocular Graft-*versus*-Host Disease: A Review. Eye Contact Lens 2015; 41(5): 256-61.
[http://dx.doi.org/10.1097/ICL.0000000000000150] [PMID: 26214529]

[18] Takahide K, Parker PM, Wu M, *et al.* Use of fluid-ventilated, gas-permeable scleral lens for management of severe keratoconjunctivitis sicca secondary to chronic graft-*versus*-host disease. Biol Blood Marrow Transplant 2007; 13(9): 1016-21.
[http://dx.doi.org/10.1016/j.bbmt.2007.05.006] [PMID: 17697963]

[19] Jacobs DS, Rosenthal P. Boston scleral lens prosthetic device for treatment of severe dry eye in chronic graft-*versus*-host disease. Cornea 2007; 26(10): 1195-9.
[http://dx.doi.org/10.1097/ICO.0b013e318155743d] [PMID: 18043175]

[20] Theophanous C, Irvine JA, Parker P, Chiu GB. Use of prosthetic replacement of the ocular surface ecosystem scleral lenses in patients with ocular chronic graft-*versus*-host disease. Biol Blood Marrow Transplant 2015; 21(12): 2180-4.
[http://dx.doi.org/10.1016/j.bbmt.2015.07.027] [PMID: 26234721]

[21] Schornack MM, Baratz KH, Patel SV, Maguire LJ. Jupiter scleral lenses in the management of chronic graft *versus* host disease. Eye Contact Lens 2008; 34(6): 302-5.
[http://dx.doi.org/10.1097/ICL.0b013e318188e205] [PMID: 18997537]

[22] Pullum K, Buckley R. Therapeutic and ocular surface indications for scleral contact lenses. Ocul Surf 2007; 5(1): 40-8.
[http://dx.doi.org/10.1016/S1542-0124(12)70051-4] [PMID: 17252164]

[23] Lin SJ, Jacobs DS, Frankenthaler R, Rubin PA. An ocular surface prosthesis as an innovative adjunct in patients with head and neck malignancy. Otolaryngol Head Neck Surg 2008; 139(4): 589-91.
[http://dx.doi.org/10.1016/j.otohns.2008.06.032] [PMID: 18922350]

[24] Greenlee EC, Kwon YH. Graft failure: III. Glaucoma escalation after penetrating keratoplasty. Int Ophthalmol 2008; 28(3): 191-207.
[http://dx.doi.org/10.1007/s10792-008-9223-5] [PMID: 18431550]

[25] Erdurmus M, Cohen EJ, Yildiz EH, *et al.* Steroid-induced intraocular pressure elevation or glaucoma after penetrating keratoplasty in patients with keratoconus or Fuchs dystrophy. Cornea 2009; 28(7): 759-64.
[http://dx.doi.org/10.1097/ICO.0b013e3181967318] [PMID: 19574912]

[26] Fraunfelder FW. Corneal toxicity from topical ocular and systemic medications. Cornea 2006; 25(10): 1133-8.
[http://dx.doi.org/10.1097/01.ico.0000240084.27663.fd] [PMID: 17172885]

[27] Konowal A, Morrison JC, Brown SV, *et al.* Irreversible corneal decompensation in patients treated with topical dorzolamide. Am J Ophthalmol 1999; 127(4): 403-6.
[http://dx.doi.org/10.1016/S0002-9394(98)00438-3] [PMID: 10218692]

[28] Carrasquillo KG, Barnett M. Scleral lens applications in unique populations. Contact Lens Spectrum PentaVision, 1 2016.

[29] Tanhehco T, Jacobs DS. Technological advances shaping scleral lenses: the Boston ocular surface prosthesis in patients with glaucoma tubes and trabeculectomies. Semin Ophthalmol 2010; 25(5-6): 233-8.
[http://dx.doi.org/10.3109/08820538.2010.518873] [PMID: 21091005]

SUBJECT INDEX

A

B

C

Melissa Barnett & Lynette K. Johns (Eds.)

G

H

I

J

K

L

M

N

O

P

R

S

T

V

W

Z

Made in United States
North Haven, CT
03 November 2026

21600176R00281